GENETICS AND THE LAW III

GENETICS AND THE LAW III

EDITED BY

AUBREY MILUNSKY, MB.B.Ch., D.Sc., F.R.C.P., D.C.H.

Professor of Pediatrics, Obstetrics, Gynecology, and Pathology
Director, Center for Human Genetics
Boston University School of Medicine
Boston, Massachusetts

AND

GEORGE J. ANNAS, J.D., M.P.H.

Edward Utley Professor of Health Law
Chief, Health Law Section
Boston University Schools of Medicine and Public Health
Boston, Massachusetts

PLENUM PRESS · NEW YORK AND LONDON

Library of Congress Cataloging in Publication Data

National Symposium on Genetics and the Law (3rd: 1984: Boston, Mass.)
   Genetics and the law III.

   Proceedings of the Third National Symposium on Genetics and the Law,
held Apr. 2-4, 1984, in Boston, Mass. and co-spondored by the American
Society of Law and Medicine and others.
   Includes bibliographies and index.
   1. Medical genetics — Law and legislation — United States — Congresses. 2.
Genetic engineering — Law and legislation — United States — Congresses. I.
Milunsky, Aubrey. II. Annas, George J. III. American Society of Law and
Medicine. IV. Title.
KF3827.G4N38   1984   344.73′0419   85-19347
ISBN 0-306-41983-1   347.304419

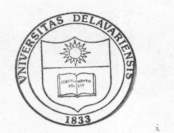

Proceedings of the Third National Symposium on Genetics and the Law,
held April 2-4, 1984, in Boston, Massachusetts. Cosponsored by the
American Society of Law and Medicine and the Boston University
Schools of Medicine, Law, and Public Health. Supported with a grant
from the National Science Foundation and the National Endowment for
the Humanities.

Plenum Press is a division of Plenum Publishing Corporation
233 Spring Street, New York, N.Y. 10013

CONTRIBUTORS

GEORGE J. ANNAS, J.D., M.P.H.
Edward Utley Professor of Health Law
Boston University Schools of Medicine and
    Public Health
80 East Concord Street
Boston, MA 02118

MICHAEL S. BARAM, LL.B.
Professor of Public Health Law
Boston University School of Public Health
80 East Concord Street
Boston, MA 02118

CHARLES H. BARON, LL.B., PH.D.
Professor of Law
Boston College Law School
885 Centre Street
Newton, MA 02159

CHARLES L. BOSK, PH.D.
Associate Professor
Department of Sociology
University of Pennsylvania
Philadelphia, PA 19104

DAVID BOTSTEIN, PH.D.
Professor of Genetics
Massachusetts Institute of Technology
56-721 77 Massachusetts Avenue
Cambridge, MA 02139

ROBERT A. BURT, J.D.
Southmayd Professor of Law
Yale University School of Law
New Haven, CT 06520

ALEXANDER MORGAN CAPRON, LL.B.
Topping Professor of Law, Medicine, and Public Policy
The Law Center
University of Southern California
Los Angeles, CA 90089-0071

JAMES F. CHILDRESS, PH.D.
Commonwealth Professor of Religious Studies
Professor of Medical Education
University of Virginia
Department of Religious Studies
Cocke Hall
Charlottesville, VA 22903

JESSICA G. DAVIS, M.D.
Associate Professor of Clinical Pediatrics
Cornell University College of Medicine
Chief of Genetics
North Shore University Hospital
300 Community Drive
Manhasset, NY 11030

BERNARD M. DICKENS, LL.M., PH.D.,
    LL.D.
Professor
Faculty of Law
University of Toronto
Toronto, Ontario, Canada M5S 2C5

REBECCA DRESSER, J.D.
Assistant Professor
Center for Ethics, Medicine, and Public Issues
Baylor College of Medicine
Texas Medical Center
Houston, TX 77030

SHERMAN ELIAS, M.D.
Director, Clinical Genetics Services
Prentice Women's Hospital and Maternity
    Center
Chicago, IL 60611
Associate Professor of Obstetrics and Gynecology
Northwestern University Medical School
Chicago, IL 60611

NORMAN FOST, M.D., M.P.H.
Professor of Pediatrics and History
    of Medicine
Director, Program in Medical Ethics
University of Wisconsin, Madison
600 Highland Avenue
Madison, WI 53978

LEONARD H. GLANTZ, J.D.
Associate Professor of Health Law
Boston University School of Public Health
80 East Concord Street
Boston, MA 02118

JOSEPH M. HEALEY, JR.
Associate Professor
Department of Community Medicine
University of Connecticut School of
    Medicine
Farmington, CT 06032

ALBERT R. JONSEN, PH.D.
Professor of Ethics in Medicine
Departments of Medicine and Pediatrics
University of California, San Francisco
1326 Third Avenue
San Francisco, CA 94143

SHELDON KRIMSKY, PH.D.
Associate Professor
Department of Urban and Environmental
    Policy
Tufts University
Medford, MA 02155

SEYMOUR LEDERBERG, PH.D.
Professor of Biology
Brown University
Box G
Providence, RI 02192

RUTH MACKLIN, PH.D.
Professor of Bioethics
Albert Einstein College of Medicine
Department of Epidemiology and Social Medicine
1300 Morris Park Avenue
Bronx, NY 10461

AUBREY MILUNSKY, MB.B.CH., D.SC.,
    F.R.C.P., D.C.H.
Director, Center for Human Genetics
Professor of Pediatrics, Obstetrics,
    Gynecology, and Pathology
Boston University School of Medicine
80 East Concord Street
Boston, MA 02118

JAMES V. NEEL, M.D., PH.D.
Lee R. Dice University Professor
Department of Human Genetics
Kresge I, Room 4560
University of Michigan Medical School
Ann Arbor, MI 48109

J. ROBERT NELSON, DR. THEOL.
Director of Institute of Religion
Texas Medical Center
Houston, TX 77025
Adjunct Professor of Medicine
Baylor College of Medicine
Houston, TX 77030

ROBERT B. NICHOLAS, J.D.
Chief Counsel/Staff Director
Subcommittee on Investigations and
    Oversight
Committee on Science and Technology
United States House of Representatives
Washington, DC 20515

STUART L. NIGHTINGALE, M.D.
Associate Commissioner for Health Affairs
Food and Drug Administration
Room 1495 (HFY-1)
5600 Fisher Lane
Rockville, MD 20857

DAVID OZONOFF, M.D., M.P.H.
Associate Professor of Public Health
Chief, Environmental Health Section
Boston University School of Public Health
80 East Concord Street
Boston, MA 02118

JOSEPH G. PERPICH, M.D., J.D.
Vice President, Planning and Development
Meloy Laboratories
Revlon Health Care
6715 Electronic Drive
Springfield, VA 22151

TABITHA M. POWLEDGE, M.S.
Senior Editor
Bio/Technology
271 Degraw Street
Brooklyn, NY 11231

PHILIP R. REILLY, J.D., M.D.
Department of Medicine
Boston City Hospital
818 Harrison Avenue
Boston, MA 02118

ARNOLD S. RELMAN, M.D.
Editor
New England Journal of Medicine
10 Shattuck Street
Boston, MA 02115
Professor of Medicine
Harvard Medical School
25 Shattuck Street
Boston, MA 02115

JOHN A. ROBERTSON, J.D.
Professor of Law
University of Texas Law School
2500 Red River
Austin, TX 78705

LEON E. ROSENBERG, M.D.
C. N. H. Long Professor
Department of Human Genetics
Yale University School of Medicine
333 Cedar Street
P.O. Box 3333
New Haven, CT 06510

MARGERY W. SHAW, M.D., J.D.
Director
Health Law Program
University of Texas Health Science Center
Fanin Bank Building
1020 Holcombe, Suite 600
Houston, TX 77030

ROGER L. SHINN, PH.D.
Reinhold Niebuhr Professor of Social
    Ethics
Union Theological Seminary
3041 Broadway at Reinhold Niebuhr Place
New York, NY 10027

I. DAVID TODRES, M.D.
Director, Neonatal and Pediatric
    Intensive Care Units
Massachusetts General Hospital
Fruit Street
Boston, MA 02114
Associate Professor of Pediatrics
Harvard Medical School
25 Shattuck Street
Boston, MA 02115

LEROY WALTERS, PH.D.
Director, Center for Bioethics
Kennedy Institute of Ethics
Associate Professor
Department of Philosophy
Georgetown University
Washington, DC 20057

INVITED DISCUSSANTS

DAVID BALTIMORE, PH.D.
Nobel Laureate
Professor of Microbiology
Director, Whitehead Institute for Medical
    Research
Massachusetts Institute of Technology
Cambridge, MA 02132

PHILIP LEDER, M.D.
John Emory Andrus Professor
Chairman, Department of Genetics
Harvard Medical School
Boston, MA 02115

WILLIAM SCHWARTZ, J.D.
Dean
Boston University School of Law
Boston, MA 02215

CONTENTS

Human Applications of Genetic Engineering—Philip Leder, Moderator

NEW WAYS OF MAKING BABIES: BRAVE NEW WORLD

Laboratories for Babies—Aubrey Milunsky, Moderator

PROTECTING THE VULNERABLE: AT WHAT COST?

TREATMENT OR AVOIDANCE OF GENETIC DISEASE

PREFACE

*It was the best of times, it was the worst of times, it was the age
of wisdom, it was the age of foolishness, it was the epoch of
belief, it was the epoch of incredulity, . . . it was the spring of
hope, it was the winter of despair. . . .*
                              —Charles Dickens, A *Tale of Two Cities*

Dickens, of course, did not have the contemporary dilemmas of modern genetics in mind. Indeed, we need to remind ourselves how short the history of modern genetics really is. Recognition that genetic traits are carried by deoxyribonucleic acid (DNA) occurred only about 40 years ago. Knowledge of the three-dimensional structure of DNA is only about 30 years old. The correct number of human chromosomes was not determined until the mid-1950s, and Down syndrome was recognized only in 1959. It was not until in 1968 that the exact location of a gene was determined on an autosomal chromosome, and the study of genes, rather than their protein products, has been possible for barely a decade.

As the writer of Deuteronomy noted, "these things" are both "the blessing and the curse." The "new genetics" has spawned problems for society that may equal those spawned by the discovery of fire. Judgment on this will be possible only in a generation or more, provided that we have not all been consumed by the new metaphorical fire. The implications are far-reaching and dramatic, involving agricultural, environmental, entomological, and, obviously, human-health dimensions. New forms of food crops—those that grow in salt water, those that no longer require traditional fertilizers for nitrogen, and those that are bred to resist environmental assault, such as frost—will someday revolutionize worldwide agriculture. The application of new molecular knowledge will facilitate the breeding of larger and more fecund food animals. Newly created microorganisms— for example, those that feed on oil spills—as well as other newly patented life forms, can be expected to assume roles hitherto undreamt of. For humans, health implications are more predictable. Life expectancy will be prolonged, if not through the cure of such scourges as cancer and heart disease, then through the detection of genetic susceptibility and therapeutic intervention. Genetic screening in the workplace may become commonplace in an effort to prevent certain occupational diseases or as a rationale for not minimizing hazards. The detection of carriers of many genetic disorders will evolve as a consequence of great strides in the mapping of genes for the already-cataloged 3,400 single-gene disorders. The opportunities for the detection of single-gene disorders prenatally will be enormous.

Biomedical research on humans continues to be governed by Health and Human Services Regulations supervised by local Institutional Review Boards and based on the Nuremberg Code. The code, which was adopted by the United Nations General Assembly in 1946, is founded on the premise that only certain types of medical experiments on human beings "satisfy moral, ethical, and legal concepts." These principles require, among other things, (1) the informed, voluntary, competent, and understanding consent of the subject; (2) a scientifically valid study based on animal testing and designed to yield fruitful results for the good of society not obtainable by other means; and (3) risks to the subject that are outweighed by the potential humanitarian importance of the study.

Notwithstanding efforts to adhere to moral and ethical standards and values, the new genetic technology has created direct confrontations with both law and theology. The potential for germ-line engineering is the latest lightning rod. Those opposed to such developments call for governmental regulation, invoking what Alex Capron has called the "supreme irony" by seeking to endow government with the very eugenic powers they wish to avoid.

Daniel Callahan reflected more than 5 years ago that genetic engineering has dominated all other issues in medical ethics. He also noted, with ambivalence, that "both the scientific community and the general public are more than ever prepared to go ahead with it" and that "those opposed to genetic engineering have not been able to mount generally persuasive arguments." These statements remain true today, as the contributions to this volume evidence. And we are still unable to move beyond the three "moral premises" Callahan identified, which seem to underpin this enthusiasm for genetic engineering: individual liberty to seek what one desires as long as it does not cause demonstrable harm to others; a risk–benefit equation that sees benefits clearly outweighing risks; and adherence to the notion of *beneficience*, that it is always better to attempt to do good than to try simply to avoid harm.

A new player has also joined the game, complicating the rules and risking other values. Corporate giants have sniffed the technological sizzle. Never shy with business incentives and actions timed to coincide with the declining research dollar, they have swiftly and decisively moved into the universities under the guise of a symbiotic relationship and without claim of directed research. Many, but not all, academic institutions have become rapidly ensnared, leaving discarded idealists muttering audibly about conflicts of interest and loss of freedom in academic research, and raising serious questions about appointments, promotion, and tenure when the denominator is profit. The corporate-academic merger is becoming a reality with the passive acquiescence of government. As these connections grow deeper and the results are applied to society, government will rear its bureaucratic, and often commissioned, head: Do we need a government-sponsored national genetics commission? Would a commission or board of the National Academy of Sciences be a wiser oversight group? And what implications flow from the involvement of National Academy members in industry? Should there be a commission or board with authority and accountability?

How, in a free society, can or should we interdict research and development within private corporations that need not answer to any government agency, possibly until they have already applied their findings to a helpless public? And how do the dual matters of conscience and loyalty of the scientist accommodate to the military-medical-industrial complex? Does biomedical research for a country's survival operate beyond the boundaries of morality, law, and rationality? Is it rational to demand that a scientist be responsible for a work product that may be applied to an anticipated or unanticipated destructive use? This responsibility seems to place an untenable burden and constraint on scientific discovery. The scientific community as a whole, however, has an obligation to develop a moral conscience in these matters. But can society depend on the scientists and the scientific community for self-discipline and restraint? What of the unscrupulous, the unethical, or the negligent? Don't we need government, with all its implications, to safeguard our survival, with perspicacity to police the present, and with prescience to protect the future?

The new ways of making babies without sex provide endless grist for the mills of moralists, theologians, philosophers, scientists, ethicists, people at large, and even lawyers. In this land, laws usually evolve in a reactive rather than a directive way. Hence, we have a flood of reproductive technologies, which include artificial insemination by donor, *in vitro* fertilization, oocyte retrieval and surrogate embryo transfer, the use of frozen embryos, ovum and sperm banks, and potential germ-like engineering techniques, without a clearly expounded public policy. We may also need to redefine maternity in a world where a child can have three mothers: a genetic, a gestational, and a rearing mother. And we should be developing policy about embryo selling and baby buying. As we write, terms like *negligence, liability, duty, wrongful life,* and *wrongful birth* have crept into the daily vocabulary of medical geneticists and obstetricians alike.

Constant attention to the fetus and the anomalous newborn continues, and foes of abortion choice attempt to force their beliefs on others. In our last volume, Rev. Joseph Fletcher advanced the concept of fetal abuse for those women who damage their fetuses by alcohol or drug ingestion, and he questioned whether fetal damage resulting from the transmission of known harmful genes should also be so construed. In this volume the debate resumes, this time centered on fetal surgery and cesarean sections.

Care of anomalous newborns remains at the height of controversy, with parents consumed by guilt and pondering moral culpability along with legal liability. Faced by Health and Human Service's "Baby Doe" regulations, an action that judicial description painted as "arbitrary and capricious," we have experienced direct government intrusion into the neonatal intensive-care nursery. These actions lack the civility, described by Judge David Bazelon, in which "human beings are the measure of value and humankind [is] the subject of enhancement," and have demonstrated an insensitivity to the complexities of decision making in this arena. The polemics surrounding the care of anomalous newborns is not about to fade: federal legislation on this subject was enacted seven months after the Third Genetics and Law Conference, and new federal and state regulations will probably be in place by the time this volume is published.

Meanwhile, the realities of environmental mutagens have dawned. Genetic susceptibility, occupational hazards, and random environmental risks have become prime public-policy concerns that remain unresolved. The roles of both government and private industry are explored in this volume.

The remarkable advances in genetic technology involve our entire society. No single element of society—be it the executive, the legislative, or the judiciary; corporate interests, physicians, or lawyers—can satisfactorily resolve the evolving dilemmas. Together, we must accommodate conflicting values and ideas and assess health priorities, given limited resources. If we are to secure the complex options of a free society, we must acknowledge and respect personal reproductive freedom, support free scientific inquiry, and fight to retain academic freedom. We can find neither solace nor security in recent history, no assurance or safety from the evanescent present, and no certainty or promise in the threatening future. We must seek each other's counsel, carefully assess our opportunities and their risks, and morally orient our policies. As with the preceding volumes, it is our hope that *Genetics and the Law III* will prove a constructive contribution to this collaborative assessment. This may not be "the epoch of belief," nor the "epoch of incredulity," but it is, hopefully, "the coming of the age of wisdom."

AUBREY MILUNSKY
GEORGE J. ANNAS

ACKNOWLEDGMENTS

We are most grateful to the National Science Foundation and the National Endowment for the Humanities for a grant that made this third national symposium possible. This meeting was held under the cosponsorship of the American Society of Law and Medicine and the Boston University Schools of Medicine, Public Health, and Law. We very much appreciate the strong support of Dean John I. Sandson, Dean Norman A. Scotch, and Dean William Schwartz of the respective schools.

We sincerely thank the Program Committee for assisting us in the planning of an outstanding symposium. In this connection, we thank Professor Alexander Morgan Capron, Professor Willard Gaylin, and Professor Margery W. Shaw.

Once again, we owe a debt of gratitude to the outstanding scientists, lawyers, physicians, theologians, sociologists, ethicists, and philosophers who shared their special insights, wisdom, and expertise, not only with the symposium participants through their presentations, but also with so many more through their outstanding manuscripts contained in this volume.

BIOTECHNOLOGY: BOON OR BANE?

THE FUTURE OF GENETIC MANIPULATION

MODERATOR: DAVID BALTIMORE

1

CAN WE CURE GENETIC DISORDERS?

LEON E. ROSENBERG, M.D.
C. N. H. *Long Professor*
Department of Human Genetics
Yale University School of Medicine
333 Cedar Street
P. O. Box 3333
New Haven, CT 06510

The question posed in this chapter—namely, "Can we cure genetic disorders?"—is straightforward. The answer is anything but simple, the best answer, in fact, being "Yes, no, and maybe." If *cure* is defined as dictionaries define it, (that is, "to restore health," or "to treat successfully," or "to succeed with a course of medical treatment"), then current approaches to some genetic disorders qualify. For instance, lifelong restriction of dietary phenylalanine in a neonate with classical phenylketonuria is likely "to restore health" and "to succeed with a course of medical treatment." Treatment of Wilson's disease with D-penicillamine and of congenital adrenal hyperplasia with adrenal steroid hormones and of diabetes mellitus with insulin are other examples of successful medical treatments of genetic disorders. But I contend that we ordinarily reserve the word *cure* for those situations in which the cause of the disorder is eliminated and treatment can be discontinued without relapse (as in the cure of pneumococcal pneumonia with penicillin or of appendicitis by appendectomy). Given this more restrictive definition, the only genetic disorders that we currently cure are those that can be managed surgically (e.g., the correction of cleft palate, the repair of a congenital heart defect, or colectomy for familial polyposis of the colon). Even in these instances, the primary cause of the disorder (i.e., the genetic factors or mutations) has not been addressed. In truth, if we use elimination of the mutant gene as the criterion defining the cure of any genetic disorder, we will never cure any of them because new mutations are occurring all the time, and because I cannot foresee being able to replace defective genes by normal ones in all cells of an affected patient— regardless of how sophisticated we become in our ability to understand and manipulate DNA.

If, however, we are prepared to use the word *cure* to refer to a single course of treatment that restores health, then I believe that modalities other than surgery qualify, and it is these modalities that I wish to concentrate on. They include organ or tissue transplantation and gene therapy. Each of these modalities can, under optimal conditions, yield permanent restoration of health for a selected group of patients for whom such modalities are appropriate. I intend to explore the rationale for these approaches, as well as their limits and problems. I will concentrate on technical and medical issues but will mention some recent developments concerning the ethics of their use as well.

TRANSPLANTATION AND GENE THERAPY

Restricted Indications

The first point to emphasize about the therapeutic potential of transplantation or gene therapy is that these modalities, at their best, are useful for only a small subset of genetic disorders. Neither will ever have any place in the treatment of disorders caused by chromosomal aneuploidy, such as Down syndrome or Turner syndrome. Neither can be directed at multifactorial traits, such as schizophrenia or anencephaly. Either modality is useful essentially only for those disorders caused by single gene defects in which the mutant gene is expressed in a single tissue or organ (i.e., blood cells), or in which damage is confined to a single organ (i.e., the liver). Both strategies (transplantation and gene therapy) seem most compelling for a small but important group of disorders affecting hematopoietic stem cells. These disorders include severe combined immunodeficiency (SCID), Wiskott–Aldrich syndrome, β-thalassemia, sickle-cell anemia, aregenerative anemia, and chronic granulomatous disease.[1] For this group of disorders, I see no major strategic difference between giving the affected patient a bone marrow transplant (i.e., using another person's normal cells) and using gene therapy (i.e., putting the normal gene into the patient's own marrow cells). The risks and problems are quite different, as will be discussed below, but the aim is the same: to provide the patient with marrow cells expressing the normal gene. Because bone marrow cells are readily accessible and can be grown outside the body, these disorders are the prime candidates for either gene therapy or transplantation.

Similarly, disorders of liver-specific gene products (PKU, glycogen storage disease-Type I, and ornithine transcarbamylase deficiency) or those affecting the liver exclusively or nearly so (Wilson disease and tyrosinemia) can theoretically be approached either by hepatic transplantation or gene therapy, provided the latter approach is made feasible by developing a means of directing the normal gene to liver cells. In the same way, both approaches could be considered for disorders affecting the kidney (Fabry disease and cystinosis).

It should be emphasized that the vast majority of Mendelian disorders—and many of the most common and serious ones (e.g., cystic fibrosis, osteogenesis imperfecta, Huntington disease, and muscular dystrophy)—will almost surely not be approached by either of these curative strategies because the disorder affects multiple tissues (as in cystic fibrosis or osteogenesis imperfecta) or because the affected organ or tissue is beyond the reach of transplantation or gene therapy (as in Huntington disease or muscular dystrophy).

TRANSPLANTATION

Problems and Limits

I have already mentioned a considerable number of genetic disorders for which tissue or organ transplantation would seem an appropriate, perhaps even optimal, therapeutic strategy. Surely, bone marrow transplantation for β-thalassemia, sickle-cell disease, or SCID, or liver transplantation for Type I glycogen-storage disease or neonatal-onset ornithine transcarbamylase deficiency would appear to offer major advantages over more commonly used symptomatic or palliative therapies. Since 1968, as reviewed by O'Reilly et al.,[1] nearly 150 patients with inherited disorders have received bone marrow transplants in curative attempts. Nearly half of these patients suffered from SCID, a group in whom successful engraftment occurred in ~60% of those treated. In two other conditions, Wiskott–Aldrich syndrome and β-thalassemia, as many as 20 patients have received marrow transplants. Single-case reports for a lengthy list of immunologic, phagocytic, and storage disorders constitute the remainder of this patient population. In addition to this small population treated with marrow transplants, a handful of patients with Wilson disease, tyrosinemia, α_1-antitrypsin deficiency, and Niemann–Pick disease have received liver transplants,[2] and another small group with cystinosis, Fabry disease, polycystic kidneys, and Alport syndrome have undergone renal transplantation.[2]

Why have so few patients with inherited disorders been treated with transplants? The first and foremost reason is that transplantation remains a high-risk procedure. Because of the need for ablative radiation and drug-induced immunosuppression, bone marrow transplantation carries with it an overall mortality of 20%–40%, and liver transplantation carries at least as great a risk. Second, transplantation programs exist at only a few centers; thus, accessibility is a real problem. Third, investigators have searched hard for less invasive therapeutic strategies, such as drug administration, transfusion, or enzyme replacement. Fourth, the metabolic basis for many of these disorders and the tissue-specific expression of the relevant gene product have been appreciated only recently.

Prospects

There is little doubt that tissue and organ transplantation will be used more widely for genetic disorders in the near future. As increased experience leads to decreased perioperative risk, as newer immunosuppressive drugs reduce the incidence of rejection, as more is learned about the control of graft-versus-host-disease, and as the likelihood of developing such modalities as enzyme replacement therapy recedes, bone marrow transplantation and liver transplantation will be tried. That trend has already begun for bone marrow transplantation in sickle-cell anemia, Gaucher disease, and other lysosomal storage disorders. It has begun as well for hepatic transplantation in tyrosinemia and Wilson disease and will soon be pursued for certain urea-cycle enzyme defects and other lethal disorders of hepatic function. How widely such transplant approaches will be used ultimately will depend on two issues: the collective and disease-specific benefit–risk experience and the rate of progress toward gene therapy.

GENE THERAPY

Scope and Definitions

It is now almost 10 years since the first human genes were cloned by means of recombinant DNA techniques. In the ensuing brief interval, an enormous amount has been learned about the structure, location, and expression of human genes. This basic information has been translated rapidly into the availability of gene probes for the antenatal and postnatal diagnosis of a growing list of Mendelian disorders in humans.[3] This capability will doubtless continue to burgeon in the years to come and will bring heretofore unavailable preventive programs with it. Such gene-cloning technology has not yet led to a single serious attempt to treat a human disease (i.e., altering genes in human cells to correct a human disorder), but such therapeutic strategies are much discussed in the scientific and lay literature.[4–7] Gene therapy has been carried out in fruit flies[8] and in mice.[9] How close are we to trying gene therapy in humans? What problems remain to be solved? Why does this matter engender such heated societal debate? I'll address these issues in the remainder of this chapter.

Somatic versus Germline Strategies for Gene Therapy

No intelligent discussion of gene therapy in humans can be undertaken without distinguishing between the insertion of genes into somatic cells and their insertion into germ cells. Somatic cells, such as bone marrow or liver cells, belong to a single individual and can undergo mitotic division only; they have no potential for affecting the individual's progeny or the human gene pool. Tampering with the genetic material of somatic cells may or may not help the individual from whom the cells are obtained, but it cannot affect anyone else. In contrast, inserting genes into fertilized eggs or early embryos carries with it the possibility that the gene will be integrated into all the cells of the developing organism—including the gonads; thus, the inserted gene may be capable of being transmitted to the initial recipient's progeny. Simply put, the inserted gene could become a hereditary trait. This fundamental distinction cannot be overemphasized. Failure to appreciate it has led to much of the cacophony regarding human gene therapy.[7] As stated earlier, I see very little difference between inserting a normal β-globin gene into the marrow cells of a patient with sickle-cell anemia and replacing that patient's marrow cells with normal cells by transplantation. Thus, I see no fundamental ethical problem with somatic-cell gene therapy. In my view, such somatic cell therapy is a rational and appropriate strategy for the treatment of those genetic disorders that meet the criteria discussed earlier. But a lengthy number of required steps must be met before this rational strategy becomes a clinical reality (Table I).

Steps in the Development of Gene Therapy for Somatic Cells

This list of steps begins with ascertaining that the benefit–risk assessment for the disorder favors gene therapy. In essence, this means that gene therapy should be considered only for serious disorders for which the current treatment is unsatisfactory. There are many genetic disorders that, unfortunately, meet the dual criteria of being both serious and poorly treatable. Hence, there are many disorders that qualify as candidates.

The second requirement involves isolating and cloning the normal gene whose mutation leads to the particular disorder being considered. It is startling to realize that this once formidable obstacle is now essentially trivial. Over 100 human genes, each potentially useful in the gene therapy for a particular genetic disorder, have already been cloned,[3] and this list grows weekly. But merely isolating the cloned gene is only the beginning.

The third requirement for somatic-cell gene therapy involves the definition of the regulatory sequences necessary for obtaining the expression of the gene in the cells. Most genes act, of course, by coding for the synthesis of a single gene product—usually a particular protein. This protein will not be produced unless regulatory sequences, called *promoters* or *enhancers*, activate the "coding" sequence.[10] Rapid progress is being made toward understanding both the composition of those regulatory elements and the means of ligating them to the coding portion of cloned genes.[10] This step will, therefore, not be a long-range obstacle to gene therapy.

The fourth requisite step involves integrating the cloned gene and the regulatory elements into the genome of the recipient cells. This is currently the greatest obstacle to

TABLE I.   Steps in the Development of Gene Therapy for Somatic Cells

1. Ascertaining that benefit–risk assessment favors gene therapy.

2. Isolating and cloning the normal gene.

3. Defining the regulatory sequences necessary for the expression of the cloned gene.

4. Integrating the cloned gene and the regulatory sequences into the genome of the recipient cells.

5. Propagating the recipient cells in appropriate tissue of the patient and providing them with the selective advantage.

6. Regulating the production of the gene product by the recipient cells.

7. Continuing evaluation for untoward effects of the treatment.

somatic-cell gene therapy and has, in no way, been solved. A variety of means are being employed to get genes into recipient cells: direct injection, bulk uptake, membrane fusion, and the use of viral vectors.[5] All strategies have significant unsolved problems. Injection, membrane fusion techniques, and bulk uptake are inefficient modes (success in only 1 in 10 million cells) and demand that the cells with inserted genes have some way of being recognized and selected for. Packaging human genes in viral vectors circumvents the efficiency problem but raises new problems, including the malignant transformation of the recipient cells and the spread of the virus particle to other cell types.[11,12] All of these delivery systems share one enormous problem, namely, the inability to control the site of integration of the inserted gene—among different cells in the same experiment, or among different therapeutic attempts. Such random integration raises the real possibility that untoward efforts may be produced in the recipient cells. The most talked-about complication is activation of a cellular oncogene. Interference with gene expression is as plausible a problem, thereby raising the possibility of rendering the recipient cell heterozygous at any given autosomal locus or even hemizygous for X-linked loci in males.

The fifth step requires that the treated cells containing the inserted gene be returned to the patient in such a way that they will grow and proliferate. This, too, is a very major problem. Even if we take the most simple example of bone-marrow-cell modification, we confront real problems. For instance, treatment of β-thalassemia by inserting a normal β-globin gene into marrow cells of an affected patient will be without value unless the treated cells have a particular selective advantage over the mass of untreated cells in the patient's bone marrow. Such an advantage may be provided by ablative radiation of the patient's marrow or, theoretically, by radiating only a small portion of the bone marrow so as to offer a suitable physical location for the treated cells to "home" to. Alternatively, cotransfection with a drug-resistance gene, followed by treatment of the patient with that specific drug, might provide the cells with an advantage.[13] For certain disorders, such as the inherited severe combined immunodeficiencies, recipient cells containing the normal gene may have a natural selective advantage over untreated cells. In my view, this makes such disorders the most immediately attractive candidates for gene therapy. For disorders involving genes expressed selectively in other organs (such as the liver), this problem is even more formidable. Means must be found to deliver the recipient cells to that organ and to enable them to grow. Hepatocytes turn over very slowly compared to marrow cells. In fact, little cellular proliferation takes place in this tissue. This slow turnover may pose an enormous obstacle to hepatic-cell gene therapy because the treated cell will not divide and share its new information with daughter cells.

The sixth required step involves the regulation of gene expression. Most inherited disorders are characterized by a synthesis of too little of a particular enzymatic or structural protein. The goal of gene therapy is to increase, above some critical value, that particular gene product. For some proteins, like hemoglobin, two different polypeptides (α and β globins) must be found, matched, and joined together if the hemoglobin tetramer is to function. Pathologic consequences occur when one or the other chain is not made in sufficient amounts. If gene therapy for such a disorder is to be clinically useful, restoration of the balance of synthesis of both chains is required. Whether this will occur with the random insertion of the particular gene into the recipient cell's genome depends on an understanding of the mechanisms used to achieve balance. Such an understanding is not at hand. For those gene products that work by themselves, the issue of feedback regulation and control of synthesis is germane as well.

Finally, we come to the seventh step, which involves long-term evaluation for untoward effects of the treatment. This step is followed after the introduction of any new experimental therapy. Each treated patient must be carefully observed for beneficial as well as harmful results of the intervention.

From the foregoing, it should be obvious that major technical problems remain to be solved before somatic-cell gene therapy is used in humans. How long will it take to overcome these problems? Which disorders are the best candidates for such treatment? Who should determine when such treatment is first to be used? I am confident that careful experiments, the use of animal systems, and the development of new technology will provide reasonable answers to these questions in the next few years. Ultimately, I see somatic-cell gene therapy as a viable strategy for a limited number of disorders affecting bone marrow cells, and perhaps for another small group of conditions affecting such other somatic cells as hepatocytes.

Problems in the Development of Germ-Cell Gene Therapy

Whatever the magnitude of the unsolved issues regarding somatic-cell gene therapy, they are minuscule compared with those involving germ cell therapy. Perhaps the magnitude of this problem can best be appreciated by looking at the same steps discussed for somatic-cell gene therapy (Table I). Immediately, we come to the crux of the difference between the two strategies, namely, ascertaining that benefit–risk assessment favors gene therapy. For which disorders is germ-cell gene therapy theoretically appropriate? In which clinical settings would it be considered? When one attempts to answer these classic questions, the limits of germ line therapy become immediately apparent. I have no problem in recognizing a number of disorders that could benefit from effective germ-line gene therapy. The general features of such disorders would be these: major clinical consequences (morbidity and mortality); the affecting of multiple tissues or a single tissue unreachable by somatic-cell gene therapy; serious damage done prenatally; and the lack of any other efective means of therapy, either currently or in future serious contemplation. Given these four criteria, such disorders as cystic fibrosis, Duchenne muscular dystrophy, and Tay–Sachs disease appear on the list of possible target conditions. But how do we identify the affected zygote? Each of the above disorders is inherited as an autosomal recessive trait (cystic fibrosis and Tay–Sachs) or an X-linked one (Duchenne muscular dystrophy). Thus, couples at risk have a 1:4 chance with each pregnancy of having a severely affected offspring. Even if we developed perfect tests for the prenatal detection of these disorders, such testing would not identify the particular embryo for which germ line therapy would be required unless the prenatal detection could be accomplished within a few cell divisions of fertilization. Because I think that capability a most unlikely one, and because it is irrational to treat all fertilized ova when only one out of four is at risk for the disorder in question, I think germ line therapy is a serious option in only a handful of settings, such as for the offspring of two people with oculocutaneous albinism or with sickle-cell anemia—all of whom will be affected with these disorders inherited as auto-somal recessive traits.

Even in these very rare circumstances where such intervention might be appropriate, all the other steps noted in Table I would need to be addressed. Because the inserted gene might find its way to all of the recipient's cells, including the germ line, this form of therapy is potentially heritable. This unique feature of germ line therapy raises very serious ethical problems. It raises as serious scientific ones, because the earliest attempts at germ-line insertion in animals suggest that lethal effects on the offspring of the recipient may be a common complication.[14,15] If additional animal studies support these dire results, germ-cell gene therapy in humans will simply be excluded as a rational therapeutic strategy.

ETHICAL CONSIDERATIONS

Clearly, the cure of inherited disorders by either organ/tissue transplantation or gene therapy raises important ethical questions that our society must consider. A number of other papers in this book address these questions in detail. I wish only to emphasize that we already have a most valuable starting point for this societal discussion. It is the report of the President's Commission for the Study of Ethical Problems in Medicine and Bio-medical Research, entitled *Splicing Life*.[16] The commission studied the social and ethical issues related to gene therapy in humans and then produced a penetrating, cogent, and readable document. Among the many contributions of this book, one concerned the prerequisites to the development of an effective public policy regarding genetic engineer-ing in humans. The commission identified four such prerequisites: (1) educating the public about genetics and about the historical context of genetic manipulations; (2) clarifying the concerns underlying simple slogans; (3) identifying the issues in ways meaningful to public policy consideration; and (4) evaluating the need for an implemen-tation of oversight within and outside government. Those of us in the scientific communi-ty who believe that the genetic manipulation of human cells may one day cure disorders and, thereby, reduce human suffering must be prepared to participate in the societal debate that has already been joined and to redouble our educational efforts toward all groups among our citizenry. Only by so doing will we quiet the public concern that gene splicing might remake human beings and reply to the worry that this technology chal-lenges deeply held feelings about what being human is.

I shall close with two brief quotes from the commission's report, which return us to the focus of this paper on medical treatment:

> As a product of human investigation and ingenuity, the new knowledge (about gene splicing) is a celebration of human creativity, and the new powers are a reminder of human obligations to act responsibly.

The aid that these new developments may provide in the relief of human suffering is an ethical reason for encouraging them.

References

1. O'Reilly, R. J., Brochstein, J., Dinsmore, R., and Kirkpatric, D., Marrow transplantation for congenital disorders, *Seminars in Hematology* 21:188–221 (1984).
2. Hirschhorn, R., Treatment of genetic diseases by allotransplantation. In Desnick, R. J. (ed.), *Enzyme Therapy in Genetic Diseases:2, Vol. XVI, No. 1. Birth Defects: Original Article Series*, New York: Alan R. Liss, 1980:429–444.
3. Shows, T. B., The human molecular map of cloned genes and DNA polymorphisms. In *Banbury Report 14, Recombinant DNA Applications to Human Disease* (C. T. Caskey, and R. L. White, eds.), Cold Spring Harbor Laboratory, Cold Spring Harbor, NY (1983).
4. Williamson, B., Gene therapy, *Nature* 298:416–418 (1982).
5. Anderson, W. F., Prospects for human gene therapy, *Science* 226:401–409 (1984).
6. Friedmann, T., in *Gene Therapy: Fact and Fiction*, Cold Spring Harbor Laboratory, Cold Spring Harbor, NY (1983).
7. Rifkin, J., in *Algeny*. Viking, New York (1983).
8. Rubin, G. M., and Spradling, A. C., Genetic transformation of Drosophila with transposable element vectors, *Science* 218:348–353 (1982).
9. Hammer, R. E., Palmiter, R. D., and Brinster, R. L., Partial correction of murine hereditary growth disorder by germ-line incorporation of a new gene, *Nature* 311:65–67 (1984).
10. Weisberg, R. A., and Leder, P., Fundamentals of molecular genetics. In *The Metabolic Basis of Inherited Disease* (5th ed.), (J. B. Stanbury, J. B. Wyngaarden, D. S. Fredrickson, J. L. Goldstein, and M. S. Brown, eds.) McGraw-Hill, New York (1983).
11. Williams, D. A., Lemischka, I. R., Nathan, D. G., and Mulligan, R. C., Introduction of new genetic material into pluripotent haematopoietic stem cells of the mouse, *Nature* 310:476–480 (1984).
12. Miller, A. D., Ong, E. S., Rosenfeld, M. G., Verma, I. M., and Evans, R. M., Infectious and selectable retrovirus containing an inducible rat growth hormone minigene, *Science* 225:993–8 (1984).
13. Cline, M. J., Genetic engineering of mammalian cells: Its potential application to genetic diseases of man, *J. Lab. Clin. Med.* 99:299–308 (1982).
14. Schnieke, A., Harbers, K., and Jaenisch, R., Embryonic lethal mutation in mice induced by retrovirus insertion into the $\alpha 1(I)$ collagen gene, *Nature* 304:315–20 (1983).
15. Wagner, E. F., Covarrubias, L., Stewart, T. A., and Mintz, B., Prenatal lethalities in mice homozygous for human growth hormone gene sequences integrated in the germ line, *Cell* 35:647–55 (1983).
16. President's Commission for the Study of Ethical Problems in Medicine and Biomedical and Biomedical and Behavioral Research, in *Splicing Life*, Government Printing Office, Washington, DC, Stock Number 83-600500 (1982).

2

REGULATING GENETIC TECHNOLOGY
Values in Conflict

NORMAN FOST, M.D. M.P.H.
Professor of Pediatrics and History of Medicine
Director, Program in Medical Ethics
University of Wisconsin, Madison
600 Highland Avenue
Madison, WI 53978

I thank Dr. Milunsky for inviting me to participate in this conference, which I do with some misgivings. It is humbling to be introduced and watched over by Dr. Baltimore, who has been at the center of the science of which we will speak and of the historic leadership taken by the scientific community in not only self-regulation, but alerting the public to the difficult ethical and social issues raised by recombinant DNA research.

I would suggest that the lessons to be learned from the recent history of the regulation of recombinant DNA research are similar to the issues involved in the regulation of other activities central to this conference, including the treatment of newborns with genetic and other handicaps and the control of new reproductive technologies. I will focus on the recombinant DNA controversy and suggest analogies with other genetic technologies.

DISTINCTIONS BETWEEN SCIENCE AND TECHNOLOGY

Distinctions between science and technology, or basic and applied research, may not be useful in discussing the social control of scientists' activities. In defending the "necessity of freedom," Dr. Baltimore, writing in 1978, conceded that

> the arguments pertain to basic scientific research, not to the technical applications of science. As we go from the fundamental to the applied, my arguments fall away. . . . [T]here are many technological possibilities that ought to be restrained.[1]

I have no criticism of the reasons cited by Dr. Baltimore for opposing restrictions on basic

15

science, because I am generally in sympathy with them. He emphasized that such restraints commonly flow from ideological bases and are more likely to be generally disruptive of science than to provide the intended specific constraint. Even if we concede that these are good reasons, in general, for allowing basic science to flourish unfettered, there are problems in starting with the view that technology or applied research warrants regulation, but science, or basic research, should be nearly immune (Figure 1).

First, the distinction between science and technology is not always clear. The distinction blurs as the interval between basic and applied research narrows. Less than 10 years elapsed between the discovery of recombinant DNA techniques and human applications, closely followed by profit-making uses. Basic and applied research are conducted by individuals who work concurrently in corporate settings and academic institutions. Sometimes, it is difficult to say whether a particular project conducted in either setting is basic or applied. I review research protocols as a member of the biosafety committee of a company and have difficulty distinguishing basic from applied research. The distinction may be largely a matter of intent. Whether or not a scientist is working on a project from a desire to understand the physical universe or from a desire to develop a patentable item cannot be determined solely by the nature of the research. Imagine a jockey on the practice track who hits a horse with a whip and claims, "I am concerned with the conduction velocity of nerves." How would one disprove his claim? There may be an analogy with the question I am asked most often as chairman of our institutional review board: "Is this project research or innovative therapy?" Regulation of the former is considerably more stringent than of the latter. Although there are some litmus tests that may clearly put a project in one category or the other, the question often reduces to one of intent, answerable only by the investigator, whose conflicts of interest may lead him or her to be a less than ideal judge of whether institutional review is needed.

A second reason that the regulation of basic science may sometimes be appropriate is that, at some point during the basic research phase, it may become impossible to prevent the transition from basic to applied. This is more clearly a problem when the techniques are inexpensive or are easily copied by people or countries beyond the reach of regulation. As we will undoubtedly hear later, artificial insemination is now widely practiced by women in their homes, using common turkey basters, with sperm donated by friends or acquaintances. I am not among those who believe that this practice demands regulation, but those who do now realize that if there was a compelling state interest in regulating artificial insemination, the time to assert it was long ago, prior to the first human

---

1. Distinction blurs as the interval narrows between basic and applied research.
2. Potential for regulation may be lost at some point during the basic research phase.
3. Doing harm is worse than failing to do good.
4. Even basic science is not value-free.

Figure 1. Reasons for regulating science and technology.

application. I share Dr. Baltimore's views regarding the covert reasons and hazards of such control. I only wish to make the conceptual point that if it is conceded that the *technology* may be so worrisome as to justify restriction, the timing of that intervention may have to be during the basic research phase.

Third, I would suggest that the harms caused by suppression of research, serious though they are, are different, in a moral sense, than the harms caused by research itself. I am using the word *harm* here in the narrow sense of physical injury. Defenders of science commonly argue that suppression may "harm" those millions of persons who die or suffer from diseases that could have been prevented if research had not been suppressed. I think this is a misuse of the word *harm*. A more accurate term would be *failing to help*. Although failing to help a person in need may be tragic, it is not generally considered as clear a moral wrong as positively harming that person. Every day we all fail to help many of the millions of starving persons around the globe. Each of us has the resources to save many lives, at very little personal sacrifice. However wrong this failure may be, including the awareness that preventable deaths occur, it is not commensurate with killing a single one of those persons. Doing harm is worse than failing to do good. This is a widely shared principle in our society, reflected in the long-standing legal principle that there is a clear duty not to harm others, but very little duty to come to the aid of a person in peril. There are, of course, exceptions, when it is reprehensible not to help. Examples would include situations in which one had promised, or contracted, to care for another, or the responsibility of a government to provide basic needs for its citizens. And avoiding harm, like any principle, is not absolute. Doing harm may be justified, for example, when there is likely to be compensating benefit or, even in the absence of benefit, when there is consent. But as Jonas put it, scientific progress is optional; the duty to avoid harm is not.[2] Maxine Singer and Paul Berg stated it more strongly: "We share the belief . . . that it is unacceptable to harm others."[3] Because the potential risks of new technologies often do not have clear or likely benefits for those at risk, exposure to risk requires something like consent. That is part of the justification for public involvement in the regulation of new technology.

Although the risks of recombinant DNA research, in retrospect, appear to have been overstated by some, the drive to limit that research may have been justified if viewed from this perspective. Had 1,000 people died from a disease-bearing *E. Coli*, escaped from a basic science laboratory, I believe it would have been considered a more serious moral issue than the 1,000 deaths that occurred from a disease whose cure was prolonged or missed because of the delays in research necessitated by regulations.

Finally, I believe that the attempt to find a distinction between science and technology may be another example of the relentless search for a distinction between value-free and value-laden activities. No activity, none, is value-free. Scientists engage in research for a variety of self-serving reasons, some of them quite innocent, some laudatory, some corrupt. Just as those who would restrict science often do so for ideological reasons, so do governments support science, in general or in particular areas, for political and ideological reason. The military-industrial complex supports much research that would be considered basic science, with motives that could not be considered value-free.

We will hear more in the next few days of government attempts to regulate the treatment of handicapped newborns, in some cases resulting in great harm to these newborns. In the final Baby Doe regulations, the federal government, while reiterating its commitment to the value of treating handicapped infants the same as nonhandicapped infants, acknowledges that, in some circumstances, it may be permissible to withhold or withdraw life-sustaining treatment. The criterion it puts forth for justifying such nontreatment is alledgedly a purely technical or value-free criterion, namely, when there is no medical benefit. As an example, the regulations explain that it would be permissible to withhold life-sustaining treatment from an anencephalic newborn, arguing that there is no "medical" benefit because the infant is dying. They are, of course, mistaken in this analysis. The medical benefit of a particular treatment—mechanical ventilation, for example—for such an infant is potentially the same as for a normal infant: it maintains respiratory functions. What the government means to say is that it isn't worth it, presumably because the infant cannot experience a psychological or social benefit from having its respiratory functions maintained. This is a value judgment with which all reasonable people would concur, but a value judgment nonetheless.

Other Concerns about Recombinant DNA Research

I have been discussing the regulation of recombinant DNA research with regard to the alleged physical risks to the community. This was the first reason for discussing the regulation of such research, but it has been displaced by other considerations (Figure 2). The potential conflicts of interest created by individuals who work for or invest in such corporations while maintaining basic research laboratories in academic institutions will be discussed more extensively later in the conference. I will make only the simple point that, although the existence of conflicts of interest does not imply that such conflicts will result in actions that are against the public interest, it does suggest that some checks or review might be appropriate. Conflicts of interest, including personal financial gain, are not new in academia. Physicians who do clinical research and collect personal fees have more obvious and immediate incentives that could interfere with judgments about protecting

---

1. Public health hazards: escape of harmful bacteria.
2. Conflicts of interest among investigators: industry in academia.
3. Human applications.
    A. Organic risks to individual subjects.
    B. Effects on evolution.
        1. Somatic cell changes.
        2. Germ cell changes.

Figure 2. Concerns about recombinant DNA research.

patients' interests, and the risks of harm to identifiable persons in such settings are greater than the likely harms from basic science research.

Finally, the concerns about human applications involve two issues. The first—protecting research subjects from risk—is currently well-regulated by extensive federal regulations through the institutional review boards. I believe that there is no serious controversy about the need for such regulation. Although federal commissions will undoubtedly continue to identify the problems and inadequacies of the IRBs, there is also consensus that they have served us all well, providing a reasonable balance between the interests of science and those of potential subjects.

The concern about effects on human evolution are twofold. First, there is the acceleration of evolution that can occur when genotypes are influenced by human choice rather than natural selection. I refer here to applications involving somatic cells, such as the replacement of specific defective genes. Because these choices will obviously be value-laden, it seems unarguable that such decisions should be made in a public way, ensuring the involvement of those who may be stigmatized. We should recognize that eugenic proposals and policies are alive and well in our society. Pamphlets in doctors, offices that advertise the availability of prenatal diagnosis for Down syndrome unavoidably imply a value-judgment about the desirability of having a child with that condition. The pejorative implications of such advertising cannot be avoided by emphasizing freedom of choice or the positive aspects of having such children. Imagine, if you will, a pamphlet in your doctor's office, paid for by the U.S. Department of Health and Human Services, informing clients that they are at risk for giving birth to a child who may be a female or a black. The pamphlet, of course, would emphasize that there are good and bad aspects of having such a child, that many people enjoy such children, and that whether or not you choose to have such a child is entirely your business. By selecting some genetically controlled physical characteristics for advertising, we declare our concern about the so-called negative aspects of those conditions.

The other concern about effects on evolution involves the replacement or alteration of genes in germ cells. This methodology obviously presents the possibility of more rapid or dramatic changes in the gene pool of successive generations. Similar questions of eugenics will arise. These strike me as quantatively but not qualitatively different from those surrounding somatic cell manipulation or other techniques that affect the gene pool, such as treating manifestations of gene activity in a way that alters the reproductive fitness of affected individuals. We have been involved in this kind of genetic engineering for centuries, and I do not think there is reasonable debate that we should stop "playing God" in this way, if that is a proper term for it.

SOME SUGGESTED GOALS

I will close by responding to Dr. Milunsky's request that I identify the values that should be considered in discussions about the regulation of science and technology. According to the theory of the ideal ethical observer,[4] an action can be considered right only if it can be approved by an ideal observer with the following characteristics (Figure 3). He or she should have access to all readily available and relevant facts; be able to vividly imagine the feelings of those who are most affected—put himself or herself in other people's shoes; should have no vested interests; should not be overwhelmed by emotions that cloud critical thinking; and should be consistent, in the sense of appealing to generalizable principles, which should result in treating similar cases similarly.

Maximizing these goals requires a public process. Opening up the regulatory process will increase access to relevant facts. Noble though the process begun at Asilomar was, it failed to gain support initially because those present did not include some of the kinds of expertise needed to make informed judgments about the risks of microbes' escaping from the laboratory, such as expertise in infectious disease and epidemiology. The Asilomar conference was also criticized because it consisted predominantly, though not exclusively, of those with vested interests. It is beside the point that the individuals involved were extraordinarily concerned with public safety, to the point of imposing a moratorium on themselves and proposing regulations that, in retrospect, were too strict. The decisions violated the procedural requirement of including those with different and competing interests. The process that eventually occurred—rowdy, hysterical, prolonged, and often foolish—did result in regulations that not only allowed the science to go on with minimal interference, but that were also acceptable to the public precisely because they came out of a public process.

CONCLUSION

In summary, I believe science, technology, and the public interest will be served by recalling a few basic principles (Figure 4). First, doing harm is worse than failing to do good. The ancient medical injunction—"First, do no harm"—is based on this principle. It implies a conservative, or cautious, approach. Second, good ethics start with good facts. This principle will always include facts and expertise that are not available to the scientists doing the research, who will not only lack important knowledge but will not know what they don't know until there is broad discussion. Finally, important decisions should not and cannot be made exclusively by those with vested interests. These are arguments for process. Some of the substantive principles that should be considered were reviewed by

---

1. Omniscient (knows all relevant facts).
2. Omnipercipient (is able to vividly imagine feelings of those involved).
3. Disinterested (has no vested interests).
4. Dispassionate (is not overwhelmed by emotion).
5. Consistent (uses generalizable principles).

Figure 3. The ideal ethical observer.

> 1. Doing harm is worse than failing to do good.
> 2. Good ethics start with good facts.
> 3. Important decisions should not be made solely by those with vested interests.

Figure 4. A few basic principles.

Callahan.[5] This strong call for public decisions on issues that involve the public interest is never pleasing to those who see the issue differently, particularly those who are understandably eager to get on with the science and its potential benefits. It only reminds them of the wisdom of the sage who said, "If all the ethicists in the world were laid end to end, it would be a good thing."

REFERENCES

1. Baltimore, D., Limiting science: A biologist's perspective, *Daedalus* 107:37–45 (1978).
2. Jonas, H., Philosophical reflections on experimenting on human subjects. In *Experimentation with Human Subjects* (P. Freund, ed.), Braziller, New York (1969).
3. Singer, M. F., and Berg, P., Recombinant DNA: NIH Guidelines, *Science* 196:186–8 (1976).
4. Fost, N., Ethical problems in pediatrics. In Gluck L (ed.), *Current Problems in Pediatrics*, 1976;6, No. 12:1–31(October).
5. Callahan, D., Ethical issues in the control of science. In *Genetics and the Law-II* (A. Milunsky and G. J. Annas, eds.), Plenum Press, New York (1980).

3

Unsplicing the Gordian Knot
Legal and Ethical Issues in the "New Genetics"

ALEXANDER MORGAN CAPRON, LL.B.
Topping Professor of Law, Medicine, and Public Policy
The Law Center
University of Southern California
Los Angeles, CA 90089-0071

A decade ago, Aubrey Milunsky and I met to discuss the possibility of a project on genetics and the law. In our meetings, I proposed that we prepare a treatise on this subject, whereas Aubrey, correctly sensing how extensive the topic is, favored a symposium with a variety of speakers. As we all know, the result has been this series of conferences, of which this one is the third.

It is remarkable to me, in looking back at the issues discussed at that first meeting—issues such as genetic screening for sickle cell, PKU, and Tay-Sachs, and liability for inadequate genetic counseling—that the issues then seen as arising in the future were not the ones that have been most central as events actually unfolded.[1] Simply put, fancy alterations in reproductive technology—up to the point of cloning and parthenogenesis—are not the major concerns of today. Even at the second national symposium, relatively little attention was paid to the issues of genetic engineering, the topic to which all of today's meeting is devoted.[2]

Nonetheless, despite the shifts in specific technologies that have been addressed, this series of symposia has served to illustrate certain recurrent issues that are posed by "the new genetics." As I see it, these four issues are

1. *Justice and fairness*, whether in ensuring equitable access to powerful new genetic tools or in redressing the burdens that result from the natural genetic lottery.
2. *Well-being and the avoidance of harm*, whether in ensuring that new methods of treatment are not employed prematurely in human beings or in keeping the

23

welfare of patients, especially the unborn or the just born, at the center of
decision making.

3. *Autonomy and choice*, whether in ensuring that genetic counseling remain
   nondirective and respectful of the values and goals of each person or in respecting the dilemmas created by the unprecedented biomedical powers as they relate
   to reproduction, from the test tube to the scalpel of a team performing fetal
   surgery.

4. For want of a better word, *the "genicity"*—that is, the genetic nature—of the
   subject.

All of these common points have important ethical and legal manifestations that
will, I am confident, reappear in many specific guises in our three days of meeting at this
third symposium. But it is the fourth one on which I have been reflecting in particular of
late because to some extent it cuts against the grain for me to recognize it. There is an
understandable tendency in bioethics to look for certain broad principles that apply as well
to one area of medicine and research as to the next. In one way or another, do we not
repeatedly find ourselves grappling with the same problems—such as the difficulty of
weighing risks against benefits, the necessity of making decisions in the face of uncertainty, the challenge of identifying the appropriate decision makers, and, above all, the agony
of allocating scarce and critically important resources?[3] Indeed, modern medicine and
research are fields of such great interest to philosophers and lawyers, among others,
because they crystallize in so notable a fashion so many of the most important issues for
society, ours or any other.

But although the general problems recur—as do the broad principles with which we
attempt to grapple with them—it seems to me that the onward march of genetic technology makes ever more prominent certain unusual, perhaps unique, features of "the new
genetics," as compared with other biomedical fields. Artificial respirators and the other
concomitants of intensive care may leave us with the problem of deciding when life ends
and death occurs. And heart transplants—or mechanical implants—may initially startle
the public and seem to pose the issue: What is a human being? And psychoactive drugs or
electrodes implanted in the brain may raise in new ways concerns about freedom and
responsibility. But the very externality of these interventions, their very separateness,
means that after the startle effect wears off, the problems raised by these techniques fall
back into our existing categories—which does not mean that they are quickly or easily
resolved, merely that they are familiar beasts with close relatives already in the bioethics
zoo.

From the very first, however, I have had the sense that the desire to fit all the
problems presented by the new genetics into this existing "zoology" was doomed to
failure. When genetic screening was increasing rapidly in the 1970s, the suggestion was
made that people were worried by the resulting identification—particularly when screening was carried on by the state or by other large organizations—because of the way it
probed people's fundamental identity, their genetic thumbprint, the taproot of their very
being.[4] Likewise, when recombinant DNA entered public consciousness with the mor-

atorium on certain experiments and the Asilomar conference, the resulting public concern could not be fully explained by the risks of laboratory mishaps with microorganisms; instead, the public debate rested on the sense (perhaps *intuition* is the better word) that the techniques posed problems different from those of ordinary safety because they could lead, intentionally or otherwise, to transformations in human genes. For this reason, the story of Dr. Frankenstein became the common metaphor[5]—though I personally feel that Hawthorne's tale of "Rappaccini's Daughter" has more to tell us of the perils involved.[6]

All of this says, however, that a technology that might peer into our genes and even transform them cuts to a deeper level of psychological significance than do others in biomedicine, however technically spectacular they may be. Though we have in common with other species not merely the building blocks of DNA but actually most of our genes themselves, we still believe that our particular collection of genes is what makes human beings unique and distinctive. And though we share this collection of genes with our fellow human beings, we also regard our particular genes—along with our particular environment—as that which makes us individuals.

The mythic qualities of this "genicity" issue, which is such an unusual and distinctive feature of that segment of bioethics and law that is the topic of this symposium, put me in mind of the poor man Gordius, who became King of Phrygia and in gratitude dedicated his wagon to Zeus. The pole of the wagon was attached to the yoke by an intricate bark knot that no one was able to untie. As you recall, when Alexander the Great came to Phrygia, he severed the knot with a single blow of his sword.

So, too, Watson and Crick announced to the world a little more than three decades ago that all life is based on an intricate, twisted, self-replicating helix, a biological Gordian knot. In the late 1960s and early 1970s, biochemists and molecular biologists— in a series of experiments associated with such names as Berg and Jackson, Davis and Mertz, Cohen and Boyer—found the restriction endonucleases that could cut through that knot and, going Alexander one better, were able to splice in more biological rope and retie the knot, giving it new functions.

I have never been entirely sure what to make of the story of the Gordian knot. Plainly, it usually signifies a dramatic solution to a perplexing problem—as, by analogy, the development of the recombinant DNA techniques that I have just mentioned. But there is also a suggestion about it of shortcuts, with resulting ill consequences. The oracle had foretold that whoever untied the Gordian knot would become leader of all Asia—and though Alexander went on to great victories, particularly in conquering Persia, he fell far short of leading all Asia, and neither he nor his empire survived for long.

And so, moving to an ethical and legal use of the symbol of the Gordian knot, I think we must acknowledge that, as individuals and as a society, we may be smart before we are wise. Therefore, we should return to the challenging task of untying the knotty issues posed by the new genetics through patient analysis rather than by attempting in a single stroke to break the knot apart. Indeed, borrowing from the example of the biologists and chemists, perhaps we could think of our task as unsplicing the knot rather than simply untying it—in other words, looking into each twisted strand, sorting it out, and putting it back together in a clearer and more useful way.

For the past decade, many people have made beginnings at this project. Because this is not a test to see who will be ruler of Asia, we can take pleasure in the progress that others have made, with no thought that any single examination will be conclusive. I like to think that the report on *Splicing Life* that the President's Commission submitted in November 1982 to the president and Congress, like the hearings that Representative Albert Gore, Jr., held on that report and subsequently,[7] helped to make the knot of ethical and social issues easier to understand, a process that will continue at this meeting.

Yet, the temptation to seek the easy solution will remain. We saw this again last June, when a resolution was announced on behalf of a large group of clergy—from Jerry Falwell to the presiding Episcopal bishop of the United States to 25 Roman Catholic bishops and archbishops—that called for a prohibition of "efforts to engineer specific genetic traits into the germline of the human species."[8] That document was based on a mistaken view of the technology and how rapidly and precisely it would enter medicine. More important, the mechanism suggested by the signatories—a federal ban on germ-line genetic engineering—would be either ineffective or, if effective, almost certainly productive of exactly the opposite results intended by the well-meaning clerics. The irony is how, once again, one sees the truth of Santayana's dictum that those who do not understand history are bound to repeat it. It is appropriate, as the theologians said, for our society to be concerned about avoiding the dangers of human eugenics, which stains more than one page of the history of this century. But it is naive not to see that a proposed ban on any genetic manipulations that affect the germ line would, in legislative hands, be transformed into a general prohibition, subject to certain exceptions as determined by some process—leading, for example, to a board with the authority to allow certain exceptions "in medically indicated cases." In other words, trying to ban a technique that will have some beneficial uses is sure to lead to a new eugenics, in which someone or some group will decide which diseases will be treated and which will not. The lesson of history that the clerics forgot was that eugenics poses no great danger until it is backed up by the power of the state, well-meaning or otherwise.

Finally, the statement last June illustrates how a simpleminded blow at a Gordian knot shatters a complex problem into a thousand little pieces without helping anyone to understand what was really causing the perplexity in the first place. The call for a ban, for example, proceeded on the assumption that inheritable changes are irreversible, which may or may not always be true. By focusing on inheritance as the key factor, it obscured what seem to me to be crucial differences between efforts to overcome manifest illnesses caused by single genes and efforts aimed at altering complex characteristics associated with many genes, particularly efforts aimed at "enhancing" certain capabilities. Such a difference can be made conceptually, and we need to ask whether, in actual practice, such a line can be drawn between enhancement and repair if sufficient care and attention is devoted to the effort. If not, we would then face the question whether that is reason enough to ban the whole field.

These are the sorts of hard questions that deserve continued attention in many quarters, including from the advisory—not regulatory—commission that would have been created under a bill adopted by the U.S. Congress in 1984, though vetoed as part of a larger NIH authorization bill.[9] The great shame of alarmist resolutions is that they divert attention and effort from the hard work that needs to be done on the ethical, social, and legal sides of this field, to match the vigorous and imaginative work being done on the scientific side.

As I said at the outset, I believe that such efforts will return to some common issues—issues that pose challenges of enormous importance:

First, can we find ways for this technology, one of the most awesome and powerful ever discovered, to make the world more just? To do so, we must, of course, ensure that those who labor in this field will reap fair rewards for their efforts and that unnecessary barriers or disincentives will not be erected that would discourage further discoveries and new useful applications of the techniques—matters that will involve finding appropriate governmental regulations and academic-industrial relations. To do so, we must also try to find ways to ensure that problems of importance to many people—not only in terms of genetic diseases, but also regarding the use of science to overcome the adverse effects of the environment, from workplace safety to adequate foodstuffs—will be addressed. It would be a great loss if efforts are directed solely to matters of the highest short-term financial return. And finally, we must be concerned with equitable access to the fruits of the process.

Second, can we find a means of honoring the ancient dictum of medicine—"Above all, do no harm"—while doing more than standing still? When the Hippocratic warning was formulated, there was little of benefit that medicine could offer; today, despite the large areas of ignorance and limited technology that remain, medicine can make a great deal of difference—for the good—for many very sick patients. Thus, too literal an application of "Do no harm" would mean, "Risk nothing, even on the probability of doing good." In my view, it is wrong to suggest that safety lies in inactivity—for as protective as that may seem for those who have the genetic lottery on their side, it is a safety bought at the expense of those deprived of a chance for a better life through a creative use of the new genetics. Of course, there is need for care to minimize the harm that could come either to individual patients or to society at large. But experimentation presents some risk, no matter how carefully planned and conducted, and we cannot afford to reject all experimentation. Thus, those charged with the responsibility for rules and regulations should be as creative in developing workable safeguards as the geneticists have been in developing the new scientific knowledge and techniques.

The third set of challenges, as I suggested at the outset, revolve around the matter of choice. All new technologies raise ethical problems because they create new possibilities for action, new necessities for decision. Sometimes, the need for choice can lead to ethical embarrassments, as Governor Richard Lamm of Colorado discovered recently when—in discussing the problems that life-prolonging technology has created for seriously ill people—he confused their *right* to avoid futile (and often very expensive) treatment, a right that in practice seems so often to be ignored, with what he is quoted as having described as their *duty* to forgo such treatment.[10] If we are to minimize such difficulties and confusions in the application of genetic technologies, we will need to spell out the ways in which ethical principles can aid in decision making, from prenatal diagnosis to the care of handicapped neonates. It is not enough to elaborate such principles as self-determination or such legal doctrines as informed consent; we must also splice in appropriate strands of such concepts as community and intergenerational responsibility, concepts that will also emerge in the presentations at this symposium.

Finally, a careful approach to our Gordian knot—rather than the simplistic swing of a sword—may help to untangle our confused but still important notions of the specifically genetic aspects of this entire field. Although this task sounds esoteric, it is ultimately a matter that should concern everyone. Some of what is found may prove, once unwound, to be less than unique. Indeed, on examination, many of the oft-repeated objections to genetic engineering as "playing God" prove merely to be concerns over particular risks rather than challenges based on the inherent unacceptability of the fact of tampering with genes.[11] Insights and illuminations of this sort provide another reason for encouraging— and supporting—broad-ranging studies by publicly accountable bodies, charged not with regulation but with examination, elucidation, and education.

This, then, is what I take our common task to be at this symposium—whether we are talking about biotechnology, new ways of making babies, or the avoidance of genetic diseases—namely, to see the ways in which our particular topics may help our society better to understand and resolve issues of fairness, of well-being, of choice, and of what is special about the subject of genetics.

REFERENCES AND NOTES

1. *Genetics and the Law* (A. Milunsky and G. Annas, eds.), Plenum Press, New York and London (1976).
2. *Genetics and the Law II* (A. Milunsky and G. Annas, eds.), Plenum Press, New York and London (1980).
3. See President's Commission for the Study of Ethical Problems in Medicine and Biomedical and Behavioral Research, *Summing Up*, pp. 71–81, U.S. Government Printing Office, Washington, DC (1983).
4. Sorenson, J., Some social and psychologic issues in genetic screening, in *Ethical, Social and Legal Dimensions of Screening for Human Genetic Disease* (D. Bergsma, ed.), *Birth Defects: Original Articles Series* 10(6):165, 174–81 (1974).
5. See President's Commission for the Study of Ethical Problems in Medicine and Biomedical and Behavioral Research, *Splicing Life*, pp. 13–17, U.S. Government Printing Office, Washington, DC (1982).
6. Capron, A., Human genetic engineering, *Technology in Society*, 6:23–35 (1984).
7. *Human Genetic Engineering*, Hearings before the Subcomm. on Investigations and Oversight, House Comm. on Science and Technology, 97th Cong., 2d Sess. (Nov. 16–18, 1982).
8. Resolution, June 8, 1983 (ad hoc group organized by Jeremy Rifkin).
9. H.R. 2350 (Health Research Extension Act of 1983), 98th Cong., 1st Sess., Title IV, Part F, Sec. 11 (vetoed Oct. 31, 1984).
10. Lamm Angers Elderly with Remark on Death, *Washington Post* (March 29, 1984), at A3, col. 5.
11. See *Splicing Life*, *supra* note 5, at 53–60.

Discussion

Dr. David Baltimore (Director, Whitehead Institute for Medical Research, Massachusetts Institute of Technology): Dr. Rosenberg, one implication of your talk was that we will not have to consider very much in the way of gene therapy, because most things that can be handled by gene therapy can also be handled by conventional transplantation. Conventional transplantation has been limited by the immunologic barriers that make it difficult to transplant from one individual to another, and the notion of gene therapy as a way around this problem is that it allows autologous transplantation. So I assume that you believe that transfer of bone marrow and other tissues between individuals is now a matter of routine medical practice and that the transplantation barriers are becoming close to zero.

Dr. Leon E. Rosenberg: No, I did not mean to imply that at all. I believe that, in the coming decade, we will see organ transplantation more widely used to cure genetic diseases in individuals. I in no way believe that that will be the ultimate therapy for those diseases. Medicine doesn't seem to have a very good way of producing ultimate remedies. We do what we can today with the expectation or the hope that something better will come tomorrow. It seems to me quite likely that appropriate gene therapy of somatic cells in the autologous fashion that you mentioned will be a better means of treatment tomorrow than bone marrow transplantation of heterologous cells is today. There are already successes with individuals who have been cured of β-thalassemia by bone marrow transplantation. I know of no example yet where we are ready to do gene therapy today. And my point in all of this is to emphasize that I truly do not believe that there is very much of a distinction between curing β-thalassemia with one's sister's bone marrow cells today and curing β-thalassemia with the administration of one's sister's β-globin gene into one's own cells tomorrow.

Dr. David Baltimore: That certainly clarifies things for me. I would like to ask about two different kinds of genetic therapy. One I would like to call *gene insertion* (into somatic cells) and the other I call *gene replacement* (designed for heritable change). The second is not something that I see as possible, and in fact, there may be some very

29

strong theoretical barriers to its use. Moreover, it is not even terribly useful, because it requires the preidentification of disease in a fertilized egg, which, if feasible, could be handled perfectly well not by abortion, as we have only a single cell, but by elimination. So I don't see what the fuss is about. Dr. Fost, why did you go to the extreme of saying that it may require putting a brake on basic research, because it is such a great danger?

DR. NORMAN FOST: No, I'm sorry, you misheard me. I did not mean to say that. What I said was that I didn't think there should be a fuss about it. I see these as being quantitative and not qualitative distinctions from all sorts of other genetic engineering that we now do. As I said, the argument could possibly be raised that you could accelerate evolution a little bit faster, but even that is exaggerated. I think that the ethical issues are the same as those involved in all research involving human subjects: risk–benefit analysis being assessed through institutional review mechanisms and proxy consent, which I think is now reasonably well-handled, and the evolutionary question. I don't see it as different from things that we're now doing in affecting the gene pool by treating the reproductive fitness of certain individuals. So I don't think it warrants a big fuss.

DR. DAVID BALTIMORE: I hope you understood that I, too, was not raising a big fuss, but identifying where some of it had been heard. Let me take the example you give and try to elaborate on what I understand to be your line of reasoning. If it were impossible to identify a mutant gene in a single germ cell without destroying it, a slight delay might be required until fertilization and division had occurred and the blastocyst stage was reached. There may be people who feel a greater repugnance at destroying even nascent life rather than undertaking risky treatment. Those people, with the aid of physicians, might say that is is better to attempt a genetic treatment than to destroy the embryo. I would also raise another issue concerning serious diseases such as cystic fibrosis. If there was a genetic treatment, some might argue for treatment only after birth. If that were done systematically by injection of the relevant gene, which the vector would carry not only to the specific malfunctioning cells but also to the gametic cells, some would simply say that that is an acceptable price to pay. Why not change the gametes, too, if that were possible? The objection is that by using this approach to cure this individual, we would be affecting future progeny. This is one of the reasons that I have such problems with the notion of a ban on anything that has to do with the germ line. What is different about the germ line? If in that case you were reasonably assured that the effect would be limited to cystic fibrosis, why not cure the grandchildren as well as the children? The next question is: If we know how to do it, can we undo it? Then, we have that additional question: Will we be able to overcome or remove whatever we put in? All these questions are fundamental. It seems to me that those are at least the questions that one would want to ask and not assume the outright answer that, if it has to do with the germ line, then it is automatically out of bounds.

DR. NORMAN FOST: I don't believe it is appropriate to make an outright ban on anything, but there is a very important distinction between the germ line and somatic cells that your discussion glosses over. In the germ line, as chromosomes are transmitted to further generations, they are segregated from one another, and so the insertion of a gene anywhere but in the place where the lesion is runs the extremely high probability that, in the next generation, it will not be there. It will be a loose cannon sent through all the rest of the progeny but would itself not be serving any purpose. Thus, I do not believe for an instant that it would be acceptable. That's why I say that it must be replacement and not insertion if it's to happen in the germ line.

DR. BERNARD DAVIS: Dr. Baltimore, you properly emphasized the importance of the distinction between intervention in somatic cells and germ line cells, and clearly, that is going to be a major source of discussion for a long time to come. I can hardly imagine that we are not going to succeed in getting permission to go ahead with the somatic line of therapy, but the germ line part is much more complicated. However, I was disturbed by how you presented it because you defined one as affecting the gene pool and the other, if I understood you correctly, as not affecting the gene pool. Now, the gene pool is the sum total of all the genes in the next generation of any species, and as J. B. S. Haldane pointed out many years ago, even a change in the tax structure affects the gene pool of the next generation if it has any effect on the differential fertility of different individuals. Now, let's take the example of someone with hemophilia who ordinarily would not have children. If you get a somatic cure in that person and that person is quite healthy, then there is every reason to expect that that person will be more likely to have progeny than otherwise, and that those progeny will carry the gene for hemophilia. You will therefore be affecting the gene pool of the next generation not in a way that I worry about, because we all know that the reservoir in recessive diseases is so huge that the increment in any one generation would be negligible. Nevertheless, you'll be affecting the next generation's gene pool negatively, whereas, if you could replace or correct the hemophilia defect in the germ line, you would also be affecting the next generation, but in a different way. I wonder if you would accept perhaps the substitution of the concept of a direct versus an indirect effect on the next generation. I have taken the trouble to spend so much time on this because this is not just a matter of trivial difference of phraseology. This is the heart of the issue with which Mr. Rifkin was able to mislead a group of well-meaning clergymen into what I think was an unfortunate position, because he painted a picture of enormous effects on evolution, playing God and all that. And so I wonder if you would accept this correction in definition?

DR. DAVID BALTIMORE: I completely accept it. In fact, I only mentioned the germ pool in that it is a theoretical fact that, if you change one gene, you change the numerator a little. But, in fact, the actual change that could be produced in the germ pool by genetic manipulation is so trivial compared to a whole variety of other effects, including the tax structure, as to fall into insignificance. I completely agree.

DR. RUTH HUBBARD: I wanted to ask Norman Fost and Alex Capron what models they would propose for opening up the public process and making it more inclusive. I've been bothered since the beginning by the narrowness of the process. Take a symposium like the one we're at right now, which is in Boston, where there are many people in the women's health movement, the disabilities rights movement, the Third World people's health movement, and yet those people, by and large, aren't here—Partly not at the podium and also excluded because of the fees that are charged—and I'd like to have your ideas of how one would open this up.

DR. NORMAN FOST: Obviously, one can always broaden the process. I myself wouldn't characterize the last 10 years of the regulation of genetic technologies as a narrow process, though. One can criticize Asilomar as possibly narrow, but that quickly gave way to everybody from the Cambridge City Council to the U.S. Congress getting into the act. At least within our own country, I don't think anyone who had something to say lacked access, that is, at least those people who have access through education and status and so on. I agree with you that there are people who always lack that access, but insofar as we have public debates on decision making in any regulatory issue in this country, we've had it on this one. I agree with you that that is an imperfect process and that we can always strive to do it better, but I don't think the word narrow can be used to describe it.

MR. ALEXANDER CAPRON: I think the concern that Dr. Hubbard raises is one that we have to keep at the forefront. The experience of the last decade has shown that this is an issue that people, once introduced to it, do not regard as something that is solely the province of scientists, or beyond our general understanding. I think we should begin by urging greater attention to the issues of human genetics as part of the biology curriculum of secondary schools. Genetics is in some ways a rather accessible subject. The basic principles can be set out, and then their social relevance can be discussed, such as the way in which genetics, unique aspects aside, ties in with medical care and access to health care. If it's a powerful technology, it raises questions about other powerful technologies, which are sometimes dollar-dependent in our society. The President's Commission, when it met, held hearings across the country, and we heard from ordinary citizens when we met in Los Angeles, Atlanta, Boston, Florida, and so forth, so that I think it is possible to have a process that is open and reaches out. I don't think it's necessarily all that has to be done through national symposia like this or national commissions. When the debate was going on in Cambridge, as messy as some people found it, there were booths on the sidewalks with people passing out literature and discussion. Dr. Fost used the word *rowdy* for some of that, and it probably was, but I think that's also healthy. So, I would suggest that we be alert, and reminders such as your own make us alert. I welcome that.

DR. NORMAN FOST: Let me say the word *rowdy* is most appropriate especially for the then mayor of Cambridge.

DR. RUTH HUBBARD: I think the Cambridge hearings were a good model because they're the only ones I'm aware of that in fact called on people other than those who usually have access to the kinds of decisions we're talking about. I am worried about the models that you are proposing and not going beyond because it seems to me that we're sticking with a process where the people who are doing the work are making the decisions.

DR. NORMAN FOST: Sorry, I didn't mean to say that by *rowdy* it was bad. In fact, it was a popular event.

A PARTICIPANT: I disagree with something that Alex Capron said regarding this issue of "First, do no harm." First, an empiric point. I would disagree with the suggestion that the chance of being benefited by a visit to the doctor is greater than 50-50. About 80%– 90% (by actual study) of all visits to the doctor for primary care are for conditions for which there is no effective treatment. Where there is no benefit in the technical sense, the risk–benefit ratio is obviously high. That's not to deny the value of other things that doctors do in the way of support, but in the technical sense, "Do no harm" is still an appropriate injunction because the possibility of benefit is still low. Second, at a more theoretical level, as I suggested, the principle doesn't just come from medicine. It's a principle basic to all societies. If you have a bunch of people together on a desert island, they would surely agree very quickly, "No harming here, no unconsented touchings, no battery." But if someone said, "I have another idea for a rule. I think you have to help people, too. I think we should have rules that compel people to find benefits and to come to the aid of those in peril." If history is any guide, it would be a reluctant rule, and most societies would not come around to it—not because it's not important and not because we don't want to encourage and nurture and avoid restricting people who want to help others, but we wouldn't compel it as we would the injunction to do no harm.

MR. ALEXANDER CAPRON: I would take issue on two levels. The first is that, although it is certainly true that most visits to the physician involve what are called "the worried well," I think that the notion of standing still and doing no harm means doing nothing. I think that's a mistake. I am amazed to hear a physician and ethicist embrace as warmly as you did, Dr. Fost, the legal doctrine that there is no liability for failing to aid someone. It is true that there is no liability. You may stand next to an 8-inch pool of water and watch a 2-year-old child drown, and the law will not impose any penalty on you if you are not the guardian or caretaker of that child. I think society at large would look at you then and make a moral judgment that is very different. I think that, in this case, we are dealing with moral and ethical judgments about our fear that we will slide down some slippery slope that is very steep and glassy, and that we should be concerned about sliding down because we have no foothold. But other times, I think our ingenuity should be applied to saying, "Let's find the foothold so that we may move forward without sliding down that slope, for those who might benefit by an intervention." We do owe them something, and even if we are not legally bound to do that, morally we do owe some remedy to those who are in need.

DR. LEON E. ROSENBERG: There is no modality that we currently have in the medical armamentarium that has been accomplished without doing harm. Whether it be surgery for an inflamed appendix or the use of penicillin to treat an infection. Every medical modality that has ever been employed has done harm on its way to doing good. It seems to me that to project this as an absolute is not consistent with the history of medicine.

DR. HENRY MILLER: I have a comment that many of you perhaps will find reassuring or perhaps unsettling or merely mundane. There is a great deal of discussion about the oversight that's necessary or desirable for gene therapy, whether somatic or germ line. I'd just like to remind you that, under existing federal statutes and regulations, there will be both local (through institutional review boards) and central (through the FDA, for example) regulation of both the processes and the products that are employed in gene therapy. The product, of course, will presumably be DNA with or without the presence of some appropriate vector, and we intend to regulate this as a biologic product analogous to vaccines or interferon. So there will be a great deal of regulation of this, a formal consideration of risk–benefit concerns, and a great deal of scrutiny in individual subjects for a variety of side effects, some of which Mr. Capron alluded to in theoretical terms.

MR. ALEXANDER CAPRON: I'll take the opportunity to respond to Dr. Rosenberg's additions to the harm–benefit debate that the principle is not an absolute one of doing no harm. An appendectomy involves harm. It involves benefit and harm, as all medical interventions do, or at least risk of it. The principle is no harm without compensating benefit. To the degree that we try to avoid harm, we obviously forgo benefits, and any restrictions on any human activity (not only research) runs the risk of precluding or delaying or reducing the onset of benefits. So there's no question about it. The question is what the proper trade-off is, and the modest point that I want to make is that you start by at least not harming people unless there's some compensating benefit. Harming them without any clear likelihood of any benefit is worse than failing to benefit them. Unquestionably, we are delaying and possibly forgoing altogether some benefits by protecting people from harm.

A PARTICIPANT: I'd like to respond to that and link it to Dr. Miller's comments. As a person who believes that there are some areas that should concern us here, although I hope in a nonalarmist way, I'm not sure that I would be fully satisfied with the notion that the FDA or local institutional review boards will be reviewing. It would be beyond the scope of institutional review boards, and I believe also, in light of our recent experience with the prenatal kits for neural tube defects and the consideration the FDA gave there, even beyond the scope of the FDA, that societal risk as a whole is the grounds for not approving an otherwise acceptable form of experimental treatment. That is to say, those bodies are not well positioned or even authorized, it seems to me, to say that they have some idea that a society in which this capability existed would be a less good society than we are today, and therefore, they do not want to allow that experiment to go forward. So, if we are concerned that that question will arise, that will need another mechanism, and we cannot simply say the FDA or the IRB will take care of it.

DR. AUBREY MILUNSKY: I did come to learn, although I did know something before I came. I knew that there was little truth in justice, and now Alex Capron has just told us that there is no morality in law. Hopefully, I'll learn deeper lessons later.

MR. ALEXANDER CAPRON: There are no other deeper lessons.

DR. AUBREY MILUNSKY: Dr. Hubbard mentioned that we had excluded the poor and others who are underprivileged. We have clearly not done that. We have provided entry fees that are much lower for representatives of neighborhood health associations and other organizations; in addition, the American Society of Law and Medicine has always responded to appeals or applications by individuals asking if they could come to a meeting if they lacked the necessary admission fees.

THE UNIVERSITY–INDUSTRY–GOVERNMENT COMPLEX

MODERATOR: DAVID BALTIMORE

4

THE ACADEMIC-CORPORATE MERGER IN MEDICINE

A Two-Edged Sword

ARNOLD S. RELMAN, M.D.
Editor
New England Journal of Medicine
10 Shattuck Street
Boston, MA 02115
Professor of Medicine
Harvard Medical School
25 Shattuck Street
Boston, MA 02115

The rapid development of molecular genetic technology in the past decade has opened up exciting new vistas for the application of this technology to the manufacture of important biological molecules, as well as to the diagnosis and treatment of inherited diseases. The enthusiasm attending this development in the research laboratories of universities and medical schools generated an equal stir in the corporate world, where the possibilities for commercial exploitation of these dramatic scientific advances were immediately appreciated.

The story of the birth and the phenomenal postnatal growth of the biotechnology industry in the United States has been told many times, and I do not wish to repeat it in any detail here. New venture companies, by the score, as well as new divisions of large established firms, have sprung up in response to a general perception that opportunities for substantial commercial profit from genetic engineering were just over the horizon.

These new enterprises have depended heavily on the technical knowledge of the academic scientists working in this field, as virtually all of the expertise initially was in the academic institutions. Faculty have been employed as consultants and, in many instances, have been allowed to share equity interests in the new corporations in exchange for their technical advice. In still other cases, faculty members independently, or in partnership with venture capitalists, have formed new companies to exploit ideas derived from their research. Patents held by faculty have sometimes been the basis for the establishment of new companies or have been offered by their owners to existing companies on a licensing basis. The medical schools and universities have also entered into arrangements with these new biotechnology enterprises through patent licensing, joint ventures, or agreements to share new information in exchange for some sort of ongoing financial support. In addition, companies have contracted with academic institutions through grants for the support of faculty research.

There is a general opinion that a very substantial fraction, perhaps half or more, of all the senior scientists working in molecular genetics in the major research institutions in this country have some industrial connection. Certainly, most of the medical schools and universities in which these scientists work have by now entered into some sort of institutional arrangement with one or more biotechnology companies, and many of the leading research institutions have multiple arrangements of this kind. However, to put this in perspective, it is important to understand that support from private industry is still a relatively small part of the funding for research in universities in the United States. Recent estimates by the National Science Foundation put the corporate contribution, from *all* sectors of industry, at only 6%–7% of the total. Although the corporate contribution is increasing, it is dwarfed by the government's share, which accounts for almost three quarters of the total university research budget. Nevertheless, as federal support of medical research begins to level out and the competition for these fixed resources continues to grow, academic institutions are increasingly prospecting for new sources of support. For this reason, the possibility of cooperative programs with the new biotechnology industry has looked very attractive to most of the major medical schools and teaching hospitals.

Industrial support of applied research and development in academic institutions is hardly new. For many decades, corporations have sponsored academic research in the physical sciences, especially chemistry, and in engineering. Faculty members in engineering schools, and in departments of chemistry, physics, and applied science, have been employed as consultants by industry, have benefited from patent licensing, have served as company directors, and have even held equity interests in businesses. Many research-oriented universities and engineering schools have long had special programs for corporations that offer access to information about new research in exchange for corporate support.

But the phenomenon we are talking about here is not quite the same thing. Whereas the older academic-industrial liaison usually involved the engineering and the applied-science faculties and tangible technological products in fields that were relatively mature, the biotechnology corporations are a brand-new industry, spawned in direct response to revolutionary basic-science discoveries in academic laboratories. Most of these new companies are highly speculative, as they have been launched primarily on the expectation, rather than the reality, of marketable products. Most of the initial profits depend on public perceptions and expectations of profitability rather than on actual new products or sales. Furthermore, the essential property of these new firms mainly consists of patent rights to new ideas or processes. There is intense competition among the companies to obtain these patent rights from the scientists working at the cutting edge of a rapidly evolving field. Every new scientific report is carefully scanned for its commercial potential, and every new graduate student, research fellow, or young faculty appointee is viewed as a potential employee. The feverish atmosphere generated by this competition is directly communicated to the university laboratories and classrooms because so many senior faculty are involved, and so many fortunes are being made overnight. All of this sets the new biotechnological academic-industrial complex apart from most of the more traditional associations between universities and industry that have existed in the past.

This new development has created serious problems for the universities, which have been described so often that no further detailed recitation is needed here. The presidents of most of the leading research universities in this country have publicly voiced their concerns about this issue, including Bok of Harvard, Giamatti of Yale, and Kennedy of Stanford. They have recognized that corporate support has both positive and negative aspects, and that universities must be vigilant to ensure that the negative aspects will not dominate the arrangements. Each of these institutions has published guidelines for avoiding some of the problems. Their major concerns are that financial arrangements between faculty and corporations may lead to secrecy, delay in communicating ideas and reporting new results, neglect of teaching responsibilities, and constraints on freedom to choose research topics.

The solutions proposed vary somewhat in their details but agree essentially in principle. No arrangement should be accepted that limits a faculty member's freedom to work on problems of her or his choice or that restricts the communication of ideas and research results. Brief delays to allow sponsoring companies a reasonable opportunity to evaluate their patent interests can be permitted, but otherwise there should be no impediment to the free exchange of information with colleagues and students. Faculty members must not spend more than a minor fraction (usually 20%) of their time working for corporations (exclusive of time spent on contracted research) and should not have an operating or managerial responsibility in any corporation. Rules about patent arrangements vary, but there is general agreement that universities ought to share in the benefits with the faculty member, that the granting of exclusive patent rights should be avoided if possible, and that it is best if universities, not faculty members, hold patents and negotiate with corporations on behalf of their faculties.

All of these general guidelines are fine as far as they go. I would like to add a few more suggestions of my own:

1. Whatever guidelines are adopted should be the result of full faculty deliberation and consent.
2. As guidelines are necessarily general, university administrations should establish standing committees to review individual arrangements and to make recommendations for the resolution of specific problems.
3. All arrangements should be fully disclosed. Faculty should disclose their financial arrangements to the university administration; university administrations, for their part, should publicly disclose any special arrangements that they may have with faculty members or business corporations.
4. In my opinion, it would be better if these arrangements (for both the university administration and its faculty) did not include the holding of equity interest in

any business venture with which the university or its faculty have been involved through research and development contracts, consultations, patents, and so forth. Through these latter kinds of arrangements, universities and business corporations can help one another in areas of mutual interest. Corporations may also see fit to assist the mission of universities by contributing to their general support, and universities may choose to invest their endowments in the purchase of equity shares in various unrelated business corporations. But in all of these relationships, the university must remain at arm's length, independent of and uninfluenced by corporate policies and objectives. Equity in corporations with which the university or its faculty are directly involved changes the university's arm's length position and raises the possibility of conflict of interest.

To maintain the confidence and support of the public, the university must be seen to be unbiased in its expert judgments and committed primarily to the public interest through the pursuit of new knowledge and the cultivation of scholarship and education. If it has a financial stake in the outcome of the research that its faculty do or in the scientific judgments that they are called on to make (which is what an equity interest would mean), its objectivity will surely be questioned. Furthermore, the university's impartiality in dealing with its faculty may be severely strained if the research programs of certain faculty members, but not of others, offer the possibility of significant financial benefits to the institution. Such problems and temptations can never be totally avoided, but contractual arrangements, clearly defined and publicly disclosed, are much less likely to subvert the university's basic philosophy than are equity-sharing arrangements.

The argument against faculty members' owning equity interests in biotechnology companies that support their research or that employ them as consultants may be more debatable than the argument against universities' owning equity in such companies, but I believe it is no less sound. Like the universities to which they belong, faculty members are expected to be unbiased and objective. This expectation is called into question when faculty members publish research dealing with products or processes in which they have a vested financial interest, or when they publicly express their professional judgment about such matters. Of even greater concern, however, is the influence that investment in a company may have on faculty members' interest in their teaching reponsibilities, their willingness to talk about their work with their colleagues, and their supervision of graduate students and postdoctoral fellows.

The problems arising from the academic-corporate merger result from fundamental differences between the parties to the merger. Universities and investor-owned corporations have different purposes and philosophies. Universities, if they are to cooperate successfully with corporations, need to have the benefit of carefully thought-out guidelines.

Beyond those guidelines, however, is a basic consideration often forgotten by hard-pressed universities as they seek additional research funding from industry: corporate support is not likely ever to be of great importance in the overall picture. The present very modest contribution of corporations to medical research will probably increase in the future, but it seems clear that university medical research will continue to be largely dependent on government grants. Charitable foundations, gifts, and endowments will probably continue as a distant second source of support, with corporations a poor third. Corporate interests are generally not consonant with the basic purposes of academic biomedical research. Except for a relatively few wealthy and enlightened corporations that are genuinely interested in supporting medical research and education as a public service, most biomedical corporations can be expected to provide only modest support at best. The new genetic-engineering companies will contribute to molecular genetic research in the schools for only as long as the industry lacks the technical expertise and the trained personnel now mainly centered in academic institutions. Once the new companies have the requisite in-house capacity, they will lose interest in the schools because they will find it cheaper and more efficient to do their own research and development. They will probably continue to use the consulting services of senior faculty, and they will always be interested in licensing commercially promising patents, but no great outpouring of industry support for academic programs in molecular genetics—or any other field of medical research, for that matter—should be anticipated in the future. Schools would be making a serious error, in my view, if they were to bend their policies in search of greater industrial support. That support will not ever be very substantial, and its single-minded pursuit may jeopardize university traditions of far greater value.

I therefore predict that the academic-corporate partnership will prove of much greater benefit to the biotechnology corporations than to their academic partners. Some academic scientists will get rich, and some of the stronger research institutions will have received substantial help for their research programs in molecular biology. Royalties from patents will be a modest source of support for a few schools. By and large, however, there will be no industrial bonanza for academic research.

When that sobering fact begins to be generally appreciated, universities and medical schools will realize that they must look elsewhere for support of their research programs. Academic scientists who have been caught up in the entrepreneurial excitement will have an opportunity to sort out their priorities. They will need to decide whether they wish to remain as full-time academicians or whether they prefer careers in industry. Values in academic life are different from those in business, and it is difficult to be a good professor and a good biotechnology entrepreneur at the same time. Few faculty members will be able to do both, and few academic institutions will allow them to try.

5

THE CORPORATE CAPTURE OF ACADEMIC SCIENCE AND ITS SOCIAL COSTS

SHELDON KRIMSKY, PH.D.
Associate Professor
Department of Urban and Environmental Policy
Tufts University
Medford, MA 02155

Commercial applications of molecular genetics and cell biology have resulted in a flurry of entrepreneurial activities among academic biologists and universities eager to cash in on the financial side of this technological revolution. The situation is not unique to biology. It is following the path of other disciplines that have formed close partnerships with industry, including nuclear and petroleum engineering, computer sciences, nutrition, electronics, and chemistry. Nevertheless, the current debate that has centered on the commercial ties of academic biologists has been more widely publicized than at any time in the past. Several hypotheses may be offered to explain this phenomenon.

The commercialization of biology occurred rapidly, and considerable media attention was given to the discoveries and the personalities involved. By the time many biologists developed commercial interests, a widely publicized controversy over the safety of recombinant DNA techniques had already taken place. The social and ethical issues associated with gene splicing provided grist for the public's concern over the commercial activities of its pioneers. The confluence of social and ethical debates with commercialization of science generated a larger public reaction to the latter.

A second explanation centers on the perceived role of biomedical science in society. Unlike other scientific and engineering fields that have developed linkages with the private sector, biological research has been closely associated with public health. The public expectations of this area of research are greater than they are of such areas as chemistry or computer sciences. Moreover, the preponderance of funding for biomedical research comes from social resources. Consequently, in the public consciousness, the conjunction of these factors—namely, the sources and goals of funding—makes the academic entrepreneurs in biomedical science accountable for their commercial activities in ways that other scientists are not.[1]

However, I would conjecture that the distinction between the goals and funding of biomedical research and those of other commercialized disciplines provides only part of the answer. The types of university–industry relationships in biology are more varied, more aggressive, more experimental, and more indiscreet than they have been in similar historical circumstances. A significant number of new firms in biotechnology have sprung directly out of academia. By contrast, in the microelectronics field, most firms were spawned directly from industries that were recipients of U.S. Department of Defense contracts.[2]

Another explanation that sets biotechnology apart from other academia–industry partnerships was advanced by Congressman Albert Gore (D. Tenn.). According to the Congressman, in the past there has always been a distinction between pure and applied research in the means by which technology is transferred from academe to industry. Gore observed that, in genetic engineering, "there seems to be no phase of applied research: the discovery of the basic scientists may go directly and swiftly from the laboratory bench in the university into a profit making venture."[3] As a result of the omission of the intermediate stage, Gore believes that an unusual set of ethical issues results.

An additional factor that helps to account for the vehemence of this issue is that our society has changed. In the post-Watergate period, we have become more sensitive to conflicts of interest. Laws have been passed to protect society from unsavory kinships between the public and the private sectors. Public interest groups monitor corporate influence on government agencies. As a consequence, the public and the media are more sensitive to allegations that public funds are being misused or that private interests are exploiting social resources. Public universities have been sued for violating their mandate to serve the general interest.[4] Recent attention has also been directed at faculty misuse of federally supported projects.

The public perception of science, by and large, still portrays the contemporary scientist as a selfless discoverer of truth, despite efforts on the part of sociologists and the media to show otherwise. The marriage of science and Wall Street portends an illicit affair to most people. Perhaps this attitude is an outgrowth of the American Puritan tradition that financial gain distorts truth and values.

Why should we be concerned about what our universities or their faculties do to raise money? For one thing, universities and their faculties are a national resource. Our government depends on the expertise in academe for public policy formation. Second, universities are recipients of substantial government support, which implies some responsibility and accountability.

Much of the debate on the commercial ties of university faculty has centered on a number of issues involving the conflicting missions of business and academe. These include the control of intellectual property, the openness and accessibility of scientific and technical knowledge, the commingling of funds, the ownership of tangible research property, the use of public research funds for private business interests, and the influence of entrepreneurial faculty on the education of students. These are serious issues, and they have been aired to some extent in media coverage, university debates, and congressional hearings.[5] Several leading universities have issued guidelines for faculty pursuing commercial interests and have established policies on contractual agreements between the university and the private sector.[6]

Notwithstanding these initiatives, there is an important side to the problem that the current debate has totally neglected. Even if all the aforementioned problem areas are satisfactorily resolved and the conflict of interests is removed, intense commercialization of biology could result in an enormous social liability. Let me summarize the principal argument in the form of a conjecture.

If a sufficiently large and influential number of scientists or engineers become financially involved with industry, problems related to the commercial applications of the particular area of science or engineering are neglected. The scientific community becomes desensitized to the social impacts of science. This desentsitization leads to a conservative shift in attitudes and behavior. The new values emphasizing science for commerce become internalized and rationalized as a public good. The disciplinary conscience becomes transformed. This transformation happens incrementally, without conspiracy or malice. Scientists or engineers with a stake in the commercial outcome of a field cannot, at the same time, retain a public interest perspective that gives critical attention to the perversion of science in the interests of markets.

We are not dealing with a threshold phenomenon. There is no clear stage in the growth of academic-corporate partnerships when the effects I have outlined suddenly become observable. That this phenomenon exists must be inferred from the psychology of individual behavior and from our knowledge of how people's values are shaped by their institutional affiliation and financial associations.

When the number of faculty involvements are small, the effects on public interest science are not likely to be important. As long as a sufficient number of scientists remain free from corporate influence, there will be a disinterested intelligentsia to whom the public can turn for a critical evaluation of technological risks, goals, and directions.

If my argument is correct, then the individual instances of faculty–industry ties are far less important than the aggregate corporate penetration into an academic discipline and the degree to which the major institutions and leading faculty are involved. It is my contention that, unless we have some quantitative information about the degree of corporate-academic interaction, we cannot appreciate the gravity of the problem.

What can be learned from a study of dual relationships in the area of biotechnology? Suppose we had before us perfect information about the commercial affiliations of academic scientists. What questions would we ask? We might want to know what percentage of faculty at leading universities have a substantial involvement in commercial enterprises. We might look at the extent to which the dual-affiliated academic population participates on public advisory committees or study panels. Unexpected results may be interpreted in several ways. Imagine that the participation is heavy. A skeptic might question whether the peer review process is being compromised by having a substantial number of commercially affiliated scientists reviewing grant proposals. It is inescapable that a diffusion of ideas will take place between reviewers and the institutions with which they are associated. On the other hand, suppose the participation is low. The same skeptic might explain this low participation by arguing that business interests have taken priority over the responsibility of scientists to participate in the peer review system.

Alternatively, there will be those who interpret the results, whatever they might be, as irrelevant to the effects mentioned. Notwithstanding problems of interpretation, I believe that there is some value in understanding the degree to which academia has financial interests in biotechnology.

To investigate the corporate relationships of academic scientists, I developed a data base of university faculty in biology, biochemistry, molecular genetics, and medicine who meet one or more of the following criteria with respect to biotechnology firms: (1) they serve on a scientific advisory board; (2) they hold substantial equity; (3) they serve as a principal in a company. Armed with this data base, which represents a lower bound of involvement because faculty connections to private firms are not ordinarily available, one can correlate this population group with other academic populations comprising leading biology departments; service on committees of the National Institutes of Health, the National Science Foundation, and the U.S. Department of Agriculture; and membership in the National Academy of Science.

This inquiry is not designed to test a hypothesis. Rather, it is designed to suggest a research program. If the degree of the corporate penetration of academic biology is sufficiently high, the next obvious question is: What are the effects of this penetration? I conjecture that these effects will reveal themselves as a shift from a public orientation of science to science for private profit. In the long run, this shift will result in the social neglect of technological abuse. Before I turn to the data, I shall offer some qualitative and historical examples that support the conjecture.

SCIENTIFIC OBJECTIVITY AND INDUSTRIAL INTERESTS

Public policy formation in a highly industrialized society such as ours is a complex affair. It frequently involves input from many areas of expertise. Scientists serve on a labyrinth of public advisory committees, review boards, and risk assessment panels throughout all levels of government. How do we ensure objectivity in the contributions of scientific experts to public issues, particularly where consensus is difficult to find? Recently, the Office of Technology Assessment (OTA) issued a report on biotechnology that made the argument that the dual affiliation of scientists in the academic and commercial worlds is actually more desirable from a public policy standpoint when expertise is needed:

> An argument could be made that because the public has supported research in universities, it has a right to know whether a particular university faculty member who is giving testimony, for example, has a consulting relationship with a company that manufactures a particular harmful chemical. The negative side of the disclosure policies is that "objective" information may be judged "subjective" because of guilt by association. If a faculty member's consulting arrangement with industry is declared openly, it is not necessarily the case that his or her testimony is biased. In fact, the

expert may have a more objective view because he or she understands both the research and development aspects of the technology.[7]

There are two arguments here. The first is that the veil of confidentiality on the commercial affiliation of a scientist testifying before a governmental body would prevent bias against the individual's presentation. According to the OTA, if the disclosure is required, testimony would not be taken on face value but would be dismissed for reasons of association. The second argument interprets objectivity to mean "multidimensionality." The implication is that the more affiliations a person has, the more objective that person can be.

The OTA analysis confuses objectivity with eclecticism. There are many advantages in having faculty link up with the private sector. Those advantages include a greater awareness of the full life cycle of science, from discovery to manufacture. But the OTA makes a serious error when it describes the financial involvement of academic scientists in commercial ventures as a contributor to objectivity. The argument fails because of the financial interest. A form of eclecticism that is independent of pecuniary interests could indeed enhance objectivity. Proposals for a disinterested and eclectic intelligentsia have been advanced by a number of social theorists, including the Greek philosopher Plato and the German sociologist Karl Mannheim, both of whom were aware that knowledge is subject to the control of economic interests.

The history of technology provides an abundance of examples illustrating the distortion of objectivity when scientific expertise is beholden to the industrial sector. The causal relationship need not be absolute. We are dealing with a statistical phenomenon that is guided by factors of social psychology. Our conflict-of-interest laws are based on assumptions of human frailty as exemplified by the aphorism "Don't bite the hand that feeds you." It is a mistake, however, to view conflict of interest in terms of conspiracy of conscious design. It is my hypothesis that a sizable academic-industrial association will slowly change the ethos of science away from social protectionism and toward commercial protectionism. The aggregate of isolated individual decisions to go commercial creates a qualitatively new effect. It should be emphasized that the discovery of a problem tells us nothing about the solution. In some cases, it might be wise to live with the problem, to understand its social consequences, and to avoid draconian measures. For the problems outlined in this chapter, I will offer a few modest social antidotes.

Let me begin with a phenomenological exercise to illustrate my thesis. Imagine that you are heavily funded by a company to engage in research. Is it likely that you would publicly embarrass the company by revealing information or posing questions about its technological direction? Most scientists with a conscience would make their viewpoints known to the firm's directors. But who wants to jeopardize his or her funding by making an issue public? The closer the relationship one has to a firm, the more propriety and self-interest dictates keeping criticisms within the corporate family.

A few years ago, I supervised a policy study involving the chemical contamination of a town's water supply. The actors included a multinational corporation; town, state, and federal officials; a public advocacy group; and technical people. I chose to do the study for several reasons. First, it served the public interest. Second, it was a useful case for instructional purposes. Third, from a public policy standpoint, it represented a milestone for the implementation of a major federal law. If I had been funded by the corporation in question, that research study would never have entered my mind because of the likelihood the company would not be shown in the best light. If my department had been heavily funded by the company, including possibly graduate student stipends and multiyear grants, it is extremely doubtful that any faculty member would have chosen to study how the department's corporate benefactor was implicated in the contamination of a water supply, unless there was reasonable assurance that the outcome would not be an embarrassment.

As the financial connections become more remote, the psychological and social factors that limit or restrict freedom of inquiry become less important. A corporate representative on the university board of trustees might have an effect on the choice of a research program or even on its outcome. However, the strength of that influence would be severely weakened as it was mediated through university channels.

When our policy study on the chemical contamination of the town's water supply was complete, a vice-president of the corporation made a personal visit to the president of my university and asked to have the study suppressed or totally disassociated from the university. It is gratifying to report that my university made no efforts to restrict my academic freedom. But the direct political influence on research has become less of a problem since the introduction of the tenure system in the aftermath of the McCarthy period.

However, the economic determinants of research and their influence on the latitude of inquiry are far more pervasive and subtle. Sometimes, this influence manifests itself in the distortion of science. At other times, it is expressed in the control of information. Most frequently, it is felt by the kinds of questions that are pursued in the areas where science and social policy intersect.

SCIENTISTS AND THE PUBLIC TRUST: SOME HISTORICAL ABUSES OF DUAL AFFILIATIONS

Periodically, a story appears in the media about an academic scientist who expresses views sympathetic to an industry position on a controversial health or environmental policy. The article may then mention the financial association between the scientist and the company that has a stake in the outcome. Considering the amount of industry consulting that takes place, the public learns only about the proverbial "tip of the iceberg" of the associations. Because the documented cases may be small in number, there is no clear way of knowing the aggregate effect that these individual associations will have on social policy formation. Given the choice, the public sector would rather place its trust in scientific experts who are not linked financially to industry. Problems arise when the pool of experts in molecular genetics who are unaffiliated with industry becomes vanishingly small.

A situation like this occurred in 1969 when close ties between the oil industry and university experts in academic disciplines such as geology, geophysics, and petroleum engineering incensed California officials and federal authorities. State and federal agencies were responsible for the environmental problems arising from massive oil leaks of the Union Oil Company's offshore well in the Santa Barbara Channel. According to the report in *Science*:

> California's chief deputy attorney general . . . publicly complained that experts at both state and private universities turned down his requests to testify for the state in its half-billion dollar damage suit against Union and three other oil companies.[8]

The explanation offered by state officials for the difficulty they had had in getting testimony from experts was that

> petroleum engineers at the University of California campuses of Santa Barbara and Berkeley and at the privately supported University of Southern California indicated that they did not wish to risk losing industry grants and consulting arrangements.

It was reported in *Science* that most petroleum engineers in academia did extensive consulting for oil companies and formed part of the university–industry "oil fraternity."

> Consulting is regarded not simply as a lucrative perquisite of the profession but as a necessary way to establish and maintain a departmental reputation and create job opportunities.[9]

Another obstacle facing public officials attempting to getting objective advice from the experts who serve on public service panels is that many own stock in the companies that are affected by their decisions.

The lesson illustrated by this case was not that petroleum engineers refused to testify. They were probably acting ethically in not testifying, as their corporate ties might have compromised their objectivity. The real problem was the scarcity of academic experts who were not affiliated with the oil industry and who could thus provide a disinterested perspective.

In some situations, research is so highly specialized that only a few scientists in the entire country may have the information necessary to render a decision on the health and safety of a new substance. Several decades ago, it was common practice for scientists to sign restrictive publication agreements with companies. Such agreements are still used today in the biotechnology industry. In one important case, information withheld from publication could have prevented a toxic pesticide from being marketed. A clinical professor of occupational and environmental medicine at the University of California at San Francisco was engaged in toxicological research on the pesticide DBCP for the Shell Development Corporation in the 1950s. He discovered that the chemical caused severe cases of testicular atrophy in test animals. As was common practice at that time, the research results were kept out of print for a period of time to protect trade secrets. Although a brief abstract of the toxicological study was published in 1956, the full results were held back from publication until 1961, six years after the pesticide had been approved for marketing.

In the late 1970s, workers in a DBCP plant were monitored. An unusually high incidence of male infertility was reported. At state hearings on DBCP, it was noted that the scientist who had studied the pesticide had testified at public hearings on other environmental health matters without disclosing his consultant work with firms that had a financial interest in the subject matter under investigation. The chairman of the panel stated:

> it is difficult to know in the cases of [such scientists] with 30 years of dual relationships with the university and with Shell where advocacy on behalf of private interests ends and where responsibility as an "objective" professor begins.[10]

A special feature of the journal *Business and Society Review* reported cases where the public received expert testimony from scientists with undisclosed relationships to companies that stood to gain from the recommendations. Michael Jacobson, Executive Director of Science and the Public Interest, described conditions in the field of nutrition:

> In the area of food safety and nutrition . . . a large percentage of experts has received industry money. Rare is the expert who accepts such funds and is an ardent defender of the public's interest.[11]

Similar examples can be found in nuclear engineering, occupational health and medicine, and ecology. Ultimately, it is socially desirable that there be a balance in the academic community. For any discipline that has a commercial offspring, it is vital that a critical mass of experts remain disassociated from industrial ties in areas related to their field of expertise. And when scientists maintain such ties, it is essential that the public understand the nature of the relationships when their expertise is sought in setting policy. But just how extensive is the problem in biotechnology?

ACADEMIC-CORPORATE LINKS IN BIOTECHNOLOGY: SOME QUANTITATIVE RESULTS

To evaluate the degree of the link between academe and the biotechnology industry, I developed a data base of scientists who are formally affiliated with biotechnology firms either as members of scientific advisory boards, as consultants on retainer, as principals in the firm, or as large stockholders. I shall label this subpopulation of dual-affiliated scientists with the term *ACIND* for "academics in industry."

The primary source for the data base was 50 public biotechnology companies. These were drawn from a pool of 250 public and private firms that have been inventoried by trade organizations in the United States. Each of the public corporations reviewed for the study publishes a list of its scientific advisory board, its management, and major stockholders in its company prospectus (the 10K report required by the Securities and Exhange Commission). Additional entries into the data base were gleaned from the trade literature and media reports. However, as private firms are not legally obligated to file reports in the public domain, it is more difficult to obtain this information.

For this study, only 20% of the total number of biotechnology firms have been systematically surveyed, although these represent the largest and most active firms. Therefore, the actual number of academic scientists involved in the biotechnology industry could run three to four times the figure of 345.

Another consideration in interpreting the data is that the number of biotechnology firms has increased at an exponential rate within the past few years. The trade magazine *Genetic Engineering News* reported that there was a handful of biotechnology companies before 1981.[12] By the next year, 184 companies were listed in its registry. That figure climbed rapidly to 220 by November 1983, and current estimates place the number of firms at 250.

One of the goals of the study is to examine a number of assumptions about the extent of corporate affiliations in biomedical science. For example, in 1982 Barbara Culliton, writing for *Science*, stated that most of the country's leading biologists are associated with biotechnology companies.[13] Under what criteria can we evaluate such a statement? I looked at corporate affiliation as a function of membership in the National Academy of Sciences (NAS), choosing membership as a proxy for "leading biologists."

Another area of inquiry is the relationship of ACIND scientists to participation on study panels and public advisory committees in major government funding agencies. The National Science Foundation (NSF) has a rigorous criterion for weeding out potential conflicts of interest on proposal review. An individual's commercial relationship is a relevant input in the review process according to NSF staff. It is expected that such information will be disclosed by mail reviewers as well as by members of study panels. The obligation of disclosure rests with the prospective reviewers and is used by the NSF in determining whether a conflict of interest or its appearance exists. In this study, we are at the stage of developing aggregate statistics. The inquiry into NSF affiliation is still in progress.

The quantitative information that we have compiled thus far can be summarized as follows. This information is based on a total data base of 345 dual-affiliated scientists in 50 biotechnology corporations and various private companies.

1. Sixty-two scientists of the 345 are members of the NAS (18%).

2. The four most relevant categories of NAS membership for biotechnology are biochemistry, cellular and developmental biology, genetics, and medical genetics. The ACIND entries in our data base constitute 25% of the NAS members in the four categories. The *percentage* of NAS scientists with industry affiliations revealed in the study represents a lower bound for the profession as a whole. The scientific affiliates of the additional 200 firms could bring the number of corporate-affiliated NAS members well beyond 50%. This percentage is particularly significant in that the NAS is frequently called on to render decisions on the social uses of science and technology.

3. In another correlation, we looked at the number of ACIND scientists who participated on NIH study panels or in public advisory groups. In this category, 40 scientists were identified in a listing of NIH groups that covered a 12-month period. That figure represents 12% of our data base.

These statistics must be understood in the context of other questions. For example, is there an appearance of conflict of interest if an ACIND scientist serves on a study panel? If the answer is affirmative, then 40 is a significant number. Alternatively, are ACIND scientists less likely than their nonaffiliated counterparts to serve on study panels? Are they being self-selected out of this responsibility because of commercial interests and are the numbers large enough to have an effect on the peer review system? To date, from our data base, ACIND scientists make up 10%, at most, of NIH sudy panels. Further studies are needed to interpret the significance of the data. Trends should be followed over a longer time period to disclose the impact of the biotechnological revolution on the social and scientific character of academic biology and the health sciences.

In addition to quantitative data, the preliminary results reveal interesting qualitative information. A number of the biotechnology firms offer stock to members of their scientific advisory boards as one means of remuneration, giving scientists direct equity in the business. Among the ACIND scientists, we found many heads of departments, chairpersons, a college president, and a former director of the National Institutes of Health (which has established the principal regulatory apparatus for the industry use of recombinant DNA techniques).

Our inquiry also revealed several types of restrictions placed on scientific advisors by the companies with which they are associated to protect proprietary information. One prominant firm requires that its academic affiliates "not perform research in competition with the Company for a period of three years after termination of the consulting arrangements."[14]

Another company states that "there is no assurance that the company's business will not conflict with the business of the institutions with which the various consultants are affiliated."[15] These are particularly troublesome signs. Several universities that have acted on potential conflicts of interest among ACIND individuals have introduced disclosure procedures that are supervised by departmental chairpersons. But if the degree of faculty linkage becomes significantly high, many chairpersons will be part of the same reward system.

In conclusion, there is much that needs to be done to improve the public's attitude toward the role of science in social policy, and particularly to enhance the image of scientific objectivity. One contribution to this end is to promote disclosure. The commercial connections of scientists with dual affiliations should be part of their résumé and open to the public record when they enter the policy realm or when they serve on public advisory committees. This is not a difficult or burdensome requirement.

A second recommednation, which is more difficult to implement, would reward scientists who maintain an independence from commercial activities. Such independence might be factored into appointments on prestigious commissions and other policymaking activities, including service on study panels, as well as preference in the competitive grants program.

Without some incentives to reverse the momentum of the ACIND phenomenon, the pure biomedical scientist may become the vestigial remains of a past generation. At risk are the foreclosure of an important agenda: the social guidance of a technological revolution and the increasing erosion of public confidence in scientific objectivity.

References and Notes

1. Weiner, C. (1984) (personal communication).
2. Office of Technology Assessment, *Commercial Biotechnology: An International Analysis*, U.S. Government Printing Office, Washington, DC (Jan. 1984).
3. Subcommittee on Investigations and Oversight, Committee on Science and Technology, U.S. House of Representatives, *Hearings on Commercialization of Academic Biomedical Research*, U.S. Government Printing Office, Washington, DC (June 8–9, 1981).
4. California Rural Legal Assistance *vs.* Board of Trustees of the University of California. Brief filed in the California Judicial Court, 1984.
5. Subcommittee on Investigations and Oversight, Committee on Science and Technology, U.S. House of Representatives, *Hearings on University/Industry Cooperation in Biotechnology*, U.S. Government Printing Office, Washington, DC (July 16–17, 1982); and *supra* note 3.
6. See *supra* note 2.
7. *Supra* note 2, at 417.
8. Walsh, J., Universities: Industry links raise conflict of interest issue, *Science* 164:411–2 (Apr. 25, 1969).
9. *Id.* at 412.
10. Cone, J. and Robinson, J. DBCP-UC Research, *Synapse*, San Francisco, CA: University of California at San Francisco, 22(9):4, 1 (Nov. 10, 1977).
11. Orr, L. (ed.), Corporate money and co-opted scholars, *Business and Society Rev.* 37:4–11 (Spring 1980–1981), at 5.
12. *Genetic Engineering News* (M. Liebert, publisher, in letter to readers) 3(6):4 (Nov./Dec. 1983).
13. Culliton, B., The academic-industrial complex, *Science* 216:960 (May 28, 1982).
14. Biogen, N. V., *Company Prospectus* (1983).
15. Centocor, Inc., *Company Prospectus* (1982).

6

THE DOUBLE HELIX AND THE RESEARCH TRIANGLE

University–Industry–Government

ROBERT B. NICHOLAS, J.D.
Chief Counsel/Staff Director
Subcommittee on Investigations and Oversight of the Committee on Science and Technology
U.S. House of Representatives
Washington, DC 20515

I welcome the opportunity to share with you some of the questions that have been raised in the Congress by the increasing commercial investments in biotechnology at universities. Although closer cooperation between universities and private companies is seen generally in Congress as desirable, particularly as a means of shortening the time between the discovery and the commercialization of a product, arrangements involving biotechnology research have received special attention because of the uniqueness and power associated with genetic engineering. Before discussing some of the concerns that have been voiced, I would like to briefly describe why biotechnology research is seen as needing to be more sensitively handled than other areas of research have been in the past.

The implications of genetic engineering are staggering. The line between fantasy and realistic end points is not now clearly understood, and with advances in science occurring rapidly, it is difficult to have any real confidence in predictions about when new products or procedures will become available. These great uncertainties frustrate efforts to assess clearly the meaning and impact of biotechnology. When the technology of celestial navigation was first systematized by Henry the Navigator, humankind did not know where their ships, so guided, would travel. Similarly, the newly discovered road map to life itself will undoubtedly lead us to new worlds of which we now have no knowledge.

Although it seems as though it has happened overnight, the revolution in biology and genetic engineering did *not* happen overnight. Research into genetics *per se* reaches back into the nineteenth century and Gregor Mendel's experiments. The most important work in this century, of course, was that of Watson and Crick. Not until the mid-1970s, however, did we begin to see the possibilities of recombinant DNA technology and the science of molecular biology.

In agriculture, medicine, energy, environment, and all the life sciences, new discoveries promise to have major effects on the way we live. In the last Congress, the Congressional Office of Technology Assessment (OTA) issued a lengthy report in which it discussed the uses—both actual and potential—of applied genetics in the commercial, industrial, and agricultural areas. The list was impressive. And, as the new OTA report on the commercialization of biotechnology[1] discusses, the rapid advance in our understanding of molecular genetics is leading to products in the shorter run.

The most alluring, yet potentially the most ethically troublesome, uses of the new recombinant DNA techniques and biotechnology relate to their human applications. This is the area in which the greatest potential—and the greatest challenges—awaits us. The human applications of genetic technology fall into three basic categories:

1. The production of pharmaceuticals, diagnostic tools, and delivery systems for the diagnosis and treatment of illness and disease.
2. Genetic screening, for both medical and employment purposes.
3. Genetic engineering to alter human beings and the human genome.

In the first category, microorganisms have already been engineered to produce human insulin, interferon, interleukin, growth hormone, urokinase (for the treatment of blood clots), thymosin (for controlling the immune response), and somatostatin (a brain hormone). The most advanced applications today are in the field of hormones. Genetic technologies also present new approaches to vaccine development.

In the second category, genetic screening presents a different set of possibilities and considerations. Scientists are seeking to develop a technology that is able to ascertain as individual's predisposition or susceptibility to diseases by examining her or his genetic structure.

The third human application of genetic technology—human genetic engineering—is easily the most far-reaching. Although it sounds like science fiction, human genetic engineering may, in a relatively short time, allow us to cure some diseases caused by a single gene defect in individuals. Some day, gene therapy may enable us to eliminate such diseases from the human gene pool. Recently, *Science* magazine reported advances in gene transfer methods using retroviruses that could bring the cure for certain inherited diseases closer to reality.[2]

Before the end of this century, the human applications of genetic engineering techniques will present society with some of the most difficult questions that have ever confronted humankind, questions about the very essence of what it means to be human. If we can develop the ability to alter our own genetic blueprints, then the potential for affecting the future of the human race, as we know it, becomes limitless.

Last year, Congressman Albert Gore introduced, and the House of Representatives passed, a bill to establish the President's Commission on the Human Application of Genetic Engineering. The commission, composed primarily of nonscientists, was established for the purpose of providing a focus for the review of the many issues raised by the application of genetic engineering techniques to humans. The bill resulted from three days of hearings on the scientific, religious, ethical, and societal issues inherent in human genetic engineering held by the Committee on Science and Technology's Subcommittee on Investigations and Oversight. The testimony presented at the hearing confirmed that our social, educational, and political institutions are currently unprepared to address many of these issues raised by the application of genetic technology to humans, and that, to a great degree, an entirely new body of ethics may need to be developed to resolve them.

In part, it is the uneasiness about the unknowns relating to biotechnology, and about our lack of preparation to find answers for these new questions that has created controversy about how biotechnology is to be developed, funded, and controlled. Almost all of these questions are confronted first in the university research community. As a result, we will all be relying heavily on universities to preview these questions with unusual sensitivity.

To keep its commitment to the advancement of public knowledge in this field, Congress has to ensure that research will be properly funded. At the same time, for universities to meet their obligations to the public, they need to maintain an institutional structure and a knowledge base that can provide neutral guidance on what we as a society should do with the knowledge and the inventions we generate. As choices become more difficult, the nature of the forum in which they are addressed will become more important.

Although in the past public funding has been the almost exclusive source of university funds for research in biotechnology, over the last few years we have seen the development of new relationships between some of our most highly esteemed research universities and hospitals and private corporations. Some of this influx of private-sector capital has been in the traditional form of short-term, limited-scope research contracts or unrestricted grants. Increasingly, however, the arrangements in biotechnology have become "big ticket" items as companies seek to acquire the advanced expertise in molecular genetics and biotechnology available almost exclusively at the university. In some cases, new academic departments financed by companies are springing up to conduct basic, but also potentially patentable, research on recombinant DNA technology. One of the best known of these arrangements is the agreement between the Massachusetts General Hospital and the Hoechst Chemical Corporation of West Germany. Under the terms of the agreement, Hoechst will provide $70 million over the next 10 years to Massachusetts General to fund a new Department of Molecular Biology at the hospital. Although researchers at Mass General will have freedom of choice in their basic research activities, Hoechst will receive, in return for its $70 million, exclusive worldwide patent rights on any discoveries that may be produced in whole *or in part* with its money. Agreements with variations on this basic arrangements and amounts have been reached by the Monsanto Corporation with Washington University in St. Louis, by the Dupont Corporation with the University of Maryland, and by Yale University with Bristol-Myers, to name just a few. In the Monsanto–Washington University agreement, which was examined in detail at the hearings held in the last Congress, great sensitivity was shown by the participants in avoiding the pitfalls of the relationship. Yet, read literally, the agreement places in

Monsanto the final control over the choice of research projects financed under the agreement.

In fairness to Monsanto and Washington University, their collective judgment, expressed at the hearing, was that the contract would be a failure if the trust so essential to the agreement were broken down to the point where anybody needed to cast the deciding vote.

It is not surprising that, in this time of decreasing federal involvement in basic research programs, universities are turning to private industry for support of important research efforts. Indeed, in many respects, this development is a very healthy one and is generally consistent with the historical amalgam of university–industry efforts that have greatly benefited society in other areas. Although such ties have substantial benefits, this trend toward increased financial ties is not without real risks to the traditional university values of freedom of choice in the selection of research topics, openness in communication, and priority of the educational role. Clearly, these issues need to be fully debated— as they now are being—and agreements need to be sensitively and flexibly drawn as all parties feel their way in this arena. In some cases, alternatives to direct arrangements may need to be explored before these new arrangements set precedents that could be injurious.

What are the concerns about these new relationships that have been voiced in Congress and elsewhere?

First, if the Congress is to grapple successfully with the unprecedented implications of recombinant DNA research, for which it is still the principle source of funding, it must have a reasonably neutral source of advice on these matters. It would be disastrous if Congress and others were unable to obtain neutral opinions from the best minds at universities and other research institutions because they were all on the payrolls of companies that had financial stakes in the outcome of the policy debates. It would be equally troublesome if truly neutral scientists could be found but they could not discuss their work because of the financial relationships that their universities had with profit-making entities.

Second, the nature and focus of departments, or potentially of research institutions themselves, could be dramatically affected by these new agreements. In hearings before two subcommittees of the House Committee on Science and Technology, distinguished scientists expressed a concern that these agreements could force changes in direction in the research priorities of institutions and could place great strains on the ethic of scientific openness that has helped to generate our greatest discoveries.

Should we not all be concerned about the potential impact on the university community of competition in academic departments for the best graduate students on the part of professors who are principals in biotechnology companies with an interest in the research conducted? Should we not all be concerned about the potential impact on the university community of giving the legal right to an outside party to require university researchers to remain silent about the work they have in progress? Should we not all raise questions about freely giving an outside party legal veto power over any substantial portion of the research projects undertaken in any university with the money they provide?

A third reason for concern about the impact of broad-scale arrangements between companies and universities is that they can create potential conflicts of interest for faculty involving the allocation of time and resources, the attribution of sponsorship or patents, the selection of graduate-student research topics, and the commingling of funds.

Fourth—and this concern is different in kind and degree from the others I have discussed—agreements between American research institutions and foreign companies have raised the spectre of undesirable technology transfer. Even people who are not particularly jingoistic or chauvinistic have expressed concern that some of these initial contracts have been with foreign firms. Regardless of our best intentions in the matter, and despite contractual niceties that attempt to respect American patent law, we may be too easily allowing basic research expertise to be converted into foreign profits by permitting a small value add-on by a foreign firm to entitle the firm to an exclusive patent. Similar concerns were echoed in the OTA report on international competitiveness in biotechnology, which concluded that "continuation of the initial preeminence of American companies in the commercialization of biotechnology is not assured."[1]

For example, in the Hoechst–Massachusetts General arrangement, where research is conducted with both public and industry funding, the Hoechst Corporation may well have profited from research that was largely funded with taxpayer dollars. In a letter to Congressman Gore, the head of the General Accounting Office indicated that "a possibility exists that Hoechst will gain title, in violation of Public Law 96-517, to inventions that have been partially funded with federal dollars."[3]

American companies should not be complacent about the prospect of competing with technologies that their tax dollars helped to fund and to which they are denied access. As a public policy matter, we need to think long and hard before we permit foreign corporations to "skim the cream" from research that the American public has supported.

To address all these concerns, we must focus on the larger issue as well: How are the conflicting goals and values of universities and corporations to be mingled together? Can we avoid the worst of the problems without denying ourselves the significant fruits of these new combinations? I think we can, but before reaching some conclusions, I want to state one additional concern. It is this: The rush of private industry into relationships with universities and research institutions—if not handled carefully—could lead to an erosion of public trust in science, on which all these enterprises depend. For example, previously, when new scientific breakthroughs were announced, there was little concern that our scientists and universities were not operating candidly and in the public interest. But today, unfortunately, there may well be skepticism. When announcements of new "breakthroughs" are made today, one must always wonder whether these "discoveries" are really new or significant or whether they are simply creations of Madison Avenue designed to boost a stock offering on Wall Street. We must all be sensitive to these concerns lest the public's support for scientific research funding be undermined.

As my comments have emphasized, as the ties between universities and industries grow increasingly closer, a balance must be struck between the intellectual independence of the scientist and the university and the industrial desire and society's need for commercial opportunity. Although there are very positive aspects to closer industry–university relations, the congressional investigation of this trend has illustrated both real and potential difficulties. The investigation has also substantiated the need to develop better contractual models for the participants and to look for some alternatives to the direct agreements being negotiated between universities and industry.

Of course, one alternative would be increased public funding of research. According to the Five Year Outlook for Science and Technology published by the National Science Foundation, 90% of the basic research in this country is still funded by the federal government.[4] Although industry support of research has grown over the past few years, cooperative research efforts between universities and industry account for only 5% of university research funding, generally, and 4% in biotechnology. Although small in comparison to governmental support, the industry share of research financing is potentially significant enough to have a dramatic impact on individual universities, particularly universities with few alternative sources of financial support. Regardless of the exact level of government funding, the government is likely to remain the primary supporter of biomedical research in the foreseeable future and thus to remain a major player in this debate. And industry interest in biotechnology—at least in the short run—is sufficiently high to allow us to believe that the trend of increased cooperation will continue.

When this debate began several years ago, there was little congressional interest in a heavy-handed regulatory approach to this admittedly sensitive area. Rather, the focus was on stimulating debate and helping to ensure that the parties to the particular agreements, and their broader communities, would focus on the potential problems and carefully consider the implications of their actions. Congressional intent in this area has not changed, largely, I believe, because of the generally constructive response by those involved.

In reply to a request by Congressman Don Fuqua, Chairman of the House Committee on Science and Technology, together with Congressman Gore, the Association of American Universities took the lead and formulated a set of very broad general principles for universities to use when negotiating agreements with industrial concerns. The AAU also established a clearinghouse for information on biotechnology commercialization arrangements.

The AAU effort is generally viewed as a positive step. Many others as well are continuing to develop better and more precise guidelines and agreements that will help protect the interests of the public, of the research institutions, and of the companies. Constructive as all this debate has been, I believe that there will continue to be congressional oversight in this important area.

By way of conclusion and summary, I would like to share with you several of the staff conclusions from the subcommittee's review:[5]

- The contractual relationships between universities and commercial firms need to be continually reviewed by university administrators and faculty, and by industry management, to determine if the expectations and interests of all parties are being satisfied and protected.
- The federal government should, on a continuing basis, assess the benefits and

problems resulting from large-scale corporate support of university research programs in biotechnology.

- Faculty should not hold equity positions in commercial ventures that coincide with their academic endeavors. I think the record developed demonstrates the problems that can arise from such a situation. General support for this conclusion has been found in both industry and academia.
- The scientific community needs to seriously address the industry–university issue. A second national conference, in the tradition of the first Asilomar gathering, should be convened for the purpose of setting some more precise guidelines than those of the AAU that could protect the interests of both the universities and the companies involved. The consensus on biosafety that was reached at Asilomar established a level of public confidence in the scientific community in this field.
- More effort needs to be devoted to exploring "middle-man" mechanisms. As an example, the North Carolina Biotechnology Foundation, established by the State of North Carolina, was set up to accept industrial contributions for university-based research. Such mechanisms may better insulate the university from commercial activities and thereby more appropriately safeguard the interests of all parties.

In the final analysis, the issues raised by closer university–industry ties and those arising from our race for technological innovation as we seek to exploit the potential of biotechnology will be with us for some time. They require thoughtful, cooperative analysis from all three sectors: government, industry, and universities.

REFERENCES

1. Office of Technology Assessment, *Commercial Biotechnology: An International Analysis*, U.S. Government Printing Office, Washington DC (Jan. 1984).
2. Kolata, G., *Science* **223**: 1376 (1984).
3. Correspondence from Elmer Statz, Comptroller General of the United States, to the Honorable Albert Gore, Jr., Chairman of the Investigations and Oversight Subcommittee, Committee on Science and Technology, U.S. House of Representatives (March 1981).
4. National Science Foundation, *Outlook for Science and Technology: The Next Five Years*, U.S. Government Printing Office, Washington DC (Nov. 1983).
5. U.S. Congress, Committee on Science and Technology, Investigations and Oversight Subcommittee, Draft Staff Paper, 98th Congress, 1st Sess. (1983).

Discussion

Dr. David Baltimore: I can echo from personal associations that the percentage of senior faculty involved in industrial connections in the major research universities in the United States is very high. It certainly is higher than 50%. Although I don't have data that are as precise as Dr. Krimsky's, I probably know more people. The second point is that the absolutist position stated by Dr. Relman that there should be no equity involvement of faculty in any corporation is a very persuasive and important position that runs counter to the policies of almost every university at present, as well as against the behavior of most academics. Yet, the logic for it is very strong, and I think it represents a very important takeoff point for discussion. I would point out that his proposal and Mr. Nicholas's proposal are different because he was talking about, if I understand correctly, the absolutist position of no equity involvement in any company with which one has either a consulting agreement or any contractual relationship for research. In contrast, the other position is that there should be no equity involvement where there is any research going on in the institution, and that's a very different perspective. The second is much easier to deal with than the first. I would also make the observation that no one in all of these discussions has actually questioned the health of today's biomedical sciences in the United States, and our efforts remain far and away the most important on a worldwide scale. There may be a variety of conflicts and difficulties, but there is also at the heart of the matter a continuing very high level of production, and much of that by people and in laboratories where these kinds of conflicts can be found. I would last point out that the desire to have neutral people on review boards and objective people on review boards is something that I thought had long ago been understood as impossible. There is no person who is neutral. There is no person who is objective. We all carry "baggage" of a variety of sorts. Public interest people carry the "baggage" of maintaining the public interest organizations and a variety of other things, and government maintains its interests. University people may be in conflict because of corporate relationships. So the real issue is openness of involvement and what that implies, rather than the search for an unfindable neutrality or objectivity.

DR. SHELDON KRIMSKY: I just want to make a comment on the last distinction, or nondistinction, that you made. I think there is an important distinction between a person who is serving on a public service panel and who is rendering a decision in an area in which that person has some financial interests, and other people who bring to that panel a whole range of "baggage" from their socialization or position in life. I think if you polled most people in the country, they would see a very clear distinction between direct financial interests in the service of society and other kinds of special interests that they might have, including their position in life. I think it's a distinction worth making, and most people would probably accept it.

MS. ELAINE LOCKE: The discussion this morning has appropriately focused on cellular-level things and laboratory research. I'm coming from a perspective where we're interested in how the physician deals with the patient directly. Several of the speakers have commented that there's a greater level of sensitivity involved when it's biotechnology than for other kinds of research. There may indeed be different ethical questions or different standards. I'd like for the panel to comment, if possible, on whether there may be another level of sensitivity and another level of concern when the discussion is extended to clinical things. For example, what about patenting surgical procedures as opposed to surgical equipment or laboratory products?

DR. ARNOLD S. RELMAN: That's an important question. My personal view is that direct health services to patients—the facilities, the procedures, and whatever's involved in direct health care—are an inappropriate object of commercial exploitation. I feel that it is not in the public interest for any aspect of personal health care to be in the commercial marketplace. I am opposed to investor-owned hospitals. I am opposed to investor-owned diagnostic laboratories. I oppose investor-owned procedures, embryo transfer procedures, CAT-scanning, Nuclear Magnetic Resonance (NMR) diagnostic facilities—you name it. I think it is undesirable and in the long run will damage society and will be counterproductive, so that I lump them all together. I am opposed to them all.

MR. ROBERT B. NICHOLAS: I think that the difference between that area and biotechnology is more one of public perception than reality. I think it's easier to define what these issues are within the context that Dr. Relman has just proposed. We can have feelings and opinions on them relatively readily. The area of biotechnology for the general public is shrouded in a mist, and even for those who are reasonably well informed, the ability to predict where the science is going is not very good. So I think that clouds the whole debate on biotechnology and makes some of these issues much more pointed in a public forum.

DR. LISA H. NEWTON: I've observed that the disinterested intelligentsia that we are seeking seem to become more personally involved the less they have outside interests, that clogging in academic procedures very often seems to come from personal things and not from these conflicts of interest, which could be objectively documented. I wonder if that isn't more serious. Second, the university itself was formed from the kind of conflicts of agendas that we seem to have here, and it seems that differences in points of view can often cross-fertilize each other. We've had three speakers talking about the dangers of commercial involvement in biotechnology, which is a fairly new phenomenon. I wonder if anybody's tried any speculation on what possible benefits might come from the joining of these two previously disparate worlds of biotechnology and academe.

DR. ARNOLD S. RELMAN: Well, I was not arguing against the commercialization of biotechnology. I was arguing the proposition that there should be clear limits on the involvement of universities and university faculty in that commercialization. I see nothing inappropriate in the commercial exploitation of products derived from genetic engineering. I think that's fine. And as I have made quite clear, with appropriate guidelines with full disclosure, I think that there is an appropriate role for academic people, academic scientists and universities, to work together with these companies within certain limits. But I draw the line at some point. I draw the line when the financial fortunes of universities and professors become intertwined with the financial fortunes and entrepreneurial goals of the companies. At that point, it seems to me that the essential functions of the university and the essential functions of a professor become compromised. That's what I argue against, and not against the commercialization of biotechnology.

DR. BERNARD DAVIS: I'd like to reinforce some of the comments that Dr. Baltimore made. I share very much the concerns expressed by Dr. Krimsky and Dr. Relman, but I am a little bit concerned about their recommendations. It seems to me that we can't possibly prevent faculty members from holding equity in corporations to which they are supplying their services. The situation, Dr. Krimsky, is worse than you think. The National Academy is a lifetime election with a large fraction of the members past retirement; for the active members, it's way over 50% that have such connections. Dr. Baltimore said that if that was as disastrous as it seems to you, you'd think that our biological sciences would be suffering enormously. As he said, they are thriving more than anywhere else in the world. The question is: How can we somehow prevent the holding of equity from having the undesirable consequences that we all recognize, and that in many cases are there. I would suggest that it's much more profitable to focus not on how terrible it is to hold equity, but on how to prevent the undesirable consequences. With respect to committees, I agree with you entirely that there should be open disclosure, and that all the members of the committee and the government officials in charge of a committee should know who has what industrial connections. I would suggest that it's up to the universities to work out mechanisms for carefully monitoring the distribution of time of their faculty, instead of trusting them as much as has been more appropriate in years past. We should protect the interests of graduate students and postdoctoral fellows, perhaps by having mechanisms for inquiry and finding out whether they feel that they are being pushed into things that they don't want to do or into being too secretive. I think the universities have a real responsibility for seeing that the holding of equity doesn't have bad consequences.

Dr. ARNOLD S. RELMAN: Dr. Davis, I agree with most of what you said, but not all. I take exception to the point that you and David Baltimore made, namely, that everything is hunky-dory with American biotechnology. We are the cutting edge. America's the center of most molecular genetics research. Therefore, as I understand the argument, the merger between American biotechnology, commercial technology companies, and American universities must be all right. It's a *non sequitur*—it doesn't follow at all. The question is: What would it be like if we didn't follow the present model? It might be much better. How do we know? And besides, the bad consequences that I'm concerned about are consequences to the soul and spirit and life of the university. Those consequences are going to become apparent only in a while. It may take a generation, so that the present domination and obvious international success of American molecular biology has nothing to do with the issues I am raising. Nothing at all.

Dr. DAVID BALTIMORE: Let me say, just to be fair, that I made that remark only because I felt we had such an unrelievedly negative view of things that at least one measure of some positive side ought to be there. But I don't disagree with anything you've said.

Dr. SHELDON KRIMSKY: Let me offer an example of where I think there's been silence when there should not be on a particular public issue. One of the principle research programs now in progress is to make food crops herbicide-resistant. Now, we just had a major national controversy over EDB, which is just one substance that's been around for quite a while, and all of sudden, people realize that it is being used pervasively and that it's more dangerous than we thought. The purpose of a research program designed to make food crops herbicide-resistant is to raise the use of herbicides in agriculture. Now, I have not seen any debate on whether we want to make food crops dependent on yet another chemical. One of the most important of the herbicides that are being considered for this is atrazine. Those of you in the audience who know more about atrazine than I do realize that there are some problems with atrazine's entering the water supply system. So we have a $4-billion pesticide market, and we have only a $2-billion herbicide market. I don't see any public debate about whether we want to see this research make our food crops dependent on yet another chemical that could, in the future, have some adverse consequences.

MR. ALEXANDER CAPRON: My question goes to Dr. Relman and Mr. Nicholas. If we are looking for the analogy, which your earlier answers suggested we were, is the analogy for the behavior of the university scientists to be that of the physician? The physician who has patients' interests at heart and was seen to have the kind of conflict that you have criticized, Dr. Relman, if she or he took a financial interest—particularly an undisclosed financial interest—in a patient's treatment? Or that of those in business, where we don't stop and say, "You are not supposed to take advantage of people"? We say as long as you fight fair you can operate in the marketplace. Which is the university scientist going to be? I think you have raised very good questions, but my problem with some of the details, Dr. Relman, is that you have suggested that it is perfectly appropriate for universities to have the patent interests that come out of the work of the scientists who are involved. If you look at the perturbations that can occur within the university and the desire of university scientists, therefore, to pursue a course that is more likely to produce the patents, it will not be a direct financial interest, which you were right in criticizing. But is it not, in effect, turning the university more explicitly into something with a business interest, which, in turn, affects the way the internal operations of the university works? I see a contradiction between the very flat rule, where you say, "No equity interest," and yet say, "Yes, contracts and commercial interests." The question as it relates to the Congress would be: Does Mr. Nicholas think there will be any reaction after the series of hearings you've held? We have recently liberalized the patent policy in a number of ways, including turning over and making more available for commercial exploitation patent rights that were generated with public monies, something that you criticized as it relates to foreign corporations. But I wonder if the Congress is looking at anything about these interests as they affect United States universities even with American corporations.

MR. ROBERT B. NICHOLAS: One of the difficulties in terms of looking to Congress to obtain some resolution of these issues is that, on the one hand, Congress is generally short-term-oriented. The buzz words in Congress for the past several years have very much been *innovation* and *productivity*. So there is a lot of general sentiment in Congress toward increased cooperation between industries and universities. Indeed, if one looks at the National Science Foundation report on industry–university relationships, it doesn't reflect very much of the healthy skepticism that many have expressed about the nature of these relationships. So, as a practical matter, I don't see, in the short run, Congress producing any legislation in this area. That's not to say that there is not concern about these kinds of issues, but I just don't think that there's enough political momentum at this point to create any legislation. Again, if things change, if there's an indication that this is a serious problem in terms of affecting a substantial public interest in a different way than the debate has been proceeding, then there might be some sentiment. But at the present time, I don't think so.

DR. ARNOLD S. RELMAN: Mr. Capron, your question about patents is a trenchant one. I don't take quite the absolute position that you impute to me. I feel very strongly about the equity interests question for reasons that I stated. I said that I see nothing inherently wrong with the patent idea, but I'm open to reconsideration. It seems to me that it is desirable and it is inevitable that universities and their faculties are going to generate commercially valuable ideas. Question: Should those ideas be given away? Who should benefit from the commercialization of those patentable ideas? Should it be given to the government for the benefit of the public? It seems to me the universities ought to benefit in the same way that faculty benefit from writing successful books. Faculty have a right to share, it seems to me, under appropriate university guidelines, in the financial benefits from those patents. If it turns out that there are widespread abuses, then I would reconsider my position. The issue should not be patents or no patents. The issue should be free universities at arm's length from all commercial involvement, from ongoing responsibilities or not. I clearly take my stand there if patents can be lived with. I think universities ought to have an opportunity to benefit. Furthermore, and finally, I don't think it's going to be very much money. I don't think many universities are going to get rich from patents. The model of Wisconsin . . . it's a fantasy, it's a myth. Wisconsin did not get rich from the patents on vitamin K. They got rich from the investments they made on the modest amount of patent royalties they won. Stanford has made a few million dollars. It remains to be seen, in the big scheme of things, whether patent income is going to be a big source of support for Stanford. I suspect not. So I don't think it's going to be a major issue.

DR. LEON E. ROSENBERG: I think we shouldn't forget the responsibility and perhaps the power of the university to modify the situation that we are all discussing today. I believe, as Dr. Relman does, that the equity situation is a great concern. Certainly, I share Dr. Krimsky's view on that as well. I think if university officials determine what it really means to be a full-time faculty member, define the guidelines for what full-time means, and therefore, for what tenure means, we will perhaps find ourselves in the situation where well-meaning scientists can decide if they wish to be full-time faculty members, with all the rights and privileges and accolades that go with that, or if they would just as soon be part of an adjunct faculty with all of the rights and privileges that go with that. I have no bias about which is appropriate, but I think defining things a bit more clearly, along the lines of what it means to be full-time, might make some difference to people in defining whether they wish to have their cake or eat it.

DR. SHELDON KRIMSKY: I don't see how holding equity in a firm would be at all inconsistent with any of the things that Professor Rosenberg mentioned, even owning three-quarters equity in the firm as long as a person were considered full-time. I wonder if Dr. Relman, when he talks about equity, could mention about how much is equity? Owning how much stock in a firm constitutes equity? Do you have any response?

DR. ARNOLD S. RELMAN: Tough question. I think enough equity to influence your behavior and your attitudes.

DR. DAVID BALTIMORE: You can't get out of it that way.

DR. ARNOLD S. RELMAN: Obviously, you can't say percentages because 5% of Hoechst makes you a multimillionaire many times over, and 5% of some little bitty company in absolute dollars might not be a lot. I can't answer that question. I don't think I have to. That's for lawyers and smart university administrators to work on. The principle is, though, that if you own enough interest in a firm so that it influences your behavior, your teaching, your attitudes, what you do is influenced because you are interested in the welfare of that firm, it seems to me it's too much. Whether it's 1% or 10% or $10,000 or $100,000. I don't know.

A PARTICIPANT: I'm afraid the only tenable position for that is zero.

DR. ARNOLD S. RELMAN: If that's the way the argument comes out, that's what I think.

DR. JACQUES LORRAINE: I would like to remind you that we in the Province of Quebec have totally socialized medicine. Everything is paid by the government. I would like to point out one of the problems that may happen. It is that whenever the government pays, they may seek total control. Also, the bureaucracy is extremely time-consuming. It does make sense to work to preserve the liberty of what you are doing here.

Human Applications of Genetic Engineering

MODERATOR: PHILIP LEDER

7

Commerce and the Future of Gene Transfer

Tabitha M. Powledge, M.S.
Senior Editor
Bio/Technology
271 Degraw Street
Brooklyn, NY 11231

Obviously, providing an overview of the vast and windy subject of the ethical issues in gene transfer is out of the question, so I'm going to be selective. I think I need spend almost no time on the immediate questions of human experimentation that will come up with the first attempts at gene transfer. There is a consensus that those attempts will present no novel ethical issues but raise the same sorts of worries about safety that attend any experimental therapies. We already have available an array of agencies from several parts of the alphabet that are supposed to deal with those questions—IRBs, FDA, RAC, and so forth—and I think we can be reasonably confident that the machinery for overseeing human experimentation will function to forestall major abuses.

Nevertheless, a lot of time and energy does go into discussing the human experimentation aspects of gene transfer.[1] Doubtless, some of it is traceable to the activities of Martin Cline, who caused so much controversy with his premature attempts to use gene therapy for thalassemia a few years ago. Although there has been a good deal of private grumbling that the government punished him too severely when it took away his grants, my sense is that a great many people who are interested in the development of this field believe that it was important to declare as publicly as possible that any tinkering with human genes should take place only under the highest ethical precepts. As a result, Cline may well have unwittingly stimulated a more exhaustive exploration of the human experimentation issues than might otherwise have taken place. Perhaps we should all be grateful to him.

But to some extent, our concentration on issues of human experimentation has been a distraction, using up energy and brain room that we might otherwise have given to some of the longer term issues that will probably arise as a result of moving genes around in human beings. I'd like to explore briefly a couple of the possibilities.

My hunch is that we will not confine genetic engineering to specific human tissues and organs, despite a certain amount of public opposition to going further. A number of individuals and groups have decried the sort of human genetic engineering that will lead to changes in the germ cells. It was mentioned in *Splicing Life*, the report of the President's Commission for the Study of Ethical Problems in Medicine and Biomedical and Behavioral Research.[2] About a year ago, a group put together by Jeremy Rifkin, professional opponent of genetic engineering, declared its opposition to germ cell changes. Nevertheless, I expect that researchers are going to be able to come up with some plausible reasons for going ahead with engineering a human embryo.

Here's one scenario, suggested by a well-known gene therapist. As a result of the genetic screening programs that we set up for newborns a generation ago, there now exist adults who are functioning normally in this society despite the fact that they suffer from phenylketonuria (PKU). PKU is an autosomal recessive inborn error of metabolism in which the amino acid phenylalanine is not broken down properly. One result is severe mental retardation, which can be averted if the sufferer consumes a special diet containing very little of the offending amino acid. Although the diet is anything but perfect, and intellectual performance appears to be slightly impaired despite the best efforts of physicians and parents, thanks to newborn screening programs and the special diet a number of babies with PKU have now grown up free of the worst effects of the disorder. Inevitably, two such people are going to meet, marry, and wish to begin a family. As far as we know, it hasn't happened yet, but very likely it will happen eventually.

Because neither one will possess a normal gene for phenylalanine hydroxylase, any child they bring into the world will have PKU, necessitating yet another generation of an unpalatable special diet, expense, inconvenience, and damaged intellect. On the other hand, any fertilized egg that this couple produced would be a perfect candidate for gene therapy. There are doubtless many researchers who would be intrigued by the notion of trying to cure PKU in a fertilized egg or a very early embryo. It would present a technical challenge, formidable, but probably not insuperable. Gene transfers are moving along rapidly, elegant new methods for accomplishing them are tumbling out of the labs, and we have even moved forward with the tricky business of getting the gene to work properly once it's in the cell.[3] In short, supplied with enough money and brains and motivation, science could probably find a way to cure PKU, and a great many other genetic disorders, at the beginning of life.

Aside from the technical challenge that finding that cure would provide scientists, there would be other rewards as well. There would, of course, be a warm glow of pride and sense of virtue in helping a couple achieve a healthy child. And then there would be a few accessory benefits: fame, plum appointments at classy universities, television appearances, book contracts, an endless supply of grant money, and, just possibly, a Nobel Prize. None of these would compare with the internal rewards of overcoming a technical challenge and extending help to fellow human beings, of course, but I am told that they have their attractions.

I spin out this scenario in an attempt to show that we are likely to proceed beyond the forms of gene therapy that scientists are working on today, and to illustrate the sorts of apparently sound moral reasons that we are going to give ourselves for doing so. An embryo produced by a couple with sickle-cell disease might also be an appropriate candidate for genetic engineering. The strictures against the sort of genetic engineering that will lead to changes in human germ cells may well be swept away by the argument that curing a genetic disorder in an embryo is no different from curing it in childhood. In fact, it may well be preferable, both medically and morally, because by changing the germ cells as well as the somatic cells, doctors can at one stroke both cure a disease and prevent it from being passed on to subsequent generations. The traditional long-term argument against permanent genetic engineering of the germ cells is that it endangers the human gene pool. But that argument will be irrelevant here. Scientists will not be proposing massive eugenics programs; rather, they will be proceeding with a handful of individuals. They will not be moving ahead with genetic engineering of the human species, but only of a few human beings. And their motives will be decent and honorable and difficult to counter.

It may be possible to draw the line on human genetic engineering with strictly medical applications, such as in my hypothetical case of PKU. On the other hand, separating the truly medical applications of medical techniques from those with other purposes can be a difficult business. It has been traditional in these discussions to distinguish between, on the one hand, getting rid of something bad—as in the case of curing a genetic disease—and, on the other hand, trying to add some genetic characteristic to the genome. A number of authorities have argued that the former is morally acceptable, whereas the latter is not. I must say that the distinction seems specious to me. For one thing, speaking strictly technically, gene therapy is currently developing by adding new genetic material to cells, not by excising the defective genes. Most authorities seem to think that the ability to do that will be a long time coming. And why bother, if they can get a cell to function adequately by putting genetic material in rather than taking it out?

It is clear that the morality of human genetic engineering does not depend on whether it involves addition or subtraction. Nor, I believe, does it reside in trying to distinguish medical from nonmedical purposes. If it would be acceptable to improve our ability to resist cancer, what would be wrong with trying to enhance certain other talents and abilities that have a genetic component? Assuming that access to the technology were equally available to all potential parents, where lies the immorality in trying to increase our children's competence in mathematics or music?

I don't mean this to sound like an argument for human genetic engineering; quite the contrary. But I do mean to point out that if the notion of human genetic engineering makes us nervous, we are going to have to come up with better arguments against it. As is usual with the moral questions growing out of science and technology, the actual techniques, when they finally develop, present us with issues that are somewhat difficult from what we thought they might be, and they render some of the previous discussions obsolete.

We are also going to have to come up with those arguments fast. The Recombinant

DNA Advisory Committee, which is the arm of the NIH that advises on the acceptability of gene-splicing experiments, expects to get its first proposal to try gene therapy in 1985. Assuming that the proposal is medically reasonable, I expect approval without much difficulty. Genetic engineering of somatic cells is upon us. And germ cell engineering is hot on its heels. As I have already indicated, there are some reasons that it might be medically more sensible to engineer an embryo. And the technical problems could be, if anything, easier to solve than those of somatic cell engineering.

For one thing, researchers are moving ahead swiftly with animal genetic engineering.[4] They have a number of purposes. One main one, particularly for those working with laboratory animals, is to sort out the myriad puzzles of regulation of gene action: what turns genes off and on at the appropriate times in a cell's life. This is basic research of the highest order, but its consequences are incalculable.

One group watching eagerly is livestock breeders, avid to find new ways of genetically engineering the animals we eat. Animal breeding is one of the oldest of human activities. Dogs did not exist until we invented them, perhaps as long ago as 40,000 or 50,000 years. The genetic engineering of animals and plants is almost a defining human characteristic, one on which our entire species now depends. This central fact of our existence is usually ignored in discussions of genetic engineering, although for me it helps explain why our dilemmas over proceeding in this direction are so painful, and why we usually opt for going ahead. Our traditional method of trial and error has met with much success, but the new genetic engineering is likely to make breeding animals and plants to specifications a much more precise, efficient, controllable process than it has been before. Furthermore, it will have a direct effect on the technical possibilities of human genetic engineering. Most of the animals in question, be they small ones like laboratory mice or huge ones like cows, are mammals, just like us. What scientists learn from them will be applicable to us.

Of course, technically speaking, there will be more to human genetic engineering than transferring the new gene into the embryo and getting it to work right. Researchers must then get the genetically engineered embyro to a safe haven for the next nine months. Mouse engineers and livestock breeders will be helpful there as well. But there is a rapidly developing set of techniques for embryo transfer in our own species, too. Thanks to television, we all know about the miracle babies created in petri dishes, and about those conceived in one woman but borne by another. In the not-too-distant future, when engineering a human embryo becomes technically possible, methods for sustaining that embryo will already be in place and functioning.

Indeed, they will be in place and functioning in a particular kind of way, which brings me to my final point. Much of the work on human *in vitro* fertilization and embryo transfer has gone on under private, not public, auspices. The federal government, after studying the issues briefly in the 1970s, has decided to deal with the topic by ignoring it. So infertile couples have lined up at places like the clinic in Norfolk, Virginia, and have paid their own money to try for a child conceived in the laboratory. Now along come the Seed brothers, who want to transfer embryos from one woman to another as a commercial service. The Seed brothers, who have been working on their techniques in Chicago since the early 1970s, were responsible for the baby born in February from an egg fertilized in one woman and transferred to another. Their success rate is low so far, but they expect improvement and will probably get it, as the success rate in cattle approaches 60%. And they have remarkable ambitions to treat 50,000 women a year at a cost of between $4,000 and $7,000 each. But they intend to go further. In an interview that appeared, appropriately, in the *Wall Street Journal*, Richard Seed made it very clear that he hopes his company will eventually genetically engineer embryos as well as simply move them around.[5]

Whether the Seed brothers have more than their name going for them is really not the issue. The point is that they have founded a for-profit company with the aim of eventually making money doing human genetic engineering. In our discussions of the possibilities of human genetic engineering in the past decade or so, we really haven't faced up to the prospect that human genetic engineering might end up simply as part of, as the financial experts say, our rapidly growing service economy. Let us, in the year 1984, cast our minds back briefly to that other classic cautionary tale *Brave New World* and contemplate how our many erroneous ideas about what it says have misled us. We have feared that human genetic engineering was going to be imposed on us by a totalitarian government, eager to breed docile workers for specific jobs. Instead, it now seems possible that genetically engineered embryos will be just another consumer product, available for a fee. A far cry from Huxley's vision of the future, but is it any more acceptable? And if we decide it is not acceptable, is there anything in this free-enterprise system we're so fond of that we can do about it? It's time to start thinking about human genetic engineering in new ways. Indeed, it's almost past time.

References

1. Friedmann, T., *Gene Therapy, Fact and Fiction*. Cold Spring Harbor Laboratory, Cold Spring Harbor, NY (1983).
2. President's Commission for the Study of Ethical Problems in Medicine and Biomedical and Behavioral Research, *Splicing Life* (1982).
3. Kolata, G., Gene therapy method shows promise, *Science* 223:1376 (March 30, 1984).
4. Palmiter, R. D., *et al.*, Metallothionein-human GH fusion genes stimulate growth of mice. *Science* 222:809 (Nov. 11, 1983).
5. Lancaster, H., Firm offering human-embryo transfers for profit stirs legal and ethical debates, *Wall Street Journal* (March 7, 1984), p. 33.

8

THE HUMAN PROBLEM OF HUMAN GENETIC ENGINEERING

J. ROBERT NELSON, DR. THEOL.
Director of the Institute of Religion
Texas Medical Center
Houston, TX 77025
Adjunct Professor of Medicine
Baylor College of Medicine
Houston, Texas 77030

WHY HUMAN LIFE IS SACRED

In their preface to *Genetics and Law II*, Aubrey Milunsky and George Annas looked ahead to the advances in genetic technology by 1984 and wrote: "Our hope is that the price will not be the diminishing of human values. Genetic progress and human values must coexist."[1] Their hope and their statement are presumably favored by all of us present—unless, by chance, some unreformed veteran researchers of the German Nazi and Japanese Manchurian death labs are among us.

It is scarcely a bold or distinctive act to declare one's support of human values in defense of human life. We all do this, and we do it with sincerity. Indeed, it gives us a sense of moral invigoration and justifiable rectitude to assert such purpose. We really do want to be on the right side of important questions about the protection and preferment of human life and human values. This is why we can enjoy the satisfaction of dealing with decisions that are unambiguous: when right is clearly right, and wrong is wrong. It is a deplorable but unavoidable fact, however, that most problems occasioned by the new genetic techniques are not that simple. Not needing to face moral ambiguity is a luxury that is denied us today. Where ambiguity exists, our consciences are sensitized; and as a result, we professional religious ethicists are enabled to make a decent living.

The application of recombinant DNA techniques to human beings is like the stuff of which fairy tales are made. In fairy tales, dwarfs become giants, beggars become princes, and ugly witches become princesses; weaklings become Herculean strongmen; even frogs become handsome youths; and magic and all-purpose healing potions abound.

The stories rely on the love of our imaginations for metamorphosis. We like to believe that ordinary people can be transfigured into persons of superior health, intelligence, strength, and beauty. The merely human in its natural state is just not good enough for our imaginations.

In this respect, religious beliefs resemble fairy tales. Of course, some iconoclasts hold that our religious beliefs are, indeed, nothing but fairy tales. Such skepticism aside, let it be noted that the transfiguration of human beings, both individually and collectively as a species and a race, is the aspiration and hope of the prevalent religions of Western civilization. Judaism and Christianity are both committed to the highest expectations of human life. They look hopefully for health, longevity, and the fulfillment of our potentials of mind and spirit while we are alive on earth, and for transcendence of mortal limitations beyond. Integral to these systems of belief is the highest regard for the enhancement of human life. Whenever dehumanizing and debasing actions have been, and are, taken in the name of religion, or when institutions and practices that degrade humanity have been, and are, tolerated, the very purpose of the religions is contradicted. Certainly, religious beliefs do not hold a monopoly on desires for human health and enhancement; but they are so fixed on the goal and the hope of betterment and fulfillment of life that the new powers of genetic engineering must be of emphatic concern to persons who hold such beliefs.

The more we learn of the powers of genetic engineering, both currently practicable and putatively potential, the more we are impelled to think about the nature, meaning, and value of human life. The statement of one prominent researcher illustrates this impulsion. In July 1982, in Washington, before the President's Commission for the Study of Ethical Problems in Medicine, Biomedical and Behavioral Research, Dr. W. French Anderson (Chief of the Laboratory of Molecular Hematology, National Institutes of Health) was expressing his views on human genetic engineering. Suddenly, spontaneously, he exclaimed,

> I want to make a statement of self-revelation, which has been occurring over the last two or three hours. . . . I finally understand, after thinking about this for . . . fifteen years or so, why I feel uneasy about the gene therapy work. . . . Is there anything unique about humans? . . . If there's nothing unique about humans—that's not a *theological* question but a very *real* one. That's what I am nervous about.[2]

As if to demonstrate the fact that Anderson's question is not only very *real* but is essentially *the* theological question, the commission members, with Dr. Morris B. Abram in the chair, found themselves discussing the theology of human life for the next hour. For, as Anderson has said, "if there isn't anything unique about humans, there's nothing wrong with doing gene manipulation."

It is not human uniqueness as such, however, that requires this warning. In terms of taxonomy, human beings *are* unique in the same sense that all other species of animal life are unique. Even if it is perceived that human uniqueness is not merely the singularity found *among* numerous other species, but that humanity has a unique identity *distinguished from* all other kinds of organisms, the particular inviolability of human life is not thus established. What is it, then, that warrants our speaking of the grounding of ethics in the unique value of human life? Or, to put the question more searchingly, how can there be appeal to what we often call the *sacredness* or *sanctity* of human life? Are these words of self-evident validity and cogency? Is life literally "holy"? The well-known philosopher and director of the Hastings Center, Daniel Callahan, thinks that sanctity of life is self-evident.[3] Likewise, the sociologist Edward Shils of the University of Chicago agrees that *sanctity* is a concept of *a priori* validity when applied to all human life. Law and ethics presuppose this value, independently of any particular religious or philosophical sources for the truth; says Shils, "If life is not viewed and experienced as sacred, then nothing else would be sacred."[4]

Persons of religious faith, whose source of knowledge and belief is the Holy Bible, should only welcome this affirmation of life's distinctive value as made by humanists. Both religiously minded and secularly minded people are often able to agree on a concept of human sanctity. This implies a basic respect for all human beings, for their civil rights, their personal rights to the care and defense of their bodies and minds, and their proxy rights for dependent relatives who are either small children or incompetent. In short, the sanctity of life as a general rule is the implicit basis of medical and genetic ethics.

Beyond this level of respect for life, however, is the religious apperception of the transcendent, metaphysical, or divinely conferred value of each human life. To affirm that all human beings are made in "the image of God" is not merely a complimentary statement about human sentience, conscience, and rational capability. It is, rather, a testimony to God's creation of each distinct individual through the physiological pro-creative process and the establishing of a personal relation to that individual. For Christian faith, this belief is most highly expressed in its fundamental doctrine, namely, that God has entered the creation and human history, from the dimension of eternity to temporality, to become identified through Jesus Christ with all humanity and with every person. It is according to this same faith that the divine will favors the optimal enhancement and fulfillment of each person's earthly existence, even while it is recognized that God's will is often hindered by the distortions and misuses of human freedom, and by the enigmatic, evil contingencies of living.

When we confront today, as we must seriously confront, the challenges of the genetic manipulation of human cells, there is no angel with a flaming sword who prevents our advance into this field of biomedical science. To be religious is certainly not to be craven or obtuse about trying something new, even when that something is so potentially disturbing and perplexing as biotechnology. Nor is it an authentically religious mentality that naively expects a good result from every new scientific technique, as though human error, as well as avarice and malice, do not frustrate and corrupt our finest hopes. No, to be religious ought to mean being utterly realistic about the conditions of life in human society, regarding every person or institution or technical process with neither illusion nor despair.

With respect to human genetic engineering, therefore, this foundation for religious ethics in the literal sanctity of human life can be well expressed in the moral motto of medicine: "Primum non nocere!" ("First of all, do not harm!") And when the indications are not quite clear concerning the effects on patients of novel procedures, the maxim is "Proceed with caution."

AVOIDING GENETIC ABUSE

Much attention has recently been given in both the popular news media and the scientific journals to the question of the ethical acceptability of human germ-line manipulation. Two kinds of distinction need to be drawn clearly if the point of this discussion is to be understood and rightly appreciated. The first, of course, is the essential, textbook difference between the somatic cells, which constitute most of the human body, and the gametic, or sex, cells found in the ova and sperm. Dr. David Baltimore is quoted as remarking, "People will never understand the difference between gene therapy of somatic cells and modification of the germ line."[5] Such pessimism may be justified. Even so, in theory, it is possible to modify either the somatic cells or the germ line cells, by means of different methods, in order to cure or eliminate certain genetic diseases. The critical difference inheres, however, in the fact that, once gametes have been changed, their altered characteristics will be irrevocable and will pass on to all future progeny, whereas somatic cells will die with one's body.

The second distinction, emphasized by Dr. Bernard Davis and others,[6] is between two kinds of expectation or purpose of genetic modification: either medical and therapeutic, or eugenic and political. One is for the correcting of disease due to certain abnormally structured genes. The other, the eugenic, is for improving the traits of individuals and, eventually, of populations. Of course, the effect of a therapeutic change could also have a slight bearing on the traits of a eugenic quality, or else of a dysgenic nature. This is the distinction that is so widely unrecognized in public discussion, the neglect of which has given rise to much sensational speculation and dispute about creating "perfect people" or engineering a "superrace." At the very least, this view fails to perceive the great difference between physical traits that are monogenetic in origin and those that are polygenetic. At the most, it exceeds the limits of scientifically considered probability and belongs to fantasy and fiction. In the judgment of Dr. Arno Motulsky, according to present knowledge, "the nature and location of most genes affecting normal variation of body structure and function are unknown."[7] Only the monogenetic diseases are subject to correction by the replacement of defective genes with cloned genes.

What are the chances, then, of this procedure's being devised for therapeutic purposes? No one is entirely sure about it. Some experts agree with Jeffrey G. Williams, who wrote in *Nature*, "it seems exceedingly unlikely that there will ever be a clinical requirement for such therapy to be applied to the embryo."[8] Dr. Richard Palmiter, who cocreated the famous "mighty mouse" by using the growth hormone gene of a rat, observed, "Germ line therapy works OK in mice, but even to consider it for humans at this time is totally unrealistic."[9]

Is it only the *time* factor that is baffling? Dr. Horace Freeland Judson judges that "we are a long way from being able to supply a patient with even a single gene whose absence causes a disease."[10] And Dr. John C. Fletcher of NIH ventures a guess of 50–100 years.[11]

In Great Britain, Bob Williamson, writing also in *Nature*, has recognized the ethical problems involved in modifying germ line cells. He considers the question hypothetical at present; and he also doubts that prospective parents would even avail themselves of such embryonic intervention, as the embryo conceived *in vitro* would probably have only a 1 in 4 chance of being adversely affected by the genes carried by the parents. Williamson declared, "it strikes me as ridiculous as a form of clinical therapy for a couple who have a 75% chance of a normal child."[12] Despite his skepticism, nevertheless, he concluded that such therapy "will be possible in the future, and it should be considered now before the headlines break on us all."[13]

In a further opinion, Motulsky was bold enough to write "that genetic manipulation of germ cells is a distinct possibility," given the acquisition of currently unknown methods for prior describing of the genotypes of ova and sperm. "Nevertheless," he added, "the animal studies raise the possibility of future genetic manipulations in humans."[14]

It is precisely this expectation that apparently persuaded Dr. Gary B. Hodgen recently to leave his position as chief of pregnancy research at the NIH and to move to Eastern Virginia Medical School at Norfolk. There he intends "to study the feasibility of gene therapy in embyros, beginning with monkeys and advancing to humans."[15]

Dr. Leon E. Rosenberg, Dean of the School of Medicine of Yale University and a prominent geneticist, admits that he has modified his skepticism about germ line interventions. "I think there is a good chance that we will see such advances during my lifetime," he said in 1982, "and that is a far more optimistic guess than any I have been willing to make before."[16]

With due reserve about predicting the timetable of embryonic germ-line modification, it seems reasonable enough for both scientists and nonscientists, being equally concerned about human life and ethical approbation, to ponder what the future might bring. If some scientists regard these questions as merely speculative, or even fictional, there are sufficient numbers of others to put us on long-range guard. We are confronted by therapeutic applications to human beings of recombinant DNA techniques, neither the timing nor the consequences of which we yet know. What is unknown need not frighten us, and it does not; but it surely constitutes a warning against reckless advance in research.

The Recombinant Advisory Committee (RAC) of the NIH is already alert to the sensitivity of the procedures by which somatic cells in the bone marrow of the human body are modified for the correction of monogenetic blood diseases. Even more serious, because of our ignorance, is the concern about safety in respect to interventions in germ line cells.

Various commentators have compared the implications of recombinant DNA technology to the effects of nuclear fission. The comparison is probably apt and warranted. And one lesson that we should learn from that pairing of Promethean techniques is the mandate of much greater alertness and caution about genetic engineering than we as a people have shown toward the releasing of atomic energy. Can we not for once learn from bad experience? How much better would be the condition of our natural environment as well as the health and life of uncounted persons *if*, forty years ago, there had been adequate caution on the part of scientists, engineers, commercial entrepreneurs, and political officials!

With the upsurge of the production of new chemical compounds and plastics four decades ago, we were promised a virtually miraculous resolution of problems in manufacturing, transportation, and agriculture. *Who* were then prophesying the present catastrophic conditions of toxic emissions and industrial waste, acid rain, polluted water, and poisoned soil?

With the explosive proliferation of pharmaceuticals, we were likewise made to expect sudden cures of all our ills. But where were the far-sighted monitors, warning against untested drugs and medicaments?

When heavy equipment for clearing fields and new machines for agriculture and agrobusiness took over the nation's land, who were predicting the present imminent and irreversible crisis of arable soil erosion?

Still more cogently, as we reflect on the potential risks and dangers of biotechnology, can we possibly explain our past blindness to the costly and lethal side effects of nuclear power plants, radioactive fallout from testing atomic devices, or the dangerous madness of nuclear armaments?

If I seem to labor these analogies, it is only because of a conviction that today, in the case of genetic engineering, we still have the opportunity and the time to exercise reason, prudence, and restraint. This is the conviction that compelled men and women to endorse the June 1983 call for a *provisional* moratorium on the experimental effort to modify human germ-line cells in zygotes.[17] Most of us, though acting for ourselves, represented diverse religious institutions; but some were known mainly for their scientific work. Some would extend either voluntary restraints or regulated curbs on any application at all of recombinant DNA to human subjects. Others, like myself, were content to limit our concern to gametic cells, at least until such time as sufficiently successful experimentation on higher animals and primates had warranted the attempts at therapeutic intervention in humans.

Meanwhile, some people see the procedure of germ line gene surgery as the most promising way of curing and eliminating the strains of some of the nearly 3,000 identified debilitating genetic diseases. They will increase the pressure of persuasion on clinical geneticists to intervene with human zygotes. Should this actually prove successful, it would surely be welcomed by all. Who can but cheer for an authenticated cure? Then, even the 25% risk factor would have been reduced to zero. But still we must ask: How long must the treated individuals have to grow up and reproduce before assurance could be given that subsequent inadvertent mutations have not caused as much distress as the genetic disease that was first avoided? Perhaps, there are a few researchers who believe that, given due time, this can be achieved safely. If so, we can only hope that they are right. In the interest of the human lives that might be affected for better or worse, we await the disclosure of evidence of their assurance.

References and Notes

1. Milunsky, A., and Annas, G. (eds.), *Genetics and the Law II*, Plenum Press, New York and London (1979).
2. President's Commission for the Study of Ethical Problems in Medicine, Biomedical and Behavioral Research; Transcript of Proceedings, Ace-Federal Reporters, Washington, DC (July 1982), 115–116.
3. Callahan, D., *Abortion: Law, Choice, Morality* Macmillan, New York (1970), 308.
4. Shils, E., The sanctity of life, in *Life or Death, Ethics and Options* (D. H. Labby, ed.) University of Washington Press, Seattle (1968), 9.
5. Cited by H. F. Judson, *Science 84* (Vol. 5, No. 3, April 1984), 88.
6. Davis, B. D., Cells and souls, *The New York Times* (June 28, 1983).
7. Motulsky, A., Impact of genetic manipulation on society and medicine, *Science* **219**:138 (1983).
8. Williams, J. G., Mouse and supermouse, *Nature* **300**:575 (1982).
9. *Newsweek* (March 5, 1984), 68.
10. Judson, H. F., idem., 90.
11. Fletcher, J. C., Moral problems and ethical issues in prospective human gene therapy, *Virginia Law Review* **69**:534 (April 1983).
12. Williamson, B., Gene therapy, *Nature* **298**:417 (1982).
13. Williamson, idem., 418.
14. Motulsky, idem., 12.
15. Scientist quits NIH post over fetal rules, *Science* **223**:916 (1984).
16. Rosenberg, L. E., Toward an even newer genetics, in *Defining Human Life* (Margery W. Shaw and A. Edward Doudera, eds.), AUPHA Press, Ann Arbor (1983), 312.
17. Scientists must not play God," *Time* (June 20, 1983), 67. See also Nelson, J. R., Genetic science: A menacing marvel, *The Christian Century* **100**:636–8 (1983); and *Genetic Engineering*, Panel of Bioethical Concerns, National Council of Churches, Pilgrim Press, New York (1984); Nelson, J. R. *Human Life* Fortress Press, Philadelphia (1984), Chap. 6.

Discussion

Dr. Bertil Wennergren: I have come here from Sweden to learn more about recent events here in the United States. I am a former parliamentary ombudsman of Sweden and now preoccupied by these new views about genetics. I think they are of enormous imporance for humankind. It is very essential for us to keep things under control. In Sweden, we have a particular commission corresponding to the President's Commission that Mr. Capron talked about this morning. In Europe, we also have a committee on human genetics in the Council of Europe. I am the chairman of the Swedish comission and I'm the Swedish member of the committee in the Council of Europe. I have a question about genetic engineering. I think the role of the gene in the cell has been exaggerated, because the gene is just a part of the cell. It is in the nucleus, but sometimes, you hear people say that the gene is in command of the cell. That's not true, because it's the cell that commands the genes. It's other components in the cells that switch off and switch on genes in the nucleus. We know little about the silent zones in the genome. I think there is very little known about what happens in the cell besides that. What I would like to ask here is: How much research is going on with regard to cell functions? Because, as Tabitha Powledge said, if we don't know what switches genes on and off in the nucleus, then we can't introduce any genes because we must be sure that they will function in the correct way. We talked about human values and human uniqueness. What is unique in the human? The pope made a statement in 1982 when there was a meeting with the Academy of Science in Rome. He said that the human being is the only being that is willed for itself. If that is what makes humans unique, what is the definition of human values?

Dr. Maurice J. Mahoney: The expression of the genetic material responds to the rest of the cell and to the environment outside the cell. That is part of the regulation of our bodies. We know that there is a huge volume of information yet to be learned about how that regulation occurs, that is, how the outside of the cell influences the nucleus, as well as how the genetic material influences what the cell does and what happens outside the cell. That dynamic interaction at the cell level we've learned to accept at the organism level, that is, the human being. We are very comfortable with recognizing

89

environmental influences and genetic influences. Those are almost certainly just as true at the single-cell level within our bodies. We don't have very many glimpses as yet into what that will mean.

DR. PHILIP LEDER: I quite agree. The gene in the absence of the cell, the nucleus, and so on is a very uninteresting structure. If you would care to address the second question, it would be entirely appropriate.

DR. MAURICE J. MAHONEY: There are certainly some things that I, either intuitively or because I have grown up in this society, believe about human values. One is the maintenance of individuality and the uniqueness of each human being. If genetic engineering attempts to blur that, I think they would be entirely misplaced, misunderstood concepts. If gene therapy means addressing an illness that has no cure or control and we watch people decline, I think it should be pursued and we should try to address that individual's problems as well as those of anyone whom we can treat in other ways.

DR. J. ROBERT NELSON: Dr. Winnergan has asked the basic question about the uniqueness and distinctness and therefore the inviolability of the human race and the human person. Many have tried to resolve this in psychological terms as a matter of rationality or of self-consciousness or the ability to judge or to, in the words of Pope John Paul, to express one's own will, all of which I think are valid. Yet, somehow, I tried to convey the conception that there are two levels on which we think of this distinctness and value of human life. One at the rather natural, almost *a priori* self-evident level, which almost everyone can share. We simply know that we as a human race are not of the same moral level as other animal forms. That's a kind of intuitional thing that's been with our culture for a long time. From the religious perspective, it is because of a faith, a belief, a conviction that, among all the species, *Homo sapiens* has been chosen as a particular metaphysical or divine favorite, so that we can boldly say that we are made in the image of God and not the reverse. In my book, I tried to struggle with this, and I've reached this conclusion, although, it's only, like everything else, provisional: The one thing that we human beings seem able to do in a way that no other creatures can do is to project hopes and aspire to the realization of those hopes, not merely expectations or anticipations but a planned future. So we live in the future, not simply in the past, even though we have to live by the accumulation of our past culture. It's a broad philosophical, theological question, and I'm glad that it has to arise in our minds when we have to face questions like genetic engineering.

DR. SHELDON KRIMSKY: I'd like to direct this question first to Dr. Leder and then to the panel. It's a question that I've thought about for a while, and I must say that I have difficulty reaching any conclusions about it: Are there any ethical thresholds that might be passed in incorporating human genes into animal systems? I understand that a single gene has been incorporated into an animal system. What would happen if more genes and, possibly even cell fusion, were to be tried? Are there any principles that you might formulate, which could be applied theoretically or ethically to these procedures?

DR. PHILIP LEDER: This is a very good question, I see it from the scientific view as, first, one in which we must be sure, from the biohazards standpoint, that, for example, no lethal or otherwise dangerous material that is infectious for humans is introduced into animals or plant cells, in a form in which they could be deleteriously expressed. So there's a scientific overlay that deserves consideration. Ethically, however, you are reaching toward the science fiction notion that we might be able by genetic manipulation to create some sort of android species that would share with humans some of their unique properties. Certainly, even as geneticists, we would agree that human beings are distinct and unique in many respects. That is such a complex scientific notion that I don't see it as a real question. So that really, beyond the biohazards consideration, see no limitations on the possibility of, for example, using yeast or bacteria to create insulin or growth hormone or any other valuable pharmacological reagent.

MS. TABITHA M. POWLEDGE: Dr. Krimsky, did you mean creating a slave?

DR. SHELDON KRIMSKY: Not necessarily. I didn't mean that at all. I think that many people would find that rather offensive. I'm just thinking of incorporating substantial amounts of genes without creating an android species, some kind of cell fusion between a human and a monkey, or something like that. Possibly good reasons exist to do that intellectually—to find out how you can do more experiments on animals than you can do on humans. The question is whether or not there are any ethical thresholds in that. I'm not talking about the extremes. I'm also not talking about the obvious case where I don't think anybody would have any trouble, and that's putting a human gene into a bacterium. I am thinking of inserting genes into an animal and getting that animal to grow to normal size. Do any of the panelists have any objections to that from an ethical point of view?

MS. TABITHA M. POWLEDGE: I guess, being a consequentialist, I would say it would very much depend on the consequences: what you intend, what was the purpose of the experiment, what you wanted to do it for. I certainly don't think I could devise any generic rules that I would want to impose on people.

DR. JANE E. COOPER: Today, we heard and discussed cautionary tales about fat cats and whether or not they still have cream on their whiskers. There is also some possibility that we might confuse skinny cats with virtue, which isn't always the case. This afternoon, we're a little close, and I'm including myself in this batch, to holy cats. The problem, as I see it as a geneticist concerned with ethics, is this: We seem to attach ourselves to one side of what we're doing at the same time that we're ignoring the other side of what we're doing. For example, gene therapy represents a genuine possibility of dysgenics in terms of the human gene pool, but so does insulin in connection with diabetes. I don't see that there's a particularly significant difference between the two in terms of the human species in its ongoing sense. Similarly, to what extent does the supposed positive change and our right to make it in connection with embryos' treatment differ from our right to make the negative decision in terms of therapeutic abortion? I'm not saying I think these things are the same, but I do think they're part and parcel of who we are as human beings and therefore of what we may and may not do.

DR. PHILIP LEDER: I would like to ask the panel if they don't believe that the question of eugenics was really decided by the end of World War II, no longer to be raised again in terms of biological breeding experiments such as were contemplated and possibly even carried out in the 1930s and 1940s, and in terms of the genetic engineering technology that exists today. Isn't that really a settled issue in moral and ethical terms?

MS. TABITHA M. POWLEDGE: I don't know whether anything is ever settled in history. Remember Santayana. It's certainly true that Hitler was the final blow to the eugenics movement, but it had not been prospering for decades before that. Historically, I don't think any question is ever settled. I also believe that we can pay so much attention to the notion that government is somehow going to impose this on us that we really don't notice that sneaking in the back door is a whole other approach that hasn't got anything to do with government at all. That was really the point of my talk, and I would like to emphasize that, because I really want us to start thinking in these commercial terms.

DR. J. ROBERT NELSON: I wish I could agree with Dr. Leder, that the eugenic movement has come to an end. I think a very clear distinction has often been made between the active and passive eugenics, where the active type is a kind of enforced regimented program for whole populations, and where the other consists of genetic counseling and simply good sense. It does appear evident that the rise of genetic engineering as putatively applicable to human beings has given a renaissance, a resurgence to eugenic thinking and has affected the mentality of our whole population in the United States to a large degree, in terms of our thinking that only so-called perfect and healthy people are genuinely human people, and that all those who are at various levels of disability somehow are inferior and ought not to be encouraged to live or to be generated. In other words, I am quite sure in my own perception that there is a eugenic mentality even though there is not a eugenic program as such in the positive sense.

DR. MAURICE J. MAHONEY: I echo the last two speakers. I don't believe that the eugenic thinking has died. In fact, I think that when we learn more about brain chemistry and learn how to improve memories and such, people will flock to those means and chemicals.

DR. PHILIP LEDER: So I think that the question I'll ask is: If that's so, is that a "Bad Thing," with a capital B and a capital T? Perhaps, we'll come back to that in a moment.

DR. DAVID BOTSTEIN: I am a professional geneticist of the old, as well as the new, style. It bothers me a little bit that Dr. Cooper's question wasn't understood. I thought I would try again. The problem here is that all geneticists who deal with real organisms—and humans are real organisms—recognize that the key to improvement or destruction or whatever of the species, to changing the species, is selective breeding. We don't read, and I don't think Huxley intended, *Brave New World* in the way that was presented. The problem with any kind of eugenics and selective breeding and genetic engineering in the sense of improvement of the species or a subspecies or a subline is that you must use force of some sort in order to make the animals that you want to breed with each other breed with each other. It's an essential consequence of the fact that we are diploid. That's not going to change anytime soon. Therefore, the rule for making horses or dogs that run very fast, or dogs that bark, or dogs that don't, has been known since the dawn of time. The same is true of cows that make lots of milk. The key is selective breeding, and *that* is not what is unacceptable. It's quite the other way around. It is unacceptable to ask some woman and some man to breed for some purpose other than that over which they have control. It is the unwillingness of this society to take machine guns and say, "You marry that one and have that many children, and those children must breed with each other." The point I wanted to make, and to emphasize very strongly, is that this issue of eugenics and improving or degrading the species has in it an element of force that is unacceptable. It is not necessarily the aim or the consequence that is so terrible.

DR. PHILIP LEDER: I just wanted to create the spectrum of the eugenics argument. What is the border between good and bad, if there is one?

MS. TABITHA M. POWLEDGE: Huxley wrote a very interesting preface to the second edition of *Brave New World*, which was published after World War II, in which he pointed out that, in his book, eugenics was not the cause but the consequence of his totalitarian society. It was the last step in a series of steps, all of which had to come before eugenics could be imposed on the population. We have to have the totalitarian government in place before we have that kind of a eugenics program. We're not going to have the program first. If eugenics programs are going to happen, they are going to happen in other ways.

DR. LISA H. NEWTON: This morning, David Baltimore told us that many attempts to modify germ cells by introducing new genes would not be carried out. He gave us the following reasons: There is a 75% chance that the cell will be normal anyway, and with that kind of statistic, you'd have to be absolutely certain that the gene you inserted would not be subject to random localization. If it inserts itself in the wrong chromosome, all kinds of horrible things may happen. You may get mutations in the next generation. You have no idea whether or not it's going to breed true. You have no idea about the outcome. Therefore, he said, we'd never do it. Now, I heard from Dr. Nelson and Ms. Powledge that these experiments may happen soon. Do you know something that David Baltimore doesn't know?

MS. TABITHA M. POWLEDGE: No. For one thing, the case I was talking about was not a 75% chance of a normal child but rather a 100% chance of an abnormal child. Also, I think he may or may not turn out to be right about the question of random assortment for some genes that may not matter, and it simply remains to be seen. I am very worried about the animal experiments, even though Dr. Leder is quite right that you can look at the Brinster–Parmenter work as a failed experiment because they didn't get the gene working just exactly right. At the same time, look at it as a successful one: They really got it to work and that's what we need to keep focusing on. We have been hearing for years, "Don't worry." I'm no longer so sure!

DR. PHILIP LEDER: Well, I don't think that anyone would say that there is no problem. Suppose you were on the recombinant DNA committee or the relevant body that will evaluate this application, which you say is on the way, to do a gene therapy experiment, let alone a germ-line therapy experiment. Knowing what we now know, and in the absence, as of today, of any evidence from animal sources that such attempts at therapy would be at all useful or effective, do you think that in good conscience this body would approve such experiments?

MS. TABITHA M. POWLEDGE: No. I don't. I think its record is quite clear.

DR. PHILIP LEDER: Or that anyone would propose them, at this juncture, in the absence of animal evidence of their effectiveness?

MS. TABITHA M. POWLEDGE: All I can tell you, Dr. Leder, is that people on the recombinant DNA committee at Pfizer expect to see such a proposal this year. I've been told so. Presumably, they expect it to be in semireasonable shape—possibly not in reasonable enough shape to be approved, that I simply don't know. At this stage, nobody is even going to bother bringing a proposal to that committee unless they can try to make a case that they have a reasonable expectation that the therapy will work and will not bring harm to the patient on whom it is tried.

DR. BERNARD DAVIS: I'd like to make two points. First, I'd like to say how pleased I was that Dr. Nelson, at the end of his talk, redefined his position on the question of germ line therapy. If I understand it correctly, your position now is that if, indeed, it could really be proved to be perfectly safe, it wouldn't be different from other kinds of genetic therapy. I think that's quite different from the statement that was made by a group of theologians, including Dr. Nelson, some time ago. The reason I think it's worth emphasizing is that, as I mentioned this morning, Jeremy Rifkin, I believe, tricked theologians into making this statement. He gained a great deal in credibility thereby. He is still going around the country influencing public opinion on this subject. We are a group of people who have met to have a serious discussion of the complex problems we're dealing with, and I think that it's important to try to neutralize the really degrading effect of his kind of discussion on this subject. I would hope that some of the theologians who signed the original paper would indeed come out with a modified statement officially. The second point is that I think Dr. Botstein was being, if I may use a word that I never thought I would ever have to apply to such a sophisticated person, naive in characterizing eugenics as depending entirely on force. There are ways of giving incentives that could really influence the gene pool. Now, the extreme case, of course, is the force that tells who to mate with whom and how many progeny to have. Let me point out that, at the moment, the city and state of Singapore either has enacted or is seriously considering enacting a law providing strong financial incentives for university graduates to have more children. That's the direction in which eugenics is going to go. I want to be sure that none of you leave with the feeling that I'm in any way in favor of it, but let me draw a scenario that I think is not very unlikely in an extremely competitive world: The Japanese or the people in Singapore decide that their success in the world depends on how clever they are in producing things. Because the level of the average IQ of the population is important, they engage in a systematic program of strongly encouraging people, not necessarily with force, to have numbers of progeny related to their intelligence, however measured. How long will the rest of the world say that's only for them?

DR. J. ROBERT NELSON: I'm pleased that Dr. Bernard Davis is glad that he finds himself in agreement with what I was saying. However, I don't believe I would have to say that it was a revocation or a radical mutation of the position held last year, but simply a clarification of what otherwise has been a very widespread misunderstanding of the views, at least of some of us, who are rather strangely called clerics by Mr. Capron. Dr. Ruth Hubbard signed the statement. I don't think she is a cleric exactly. Nevertheless, it is true that the majority represented religious institutions. There is a good deal of obfuscation about our intentions. I think my word *provisional*, which I stressed so much in my presentation, has to be taken quite seriously. We're not asking for permanent bans, but very great caution, which Leon Rosenberg has also advocated.

DR. RUTH HUBBARD: The discussion of eugenics, to this point, has missed the central point. When Francis Galton coined the term, he coined it to mean "racial betterment of humanity, of humankind." The issue is that we have no social mechanisms that I'm aware of to judge or ascertain what is better and what is worse. It's not whether force is going to be involved or not, or to what degree, or at what point. Whether it's going to be the egg, the zygote, or the sperm, the issue is: Who is there in this society, or any society that we know of, that we would trust to make the decisions about what should and shouldn't be considered an improvement?

9

Mapping the Human Genome Using Restriction Fragment Length Polymorphisms

David Botstein, Ph.D.
Professor of Genetics
Massachusetts Institute of Technology
56-721 77 Massachusetts Avenue
Cambridge, MA 02139

Introduction

It is a truism that people, like all living organisms, are the products of their heredity, their environmental history, and the interaction between their heredity and their environment. This truism applies, of course, to any pathology that an individual may display. The difficulty with the truism is that the degree to which hereditary and environmental influences can contribute to disease states is variable in the extreme. Some disease states are entirely of environmental origin; in most instances, the genetic contribution to, let us say, a broken leg is negligible. Other disease states are demonstrably hereditary; the environmental contribution to beta-thalassemia is likewise negligible. Most disease states, however, fall into the spectrum in between; evidence for hereditary as well as environmental influences can be found.

Virtually all the diseases classified as clearly hereditary show simply Mendelian inheritance: they are the result of changes in a single gene. Sometimes, the disease phenotype is simply *dominant*; that is, if one inherits a single copy of the disease gene from one parent (the other parent contributing a normal allele), one manifests the disease state. Other disease phenotypes are *recessive*: one needs to have inherited the disease gene from both parents in order for the disease to become evident; heterozygotes are not affected, although they can transmit a disease gene to their offspring and are thus called *carriers*. In-between cases ("partial dominance" or "incomplete penetrance") are also known. Simple Mendelian inheritance is usually easy to detect by examination of the pattern of appearance of the disease phenotype in family pedigrees.

The inheritance of phenotypes determined by more than one Mendelian gene, however, is extremely difficult to follow in human families. Because the polygenic inheritance of phenotypes is common in other organisms, it is to be expected in humans as well. Genetic analysis that can demonstrate polygenic inheritance in other organisms is done by crossing organisms at will and thereby following inheritance; this technique is, for obvious reasons, unavailable to human geneticists. The difficulty of following even a two-gene system in human families leads to a bias in the assessment of the hereditary nature of diseases: when two or more genes determine the disease state, the disease cannot be classified, by family pedigrees, as being of purely hereditary etiology even if it is so. Because the environmental contribution is also difficult to assess, such diseases will necessarily appear to have an ambiguous etiology.

There are, however, statistical techniques that have evolved from the theories of population genetics that can be used to try to detect and to measure the hereditary contribution to disease phenotypes. These include the study of the relative concordance (coincident appearance of the disease) in monozygotic and dizygotic twins and the statistical clustering (without an interpretably Mendelian pattern) of the disease in families. From such studies, strong arguments can sometimes be made that the hereditary contribution to the appearance of a disease is substantial. Nevertheless, even these arguments are not definitive, as every aspect of environmental influence can never fully be assessed. In addition, the statistical methods are extremely sensitive (more than pedigree analysis) to heterogeneity in the cause of a phenotype: if the disease state can have two or more different causes (even if one is not primarily hereditary), then the statistical analysis will give results that are only vaguely interpretable or are even misleading. Quite understandably, therefore, clinicians view even the strongest statistical cases for hereditary etiology as still ambiguous and/or controversial.

Improvements in the power and the resolution of genetic analysis in human families could result in a corresponding improvement in our ability to define the hereditary components in the etiology of diseases such as epilepsy. Recent advances in the area of molecular biology, especially the so-called recombinant DNA methods, have the potential to provide tools that will allow human geneticists to follow the inheritance of all parts of the human genome from generation to generation. The basic idea is that, if one could follow the inheritance of marker genes spaced evenly over human chromosomes, then one could tell which segments of those chromosomes had been inherited from each parent and grandparent. The correlation of the inheritance of a particular segment with a predisposition to a disease would indicate that the gene conferring such a predisposition is located physically near the markers defining the inherited segment. Geneticists call this principle *linkage*, and the tool we propose to construct is a linkage map of the human genome. Experience with other organisms (where linkage maps have been made by classical techniques) indicates that having such a linkage map will allow the definition, genetically, not only of single-gene Mendelian inheritance, but also of two-gene and, possibly, even of three-gene systems. A genetic linkage map of the human genome might thus enable the definition of genetic models for human diseases that are inherited polygenically. The consequence would then be that the inheritance of such a disease could be followed and predicted in the way that sickle-cell anemia and phenylketonuria are now.

Naturally, the application of such technology will result in a substantial increase in our knowledge of the etiology of inherited diseases. However, it should also be realized that the application of the genetic linkage map to individual families will result in the acquisition, by the physician at least, of information about a predisposition to disease in the families under study. This information may be of great value in devising therapeutic strategies well in advance of disease onset and in making informed reproductive decisions. Presumably, genetic diagnostic systems will be used primarily for these reasons. Unfortunately, the information may also be sought for other reasons that are more controversial. For example, the knowledge that an individual is heterozygous for a gene that confers a predisposition toward early heart attack could reasonably be sought by a patient's insurance company. Genetic diagnostic systems will raise ethical and legal problems to the degree that they are indeed successful; most of the practical difficulties will lie in the area of privacy, that is, who is entitled to have and to use the information gained by physicians about the genotypes of the patient and his or her relatives? As it is likely to be many years before the human genetic linkage map is in general use, there is time for thought in advance of the problem.

CONSTRUCTION OF A GENETIC LINKAGE MAP OF THE HUMAN GENOME

Human genes, like those of other organisms, are carried on chromosomes. The genetic information in chromosomes is encoded in DNA, and each chromosome can be thought of as a long DNA molecule encoding different genes, one after the other, in the same way that a magnetic tape contains information. Changes in genes are changes in the DNA. Each individual has two copies of each chromosome (i.e., two copies of each gene), one inherited from each parent. Thus, parents donate to their offspring one of their two copies of each gene. Suppose (see Figure 1) that a child is the issue of a marriage between two individuals who are heterozygous for three genes, A, B, and C, so that one parent has alleles (forms of a gene) A1/A2 for gene A, B1/B2 for gene B, and C1/C2 for gene C, and the other parent has alleles A3/A4 for gene A, B3/B4 for gene B, and C3/C4 for gene C. If genes A and B reside on different chromosomes, the 16 possible genotypes of the progeny (A1/A3 and B1/B3; A1/A3 and B1/B4; A2/A3 and B2/B3; A2/A3 and B2/B4; A1/A4 and B2/B3; A1/A4 and B2/B4; A2/A4 and B1/B3; A2/A4 and B1/B4; etc.) are equally probable, as chromosomes assort independently. However, if two genes are close to each other on the same chromosome, then they will be inherited together. In this case, the arrangement of alleles on the chromosomes in the parents (called the *linkage phase*) makes a difference, so not only do we imagine (Figure 1) that genes B and C are near each other, but we also specify that one parent has the genotype B1-C1/B2-C2 and the other the genotype B3-C3/B4-C4. Then, the progeny genotypes B1-C1/B3-C3; B1-C1/B4-C4; B2-C2/B3-C3; and B2-C2/B4-C4 are common, and all others (involving, for

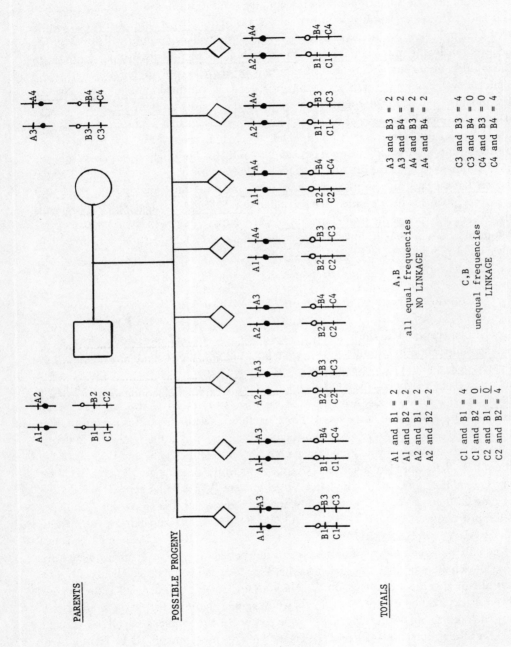

Figure 1. Possible progeny of parents and totals of linkage versus nonlinkage with distribution of equal and nonequal frequencies.

example inheritance of B1-C2 from the first parent or B4-C3 from the second) will be rare. The reason is that the common genotypes retain the arrangement in the parental chromosomes, and a crossover event (or recombination event) is required to produce the rare arrangements. This is how geneticists define *linkage*. The degree of linkage is variable, and it increases as the physical distance between the genes increases.

In the example given, all four parental chromosomes had alleles for each of the genes A, B, and C, which were distinguishable from each other. This characteristic (called by the geneticist *polymorphism*) is essential for the example given, as the only way in which one can tell that there has been a crossover between gene B and C is if B1 can be distinguished from B2 and C1 from C2. Therefore, if markers are to be useful in genetic mapping, they must be polymorphic. Ideally, the markers must be sufficiently polymorphic so that the parental alleles can usually be distinguished in a random marriage. Only if there are several (four or more) alleles, each with a high frequency in the population, will this ideal be approached. Before the development of recombinant DNA technology, only a few genes were known with usefully high polymorphism; the best of these are the HLA (histocompatibility) loci.

The ability to "clone" (in the molecular sense, that is, to isolate and propagate in a bacterial cell) single-copy human DNA sequences has made possible a new and general way of developing highly polymorphic genetic markers. These markers are called *restriction fragment length polymorphisms* (RFLPs, for short). A single-copy fragment of DNA carried in a bacterial plasmid labeled with radioactive phosphorus is used as a probe in a gel-transfer hybridization experiment using total human DNA extracted from a small blood sample. This DNA is digested with a "restriction endonuclease," which cuts the DNA at specific sequences characteristic for that endonuclease. This process produces many thousands of DNA fragments of differing length, as the distance between the restriction endonuclease cleavage sites varies depending on the nucleotide sequence of the DNA. The fragments are separated according to length by electrophoresis through an agarose gel. The fragments are transferred by blotting them onto filters, and finally, the filters are placed in a solution containing the probe. The probe DNA hybridizes and produces a radioactive band when it recognizes its complementary sequence. The band has a unique position (because of its unique length) because the sequence is represented only once in the genome. However, in some cases, the probe hybridizes to two bands in some individuals, because of polymorphism in the DNA sequence for which those individuals are heterozygous (Figure 2). This polymorphism could be due to single base alterations at a restriction endonuclease recognition site, or it could be the result of rearrangements (deletions, insertions, transpositions, and so on) of the DNA. In either case, the RFLP should be heritable, easily demonstrated with a small sample, and therefore potentially usable for genetic mapping.

The technology of finding single-copy human DNA fragments that, when used as probes, reveal RFLPs is straightforward.[1] One screens recombinant DNA libraries for single-copy DNA fragments, makes these radioactive, and carries out gel-transfer experiments[2] using the DNA from about 10 unrelated individuals. When heterozygosity (two bands in the DNA of one or more of the individuals) is observed, one has found a

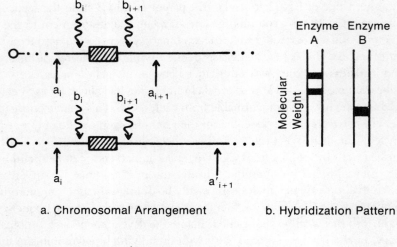

a. Chromosomal Arrangement   b. Hybridization Pattern

↑ = restriction endonuclease A

⌇ = restriction endonuclease B

▨ = probed single copy region

Figure 2. Cuts made in a pair of homologous chromosomes by enzyme B. (b) Hybridization pattern of enzymes A and B given cuts of (a). From D. Botstein, R. L. White, M. Skolnick, and R. W. Davis. Construction of a Genetic Linkage Map in Man Using Restriction Fragment Length Polymorphisms, *Am. J. Hum. Genet.* **32**:314–31 (1980).

polymorphism; when heterozygosity is frequent and/or one finds bands of several different lengths among the 10 individuals, the polymorphism can be used as a genetic marker to make the map.

When the idea of constructing a genetic linkage map using RFLPs was first proposed,[3] a major question concerned the degree of polymorphism in the genome. Within a few months, Wyman and White found the first really extensive polymorphism (Figure 3), which has about 15 alleles of different lengths, all of which are relatively common.[1] Several more really good polymorphisms have been found, and many more (more than 100) two-allele systems have been described. Many of the two-allele systems have been found to have additional associated polymorphisms when additional restriction endonucleases were tested or when DNA adjacent to the original probe was cloned.[4]

An important question concerning the practicality of making a linkage map of the human genome using RFLPs concerns the number of different RFLP loci that one needs to "cover" (that is, be within detectable linkage distance) the entire genome. This number depends in part on the amount of recombination one finds on human chromosomes and also on how polymorphic the markers are. Given highly polymorphic markers and using the estimate that the total genome is 33 morgans (a unit of recombination), this number comes out to be somewhere between 300[3] and 1,000.[5]

Once many polymorphisms have been found, they can be tested for linkage to each

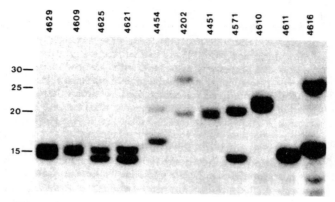

Figure 3. Polymorphisms in human DNA restriction fragments homologous to pAW101. Five micrograms of DNA from each individual was digested with *EcoRI*, subjected to electrophoresis through a 0.4% agarose gel, transferred to diazobenzyloxymethyl-paper, and hybridized with a nick-transplanted probe prepared from the recombinant plasmid pAW101. Numbers above each lane indicate the individual within a large Utah pedigree; numbers to the left indicate length of DNA in kb. From A.R. Wyman and R. White. A Highly Polymorphic Locus in Human DNA, *Proc. Natl. Acad. Sci. USA* 77:6754–8 (1980). Reprinted by permission of the authors.

other by specially designed family studies. They can also be assigned to chromosomes using human-rodent somatic cell hybrids[6] or *in situ* hybridization.[7]

Making the genetic map of the human genome is, then, a matter of applying current technology. In terms of the labor involved, however, finding and mapping many hundreds of RFLPs is a massive undertaking, the end of which is not yet in sight. Nevertheless, the undertaking is finite, and the uncertainties are few. There now seems to be little question that a genetic linkage map can (and will) be constructed within the next decade.

Using the Linkage Map

The use of the linkage map is simple to imagine in the case of single-gene Mendelian traits. A family that exhibits the trait is found, blood samples suitable for DNA extraction are obtained from as many members of the family as possible, and all the markers on the map are followed through the family tree. A correlation of inheritance of the trait and of particular RFLP loci is then sought. The only problems are statistical; in order to verify linkage, one must observe coinheritance of only one chromosomal segment. To ensure that only one segment will be implicated, one must look at enough cases so that the probability of an association by chance becomes extremely small. This number can be calculated and is of the order of 20 individuals in a single family of appropriate structure for a dominant trait.[3]

Once one identifies one or more RFLP loci tightly linked to a disease gene, one can carry out tests for inheritance using only the relevant loci; such tests will allow the diagnosis of the inheritance of disease genes, given information about the marker alleles and the linkage phases in the parents. In other words, a simple family study will allow the prediction of the inheritance of diseases by linkage, even when nothing is known about the disease gene other than the mode of its inheritance. For some diseases (Huntington's disease[8] and cystic fibrosis are notable examples), it appears likely that such linkage tests will be the major form of prenatal diagnosis, as it seems at present unlikely that enough will be learned about the disease gene itself to make possible the direct cloning of the gene.

It is important to note that some diseases of an uncertain mode of inheritance will be easily clarified if one has a map. For example, hemochromatosis is a simple Mendelian disease for which it was difficult to decide whether the gene was a dominant with incomplete penetrance or a recessive that showed some intermediate phenotype (but no pathology) in heterozygotes. The matter could be resolved simply because it turned out that the disease gene is linked to the major histocompatibility locus, a highly polymorphic gene that is most suitable as a marker. Given the linkage, the ambiguous heterozygotes could be classified, and it became clear that hemochromatosis is indeed a recessive disease.[9]

ETHICAL AND LEGAL IMPLICATIONS

As mentioned above, the promise that the genetic map holds is primarily a great improvement in the amount and the precision of information that can be obtained about the genetic factors that predispose to disease. In the cases of simple Mendelian diseases with dread consequences, diagnostic tests will become available that will be used to make informed reproductive decisions. The legal and ethical problems for, let us say, a reliable test for cystic fibrosis seem quite similar to the very real problems already posed by the existence of a reliable indicator for Down syndrome.

In the case of major diseases like diabetes, schizophrenia, epilepsy, and manic depression, when the mode of inheritance is not clear and the consequences of having the disease are less disastrous, the development of diagnostic systems based on a genetic map may allow improved therapy. For each of the listed diseases, arguments can be made that knowing in advance of symptoms that a person is at risk will be helpful.

Despite all these attractive consequences, there are also clear dangers. The information that one is predisposed to (or even a genetic carrier of) a disease is not neutral information that can be bandied about like one's age or gender. In many instances, the consequences of the label may be worse than the disease. Many precedents (not all favorable) already exist in the cases of diabetics and epileptics: the advent of genetic diagnosis will increase greatly the number of citizens who will labor under the knowledge (hopefully confidential) that they are predisposed to some illness. These are fundamental issues of privacy and confidentiality that do not seem very different from problems already faced by people with chronic diseases. The advent of genetic diagnosis on a large scale will increase, however, the number of citizens with such problems.

Another set of problems has to do with the cooperation of family members, which is essential for linkage studies. For example, in the interests of an unborn child, can one compel one's relatives to donate samples for analysis? What happens to the information about the relative that is inevitably obtained?

Finally, there are potential issues associated with the keeping of records. From the point of view of the physician and the geneticist, the patient's health interest is clearly served by the keeping of good permanent records. Such information will be cumulative, and of direct usefulness to offspring and other relatives in future genetic diagnoses. On the other hand, the existence of such records, even in a purely medical circumstance, opens up the possibility of abuse of the privacy of the patients and their relatives. Should physicians keep records so that the next determination will no longer require family samples? If so, how should the confidentiality of these records be protected?

In conclusion, it is clear that ethics and laws about proper limits on the distribution of information about one's genotype need to be established soon, lest the good that might be done by genetic diagnosis be outweighed by the damage done by foreknowledge in the wrong hands. We are now in the position of being able to anticipate certain problems, and of having the opportunity of doing our ethical and legal homework in advance of the arrival of the new technology.

REFERENCES

1. Wyman, A. R., and White, R. A highly polymorphic locus in human DNA, *Proc. Natl. Acad. Sci. USA* 77:6754–8 (1980).
2. Southern, E. M., Detection of specific sequences among DNA fragments separated by electrophoresis, *J. Mol. Biol.* 98:503–17 (1975).
3. Botstein, D., White, R. L., Skolnick, M., and Davis, R. W., Construction of a genetic linkage map in man using restriction fragment length polymorphisms, *Am. J. Hum. Genet.* 32:314–31 (1980).
4. Antonarakis, S. E., Boehm, C. D., Giardina, P. J. V., and Kazazian, H. H., Nonrandom association of polymorphic restriction sites in the B-globin gene cluster, *Proc. Natl. Acad. Sci. USA* 79:137–41 (1982).
5. Lange, K., and Boehnke, M., How many polymorphic genes will it take to span the human genome? *Am. J. Hum. Genet.* 34:842–5 (1982).
6. DeMartinville, B., Wyman, A. R., White, R., and Franke, U., Assignment of the first random restriction fragment length polymorphism (RFLN) locus (D1451) to a region of human chromosome 14, *Am. J. Hum. Genet.* 34:216–26 (1982).
7. Harper, M. E., and Saunders, G. F., Localization of single copy DNA sequences on G-banded human chromosomes by *in situ* hybridization, *Chromsoma* 83:431–9 (1981).
8. Gusella, J. F., Wexler, N. S., *et al.*, A polymorphic DNA marker genetically linked to Huntington's disease, *Nature* 306:234–8 (1983).
9. Kravitz, K., Skolnick, M., Cannings, C., *et al.*, Genetic linkage between hereditary hemochromatosis and HLA, *Am. J. Hum. Genet.* 31:601–19 (1979).

10

Mapping the Human Genome
Problems of Privacy and Free Choice

Ruth Macklin, Ph.D.
Professor of Bioethics
Albert Einstein College of Medicine
Department of Epidemiology and Social Medicine
1300 Morris Park Avenue
Bronx, NY 10461

Revolutionary progress in genetic theory and its applications has led to the ability to map the human genome. As with numerous other recent advances in biomedicine, these new capabilities in genetics bear the unfortunate consequence that ever new ethical problems and moral dilemmas accompany the positive fruits of scientific research. But are the ethical problems raised by the ability to map the human genome really new? Or are they variants of concerns already familiar in genetic screening and counseling, and in other areas of medicine?

To answer this question, we need first to identify the ethical values thought to be endangered by the new capabilities. Next, we need to explore whether those concerns are merely different in degree, or whether they differ in kind from already familiar ethical dilemmas. Only then can we determine whether the new diagnostic and therapeutic techniques in genetics, so often termed *revolutionary*, are cause for greater worry than earlier advances in genetics or similar ethical concerns in other branches of medical research and practice. In either case, the approach to resolving these problems must inevitably appeal to long-standing, widely accepted moral principles. As always, however, ethical dilemmas emerge when two or more such principles come into conflict. The focus in this chapter is on problems of privacy and free choice stemming from the ability to map the human genome.

The prospect of mandatory screening programs is probably the most obvious threat to the free choice of citizens in a society that so highly prizes the value of individual liberty. But the most obvious threat need not be the most probable one. Whether compulsory genetic screening programs can be ethically justified depends chiefly on the purpose for which screening is mandated and on the potential benefits to the individuals required to undergo the screening. Also important, but secondary, are the safeguards employed to prevent the disclosure of sensitive genetic information to third parties.

A wide range of ethical issues related to genetic screening has been thoroughly studied by the President's Commission for the Study of Ethical Problems in Medicine and Biomedical and Behavioral Research. It would be redundant to rehearse that examination here, but it is worth repeating several of the points made in the commission's report entitled *Screening and Counseling for Genetic Conditions.*[1]

On the issue of compulsory versus voluntary screening programs, the commission's report identified two main questions: "Should participation in screening and counseling programs always be voluntary? Should treatment of genetic diseases detected through screening always be voluntary?"[2] Resting its argument on an appeal to the principle of autonomy, the commission concluded that only one consideration could justify compulsion: the protection of those unable to protect themselves. And even that factor warrants compulsion only under special circumstances. The report asserts that "the Commission finds no basis in the maximization of social utility that justifies compulsory participation in genetics programs."[3]

The commission's report covers genetic screening capabilities in the areas of newborn testing, carrier screening, and prenatal diagnosis, describing the specific techniques employed in each of these categories. It does not, however, address the question of whether ethical problems arise that are peculiar to the procedures of gene mapping. We need to ask, therefore, whether there are any grounds for holding that the commission's carefully drawn conclusions and recommendations should not straightforwardly apply to the more precise, more numerous, and more effective screening capabilities afforded by genome mapping.

Does it matter ethically whether the genetic screening of individuals by these techniques would be mandated by the government, by employers, or by insurance companies? Whatever agency may require screening, the same threat to privacy and free choice is bound to exist. Yet, the purpose of these different agencies may vary considerably: The state may require screening by means of genome mapping in order to identify heritable conditions and to supply individuals and families with valuable information, thus increasing their ability to make health-promoting lifestyle choices, and in cases where treatment is possible, enabling them to choose early intervention or to take preventive steps. Although the compulsory aspect remains, thereby eliminating free choice and invading privacy by gathering intimate details about a person's genetic makeup, the avowed purpose is to benefit the individual by widening options and enabling wise life choices and decisions.

In contrast, insurance companies may require prospective customers to submit to genome mapping in order to be eligible for, say, life insurance or health-related benefits. The basic premise behind insurance companies' rates lies in the use of actuarial tables that assign risks to different populations or groups. A company could deny insurance altogether to individuals at risk for early death from one or another genetic disease, or it could set rates differentially in accordance with different people's likelihood of contracting particular diseases for which they are found to be at risk. The same information that is fruitful in the genetic counseling situation can be devastating in the hands of insurance companies or prospective employers, for example, the identification of gene carriers of late-onset autosomal-dominant disorders before clinical manifestations have appeared. People found through genome mapping to be susceptible to emphysema could be denied employment by firms in which the workplace environment is hazardous to those having lung disease. Yet, that same information in the counseling setting can aid the individual in making choices on a voluntary basis.

Unlike the case in which genome mapping is mandated by the state, a person may decline to have her or his privacy invaded and her or his freedom compromised by an insurance company requirement and may simply refuse to apply for the insurance. But that is what William James called a "forced choice"—one in which there appears to be an option but, given the possible consequences, in which genuine choice in the matter is only apparent.

The same could be said of industry's screening requirements: A person could always choose to work elsewhere—in a different company, a different field of employment, or a different type of work. But practically speaking, such options are not usually available to people constrained by poverty, low educational level, lack of skills, limited geographical mobility, and other factors. Furthermore, if one insurance company or industrial concern establishes mandatory screening for susceptibility to genetic diseases as a condition of employment, all are likely to follow. A survey conducted by the Office of Technology Assessment in 1982 revealed that half-a-dozen major American corporations already use genetic testing to identify employees susceptible to adverse reactions from toxic substances in the workplace. And another 59 companies said they were considering adopting such policies within the next five years.[4] Market forces could well lead to the universal adoption of such programs, in order for companies to remain competitive. Those prospects, however, will themselves be governed by cost–benefit considerations, as companies weigh the costs of mounting screening programs to detect genetic susceptibility among employees against the costs associated with paying for health benefits or compensation to workers who fall ill.

Do these market considerations morally justify overriding the highly cherished values of individual privacy and free choice? Although my own reply to this question is an emphatic "no," others may respond differently. Ultimately, in weighing these and other morally relevant considerations, the answer will depend on just which moral principle is selected as a basic premise in the argument. The application of a utilitarian moral principle, using a cost–benefit analysis as in the examples of insurance companies and industry noted above, will yield one result in a moral argument, whereas an appeal to the primacy of individual rights of privacy and liberty will yield another. Attempts to resolve such conflicts of moral principles are usually futile in applied and professional ethics, as the parties to a dispute come already committed to one or another fundamental principle, on which they build their arguments. But the futility of solving the most profound problems at the foundations of ethics should not deter efforts to find practical, moral solutions to the problems posed by human genetics, as elsewhere.

If the ethical justifiability of mandatory screening by insurance companies and industry rests on determining whether the goal of maximizing profits or containing costs should supersede the values of freedom and privacy, the same cannot be said simplistically for genome mapping that may be required by the state. Government, like industry, may be acting on fiscal motives, in the belief that the early detection of an increasing number of genetic conditions will result in prevention or treatment and, therefore, in reduced third-party payments for afflicted individuals who qualify for state-sponsored reimbursements. Federal and state governments, like private insurance companies, aim to lessen the amount paid out. But unlike agencies in the private sector, the state has an interest in protecting the lives and health of its citizens. That long-established interest, as expressed in statutes and regulations and in the common law, has given rise to quite a number of paternalistic acts and programs, justified by the benefits that accrue to those who have been "coerced for their own good."

This is not the place to debate the merits and shortcomings of government paternalism, but it is worth asking whether that concept strictly applies in the present context. The rationale behind compulsory screening in the form of gene mapping, as well as other types, fits better under a public health model than it does under a paternalistic conception. It is, after all, not solely for the benefit of those who undergo screening that such programs would be mandated. The benefits accrue to the offspring of those with heritable diseases as well as to the individuals themselves. Benefits may come in the form of informed reproductive choices that succeed in preventing the birth of an afflicted fetus, or even its conception in the first place. Benefits may also exist in the form of gene therapy, as those techniques become increasingly effective and more widespread.

Just as the public health model can justify the coercion of individuals by requiring vaccination, inoculation, or quarantine to avoid the spread of infectious diseases, so might it take steps to reduce the incidence and prevalence of genetic diseases. Whether the public health model can serve to justify the enforced treatment of genetic diseases, in the form of gene therapy made possible by mapping the human genome, is a separate question that deserves sustained inquiry. In all likelihood, any attempt to justify gene therapy will have to appeal to moral principles other than those that underlie the public health model. The precept underlying public health justifications for coercive measures is the utilitarian principle: Maximize beneficial consequences and minimize bad ones, where benefits and harms are construed in terms of health or well-being as against disease and impaired functioning. Although that principle can probably be used to support mandatory screening programs, it is not sufficiently strong to justify overriding individual rights of autonomy in the form of mandated gene therapy for afflicted individuals.

Although the greatest worries about restrictions on individual freedom and invasions of privacy stem from the prospect of compulsory genetic screening, some ethical concerns exist, as well, in voluntary programs. Screening that relies on the linkage principle requires studies of the genes in a family. In order to interpret the meaning of the DNA pattern in a child, it may be necessary to study both parents and sometimes other relatives, as well.[5] Leading researchers in genetics are already envisioning "tremendous implications for clinical genetics."[6] The use of the linkage principle for both prenatal diagnosis and premorbid diagnosis are hailed as promising developments.[7] McKusick cited the linkage of hemochromatosis and HLA-A, claiming it to be "a useful way to identify relatives who should be protected against iron overloading."[8]

Now, what if these relatives do not wish to be so identified? We may believe that it is irrational or foolish for people to choose to remain ignorant about information likely to be valuable for their own present or future health or that of their children, but ample evidence exists of individuals resistant to having such information themselves, quite apart from their unwillingness to have others learn about it. One has only to consider the health-risking behavior of the many individuals who smoke tobacco, eat cholesterol-laden foods, and drink alcohol to excess, or whose lifestyle choices are demonstrably unhealthy, to conclude that, even when people have sufficient information about practices that are dangerous to health, they nonetheless persist in those activities. The identification of relatives found through genome mapping to be at risk for genetic disease may result in inflicting unwanted information on those individuals.

Furthermore, once the carrier state in a relative is determined, those privy to that information (the clinical geneticist and the individual whose genome is mapped) know something about a third party that that person does not (yet) know. Does the possession of genetic information about third parties constitute an intrusion into their privacy? If that information were to be disclosed to others, should it be construed as a breach of confidentiality? The techniques that enable the human genome to be mapped raise conceptual questions like these, as well as ethical and potential legal questions. How the conceptual questions are answered will have implications for the ethical problems, as well.

These last considerations raise a broader question, one about the "ownership" of genetic information: Should that information be construed as simply a more detailed account of an individual's vital statistics? Or are the details of a person's genetic constitution information that should be treated as intrinsically private, not to be sought or disclosed without the explicit consent of the person whose statistics they are? Here again, the answer depends on which model is appropriate for conceptualizing the situation and drawing normative conclusions. If we adopt the prevailing model of the clinical practice of medicine, then genetic information, just like any other information about an individual's past or present diseases, should be held in strictest confidence except when disclosure is required by law or when there are morally compelling reasons to divulge the facts. According to the public health model, however, invasions of privacy and breaches of confidentiality are justified by the probable harm resulting from nondisclosure, a calculation that makes overriding individual rights ethically permissible. Venereal disease reporting and the notification of sex partners, the maintenance of centralized records of infectious diseases, and other public-health measures rely on a utilitarian moral principle and the use of risk–benefit calculations, relegating individual rights of privacy, confidentiality, and even liberty to second place.

It is not an easy exercise to determine which model is more appropriate to moral guidance on the problems of privacy and free choice posed by the ability to map the human genome. Under the model that prevails in the clinical practice of medicine, the physician's obligations are primarily (exclusively, according to some) to the patient: to act in the patient's best interest and to respect the patient's rights in the physician–patient relationship. When the practice of clinical genetics yields information about other family members at risk, this model would appear to dictate nondisclosure unless explicit permission is given by the patient. Happily, of course, most people have their relatives' best medical interests at heart and will readily grant permission for genetic information about themselves to be disclosed to family members who stand to be affected. Yet, sufficient evidence exists from cases in which Huntington disease has been diagnosed to indicate that, even when the disclosure of genetic information is clearly in the best interest of relatives, patients may nonetheless object strenuously to revealing that information.

A well-known distinction exists in philosophical ethics between actions that are morally permissible and those that are obligatory. It would be hard to produce a sound argument having the conclusion that physicians or genetic counselors have a moral *obligation* to contact relatives and to reveal to them that they are at risk for genetic disease. But a successful argument could be mounted to the effect that it is ethically *permissible* for physicians or counselors to do so. That argument can be supported either by a consequentialist justification or by an appeal to the "respect-for-persons" principle, a principle that embodies the notion that every person has an intrinsic dignity and autonomy worthy of respect.

"Respect for persons" is the principle that underlies the need to gain freely granted, informed consent from patients for research or treatment. Without adequate information, people cannot make informed choices and decisions related to their own health and well-being. It is evident that those at risk for late-onset genetic disease, or those whose reproductive choices might be affected by genetic information, cannot engage in informed, rational decision-making if crucial information is withheld from them. Although the "respect-for-persons" principle is usually invoked in support of the rights of the patient in the physician–patient relationship, it can be extended to cover the health-related rights of relatives, as well. Thus, although it may not be morally *obligatory* for physicians to inform relatives of their at-risk status, it is ethically permissible based on the "respect-for-persons" principle. If this conclusion appears to violate the patient's rights of confidentiality in the physician–patient relationship, it should be recalled that no rights are absolute. Physicians have a *prima facie* obligation to keep confidentiality, but that *prima facie* obligation can be overridden by stronger moral presumptions.

The consequentialist justification for disclosure to relatives is more straightforward, yet it requires accurate empirical information about the benefits and harms likely to result from revealing facts learned as a result of genome mapping. If the consequences of withholding genetic information from relatives are likely to produce more harm than good, then a consequentialist or utilitarian principle would permit disclosure. Indeed, according to utilitarian theory, a physician would probably be morally required to disclose the information, as that theory holds that the morally right actions are those that result in better consequences than all available alternatives. The application of a consequentialist or utilitarian principle relies on the ability to assess the probable benefits and harms of a contemplated action, and that assessment is often difficult to make. But as in any other area of moral decision-making, good ethics begin with good facts.

Even under the clinical practice model, or under conditions where genetic screening is voluntary, abuses may occur. The potential always exists for the witting or the unwitting disclosure of information to third parties who have a stake in that information. The recent discovery of genetic susceptibility to emphysema yields information valuable to those who may then choose not to smoke, to avoid spending time in polluted environments, or to seek certain types of employment rather than others. The screening can be voluntary, and so can the individual's choices. But that same information in the hands of employers could lead to the denial or the termination of employment, and insurance companies in possession of such facts about the insured may assign higher rates or deny them insurance altogether. A similar scenario could arise for those discovered to have a genetic susceptibility to arteriosclerosis and other conditions that remain asymptomatic until later in life. Without doubt, the ability to map the human genome yields information about susceptibility that is more precise, more certain, and potentially more threatening to individual freedom and privacy than earlier methods of presymptomatic diagnosis and vague hypotheses about "familial" traits.

It is one of the ironies of social life that information about people that is valuable to them can at the same time, if it falls into the hands of others, have the potential to harm their interests. But the prospect of the abuse or the misuse of genetic information does not, by itself, warrant a restriction of the procedures or methods by which that information is gained. As in other situations subject to abuse, the need exists for procedural safeguards to ensure that genetic (and other medical) information about individuals will be protected and kept confidential to the fullest extent possible.

Several factors are relevant in the effort to determine whether the public health model or the clinical practice model is most suited to give ethical guidance for problems of privacy and free choice. These factors are the severity of the genetic disease, the probability that relatives will become afflicted, the prospects for successful intervention of some sort, and the question of whether having children afflicted with the genetic defect can be avoided by the discovery of carrier states in the relatives of an individual who has undergone diagnostic tests by gene mapping. Just how these several factors ought to be weighed, what counts as sufficient severity of a genetic condition, and other questions are matters that need to be fully worked out. One cannot simply assume that either the public health model or the clinical medical practice model is the correct one to apply, as the consequences of adopting one or the other model are significant in the ethical problems of privacy and free choice.

In conclusion, the ability to map the human genome does not raise significant problems of privacy and free choice that are entirely new. Although the new diagnostic and therapeutic techniques are more powerful than previously existing capabilities in human genetics, and although they are able to yield a great deal more information about susceptibility to genetic disease than earlier screening techniques, the problems are the same, in principle. Mandatory screening programs, both newborn and carrier screening, have already been introduced. We have witnessed first the adoption and then the quick abandonment of compulsory screening for sickle-cell carriers, and some of the states that have had mandatory PKU screening at birth have now begun to abandon those programs because of cost–benefit considerations. Questions about the propriety of seeking or disclosing information about an individual's genetic makeup bear strong analogies to other biomedical contexts in which the ethics of invading privacy and breaching confidentiality have been debated, and the issue of what information insurance companies and employers ought to have access to is a long-standing debate among civil libertarians and other proponents of individual rights, business executives and spokespeople for management and labor, and those in the field of bioethics and health law.

This is not to imply that the ethical dilemmas in those areas have been finally settled, or that they should stand as precedents to follow uncritically in the newer areas opened by contemporary genetic research and practice. It may be of some comfort to recognize that problems of privacy and free choice raised by the ability to map the human genome have ample analogies and that they have been addressed at length by the President's Commission, as well as by many individual scholars. But that comfort should not create the misleading impression that the issues have been resolved, or that they cannot profit from continued careful analysis and debate. The price of ethical decision-making is renewed inquiry and constant vigilance.

REFERENCES AND NOTES

1. President's Commission for the Study of Ethical Problems in Medicine and Biomedical and Behavioral Research, *Screening and Counseling for Genetic Conditions*, U.S. Government Printing Office, Washington, DC (1983).
2. *Ibid.*, 47.
3. *Ibid.*
4. McAuliffe, K., and McAuliffe, S., Keeping up with the genetic revolution, *The New York Times Magazine* (Nov. 6, 1983), 95.
5. President's Commission for the Study of Ethical Problems in Medicine and Biomedical and Behavioral Research, *Splicing Life*, U.S. Government Printing Office, Washington, DC (1982), 40.
6. McKusick, V. A., The human genome through the eyes of a clinical geneticist, *Cytogenet. Cell Genet.* 32:21 (1982).
7. *Ibid.*
8. *Ibid.*, 22.

11

GENETIC ALTERATION OF EMBRYOS
The Ethical Issues

JOHN A. ROBERTSON, J.D.
Professor of Law
University of Texas Law School
2500 Red River
Austin, TX 78705

Sometime in the next two years, clinical trials with human gene therapy will begin.[1] The trials will be aimed at two rare, very serious single-gene defects. One is Lesch–Nyhan syndrome, a serious and nontreatable disesase characterized by mental retardation, cerebral palsy, self-mutilation, and an accumulation of uric acid in the body. The other is adenosine deaminase deficiency, a disease of the immune system that leads to early death. Like most single-gene defects, they cause their ill effects because the gene essential to turning on the production of a crucial enzyme is missing.

Rapid progress in recombinant DNA techniques has made clinical trials with human gene therapy a possibility. Scientists have identified the missing genes for these diseases and have cloned them in the laboratory through recombinant DNA techniques. Geneticists have also developed techniques for transferring the cloned gene into chromosomes in the nucleus of bone marrow cells. In studies with animals, the inserted gene appears to "turn on" or express itself at the right time to produce the missing substance without damaging other cells. The missing gene has also been successfully introduced into the nuclei of bone marrow cells removed from a person with the disease and has apparently turned on the mechanisms of enzyme production.[2] Although more research with animals is needed to ensure that the inserted gene will produce a therapeutic amount and not disrupt other functions of the cell, the next step will be to return bone marrow cells treated with the cloned gene to the body, to see if it will cause the cell to function properly and relieve the underlying disease. This is the step in the clinical trials that are under consideration.

The start of clinical trials is an important step in the application of genetic knowledge touched off by Watson and Crick's discovery, some 30 years ago, of the double-helix structure of DNA. But it is a mistake to think that human applications of genetic engineering to root out even single-gene defects, much less for incredibly more complex multifactorial and polygenic traits, is just around the corner. Many problems remain to be worked out before the human trials actually begin, and before gene therapy becomes widely available, even for rare and lethal single-gene defects. Although the ability to introduce cloned genes into cells has been greatly advanced by developments with retroviruses, there is still little control over where the cloned gene will lodge after it is introduced and hence over whether it will be expressed at the right time.[3] Expression at the right time and in the right amounts is essential for the genetic therapy to work. More work with animals is needed to establish that the expressed gene will produce sufficient quantities of the cell product at the right time to prevent the disease, while not overproducing or otherwise interfering with cell metabolism. Indeed, the physicians undertaking the first trials probably do not expect to cure the disease immediately. Rather, they hope to test out techniques and learn more about basic structure that will eventually prove useful.[4]

At this stage, the most significant ethical issue in human gene therapy is whether it is ethical to impose on subjects the risks of reinserted bone marrow cells that have been treated with the cloned gene, in light of the risks and benefits reasonably to be expected. The uncertainties that will attend the first human uses make this judgment difficult, but the same ethical issue arises in most clinical research.

In the case at hand, the risks of the research now appear to be outweighed by the study's benefits for the subjects and for society, making the study more acceptable than Martin Cline's use of cloned genes in 1981 to treat beta-thalassemia.[4a] The researchers will be seeking to treat a lethal, incurable disease. Previous experience with cloning genes and inserting them into animal and human cells suggests that the inserted genes will be expressed without deleterious side-effects. As only a small amount of the enzyme produced by any cell in the body will prevent the disease, there is a reasonable probability that the reinserted bone marrow could produce enough of the enzyme to prevent Lesch–Nyhan or adenosine deaminase deficiency. However, it is not clear whether successful gene insertion will produce enough of the substance soon enough to reverse the damage that has already occurred. The reasonableness of this assessment of risks and benefits has been affirmed by the institutional review boards (IRBs) at the institutions conducting the research and is likely to be approved by the NIH's Recombinant DNA Advisory Committee, when it reviews the question.[5]

The long-run potential of gene therapy is, of course, stupendous. Paralleling the rapid development of gene transfer techniques has been rapid progress in mapping the human genome.[6] This allows genetic markers for a wide range of diseases (e.g., diabetes, heart disease, and cancer) to be identified. Uncovering the genetic components of such diseases may drastically alter our approaches to them. Rather than the treatment of symptoms, effective prevention will be possible. Physicians will conceivably be able to prevent many diseases not now thought of as genetic by identifying those persons at risk from the predisposing genes and inserting the absent genetic material.[7]

Such prospects are dizzying. We should not be surprised that discussions of human gene therapy often excite profound, even religious, feelings about nature and human life. The feelings generated are usually more full of fear than joy and may be animated by more pervasive qualms about the march of technology. To date, much of the debate and discussion about gene therapy has centered on that topic. The insightful analysis of the President's Commission for the Study of Ethical Problems in Medicine[8] and the hearings in 1982 before Representative Albert Gore's subcommittee[9] have sufficiently aired the issue to establish that meddling with the human genome is no more unnatural or artificial than the other meddling that goes on in a wide range of accepted human pursuits.

The discussion has also disposed of the slippery-slope claim that benign therapeutic uses of gene transfer will set us on an ineluctable course to far more dangerous and intrusive interventions in the human genome. We know that slippery-slope arguments generally do not work. The mere fact that we do X, a necessary condition to doing Y, does not mean that we will inevitably do Y. Even if the technical hurdles to stage Y can be overcome, a decision to seek Y, with its different array of costs, benefits, and probabilities must be made. Thus, the ability to correct single-gene disorders does not mean that we will ever be able or willing to engineer multifactorial traits, such as beauty, intelligence, and height. Indeed, acquiring that capacity will require scientific leaps of such an order that we may more fruitfully compare gene therapy for serious diseases to the first step of a long, arduous climb up a mountain, the contours of which are only dimly seen, rather than to a slide down a slippery slope to the fabrication of human beings.[10] The fear is far too insubstantial to justify stopping or not investing in gene therapies, which, if effective, have such a great potential for eliminating disease and suffering.[11]

The development of effective gene therapies, nevertheless, does raise difficult and novel issues, even if we meet and overcome the slippery-slope and the defilement-of-nature arguments. Rather than cataloging and discussing solutions to all the potential ethical issues that could be listed, I would like to focus on two ethical problems that arise when gene therapy or gene transfer is applied to the newly fertilized egg or embryo.

As Clifford Grobstein has articulately pointed out,[12] the long-range significance of *in vitro* fertilization (IVF) is the window that it provides on the genome and the developing human embryo, rather than the stimulus that it gives to new forms of family. External fertilization offers an opportunity to identify and alter the genetic makeup of the fertilized egg and the person that it may become. As the ability to map and alter the genome grows, reasons for altering the genetic makeup of the embryo will also grow. Gene transfer in embryos allows all the cells of the body to receive the missing gene, thus assuring proper expression in particular organs. In addition, the gene defect is corrected before embryo development begins, a process thus assuring that it will turn on in time to prevent damage from its absence. The effects of gene transfer to embryos is especially powerful, for it will inevitably affect the germ cells as well. Thus, the transferred gene will not die with the individual organism, as occurs with somatic cells (including gentically altered somatic cells), but can be passed on to many later generations. Finally, the genetic manipulation of embryos raises profound questions about the legitimacy of research on embryos, and about the rights and duties that we have regarding them—issues not yet fully resolved in research contexts not involving genetic manipulation.[13]

These possibilities are close enough to reality to warrant discussion. After discussing more thoroughly why gene therapy at the embryo level is likely to occur, I want to discuss two ethical problems thought to arise with gene transfer to embryos. In my opinion, neither is sufficient to prevent the gene alteration of embryos.

THE NEED FOR GENE THERAPY ON EMBRYOS

As gene therapy techniques develop, we can expect that they will be applied to earlier and earlier stages in the life cycle. For example, newborn infants suffering from Lesh–Nyhan syndrome or adenosine deaminase deficiency will be treated early in life because those diseases take a toll in infancy. Indeed, genetic treatment of the fetus may also become possible in the future. If a prenatal diagnosis shows that the fetus has a serious single-gene defect and the mother opposes abortion, prenatal genetic treatment may be essential to prevent the damage that will occur when a gene necessary for normal development is missing. If the bone marrow of the fetus can be removed, treated *in vitro* with clones of the missing gene, and then reinjected in the fetus, where the new gene will be properly expressed, prenatal genetic therapy on the fetus will be possible.[14] In that case, the parents would be free to apply the prenatal genetic therapy to the fetus in order to protect the child that they are bringing into the world. Indeed, if the parents have decided against abortion there is even an argument that they have a legal duty to provide an established genetic therapy to the fetus *in utero*, if necessary to prevent serious harm to the offspring.[15] Otherwise, they will have brought an avoidably defective child into the world.

A more likely scenario than the application of gene therapy *in utero* to the fetus will be application at the embryonic level. Gene insertion after birth or even during pregnancy may come too late to prevent damage from lack of the necessary gene. Insertion in the embyro would also solve the problem of having the inserted gene reach the right organ and thus be available to express itself at the time and place needed. Introducing DNA into the fertilized egg will introduce the gene into all cells of the body (including germ cells), with such efficiency that it will be preferable to do it then, even if postnatal gene transfer is possible.

Embryo interventions pose special problems, however. One problem concerns the justification for embryo manipulation. A second problem is the likelihood of affecting the germ line, and hence future generations. Do these problems present a barrier to gene transfer in embryos?

CAN GENETIC MANIPULATION OF EMBRYOS BE JUSTIFIED?

The possibility of gene transfer in embryos raises several potential problems because of uncertainty about obligations to embryos. Experimental access to embryos is still so new and the moral status of the embryo is still so unsettled that the ethical limits on embryo experimentation are unclear. However, a consensus among informed laypersons, scientists, and ethicists may be emerging in the reports of the several commissions and boards that have considered the question.[16] They draw a line between experimentation when the embryo experimented on will be transferred to a uterus and hence may be brought into being and when it will not be. In the former case, where the manipulated embryo will be transferred to a uterus, the research must be beneficial or therapeutic to the potential offspring. In the latter case, research is possible, for good cause, as long as the embryo is not maintained for more than 14 days after fertilization, the time when differentiation of a nervous system and hence the possibility of sentience begin.[17]

Under these developing guidelines, gene therapy on the embryo can be ethically justified. The 14-day period for experimentation when no transfer to the womb is planned gives ample room to perfect screening and gene transfer techniques in embryos (assuming the embryos are available by the consent of the gamete providers). Proceeding further and transferring the genetically altered embyro to the uterus, so that it may be brought to term, can also be justified. If the embryo has been identified as having a gene defect, which will lead to it being discarded or born damaged if carried to term without treatment, then gene alteration of the embryo with the intent of transferring it to a uterus and bringing it to term is therapeutic and beneficial in intent. If there is a reasonable basis for thinking that the gene alteration could succeed, even an experimental operation, as well as one established as safe and effective, would satisfy the principle of respect for the embryo and the future offspring that underlies the rule.[18]

However, Bayles[19] and Williamson[20] have argued that it is unethical to alter embryo genes and then transfer the embryo to a womb, despite a beneficial or therapeutic intent, because of the risk that the embryo and the future child will be damaged by the experimental gene alteration. Rather than risking damage to future children, affected embryos should be discarded, and only genetically healthy ones should be transferred to the uterus.

To assess this argument, let us step back and consider the matter from the perspective of the couple confronting the need for gene transfer to correct defects in future offspring. For them, the question of gene therapy arises only if the couple knows, because of carrier screening of the prior birth of a child with the defect, that they are heterozygous carriers of the trait.[21] If they are, they would have a 1 : 4 chance of having a child with the defect. This knowledge gives them several options. They can give up the idea of having children altogether. They can seek an adopted child. Or they may choose to substitute the unaffected sperm or egg of a third party for the gametes of one of them. With some diseases, they have the additional option of conceiving and then having a prenatal diagnosis to determine if the fetus is affected. If a prenatal genetic therapy is not available, they can abort the affected fetus and try again, or they can turn to the other options. Postponing treatment until after birth is not an option where the genetic damage is done during *in utero* development.

A final option—pretransfer screening of embryos—is not now available but probably will be in the future.[22] This option would allow the couple to conceive externally through *in vitro* fertilization, to screen the embryos for the genetic defect, and then to transfer to the uterus only those embryos that do not have the defect. The logic of amniocentesis and selective abortion is carried back to an earlier stage. Although the method of conception is more difficult and presumably less pleasurable, the process of screening and selective termination is much easier. One discards a drop of fluid containing the affected embryo more easily than she or he invades the uterus and removes the fetus that has been attached for several weeks or months.[23] Although most couples who conceive externally in order to screen embryos for defects would probably discard the affected embryos, the ability to screen opens the possibility of inserting new genes in the embryo and bringing it to term. Just as *in utero* fetal therapies provide an alternative to abortion when prenatal diagnosis reveals a defect, gene therapy on the embryo provides an alternative to the destruction of the affected embryo.[24] There are, of course, differences in the two cases that undercut claims of a duty to treat such an embryo. Discarding the embryo is less traumatic than abortion after prenatal diagnosis, and it permits reproduction to occur by transferring the unaffected embryos, as external conception usually involves several fertilized eggs. If one is discarded because of a gene defect and others remain to be transferred to the uterus, the chance of achieving pregnancy and live birth is unaffected.

Would it be unethical to perform gene therapy on an embryo and to transfer it to a uterus when unaffected fertilized eggs can be transferred? Would not the genetic intervention risk harming the child to be, when a healthy child can be born from the other eggs available? Contrary to the arguments of Bayles and Williamson, the possibility of harm in the offspring does not foreclose couples and physicians from doing gene therapy on the affected embryo. In the first place, it may not be irrational to treat the affected embryo and to bring it to term. Persons who believe that embryos deserve respect and should be transferred to a uterus rather than merely being allowed to die would find gene therapy an acceptable and possibly an obligatory option.[25] In other cases, there may not be sufficient unaffected embryos available; for example, the laparoscopy may have yielded only a few eggs, each fertilized egg may be affected, and the woman may be unwilling to undergo further surgery to retrieve others. The possibility of freezing and then thawing embryos allows us to imagine other scenarios.[26]

Nor would attempting gene therapy wrong offspring who are born damaged as a result. The danger, particularly at the experimental stage when the risks are unknown, is that the intervention will damage the offspring, either enabling them to survive handicapped when they would otherwise have spontaneously aborted, or producing toxicities that cause damage in the offspring. Yet, it can be argued that bringing a damaged child into the world who could not have been born in an undamaged state does not wrong her or him. A wrong to such a child would arise only in the extreme case where existence itself is so painful and so bereft of meaning that it is a wrong to allow someone in that state to live.[27] In such a case, the wrong can be minimized by withholding treatment or even nourishment from the child. If its life is truly wrongful, these omissions are permissible and indeed, may even be obligatory.

I conclude that the possibility of *in vitro* screening of fertilized eggs for genetic defects does not bar gene therapy on the affected embryos. If parents desire to preserve embryos and bring them into the world in a healthy state, gene therapy on the embryo when there are reasonable grounds for trying it, when the parents have been fully informed, and when institutional review requirements have been met is an ethically acceptable option that general principles of civil and criminal law would not prohibit.

Can the Germ Line Be Affected?

If every footfall, as it is said, resounds through history, some clearly have a heavier thud than others. Successful somatic genetic therapy, like other successful medical therapies, will have a strong thud because it will enable people to survive and pass their genes to others. Gametic therapy, on the other hand, has potentially an even more pronounced thud, for it removes genes from the gene pool or adds new ones. This process may affect the supply of genes and their availability for future generations.

For this reason, gene insertion affecting germ cells is thought to be improper. People who raise this point question whether it should intentionally be done, and even whether it is acceptable as an inevitable by-product of gene therapy done on the embryo to affect the somatic cells of one's future child.

The concern about germ line alterations reflects the discomfort aroused by the tremendous power that gene manipulation potentially offers. On closer analysis, however, there appears to be no compelling reason not to remove a deleterious gene from future generations, either intentionally or as a by-product of somatic therapy. Indeed, several witnesses at the Gore hearings on gene therapy in November 1982 cautiously supported gametic therapy.[28] In addition, the Parliamentary Assembly of the Council of Europe has recently passed a resolution approving the use of germ cell modification for serious gene disease.[29]

Two arguments can be advanced against germ line alterations, neither of which stands up to analysis: (1) the gene may become adaptive again, and (2) gametic therapy would violate the rights of future offspring.

Preventing Future Harm

The first argument against germ line alteration is that the "deleterious" gene being removed may later prove to be adaptive. Removing it from the germ line will deprive future persons of the gene, thus causing them harm, if changing conditions make the gene useful. This argument is based, at bottom, on a view that Stephen Stich has summarized:

> The current constitution of the human gene pool . . . is no accident. We got to be the sort of creatures we are as the result of millions of years of natural selection. During those millions of years, many genes disappeared from the gene pool because the characteristics they impart to the organism were less adaptive than the surviving alternatives. Thus there is a sense in which the current genetic make-up of humankind stores a great treasury of information about the sort of design that can flourish in our

environment. It is folly, this argument concludes, to fiddle with the hard-won "evolutionary wisdom" that has been bequeathed to us in our gene pool. [30]

The argument is that a gene that has survived this long must have some adaptive advantage, even if it is nonadaptive in present circumstances, and thus should be retained because it may prove adaptive again. In fact, the sickle-cell-anemia gene is adaptive in the malarial regions in which people with it or their ancestors once lived. Migration from those regions and medical and engineering advances within them have made the gene maladaptive. Eliminating the gene altogether, rather than dealing with it anew each time it appears, could ultimately prove maladaptive, if new strains of malaria develop or other conditions change.

Yet, this concern does not justify the potential harms that would occur if germ lime alterations were prohibited. Such a ban would mean that somatic gene therapy directed at the next generation—at the couple's children—could not be done if it would affect the germ line. Yet, the only effective site for somatic therapy may be on the embryo, which carries the risk of gametic alteration as well. Prohibiting gametic therapy would also limit the parents' liberty. They could not choose to eliminate the disease in their offspring and their offspring's offspring by direct alteration of the germ line. Finally, genetic disease would have to be treated anew (presumably by gene therapy) in each generation. Inevitably, some persons will be missed and thus will suffer from a disease that could have been prevented earlier.

The harms from not eliminating the gene seem to be much greater than the speculative fear that a currently deleterious gene may at some unknown future time prove to be adaptive. Indeed, the harms tolerated would accrue over the course of the many years that it would have taken to eliminate the maladaptive gene from the gene pool. Moreover, the fear of "elimination from the gene pool" is not totally accurate. The recombinant techniques that allow gene therapy can permit us to copy and store the gene, and replace it later if conditions make it adaptive again. [31] If the gene later proved adaptive, deaths and suffering would occur while it is being replaced. But there is no reason to prefer prevention of such highly speculative deaths over the sure deaths that will occur if gametic therapy is barred. In sum, the case for tolerating these harms in order to avert speculative, distant harms is not persuasive.

The Rights of Future Offspring

A second argument against gametic therapy has not been well articulated but may be pieced together as a claim that depriving future generations of genes that may later prove to be adaptive violates their right to have the gene. Let us examine this claim by distinguishing the rights of immediate and future offspring to a particular genome.

IMMEDIATE OFFSPRING. The application of genetic therapy to one's gametes or the gametes of one's future child, as in embryo alteration, benefits the child somatically by preventing the expression of the disease in her or him. Because the application would also alter the child's gametes, it prevents the child from passing the deleterious gene to her or his children. Have the child's procreative or other rights or interests been violated by depriving her or him of a gene to transmit to future generations?

The answer is no, as it is difficult to find a right to have a particular genome so that it may be transmitted to descendants. The notion of a right to a particular genome is cogent when a genome harmful to the child could be altered to make her or him healthy. The "right" of a child to be born healthy, if steps to avoid harm are reasonably possible, would include the right to gene alteration essential to health. Refusing to apply an established genetic therapy to an embryo or a fetus that will be brought to term wrongs the resulting child as much as withholding any known prenatal therapy would.[32] In this case, the right to be born with a particular genome is violated because that genome is available through gene therapy and will prevent the severe handicap that will otherwise occur.

The claim of a right to a particular genome in order to transmit it to offspring is a claim of a different order. Here, the genome is claimed not in order to assure somatic health, but to fulfill a desire concerning the genes that the person transmits to offspring. Denying people this wish by denying them a gene to transfer could be a wrong or harm to them only if the ability to transmit those genes was so central to their identity or life plan that they should be granted a right to have that experience.

There are several problems with the claim of such a right. At the present time, the extent to which a person's procreative rights include the right to transmit genes aside from gestation and rearing is unclear.[33] Even if the right to transmit genes existed against the state's or third parties' interfering with it, it would not follow that there was a right against one's parents to have any particular set of genes to transmit (aside from the healthy genome that one is entitled to).

Suppose, however, that we believe that a person should have some control over the genes that he or she transmits to future generations, including the right as against his or her parents to be given the genes that he or she is likely to want to pass on to his or her offspring. We would recognize such a right only if we found that the ability to pass on a certain set of genes was a source of personal meaning or satisfaction central to identity. As implausible as such a right might sound, if such a right existed, it would arise only with genes that are beneficial to offspring, because only they would yield the satisfaction that grounds such a right. Depriving parents of the ability to pass on a harmful gene, the ill effects of which they themselves have escaped, would not violate our putative right, if the parents' intent was to harm future offspring, for the satisfaction of harming would not support such a right.

The only basis for a right to have parents retain the deleterious gene so that their child would have it available to pass on to his or her offspring would be the child's interest in having his or her offspring have it available if it later proves adaptive. But the chances of its being adaptive in the next generation are almost zero. In fact, it is almost certain to be maladaptive in that generation. Indeed, the parent might have a duty to prevent its ill effects, most likely by somatic gene therapy. Thus, depriving one's children (and their offspring) of such a gene by doing gametic rather than somatic gene therapy to eradicate it can hardly be considered a violation of a right to have a particular genome to transmit, even if such a strange right were recognized. The most plausible conditions for recognizing such a right would not exist in the case of a deleterious gene.

In fact, gametic gene therapy benefits the child (and his or her offspring) more than it harms. Now he or she will not have to worry about passing on the trait during reproduction, either doing nothing and ending up with an affected child, or having to deal with all the dilemmas and problems of treating the genetic disease of his or her child, including the choice of gametic or somatic therapy. The risk that such a need will arise may be small, as the offspring, or the offspring's offspring, would have to reproduce with another carrier for the need for somatic gene therapy in their offspring to arise. Yet, that risk is great enough to outweigh the slight harm to reproductive choice that gametic intervention denies the child in the generation under discussion. In addition, the person claiming the right to such a gene always has the option of inserting it in her or his offspring, if that would not otherwise wrong them.[34]

FUTURE OFFSPRING: LATER GENERATIONS.   A similar analysis applies to an individual in any later generation who himself or herself has been protected from the genetic defect but lacks the ability to pass the deleted gene on to others. Not only have they been benefitted, but no right of theirs to have a certain genetic constitution in order to transmit it to their descendants has been violated. As we have just seen, no such right exists against one's parents. A *fortiori*, no such right exists against one's more distant ancestors.

However, what if the harmful gene turns out, because of later changes, to be once again adaptive? A new strain of malaria develops from genetic engineering that conventional therapies cannot deal with, but that persons who still have the sickle-cell trait can withstand. Have those deprived of the trait been harmed or wronged by the ancestor who removed the gene from his or her blood line?

I think not. At the time the person underwent gametic therapy, he or she had reason to think that he or she was protecting his or her children and their offspring and later descendants. The small hypothetical risk that the gene might become adaptive was outweighed by the larger, more certain benefit of elimination. Moreover, it is hard to see how any right was infringed. Any "right to have a healthy genome" would exist only if it is reasonably possible to provide a person with one and the parent negligently or intentionally fails to do so. But at the time the parent opted for a germ line alteration, the risks of later harm appeared small by comparison to the risks of not doing so.

In any event, if the gene is now desirable, it is possible that it can be replaced. A technology advanced far enough to excise specific genes from the germ line, while also curing disease, may be able to reverse the process when the missing gene becomes valued. Thus, preventing harm to later generations would not be an adequate reason to prevent a parent from excising a deleterious gene in his or her children and their descendants.

PROCREATOR'S FREEDOM TO SELECT OFFSPRING CHARACTERISTICS.   One further ethical dimension merits discussion. Depending on how one resolves the moral issues, the question of public policy on the matter remains. Questions of the prohibition or the strict regulation of the gene alteration of embryos could arise. The extent of the state's power to curtail the development and use of biotechnologies is important in many contexts beyond the gene alteration of embryos. We see here the general structure of the argument against state prohibition. Although the state could choose not to fund research in gene therapy (as it now treats IVF research), the prohibition would have to meet a high standard of need, beyond moral distaste, because prohibition would violate a fundamental right.[35] The state would have difficulty meeting the high standard of scrutiny necessary to justify such an infringement.

The constitutional difficulty arises because gene therapy on the embryo is closely tied to procreative choice. The scope of the right to select offspring characteristics is just emerging as an issue and is far from being settled. A court could reasonably adopt the view that a person has the right to try to prevent suffering in her or his descendants by removing a potentially lethal gene from the germ line. Without accepting a total freedom to engineer or enhance traits (a complicated issue beyond this chapter's scope), we can recognize a right to prevent harm in one's offspring and their descendants. We have seen that offspring may have a right to gametic therapy from the parents when essential for a healthy genome.[36] The U.S. Constitution, it may cogently be argued, gives the parent the right to provide his or her children and their descendants with a healthy genome.

The cogency of the argument for such a right has not yet been fully appreciated, so the steps of the argument are worth repeating.[37] Procreative freedom includes the freedom to avoid procreation and the freedom to procreate. The latter must include some measure of freedom to select or control the characteristics of offspring, such as to prevent harm to them. The extent of this freedom when the purpose is enhancement or improvement is unclear and beyond the scope of this chapter. But it must, at a minimum, include the freedom to prevent, either by abortion or by treatment before birth, the birth of a child with harmful genes. If it is permissible—indeed, even obligatory—to treat the child's condition after birth or prenatally, it should be permissible to treat the condition at the embryo or preconception stage as well, for it will save the offspring and their descendants the burden of doing it later. Indeed, the child might not otherwise be born, if the parents are limited to postnatal remedies. Properly understood, the argument concludes, the right to procreate includes a right to practice negative eugenics—to deselect harmful characteristics from future generations.

If procreative freedom is at stake, then the state must show substantial nonmoralistic grounds for restricting its exercise. But the interests of offspring and future generations are not threatened here, and are even benefitted, because the burdens to any individual of having the gene are greater than the burdens of not having it. Any regulation prohibiting gametic therapy to protect future persons must be justified on nonreligious or nonmoral public policy grounds. If only religious or moral objections remain, they are insufficient to justify limits on the exercise of the fundamental right to procreate.

CONCLUSION

Human gene therapy lies on the near horizon. Its nearness rightfully gives us pause, for gene manipulation is potentially a very potent and very precise tool. We need to proceed with deliberate care, as we largely have proceeded, until we have a clearer sense of its dangers and benefits.

As the issues are studied and scientific progress occurs, the question of gene therapy at the embryo level will arise. In this chapter, I have tried to show how some of the issues should be resolved. Debate is just beginning and will continue as the technical capabilities grow. We need more grappling with these issues in all the varied settings in which society's moral consensus is forged to come to terms with the new genetics.

REFERENCES AND NOTES

1. Schmeck, H., Treatment of genetic defects is nearing, *New York Times* (Apr. 10, 1984), 17; Grobstein, C., Gene therapy: Proceed with caution, *The Hastings Center Report* (Apr. 1984), 13.
2. Schmeck, n. 1, *supra.*
3. Kolata, G., Gene therapy method shows promise, *Science* **223**:1376–9 (1984).
4. Schmeck, n. 1, *supra.*
4a. An account of the Cline affair is presented in the Gore Hearings, pp. 442–460. *See* n. 9, *infra.*
5. Schmeck, n. 1, *supra,* reported that the IRB at the University of California at San Diego has approved a trial in carefully selected patients. The Recombinant DNA Advisory Committee of NIH has not yet approved the research but has announced plans to begin reviewing gene therapy on humans. *Chronicle of Higher Education* (January 4, 1984) 17.
6. McKusick, V., Diseases of the Genome, *JAMA* **252**:1041 (1984); Bishop, J., Scientists are focusing on genes predisposing people to illnesses, *Wall Street Journal* (Sept. 12, 1984), 1.
7. Of course, prevention by means other than gene therapy could occur (e.g., exercise or diet) once the predisposing gene is identified.
8. *Gene Splicing* (1983).
9. Human Genetic Engineering, Hearings before the Subcommittee on Investigations and Oversight of the Committee on Science and Technology, U.S. House of Representative, Nov. 16, 17, 18, 1982 (hereinafter, *Gore hearings*).
10. Harsanyi, I., Gore hearings, 231–2.
11. Friedmann, T., Gore hearings, 275–7.
12. From Chance to Purpose: An Appraisal of External Human Fertilization, (1981), 116.
13. Despite the Ethical Advisory Board's recommended guidelines for research with embryos, 44 *Fed. Reg.* 35033 (June 18, 1979), several witnesses at the Gore hearings on human embryo transfer in August 1984 continued to list experimentation as a major unsolved issue.
14. The idea of extracting and reinjecting fetal bone marrow is not very different from many other fetal interventions that now occur.
15. Robertson, J., The right to procreate and in utero fetal therapy, *J. of Legal Medicine* **3**:333–62 (1982). But see *contra.,* Annas and Elias, "Fetal Surgery" chapter, this volume.
16. Ethical Advisory Board, 44 *Fed. Reg.* 35033 (June 18, 1979); Report of the Committee of Inquiry into Human Fertilization and Embryology ("Warnock Committee") (July 1984); Waller Committee Report.
17. *Id.*
18. If the damage of Lesch–Nyhan disease occurs during pregnancy, it would be a candidate for gene therapy on the embryo.
19. Bayles, M., *Reproductive Ethics,* Prentice Hall, NJ (1984).
20. Gene therapy, *Nature* **298**:416 (1982).
21. The importance of viewing gene therapy at any level as one component of a large system of identification and treatment is also discussed by Dr. Harsanyi, n. 10, *supra.*
22. Several technical problems now make it impossible to screen the embryo, but these undoubtedly will be removed in the future. Until embryo screening is perfected, a heterozygous couple reproducing by means of IVF could insert the missing gene in all fertilized eggs, as a way of being sure that a defective one is not implanted. Alexander Capron, Remarks at Genetics and Law Conference, April 4, 1984. Although this option may prove risky to the unaffected embryos, it may be that the extra gene will not harm them. The absence of harm would first have to be established by animal studies before it would be ethical to try it on humans.
23. This is true even if chorion villi sampling allows prenatal diagnosis of the fetus to occur at 8 weeks, rather than at the 15–18 weeks now required for amniocentesis.

24. Remarks of John Fletcher and Richard McCormack concerning the effect of the emergence of fetal therapy on our perception of the status of the fetus and our obligations to it are applicable here as well.
25. One may take this position either because he or she believes that the embryo is a moral entity in its own right or because he or she finds its potential to become a person deserving of respect. For a fuller exposition of these points, see Robertson, J., *Procreative Liberty and Embryo Transfer* (unpublished paper, available from the author).
26. We can imagine a scenario where four eggs are removed and fertilized. Three are implanted and one is frozen. The three do not implant, and the frozen one, on inspection, is found to have a single-gene defect that could be corrected before transfer to a uterus.
27. The position asserted here is that true wrongful life claims are in principle plausible but, in actuality, arise in very small percentage of handicapped births. Although there is much room for debate, as the Baby Doe controversy indicates, about whether a given handicap amounts to wrongful life, the courts have almost uniformly rejected wrongful life claims asserted on behalf of unavoidably handicapped children. The recent acceptance of limited wrongful-life claims by the California, Washington, and New Jersey Supreme Courts is only apparent. The claim has been recognized in those cases to ensure that the tortfeasor will bear the full medical and educational costs of the handicapped child. They firmly reject the claim of the child to damages for pain and suffering, which should be awarded if they adopt the position that the child has been wronged by being brought into existence.
28. These witnesses included Dr. Leroy Walters, pp. 388–9, and Dr. Bernard Davis, pp. 507–9.
29. Gore hearings, 389.
30. *Id.* at 539.
31. Dr. Leroy Walters, Director of the Kennedy Institute of Bioethics, made this point at the Gore hearings, 388–389.
32. See n. 19, *supra.*
33. See the analysis of this issue in Robertson, J., *Procreative Liberty and Embryo Transfer*, n. 25, *supra.*
34. Because the technology must be very advanced for this issue even to arise, the person claiming the right would probably be able to replace the gene herself or himself. Should not she or he, rather than her or his parents, have the duty of doing so, if it is so important to her or him?
35. Abramowitz, S., A stalemate on test-tube baby research, *The Hastings Center Report* 14:5 (1984). See also *Maher v. Roe*, 432 U.S. 464 (1977); *McCrae v. Harris*, 448 U.S. (1980).
36. The right to a healthy genome could be satisfied by somatic therapy, but in many cases, the therapy will affect the germ line. There is also the question of one's duties to a future generation.
37. This paragraph recapitulates the argument made at greater length in Robertson, J., Procreative liberty and the control of conception, pregnancy and childbirth, *Va. L. Rev.* 69:45 (1983).

Discussion

Ms. Penelope Alderdice: Few people have said anything about cost and benefit. I think that when we start talking as we do, we completely ignore cost and benefit. I would like to suggest that if we are going to talk about respect for the fertilized egg, we might go back to the sperm and to the egg, unfertilized, and if we want to deal with the recessive disease, you find a way to eliminate the sperm carrying the recessive allele. Then we won't have the problem of identifying the fertilized egg carrying that double dose.

Mr. John A. Robertson: I agree that cost–benefit considerations are relevant and need to be factored in here as well. It may be that genetic therapy for single-gene defects would be most effective at the egg or sperm cell stage, before the fertilized-egg stage. If that's not possible, it may still be acceptable within the discretion of the parties to do therapy at the fertilized-egg stage.

Dr. David Botstein: We were talking earlier about the whole issue of selective breeding. If you were to genetically segregate particular classes of sperm and eggs and prevent them from being fertilized or fertilizing, then you would be, in the real sense doing a class of selective breeding that could, in fact, reduce the gene pool. So, in many ways, at least in my view, changing a gene here and there for therapeutic benefit seems like a much less Draconian measure than systematically eliminating a particular sperm or some property or other.

Ms. Helen Holmes: It seems to me that the PKU child who is being treated by diet is allowed to live and have a reasonably normal life. So it might even be considered a duty to give this diet and force her or him to eat it, even though it's very unpleasant. However, if you could change the genes ahead of time you wouldn't have to force her or him to eat this diet, and so, at first glance, it may be far better than the current therapy. I've been looking at published work on gene transfer in mice causing increased growth to see what is hinted at between the lines. It's hard to pull it all together, but I have reached the conclusion that, for about 1,000 mouse eggs that are microinjected, approximately 15 baby mice are born who can be shown to have the DNA that was injected and to express the gene. Some of them have the DNA but don't express it. Well, if you were doing that with the eggs from PKU parents, where would you get 1,000 human eggs to work your experiment out in the first place? My question is that I wonder whether we're tilting at windmills.

MR. JOHN A. ROBERTSON: Yes, again. But of course, that's one of our purposes here. This is the Genetics and the Law Conference, and we can speculate a little about some of these issues even though I think that the scientific side of this conference has made it clear that some of them are not in the offing. We need to begin thinking about the distinctions that are relevant and to see that the issues change when we start going back to the very stages at which the manipulations can occur.

DR. DAVID BOTSTEIN: I think that the kind of calculation that the previous questionner made and the attention given to the apparently arcane details of these things are very good practice and should very strongly be encouraged. It is misunderstandings of those kinds that so often cause a rift between the scientifically minded people and the humanistically minded people who are interested in this problem.

DR. PHILIP LEDER: In the course of these discussions this afternoon and in other discussions elsewhere, fiction has played a major role in the analysis and the examples given in the form of scenarios. This is a set of issues that does have a scientific base that is quite hard and ample. I think that there is really no need to delve into the realm of fiction to cite our examples, because the public mind too easily confuses "the Andromeda strain" with a real epidemic that actually occurred. That's just a warning that I would like to offer.

DR. MARGERY W. SHAW: Could Dr. Botstein give us an overall fast history and update of when the first restriction fragment-length polymorphism was discovered? How many have been discovered in humans? How many have been mapped to the human chromosome? How many have been linked to a disease gene?

DR. DAVID BOTSTEIN: I'll do the best I can. First, one has to distinguish between truly informative markers and two allele systems. There is an uncountable number of the latter that, at least in principle, in some family or other, could be useful. Let's limit ourselves to strong systems. My understanding is that the first polymorphism discovered at the DNA level was Y. W. Kahn's marker associated with globin, which is a two-allele system and is of limited diagnostic value by itself. A very large number of polymorphisms at the globin locus are now known. The globin locus can be determined with reasonably high information content, although it's not very high because of linkage disequilibrium. In terms of random polymorphisms, I think there are about 30 that are really useful, and as you know, we need somewhere over 300–1,000 to have a really fully informative map. We are 10% of the way there. At the moment, there are no markers by linkage that would be useful as a diagnostic test. The Huntington marker isn't very informative yet. It's only a three-allele system, and about half the people are homozygous. Of course, the polymorphisms that derive from the diseased gene itself, like globin or PKU, can be used for diagnosis.

DR. JACQUES LORRAINE: I would like to ask Dr. Macklin if it is possible in socialized medicine to avoid giving information to the government? If the doctor is to be paid, information must be given about the diagnosis and the treatment provided for the patient. At the present time, Canadian socialized medicine has continued for at least 13 years, and the Canadian government knows all private health details on every citizen. I'm concerned about the information that the government may gather in the genetic context.

DR. RUTH MACKLIN: That's a good question, and it bears on the disclosure of data of this type to any third party and any organization. In fact, with regard to questions of confidentiality, I don't see any difference in principle between the practice of medicine under a system of socialized medicine and practice under a mixed system, such as we have in the United States. The majority of people in the United States are covered by some form or other of insurance, whether by the government or by private insurance carriers. An unfortunate number of underinsured or uninsured people may not seek these particular techniques. Is it possible to keep that information from the government? It seems to me that arrangements could be made. An enlightened government, which, in principle, should have no need of particular genetic data about individuals, might be satisfied, let us say, with a diagnosis of a genetic disorder, which would be sufficient for the purpose of reimbursing physicians. Another possibility would be to have some kind of procedural safeguards. In that case, the government may have detailed genetic information or a genetic profile of individuals, but there might be some safeguards on the storage of that information or on who might have access to it. Your question concerns abuses of data. If it's simply in the hands of government and nothing further will be done with that information, then it's not clear to me what the problem would be, quite apart from the important question of whether or not individuals want that information disclosed. I think that the key here becomes the uses to which such information might be put, whether it's in the hands of the government or in the hands of insurance companies. It's very difficult to make public policy or social policy based on possible or potential abuses.

DR. PHILIP LEDER: Dr. Macklin, I have wondered if we, as modern molecular geneticists, are not a little paranoid about our endeavors. That paranoia arises from the fact, I think, that there is a very special concern and a particularly high level of controversy when it comes to dealing with the applications of genetic techniques in medical screening programs. For example, we could say that all the people in this room, as a condition of leaving the room, have to provide us with 30 milliliters of blood and allow us to do a restriction-fragment polymorphism profile so that we can eventually analyze the repertoire of genetic diseases that some of them are inevitably carrying around. That requirement would be regarded as unacceptable, highly controversial, and terrible. On the other hand, we might put a small 25-cent blood-pressure machine outside the door and ask everybody to pass through, to get a blood pressure reading, and to get a little pink or green card. Those with the pink card would be treated for a disease that is deleterious and the end result would be to increase the longevity of 10% of this audience. That procedure might be regarded as less controversial. Would you tell us what you think the basic difference is and whether we are being picked on here unnecessarily?

DR. RUTH MACKLIN: I think the question of being picked on may very well be a function of the new genetic information and its application. It may hinge on people's willingness to divulge information about themselves where there may be some benefit in return. There still may be individuals who don't want others to have that information, even if it would be beneficial to them. These things need to be sorted out, in terms of both what's possible and whether the information could benefit the individual. Whatever we may have now as fears may go away as we become more comfortable with these applications. Like any other information, some of it can be stigmatizing when it falls into the hands of others, and that's probably what people worry about.

DR. PHILIP LEDER: I think you'll find also that a substantial number of patients do not want the information, even if they are the only ones to receive the information.

MR. JOHN A. ROBERTSON: Is one a case of voluntary choice, the other of coercion?

DR. PHILIP LEDER: Let's put it a little differently. I meant that both are coerced in the sense that, if you want to get an insurance policy, you would have to get your blood pressure taken. Now let's say that, if you want to get an insurance policy, you have to submit to some kind of a genetic test. What's fundamentally different? I don't think there's really very much difference, but there's much greater concern about the latter question than about the former.

MR. DANIEL AVILA: Our organization has long opposed legalized abortions, so it should not be surprising when I say that I'm quite disturbed by Dr. Robertson's comment that we do have an option here between carrying the defect and discarding the defective. The question is: Is the second option, discarding the defective, a necessary part of genetic intervention? Will there ever be a point where we can successfully treat the defective?

MR. JOHN A. ROBERTSON: It probably will be the main option, but there could be cases where people will not want to discard the fertilized egg. It is important that the new reproductive technologies that allow external fertilization and embryo transfer actually may improve the chances of some embryos surviving if someone other than the egg donor could be found to bear the child. So there is that possibility. I think that there will be much discarding of fertilized eggs found to have a genetic defect. The abortion, if you will, will occur at an earlier stage than it now does with the conventional prenatal screening of fetuses.

A PARTICIPANT: I would like to come back to your question of whether there is a difference. On the one hand, we have an interest in playing the difference down in order to make the genetic information less mysterious and in order not to mystify genetics, because there are all kinds of genetic ideologies that say that the gene will determine much of human fate. We shouldn't really concentrate on genes, gene therapy, and genetic prevention and neglect other strategies that may be very important socially. Still, genetic information about humans is different from information like blood pressure, because it predicts what may happen to the individual. All this kind of prediction is dangerous in itself once it comes into the hands of people who use this information. Safeguards against the manipulation of human beings has to be the first emphasis. We may also try to prohibit investigations into things like blood pressure because they can also be predictive, and insurance companies and employers may have interests in calculating risks better by using all kinds of predictive indicators. There, the right not to know for the individual and especially the right not to give away the information to others must be the first principle.

DR. PHILIP LEDER: I wonder if you think that the fundamental genetic difference, with which we are all familiar but little understand, is the difference between men and women. It has been suggested—and I don't know the status of the law now on the issue—that this difference can no longer be used as a criterion for determining annuity payments. So, by a stroke of law, we have eliminated a major difference that's clearly observable and does have predictive value. All those criteria that we have discussed have enormous predictive value, such as blood pressure and alpha-1 antitrypsin in lung disease. They can be eliminated with the stroke of a wand, but do we really want to eliminate them?

DR. JOHN A. ROBERTSON: I'd like to underscore what Dr. Leder just said. To some extent, the vast increase in the amount of predictive information that one might anticipate from the genetic technology is really a quantitative, rather than a qualitative, difference. Information of this kind already exists, is tabulated, and is already in the hands, in some cases, of employers and insurance companies. The civil law can, in fact, change the environment in which this information is seen. Our first turn should not be to the question of whether we should learn these things, whether we should map the human genome, and whether we should use this information for the benefit of individual patients, but to how the civil law should react in such a way that the obvious injustices won't occur. In many ways, it is more rational, because circumstances have changed, to change the law, rather than to say that the law is immutable. There are many precedents for going about it that way, and that's what I hope most reasonable people would agree needs to be done.

NEW WAYS OF MAKING BABIES:
BRAVE NEW WORLD

Laboratories for Babies

MODERATOR: AUBREY MILUNSKY

12

LEGAL REGULATION OF ARTIFICIAL INSEMINATION AND THE NEW REPRODUCTIVE TECHNOLOGIES

The Search for Clarification Continues

JOSEPH M. HEALEY, JR.
Associate Professor
Department of Community Medicine
University of Connecticut School of Medicine
Farmington, CT 06032

Concerns about the legal aspects of the new reproductive technologies—artificial insemination, *in vitro* fertilization, and ovum and zygote transfer—are part of the continuing public and professional discussions about what our societal policy toward these technologies ought to be. The concerns are many and varied and include the desirability and availability of the technologies and the potential liability of those who use them. The desire for a clarification of legal responsibility is especially fueled by a heightened fear of liability, which has contributed to the pressure for straightforward legal answers and for a clear, comprehensive public policy dealing with these technologies. Lawyers know all too well the impatient cries of "Tell us the law, not philosophy." With respect to one of the technologies, artificial insemination with donor sperm (AID), the search for legal answers during the past two decades has produced a substantial body of law. Yet, even in this area, many gaps remain. More important, there has not emerged a clear public-policy framework within which alternative forms of reproduction can be evaluated. Though this lack of a framework is frustrating to those who want clear legal answers, it is not unexpected and is not entirely bad.

The legal issues involved in the development and use of these technologies are complex, involving fundamental questions of personal and societal values. The desire for legal answers must be balanced against a recognition of the difficulty of obtaining such answers. The experience with AID should be instructive for those interested in legal regulation of the other new reproductive technologies. My task in this chapter is to review the legal questions surrounding AID and the body of law that has developed in response to them. The factors contributing to the absence of a comprehensive legal framework will be discussed, and their implications for further development of the law will be examined. In this way, I hope to address the concerns of those who are frustrated by the many areas of legal ambiguity and uncertainty, and to provide a backdrop for those who will discuss these other technologies in greater detail.

LEGAL REGULATION OF ARTIFICIAL INSEMINATION

At the initial Genetics and the Law Conference in 1975,[1] five major areas of legal concern about AID were identified and discussed. The first area involved the legal status of a child conceived by AID. Because the Anglo-American legal system has traditionally attached great significance to the concepts of legitimate and illegitimate offspring, the use of a method of reproduction in which the biological father is not the husband of the biological mother raised threshold questions about the legal status of such a child. The second area involved the legal status of AID as a procedure. At issue was the extent to which AID was a procedure that constituted the practice of medicine and whose performance should be limited to physicians. The third area involved the consent process: Whose consent was needed? What disclosure was necessary for an informed, voluntary, and competent consent? The fourth area involved the donor of sperm: To what extent were special duties imposed on those performing AID with respect to donor selection and donor screening? The fifth area involved the various types of potential civil and criminal liability for those using AID. These five areas attracted the attention of legal analysts.

George Annas pointed out the narrowness of this focus at the Second Genetics and the Law Conference:

> Most commentary on AID has concentrated on theoretical legal problems without paying attention to real psychological problems. Indeed, most of the legal literature reads like an answer to the following final exam question: "Review all of the case law and statutes relating to AID and discuss all possible lawsuits that any participant or product of AID might have against anyone. If time permits, suggest a statutory scheme that might minimize these problems."[2]

He suggested a second level of legal issues that needed to be addressed:

> Current AID practices are based primarily on consideration of protecting the interests of practitioners and donors rather than recipients and children. The most likely reason for this is found in exaggerated fears of legal pitfalls. It is suggested that policy in this area should be dictated by maximizing the best interests of the resulting children. The evidence from the Curie-Cohen survey is that current practices are dangerous to children and must be modified. Specifically, consideration should be given to the following: (1) removing AID from the practice of medicine and placing it in the hands of genetic counselors or other nonmedical personnel (alternatively, a routine genetic consultation could be added for each couple who request AID); (2) development of uniform standards for donor selection, including national screening criteria; (3) a

requirement that practitioners of AID keep permanent records on all donors that they can match with recipients; I would prefer this to become common practice in the profession, but legislation requiring filing with a governmental agency may be necessary; (4) as a corrollary, mixing of sperm would be an unacceptable practice, and the number of pregnancies per donor would be limited; (5) establishment of national standards regarding AID by professional organizations with input from the public; (6) research on the psychological development of children who have been conceived by AID and their families.[3]

In 1975, at the time of the first Genetics and the Law Conference, only seven states had statutes dealing with AID. By 1984, at least 26 states had such legislation.[4] In 1975, there were a small number of cases from England, Scotland, Canada, and the United States dealing with AID.[5] Most were older cases of little apparent value as precedent. By 1984, the number of reported cases remained small, though there were several more recent cases.[6] The major source of clarification was legislative. Virtually all statutes acknowledge the legitimacy of a child conceived by AID following the informed consent of the mother and her husband. Several statutes eliminate any rights for the sperm donor. Several statutes identify AID as the practice of medicine. Only one (Oregon) explicitly deals with constraints on the sperm donor:

> 677.370 Who may be donor. No semen shall be donated for use in artificial insemination by any person who: (1) Has any disease or defect known by him to be transmissible by genes; or (2) Knows or has reason to know he has a venereal disease. [1977 c.686 §4][7]

Judicial review of AID remains isolated and sporadic and has not contributed greatly to the development of this body of law. As Wadlington has pointed out:

> Expanded use of these proliferating techniques for artificial conception may strain the capacity of the judiciary to produce a consistent approach to the complex issues of parental rights and obligations presented by this new technology. An examination of the body of case law developed to date confirms this suspicion. Courts often find themselves bound by policies and statutes adopted to resolve unrelated past problems and are, as a result, unable to reach appropriate conclusions. Old legal categories often constrict courts confronted with problems that arise from new technology and limit their efficacy in attempting to find creative solutions. The following discussion of typical precedent underlines the need for legislative reform in this area.
> In a peculiar body of cases, the earliest arising a little over a half century ago, American and British Commonwealth courts have encountered various problems centering on artificial insemination. Only a few cases, however, have reached appellate tribunals, and many of the reported opinions are known less for their substantive law implications than for their colorful dicta.[8]

The trends in the law seem clear. The policy of the presumed legitimacy of a child born during a marriage has been bolstered by the explicit recognition of the legitimacy of a child conceived by AID. AID is generally viewed as a medical procedure that may be performed by a physician who has obtained the informed consent of the woman and her husband. The sperm donor is not considered legally the "father" of the child and does not under ordinary circumstances have rights with respect to the child. Despite these trends in legislation and case law, there remain many unanswered questions. For example, one area of increasing interest, the insemination of single women, is not expressly dealt with. Even more importantly, only approximately one half of the states have passed such statutes. The result is an incomplete picture with respect to the legal regulation of AID. The reasons for these gaps have important implications for the legal regulation of the other new reproductive technologies.

THE DEVELOPMENT OF CLEAR PUBLIC POLICIES: FACTORS AND FORCES

The reasons for the gaps in the legal regulation of AID and for the absence of a comprehensive policy are complicated. To a certain extent, concern about legal liability may have decreased or may now be viewed as less pressing. To a certain extent, frustration over legal intrusion may have led some to ignore the law and to press less enthusiastically for clarification. I think these are minor factors compared with two others:

1. We are in an era of technological, cultural, and legal transition, and the setting for developing a clear comprehensive policy remains unsettled.
2. The issues at stake involve fundamental personal and societal values about which there remains significant disagreement, resulting in a profound absence of consensus about what the legal resolution ought to be.

We live in an era of transition that involves technological, cultural, and legal dimensions. The technological dimension reflects the changes that have occurred in medicine's ability to confront the major sources of morbidity and mortality. In many areas of our lives, we have moved from chance and fate to choice and freedom.[9] Medical innovations make possible the exercise of choice, whereas formerly only submission to fate was possible. The development of reproductive options for those who formerly were prevented from participation in parenthood represents a major example of this transition. Professor Dickens has described 23 reproductive options, ranging from normal conception to posthumous *in vitro* fertilization and embryo transplantation.* Concerns about the nature and extent of the choices available contribute to a societal unease about this era of technological transition. As McCormick noted:

> there comes a point in the moral discourse surrounding reproductive interventions when one must step aside from the casuistry of individual interventions and view the future possibilities and directions in aggregate and in the light of over-all convictions about what the "human" is. When that is done, some of the following questions arise. Will such reproductive interventions, even if they provide certain short-term remedies or advantages, actually improve the over-all quality of human life? If so, how is the improvement to be specified? What is the notion of the human that functions in the description of an "improvement"? And who decides this? If the development and application of such technology are likely to be humanly destructive, why will they be such? And if the more advanced forms of reproductive technology threaten some

*See Dickens, B., Ed. Note.

profoundly cherished human values and institutions (parenthood, marriage, the family), and are therefore something to be avoided, or at least stringently controlled, how are these values threatened, and where was the first wrong step or threatening one taken? Those are the questions that will be asked for decades as technology becomes increasingly sophisticated.

If the questions surrounding basic values are not asked, not asked seriously, not asked publicly, not asked continually, and in advance of the use of reproductive technologies, the danger is that we will identify the humanly and morally good with the technologically possible. That is why so much is at stake in reproductive interventions—not only in the conclusions that are drawn, but also in the criteria and form of moral reasoning involved.[10]

The cultural dimension reflects the changing view of the meaning of family and of parenthood. Whether through choice or through divorce, single-parent family units have become more commonplace. The availability and increased use of alternative methods of conception, childbearing, childbirth, and child rearing have also become more commonplace. The increased availability of options and the increased utilization of options have influenced the cultural acceptance of these alternatives. There remain, however, major differences of opinion about this aspect of cultural transition, and there is substantial ambivalence about it.[11] One other aspect of the cultural transition is the increased commercialization in health care. Of particular concern are the financial rewards associated with the sale of organs or body parts.[12] There is significant ambivalence about the effects of this commercialism on societal values. Finally, we are in a period of legal transition. At stake is the law's role in regulating reproductive choice and in recognizing reproductive rights and duties. The search for the proper balance between social norms and individual choice has led to concern about the law as the protector of societal and individual values. For example, one area of interest is the extent to which reproductive rights and duties should be established by contractual relationships, as well as traditional familial relationships.[13] The impact of these three dimensions of our age of transition is a high degree of uncertainty and ambivalence about what our policy should be. The result has been an unsettled context for the development of a comprehensive public policy.

To parallel the ambivalence and uncertainty about the new reproductive technologies, there is also an absence of consensus about the fundamental personal and societal values that underlie their development and use and about the extent to which these options enhance or violate these values. To some, the new technologies enhance the human condition and make possible more complete human lives. To others, the technologies represent unwise and undesirable intrusions into areas beyond responsible human behavior. These views reflect an ambivalence within our society about what values should guide the development and exercise of reproductive options. The result is the absence of a clear consensus about what societal policy ought to be.

IMPLICATIONS AND FUTURE DIRECTIONS

The implications of the incomplete legal regulation of AID and of the absence of a clear, comprehensive framework for societal policy dealing with new reproductive technologies for the future are important. The issues are too complex, too divisive for us to expect clear-cut resolutions in a short period. The issues must undergo a process of identification, clarification, and consideration that will take time.[14] Prolonging the process will be the impact of the era of technological, cultural, and legal transition and the social debate over the underlying value issues. As a result, it is likely that slow, piecemeal progress through legislation, primarily, and through litigation, on occasion, will continue. This slowness is not much consolation for those engaged in developing and using these new technologies, but it represents a more accurate view of what the law is and how public policy develops. Many people in our society assume that the law is a collection of easily obtained answers. One simply has to frame the question properly to have access to the answer. In fact, the number of situations in which such answers exist is relatively small. More accurately, the law is a series of value preferences, principles, and processes that are employed in the resolution of conflicts and in the development of public policy. For the foreseeable future, we must live with large areas of legal uncertainty, while working to shape the growth and development of legal policy in these areas.

REFERENCES AND NOTES

1. Healey, J., Legal aspects of artifical insemination by donor and paternity testing in *Genetics and the Law* (A. Milunsky and G. J. Annas, eds.) Plenum Press, New York (1976), 203.
2. Annas, G., Fathers Anonymous: Beyond the best interests of the sperm donor, in *Genetics and the Law II* (A. Milunsky and G. J. Annas eds.), Plenum Press, New York (1980), 331.
3. Ibid. at 338.
4. Arriving at a complete current list of state statutes is not an easy task. Three recent attempts did not result in identical lists. My own review produced at least one statute not cited by any of the other three authors. See Wadlington, W. Artificial conception: The challenge for family law, *Virginia Law Review* 69:465, 483 (1983); Smith, G., The razor's edge of human bonding: Artificial fathers and surrogate mothers, *Western New England Law Review* 5:639, 642 (1983); Andrews, L. The stork market: The law of the new reproductive technologies, *American Bar Association Journal* 70:50, 54–5 (1984). From these three sources and my own research, the following list has been compiled:

   Alaska Stat. Sect. 25.20.045 (1982)
   Arkansas Stat. Sect. 61-141(C) (1983)
   California Civ. Code Sect. 7005 (1982)
   Colo. Rev. Stat. Sect. 19-6-106 (1978)
   Conn. Gen. Stat. Sect. 45-69F-W (1981)
   Fla. Stat. Ann. Sect. 742.11 (1984)
   Ga. Code Ann. Sect. 19-7-21 (1984); Sect. 43-34-42 (1984)
   Ill. Ann. Stat. Ch. 40 Sect. 1451 (1983–4)
   Kan. Stat Ann. Sect. 23-128 to 23-130 (1983)
   La. Civ. Code Ann. Art. 188 (1983)
   Md. Est. and Trusts Code Ann. Sect. 1-206(B) (1983): Health Code, Sect. 20-214
   Mass. Gen. Laws Ann. Ch. 46, Sect. 4B (1984)
   Mich. Comp. Laws Sect. 333. 2824; Sect. 700. 11 (1980)
   Minn. Stat. Sect. 257. 56 (1982)
   Mont. Code Ann. Sect. 40-6-106 (1983)
   Nev. Rev. Stat. Sect. 126. 061 (1979)
   N.Y. Dom. Rel. Law Sect. 73 (1983–4)
   N.C. Gen. Stat. Sect. 49A-1 (1976)

Okla. Stat. Tit. 10, Sect. 551–553 (1983–4)
Or. Rev. Stat. Stat. Sect. 109.239–109.247; Sect. 667.355 to 677.370 (1984)
Tenn. Code Ann. Sect. 53-446 (1982)
Tex. Fam. Code Ann. Sect. 12.03 (1983)
Va. Code Ann. Sect. 64.1-7.1 (1984)
Wash. Rev. Code Ann. Sect. 26.26.050 (1984–5)
Wis. Stat. Ann. Sect. 891.40 (1983–4); Sect. 767.47(9)
Wyo. Stat. Sect. 14-2-103 (1984)

5. See Healey, notes 13, 15, and 16, and Wadlington, pp. 477–479.
6. See, for example, *C.M. v. C.C.*, 170 N.J. Super. 586, 407A2d. 849 (Juv. and Dom. Rel. Ct. 1979).
7. Oregon Revised Statutes, Section 677.370 (1984). The issue of screening sperm donors was addressed by the President's Commission for the Study of Ethical Problems in Medicine and Biomedical and Behavioral Research in its report *Screening and Counseling for Genetic Conditions*, pp. 68–70, U.S. Government Printing Office, Washington, DC (1983). See also Should sperm donors be screened for sexually transmitted diseases? *New England Journal of Medicine* **309**:1058 (1983).
8. Wadlington, pp. 476–7.
9. For medical examples, see Van den Berg, J., *Medical Power and Medical Ethics*, W. W. Norton, New York (1978).
10. McCormick, R., *How Brave a New World?* Doubleday and Company, Garden City, NY (1981), 334–335.
11. For a general discussion of the impact of an increase in the available options upon society, see Berger, P. *The Heretical Imperative*, Anchor Press/Doubleday, Garden City, NY (1979), 1–31. For a contrasting view of the desirability of various reproductive options, see Ramsey, P. *Fabricated Man*, Yale University Press, New Haven, 1970. Hanscombe, G. The right to Lesbian parenthood, *Journal of Medical Ethics* **9**:133–135 (1983), and Kern, P., and Ridolfi, K., Note: The fourteenth amendment's protection of a woman's right to be a single parent through artificial insemination by donor, *Women's Rights Law Reporter* **7**:251–284 (1982).
12. See Annas, G., Life, liberty and the pursuit of organ sales, *The Hastings Center Report* **14**(1):22–23 (1984), and Scott, R., *The Body as Property*, Viking Press, New York (1981).
13. See Robertson, J., Procreative liberty and the control of conception, pregnancy and childbirth, *Virginia Law Review* **69**:405–464 (1983).
14. A valuable framework for the development of a comprehensive public policy has been offered by Wadlington, at pp. 487–515.

13

Social Policy Considerations in Noncoital Reproduction

George J. Annas, J.D., M.P.H.
Edward Utley Professor of Health Law
Boston University of Schools of Medicine and Public Health
80 East Concord Street
Boston, MA 02118

Sherman Elias, M.D.
Director
Clinical Genetics Services
Prentice Women's Hospital and Maternity Center
Chicago, IL 60611
Associate Professor of Obstetrics and Gynecology
Northwestern University Medical School
Chicago, IL 60611

Nineteen eighty-four witnessed significant scientific and societal developments in noncoital human reproduction. On the scientific side, the year saw the first birth from surrogate embryo transfer (SET)[1] and the first birth from a frozen embryo.[2] On the societal side, the year saw reports by government-appointed panels on noncoital reproduction in the United Kingdom (the Warnock Report)[3] and Australia (the Waller Report),[4] and Congressional hearings on the subject in the United States.[5]

Techniques for noncoital reproduction close a circle opened with the introduction of effective contraception that made sex without reproduction dependable. Society seems as supportive of the new techniques of creating children as it was of contraception, but more anxious about the implications that these techniques raise, and consequently more interested in public regulation of them. As with *in vitro* fertilization (IVF) and surrogate motherhood, the major argument in favor of using these new techniques has been the resulting infants. Their pictures have appeared in newspapers and magazines around the world, and *People* magazine even named the world's first IVF child, Louise Brown, one of the 10 most prominent people of the decade, one who dominated it "by simple being."[6]

With developments occurring rapidly in noncoital reproduction, especially in the United States, Australia, and England, it seems prudent to reflect on the societal issues raised by these techniques and to assess their future. The policy problem is how to deal effectively "with a series of sequential challenges" to current clinical practices.[7] It will often be critical to make distinctions, usually previously irrelevant, between the genetics, the gestational, and the rearing parents when sorting out individual rights and responsibilities.[8] Indeed, it is now possible for a child to have five parents: a genetic and rearing father and a genetic, gestational, and rearing mother.[9]

Although it would be possible to explore all of the potential methods of noncoital reproduction, including artificial insemination by the husband (AIH), ovum donation, and the various combinations possible, such as IVF, SET, and frozen embryos with implantation in a surrogate mother (so-called full surrogacy), we have chosen to concentrate on the methods that present society with the most difficult generic problems. AIH, for example, poses no problems of identifying the rearing parents or any issues regarding the sperm donor, and so it is *much* less problematic than artificial insemination by a donor (AID) itself. Similarly, the issues involved in ovum donation are so analogous to those involved in AID, that a separate consideration would be redundant. The issues involved in the myriad of possible combinations can likewise be addressed by looking at the individual methods themselves.

In reviewing the social policy issues raised by these methods, we have found it useful to construct a table that summarizes them (Table I). In this table, we list the most important policy issues raised by these techniques, and in the cells, we assign values to their importance. The values assigned represent our view of the normative importance of each issue in the context of a specific noncoital method of reproduction. We do not contend that these values are unambiguous or incontrovertible, but we believe that the attempt to quantify provides a useful impressionistic model to compare and contrast the relative social importance of the issues raised by each technique. A cursory examination of the table explains, for example, why we begin our discussion with IVF rather than AID.

In Vitro Fertilization

Although IVF requires highly sophisticated biomedical technology, when confined to married couples (using an ovum of the wife and the sperm of the husband) IVF actually presents far fewer societal problems than AID, because the genetic, gestational, and rearing parents are identical. Accordingly, IVF rather than AID should be used as the starting point for any analysis of the social policy implications of noncoital reproduction. Nonetheless, because the ovum is obtained either by laparoscopy or percutaneous transcystic follicle aspiration (both entailing risks), and because of the extracorporeal fertilization of the ovum and the temporary *in vitro* development of the conceptus, new issues are

TABLE I. Index of Relative Importance of Societal Issues in Noncoital Reproduction

	AID	Surrogate mother	IVF	SET	Frozen embryo
Potential for noninfertility use	2	2	2	2	3
Protection of embryo	0	0	3	3	3
Identification of mother	0	3	0	3	3
Identification of father	2	2	0	2	3
Donor screening	2	2	0	2	3
Donor anonymity	2	2	0	2	2
Opportunities for commercialization	1	3	0	3	3
Total	9	14	5	17	19

Note: 1 = of societal concern, but not sufficient to require uniform guidelines. 2 = of sufficient societal concern to require uniform guidelines. 3 = of sufficient societal concern to justify prohibiting or discouraging the procedure altogether if reasonable uniform guidelines cannot be agreed on and enforced. *Potential for noninfertility use:* use of the technology to gain access to the embryo for research or genetic manipulation; avoidance of pregnancy for "convenience" of the genetic mother; use of technique for eugenic purposes. *Protection of the embryo:* exposure of the embryo to (1) the potentially hostile laboratory environment; (2) research that would not directly benefit *that* embryo; and (3) use that would devalue the embryo and human life. *Identification of mother:* difficulty in distinguishing between the genetic mother and the gestational mother and determining who will be legally identified as the presumptive rearing mother. *Identification of father:* difficulty in distinguishing between the genetic father and the rearing father and determining who has legal responsibility for rearing the child. *Donor screening:* requirements for gamete donors and method of ensuring compliance. *Donor anonymity:* what records should be kept and by whom, and how access can be gained to them by the child. *Opportunities for commercialization:* buying and selling gametes, embryos or children, and the implications for society.

presented. The most controversial has been defining the steps that should be taken to protect the embryo. The former federal Ethics Advisory Board found the embryo "worthy of respect," and in at least two states, Massachusetts and Illinois, IVF was not done until local district attorneys indicated that they would not prosecute physicians under state fetal research laws as long as the physicians reimplanted all embryos.[11]

ARTIFICIAL INSEMINATION BY DONOR

Artificial insemination by donor (AID) has become widely accepted, and there are an estimated 250,000 AID children in the United States alone.[10] But familiarity has not resolved the societal issues raised by this technique. About half the states have enacted laws making the consenting husband of the woman inseminated the lawful father of the resulting child, but half have not. Controversy continues regarding the methods of selecting and screening donors, the use of single women as recipients, the types of records kept, and to what information, if any, the children should have about their genetic father. Nonetheless, AID is the accepted paradigm for all other methods of noncoital reproduction, as evidenced by commissions like those of Warnock and Waller.[3,4] It is an unfortunate paradigm, however, because it places the private contractual agreement among the participants regarding parental rights and responsibilities above the "best interests" of the child, and because it raises a series of societal issues, such as about legitimacy, lineage, and individual identity, that remain unresolved.[9,10]

SURROGATE MOTHERS

Surrogate motherhood, which relies not on new medical technology, but on lawyers as brokers, has received increased media attention in the past few years. This method employs a fertile woman who is artificially inseminated with the sperm of the husband of an infertile woman. The surrogate agrees to bear a child for the infertile couple and to turn it over to them at its birth, either by giving the child up for adoption or by relinquishing her parental rights.

This is a much more socially problematic practice than either AID or IVF because it raises new issues of maternity (the identity of rearing mother) and commercialization, as well as the older AID questions of paternity, donor screening, and donor anonymity. The maternity issue (i.e., identifying the woman with the legal right to rear the child) involves the surrogate's ability to change her mind and keep the child, and perhaps even to successfully sue the sperm donor for child support. The commercialism issue involves paying the surrogate for her "services," and whether or not such payment is properly seen as compensation for gestational services, or as "baby buying," an activity prohibited in almost all states.[11] Contracts with surrogates are not likely ever to be specifically enforceable against the surrogate, although a suit against her for money damages, should she change her mind and keep her child, might be successful. The lack of legislative or judicial recognition of the surrogate mother contract has been one of the major obstacles to increasing the popularity of this method. We believe that the potential problems, involving the protection of the child and the exploitation of all parties, are so critical that this inhibition should remain.

SURROGATE EMBRYO TRANSFER

The latest development in noncoital reproduction is surrogate embryo transfer (SET), and this technique provides a useful model for examining all of the social policy implications of noncoital reproduction. SET involves the nonsurgical recovery of an embryo by uterine lavage from a surrogate who has been artificially fertilized with the sperm of an infertile woman's husband, and the subsequent transfer of that embryo into the uterus of the infertile woman.[1] SET raises almost all of the issues of IVF and surrogate motherhood combined. We say "almost all" because the bonding and likelihood of the embryo donor's refusing to undergo the lavage procedure and retaining the pregnancy (should one result) is much less likely than the risk that a surrogate mother who carries the child to term will opt to keep it.[12] SET directly presents all of the other issues: indications, protection of the embryo, maternity, paternity, donor screening and anonymity, and commercialization.

Potential for Non-Infertility Use

SET has been introduced when there is the same indication that is used for the initial IVF trials: infertility in married couples due to irreparable fallopian-tube disease. Should the indications for noncoital reproduction remain strictly "medical" (i.e., the treatment of a disease or a dysfunction) or should they be available to anyone who wants to make use of them for their own purposes (e.g., because of being single woman or for convenience)? The use of noncoital reproduction for nonmedical reasons must be resolved on a broader base than medical practice, as the value of the traditional family unit and the relationship of childbearing to child rearing are not medical issues. Use of the traditional family unit to justify limiting these procedures to married couples may also be misplaced, as the "family unit" now includes multiple models, and society may want the indications for noncoital reproduction to conform to the real world rather than to the traditional ideal.

Protecting the Embryo: Parental Rights and Duties

We can assume that the embryo, once transferred into an otherwise infertile woman, is highly regarded by both the woman and her husband. In IVF, there would be no embryo without the *in vitro* beginnings and development, but SET actually jeopardizes the well-being or survival of an existing embryo by removing it from its "safe harbor" (i.e., the donor's uterus). The justification is that the embryo donor had no intention of having the child herself, and that the removal is just part of a larger procedure to attempt a pregnancy that otherwise would not have occurred. This justification simply restates the argument that "All we are doing is making babies," a laudable objective, but not an end that justifies any means, such as kidnapping, polygamy, or exposing the embryo to teratogens.

Who should have the authority to make decisions concerning the extracorporeal embryo? The understanding is that the embryo, once removed from the donor, will be transferred to the infertile wife. However, even with such a contract, the donor maintains the ability to continue the pregnancy. Once the embryo is transferred, the recipient contributes the gestational site and assumes the medical risks of pregnancy, and she should therefore have the final decision-making authority over the embryo. Because of her greater contribution and risk, and to provide certainty of identity and responsibility, at the time of birth the gestational mother (rather than the genetic mother) should also be deemed the child's legal mother for all purposes. [11]

The period of embryonic life that has received the greatest attention has been its brief extracorporeal existence. This *in vitro* period exposes the embryo to an artificial and potentially teratogenic or lethal environment and provides an opportunity for genetic engineering. The locus of decision-making authority during this period is undefined. An

Illinois statute requires the physican who performs IVF to assume the "care and custody" of the embryo, subject to the penalties of the child abuse statute should any harm befall it (Ill. Rev. Stat. Ch. 38 S 81-26(7), 1981). Presumably, this statute would also apply to the *in vitro* period of SET. Although ethically bound to follow through with transfer, the physician could destroy the embryo or transfer it to a woman other than the sperm donor's wife. It is our opinion that authority over the extracorporeal embryo should be with the sperm donor because he has contributed half the genetic complement and presumably has a higher regard for it as his future child than anyone else involved. Because his wife's pregnancy is the only justification for SET, only the sperm donor should have authority to do those things to the embryo that would promote this objective. Research and donation to another woman would not, so these activities would be beyond his authority.

Donor Selection

Donor selection has always been the most discussed issue in AID and remains a central issue in all forms of noncoital reproduction (except IVF with a married couple). When donors are selected on the basis of some particular trait or set of traits (e.g., medical students), we are making eugenic decisions. The question is how such decisions should be made. A Nobel Prize sperm bank has already been established, and a counterpart panel of ovum donors can be envisioned, as can catalogs of frozen embryos. Because most desirable genetic traits are polygenic and multifactorial, however, such banks are unlikely ever to be very popular or effective in producing individual traits in offspring, at least until the technology exists to clone specific embryos.

How should the women who will be used as donors in SET be selected? Fertility is obviously an important aspect, but should they already have had children? Should they be married, single, or divorced? What should their economic and social status be? What medical and genetic characteristics should rule them out as donors? What types of genetic and psychological screening tests should be performed, and who should perform them? What kinds of agreements regarding retained pregnancies and abortion should they be asked to make prior to the procedure? What relationships, if any, should the donor have with the child? None of these questions have self-evident answers, and all should be resolved before SET is made widely available.

Donor Anonymity and Record Keeping

The basic thrust of current AID policy is to protect the sperm donor from any claims that the resulting child might have on him.[10] This protection has been almost obsessional, and as a result, the interests of the child are usually given a lower priority. In SET, the issue is analogous: Does the child have a significant interest in knowing how it was conceived and implanted and, more important, who its genetic mother is? This is a difficult issue, but as the child has no voice in the matter, and as it may turn out to be an extremely important genetic and psychological issue to the child seeking information about his or her genetic heritage, records should be kept of all births in such a way that they can be matched with donors. We think that medical professionals should maintain these records. But if they refuse, legislation may be needed to require the deposit of these records with a court of relevant jurisdiction. The donor can effectively waive any right to access to such records, but no one should be able to effectively waive the child's future access to genetic, medical, and perhaps even personal information about the donor.[18] The objection that such a practice might make AID impossible seems misplaced. The only survey of donors that we have been able to locate found that 60% would donate even if their identity was made known to the resulting children.[13]

FROZEN EMBRYOS

It seems reasonable to freeze the embryo in SET, if the donee becomes ill or has an accident immediately before the planned transfer, or, in IVF, to preserve multiple embryos for use in subsequent cycles. In IVF, this procedure would eliminate the need for repeated laparoscopies to recover more ova should the initial pregnancy attempt fail. Freezing embryos, however, forces us to reexamine all of the issues raised by noncoital reproduction (see Table I), not because of freezing *per se*, but because freezing raises the possibility of transferring the embryo to a multitude of potential donees over an extended period of time. The recent case of a wealthy U.S. couple who died leaving two frozen embryos in Australia caused an international debate about the embryos' legal status and what should be done with them, including their possible implantation in a surrogate.[4,14] Other potential problems include the confusion of parental identity because the embryo may not be genetically related to either of its rearing parents; because frozen embryos could be implanted in surrogates for convenience; because embryos could be maintained for generations (raising the possibility of a woman's giving birth to her genetic aunt or uncle); because siblings could be born from different sets of parents; and because embryos could be removed from any women by means of the SET embryo-removal procedure and (when the technology is available) karyotyped, examined for nonchromosomal genetic defects, and discarded, treated, frozen for reimplantation during the woman's next cycle or at some future time, donated to another woman, or sold.

The possibility of frozen embryo banks, in which embryos are produced to order by matching the sperm and ovum of "ideal" types and are then sold to parents for genetic or eugenic purposes, raises concerns of commercialism. Even if we accept paying a surrogate mother for the "work" of pregnancy, we could still reject traffic in embryos because, in this case, there is absolutely no ambiguity about what is being bought and sold. We may even wish to go further and to require procedures similar to those used in the adoption of children when frozen embryos are used in "prenatal adoption," when neither prospective parent has contributed genetically to the embryo, although this seems extreme and confuses notions of "what will be" with "what is."

Before launching a regulatory initiative in the United States, however, it is useful to review steps taken recently on these issues in the United Kingdom and Australia.

GEORGE J. ANNAS AND SHERMAN ELIAS

United Kingdom

In July of 1984, the government-sponsored Warnock Commission, named after its chairperson, Dame Mary Warnock, issued its report, which made 63 specific recommendations: 33 involved a proposed licensing board to regulate clinical services and research; 7 involved the national health service's infertility program; and 23, for new British laws, included seven new crimes.[3] This approach is legal overkill, as it is at least premature to outlaw as criminal so many aspects of noncoital reproduction. The Warnock Commission, for example, proposed outlawing all aspects of surrogate motherhood, including for both profit and nonprofit organizations, and professional activities designed to "knowingly assist in the establishment of a surrogate pregnancy."

The commission was also upset about payment to sperm donors, ovum donors, and embryo donors but adopted a much more cautious approach to this problem. It recommended that legislation be "enacted to ensure there is no right of ownership in a human embryo" but stopped short of suggesting that the purchase and sale of genetic materials be outlawed, apparently because it believed that such a move would threaten the sperm supply for AID. Accordingly, its official recommendation was that "*Unauthorized* [by the state licensing authority] sale or purchase of human gametes or embryos should be made a criminal offence."[3] The commission did not suggest what guidelines the licensing commission should adopt, or if it should become involved in price setting for gametes and embryos. This matter awaits resolution.

Australia

The Australian Commission for the State of Victoria was, if anything, more aggressive than its British counterpart. Under the direction of law Professor Louis Waller, the commission issued reports in August 1983 and August 1984. These reports made a total of 54 recommendations, many of which were written into laws dealing with the status of children (passed May 15, 1984), and infertility (passed November 2, 1984). These laws continue the Australian ban on the sale of human tissues, including sperm, ova, and embryos, and they outlaw cloning, the fertilization of a human ovum with an animal gamete, the use of children's gametes, the mixing of sperm in AID, and all commercial forms of surrogate motherhood.

The infertility legislation also sets up a system of state regulation for AID, IVF, freezing and experimenting on embryos, counseling of participants, and required record keeping. In addition, a standing committee is created to study and report to the government about new developments in this field. One of the issues not yet considered in Australia by either the government or the Waller Commission, for example, is SET (which the Warnock Commission recommended "not be used at the present time"). The status-of-children legislation creates an unrebuttable presumption that the woman in whose womb a child gestates is the mother of that child. This, of course, will prove helpful to those engaged in SET but could be very discouraging to those who wish to foster surrogate motherhood.

On the issue that has received the most press coverage, the disposition of frozen embryos, the Warnock and Waller Commissions diverged considerably. The Waller Commission recommended that in the absence of specific instructions from the gamete donors, frozen embryos in storage should be destroyed on the death of the gamete donors. Warnock, on the other hand, recommended that their fate be determined by the storage facility, that they, in effect, be treated like unclaimed luggage. Although there are problems with both "solutions," the Waller approach seems more reasonable, as the interests of the gamete donors are superior to those of the storage facility.

THE UNITED STATES

We have no national commission like the Warnock or the Waller Commission in the United States, and the most recent attempt to set one up was vetoed by President Reagan in October 1984. On the other hand, our laws relating to parenthood and reproduction, like Australia's, and unlike the United Kingdom's, are primarily state laws. Accordingly, the debate about the appropriate legislative responses to the challenges of these noncoital methods of reproduction is already under way in many state capitals.

It is premature to attempt to answer all of the issues raised by these techniques, as they have not been adequately debated in public; but it is foolish not to act on those that can be relatively easily resolved. Of the three issues that generate the most concern (see Table I), two are capable of legislative solution now: identification of the mother and commercialization.

Identification of the Mother

Identification of the mother gets a higher "point value" in Table I than identifying the father because the mother plays a much more significant role than the father in the gestation and birth of the child. Unlike the father, for example, the gestational mother will always be present and easily identifiable at the moment of birth. The social policy issue is, as between the genetic and gestational mother, which will be *legally* presumed to have the right and obligation to rear the child. This situation will arise in SET, the use of surrogate mothers generally, and the use of donor (usually frozen) embryos. We believe that it is critical for the protection of both the mother and the child that the rearing mother be identifiable at the time of birth. Given this need for certainty, and the biological and psychological investment of the gestational mother in the child, we think that the Victoria Parliment was correct in codifying the traditional legal presumption: the gestational mother should be unrebuttably presumed to be the child's legal mother for all purposes. She may later agree to give the child up for adoption or otherwise relinquish her parental rights, but that decision is one that she will make as the child's legal mother. A state statute codifying this traditional legal presumption, and making it irrebutable, would be protective of both mother and child.

Commercialization

Surrogate motherhood has enough potential legal and personal problems surrounding it so that it is unlikely ever to become popular unless laws are passed that encourage it by clarifying its legal status. If the British and Australian commissions' conclusion that commercial surrogacy is likely to create more problems than it can possibly solve is correct, such laws should not be passed. On the other hand, laws banning surrogacy altogether seem both unnecessary and unwise. There should be no legal objection to a friend or relative's acting as a surrogate mother out of love or compassion; such a gift would remain priceless, and such altruism cannot be practically or reasonably prohibited in a pluralistic society that values autonomy and privacy. [15]

Similarly, it seems reasonable to permit embryo donation, but commerce in embryos seems wrong. There is an almost universal consensus that kidneys should not be bought and sold, and this consensus has recently been codified in federal law. [16] The arguments against the sale of human embryos are even more compelling. A commercial market in prefabricated, selected embryos would encourage us to view embryos as things or commodities that are simply a means to whatever ends we design, rather than as human entities without a market price. Ian Kennedy has argued that we know intuitively that a human embryo is more valuable than a hamster or some other experimental animal, and that is why we have trouble permitting experiments on human embryos. [17] Likewise, we know intuitively that the human embryo is more valuable than a kidney and of much more symbolic importance regarding human life: that is why we believe embryos should not be the subject of commerce.

Embryos, like babies from surrogate mothers, will be bought or sold, if at all, on the belief that they will produce a healthy child and, possibly, one of a certain physical type, IQ, stature, and so on. When the child is not born as warranted or guaranteed, what remedies will the buyer have against the seller? To accept it, to reject it, to return it for a refund or another "item"? The problem with commerce in human embryos is that the sale of human embryos can quickly become confused with the sale of human children. Accordingly, it seems reasonable to outlaw the sale of human embryos. The sale of sperm and ova does not present the same problem, but the Warnock and Waller Commissions may well have been on the right track in discouraging commerce in gametes, and in limiting payment to out-of-pocket and medical expenses. It may be time to experiment with other methods of recruiting sperm donors in the United States besides money. For example, couples who use AID could be required or requested to find one or more of their friends to act as sperm donors for other couples.

Other Issues

No commission (or any two authors) can solve all of the social policy issues raised by noncoital reproduction. Nonetheless, previous work and this discussion demonstrate both that noncoital reproduction decisions cannot survive in the private domain of infertility specialists, and that the AID–private contract paradigm is outdated and inadequate. We will need new guidelines, and even some new laws. These guidelines can and should be developed by professional associations with public participation, and a reasonable start has been made.[20,21] Both the courts and the legislatures are likely to look with favor on well-thought-out guidelines in this area. In formulating more comprehensive guidelines, we suggest the following as useful foundations:

- To protect the interests of the resulting children and the integrity of noncoital reproduction, primary consideration should always be given to the welfare and the "best interests" of the potential child, rather than to the donors, the infertile couple, or the physician or clinic.[10,11,18,19]
- To protect the interests of the resulting children, complete and accurate records should be kept of all participants, including the donors, so that the donors can be matched with offspring. These records should be kept confidential, but in a manner that makes future access by the children possible if this is determined to be in their best interests.[10]
- To protect all participants, uniform and complete standards for donor selection and screening, including genetic screening, should be developed and made public.[10,22]

CONCLUSIONS

Action on three levels is warranted: (1) a model state law designed to clearly define the legal identity of the rearing mother and father of all children, including those born to other than their genetic parents and to outlaw the sale of human embryos should be drafted, debated, and enacted; (2) professional organizations, with public participation, should develop and promulgate guidelines for sound clinical practice; and (3) a national body of experts in law, public policy, science, medicine, and ethics should be established to monitor developments in this area and to report annually to Congress and the individual states on the desirability of regulation and legislation.

At all levels, the primary focus of social policy formation should be on protecting the best interests of the children, even if their protection sometimes comes at the expense of some infertile couples and some gamete donors or sellers. This general policy is one that should help to protect basic societal values, and can provide noncoital reproduction itself societal legitimacy.

ACKNOWLEDGMENTS

The authors acknowledge the kind and thoughtful suggestions of Professors Leonard H. Glantz and John A. Robertson.

References

1. Bustillo, M., Buster, J. E., Cohen, S. W., *et al.*, Nonsurgical ovum transfer as a treatment in infertile women: Preliminary experience, *JAMA* **251**:1171–3 (1984).
2. *NY Times* (April 11, 1984), A16.
3. Department of Health and Social Security: Report of the Committee of Inquiry into Human Fertilization and Embryology, London (July 1984).
4. Committee to Consider the Social, Ethical and Legal Issues Arising from In Vitro Fertilization: Report on the Disposition of Embryos Produced by In Vitro Fertilization, Melbourne (Aug. 1984).
5. U.S. House of Representatives: Hearings on the Extracorporeal Embryo before the Investigations and Oversight Subcommittee of the Science and Technology Committee, August 8–9, 1984, U.S. Government Printing Office, Washington, DC (1984).
6. *People* (March 5, 1984), 73.
7. Grobstein, C., Flower, M., and Mendeloff, J., External human fertilization: An evaluation of policy, *Science* **222**:127–133 (1983).
8. Robertson, J. A., Procreative liberty and the control of conception, pregnancy, and childbirth, *Virginia Law Rev.* **69**:405–464 (1983).
9. Andrews, L., *New Conceptions*, St. Martins Press, New York (1984).
10. Annas, G. J., Fathers anonymous: Beyond the best interests of the sperm donor, *Family Law Q.* **14**:1–13 (1980).
11. Annas, G. J., and Elias, S., In vitro fertilization and embryo transfer: Medicolegal aspects of a new technique to create a family, *Family Law Q.* **17**:199–223 (1983).
12. Blumberg, G. G., Legal issues in nonsurgical human ovum transfer, *JAMA* **251**:1178–81 (1984).
13. Rowland, R., cited in Singer, P. and Wells, D., *The Reproductive Revolution*, Oxford University Press, New York (1984).
14. *Time* (July 2, 1984), 68.
15. Callahan, S., Callahan, D., eds. *Abortion: Understanding Differences.* Plenum Press, New York (1984).
16. Annas, G. J., Life, liberty and pursuit of organ sales, *Hastings Center Report* **14**:22–23 (1984).
17. Kennedy, I., Let the law take on test tube, *London Times* (May 26, 1984), 6.
18. Brahams, D., In-vitro fertilization and related research: Why parliament must legislate, *Lancet* **2**:736–739 (1983).
19. Wadlington, W., Artificial conception: The challenge for family law, *Virginia Law Rev.* **69**:465–514 (1983).
20. American Fertility Society, Ethical statement on in vitro fertilization, *Fertility and Sterility* **41**:12 (1984).
21. Royal College of Obstetricians and Gynecologists, Report of the RCOG ethics committee on in vitro fertilization and embryo replacement or transfer, London (March 1983).
22. Fraser, F. C., and Forse, R. A., On genetic screening of donors for artificial insemination, *Am. J. Genetics* **10**:399–405 (1981).

14

SOCIAL JUSTICE IN NEW REPRODUCTIVE TECHNIQUES

REBECCA DRESSER, J.D.
Assistant Professor
Center for Ethics, Medicine, and Public Issues
Baylor College of Medicine
Texas Medical Center
Houston, TX 77030

A woman hoping to conceive and bear a child learns from her physician that she is infertile. She undergoes corrective surgery, but the procedure is unsuccessful.[1] *In vitro* fertilization (IVF) offers this individual the opportunity to carry and deliver a child who would be genetically her own. Yet, she faces several obstacles to obtaining the procedure: a clinic waiting list of 3,000 patients[2]; approximate costs of $5,000–$7,500 for a 10%–20% chance of successful pregnancy[3]; complete or partial lack of insurance coverage for the service[4]; and the clinic's eligibility requirement that she demonstrate her sincere interest in parenthood and her membership in a stable marriage.[5]

Besides the practical hurdles, she must cope with the physical, social, and emotional components of infertility. She has become a member of a "silent minority" whose lives are dominated by "the burden of . . . involuntary childlessness."[6] As one infertility patient poignantly described the experience:

> Infertility is a blow to one's self esteem, a violation of one's privacy, a final exam on one's ability to cope, an affront to one's sense of justice, and a painful reminder that nothing can be taken for granted. Infertility is above all a wound—to one's body, one's psyche, to one's soul.[7]

This woman's predicament is shared by a substantial number of infertile individuals and couples who seek medical attention in hopes of overcoming their inability to reproduce.[8] In one sense, these people are fortunate. The health care system has responded to their demand for services by developing a broad array of methods for correcting infertility. Besides an expanded range of surgical and medical techniques,[9] artificial insemination, *in vitro* fertilization, and embryo transfer (ET) now enable certain infertile men and women to reproduce.[10] Other procedures, such as ovum donation, surrogate embryo transfer, and womb donation, are now technically feasible and may soon be available on a broader scale.[11]

But the advances in reproductive technology remain out of reach for a large percentage of the infertile. Diagnosing and correcting infertility can be an expensive endeavor, beyond the financial means of many individuals. And among those who can afford it, the demand for these services far exceeds the supply. Persons seeking access to the new reproductive technology must contend with cultural ideas on reproduction and child rearing that exert influence over allocation choices. Such attitudes play a significant role in determining the monetary support available for developing and providing this technology. They affect society's views both on the importance of experiencing genetic transfer, childbearing, and childbirth, and on the extent to which traditional adoption, with all its shortcomings, meets any societal obligation to assist individuals in becoming parents. They influence as well how resources are divided between such services as prenatal care for pregnant adolescents and the new interventions for correcting infertility.

Given the existence of new methods enabling infertile individuals to participate in various components of procreation, physicians, clinics, hospitals, insurance companies, and government agencies will inevitably set policies determining which persons, if any, may obtain the benefits of these techniques. These decision makers face the moral challenge of constructing a just system for distributing a scarce medical resource, which is, on the one hand, passionately desired by thousands of people in this country, yet, on the other, costly and of questionable rank in the hierarchy of urgently needed health-care interventions.

Do ethical principles of justice and fairness demand that we pursue the new technology with the goal of making it accessible to any infertile individual seeking to reproduce? Or do these considerations, instead, mandate forgoing such a policy in favor of one aimed at improving preventive and crisis medical-care programs? To investigate these questions, this chapter analyzes three subjects: (1) the place of the new reproductive techniques within the societal obligation to furnish health care; (2) systems of rationing the new techniques; and (3) the role of the government in setting policy on this matter. I refer most often to IVF and ET because the present allocation, rationing, and regulation of these procedures raise the chief issues relevant to social justice in health care distribution.

In this discussion, the term *societal obligation* refers to a general ethical responsibility shared by the community as a whole, including both public and private entities.[12] The term *allocation* refers to the distribution of resources to health-care programs at the aggregate level; *rationing* is the process by which individuals are selected as recipients from among a larger group of candidates seeking the services of an existing health-care program.[13]

Justice in Health Care Allocation

Social justice is rendered when people receive the burdens and benefits that they deserve or are owed.[14] A fundamental principle of distributive justice is to treat like cases alike and different cases differently in proportion to the relevant differences between them.[15] According to this principle, a just health-care system differentially distributes its resources solely on the basis of morally acceptable differences among individuals. Ethicists disagree on what constitute defensible criteria for the unequal distribution of health care goods. The matter is complex, but I will attempt to articulate the positions dominating the contemporary debate over justice and access to health care and to explain how at least one proponent of each of the general theories might describe a just system of access to the new reproductive techniques.

Utilitarians equate justice with utility.[16] Thus, it is just to pursue whatever social programs produce the greatest overall good. The question is empirical: If research demonstrates that health-care services satisfy human needs and desires comparatively more than do alternative social programs, then a just society will supply those services.[17] In this framework, unequal treatment of individuals is morally permissible if the aggregate harm that such treatment produces is less than the aggregate benefit that it produces.[18]

To ascertain whether justice requires health-care programs to include the new reproductive techniques, the utilitarian will seek empirical data: If utility is maximized through providing this form of health care to individuals, then a just society will make the new reproductive techniques available.[19] Cost–benefit and cost–effectiveness analyses furnish means by which researchers might compare, for example, the utility of supplying dialysis to all persons with end-stage renal disease with the utility of providing the new reproductive techniques to the infertile.[20] Without the requisite empirical study, it is impossible to know whether utilitarianism would support making the new reproductive technology available, but such an outcome is certainly possible, in light of the strong preferences held by many individuals to conceive and bear children.

Persons rejecting the utilitarian approach cite the presence of obvious measurement difficulties, especially those inherent in attempts to compare among individuals the degrees of utility that they obtain from various health-care and other social programs.[21] Critics of this approach argue as well that, although the utility principle may be helpful in determining the relative value of social goods, the special status of health care requires society to protect more carefully the interests of individuals when it allocates resources in this area.[22]

Libertarian theories of justice hold paramount the right to dispose of one's property freely and without coercion. This freedom overrides any conflicting societal interest in providing equal access to health care. For libertarians, the free market and its attendant inequities reign in a just health-care system.

The libertarian who formulates standards for just distribution of the new reproductive techniques will make three major points. First, as with health care in general, individuals who possess the resources to purchase access to this technology should have the freedom to do so.[23] Hence, it is unjust to limit the consumer's ability to use his or her surplus funds to buy whatever technology public or private development makes available. Second, health-care providers must be free to offer infertility services as they wish, without being hampered by external constraints such as licensing laws.[24] Government regulation ought to be limited to the minimum necessary to prevent fraud, injury, and abrogation of contracts.[25] Third, it is "literally theft" for the state to impose a system of taxation to support programs furnishing any sort of medical assistance to those without funds to purchase such services. [26]

Proponents of the remaining three perspectives on access to health care believe that a just society is obliged to supply all residents with some level of health-care services, notwithstanding the disutility or coercion that such a program might entail. Charles Fried, among others, endorsed a less extreme version of the libertarian position in his proposal for a system of limited coercive taxation to make available to all people a "decent minimum" of health care. [27] This approach accepts as just some inequality in health care, as it preserves for persons possessing surplus resources the opportunity to buy health care for themselves above the minimum level. Consequently, this sytem would always enable individuals with the necessary wealth to purchase the new reproductive techniques.

Would the decent minimum include access to the new reproductive technology? Fried believes that consumers are the best people to determine the content of the decent minimum. [28] He advocates creating a voucher system in which all individuals would receive a fixed sum to buy whatever health care they preferred. Given the fervent desire of many individuals to conceive and bear children, a number of people might well choose to spend their limited funds on infertility services rather than other forms of health care. Critics of this system point out the moral dilemmas that will inevitably arise when individuals who have depleted their resources need life-sustaining care. [29] As a result of this problem, writers adopting other perspectives grapple with the task of defining more objectively an acceptable level of universally available health care.

John Rawls's social contract theory is usually interpreted as assigning a high value to health-care access, but his work fails to specify clearly the priority of health care relative to other important social goods. [30] Other philosophers, however, have applied the theory to support the existence of a societal obligation to provide certain forms of health care. Norman Daniels has asserted that the Rawlsian principle of fair equality of opportunity should govern the availability of health care. [31] Opportunities open to disabled and diseased individuals are more restricted than "the normal opportunity range." [32] A system of health care should thus attempt to minimize such restrictions. To Daniels, disease and disability are "deviations from the natural functional organization of a typical member of a species." [33] Moreover, the normal opportunity range encompasses the various "life plans" that reasonable members of a society would select. [34] Health-care needs are ranked according to the constraints that they place on the normal opportunity range. [35] Because reproduction is a species-typical function and an essential component of the life plans of most people, Daniels's proposal counts infertility as a disease [36] and its treatment as among those that a just delivery system would offer. [37] His work, however, leaves unclear the exact rank of these techniques among the types of health care mandated by the fair-equality-of-opportunity principle.

Egalitarians believe that a just health-care system provides equal access to all persons. [38] In their view, the presence and types of disease or disorder are the only significant differences that justify administering different levels of health care to individuals. [39] For egalitarians, the importance of guaranteeing accessibility to all is great enough so that society may tax the wealthy to achieve this goal. [40]

To attain the egalitarian objective, policymakers must set the universally available level of health care either as high as is technologically feasible, which would drain the resources available for other social goods, or at some lower level, which would forbid or discourage the use of surplus wealth to develop and provide services above that level.[41] Egalitarians who acknowledge the constraints imposed by limited health-care resources agree that not every medically treatable condition can be included within the universal level of care.[42] Therefore, the relevant inquiry concerns whether or not access to the new reproductive techniques is an appropriate element of the health care that society is morally obligated to provide.

There are suggestions in the egalitarian literature that the new reproductive technology would receive a low rating compared with other health-care interventions. One egalitarian, Gene Outka, claimed that it is preferable for a society with finite health resources to discriminate based on illness categories rather than on ability to pay.[43] Categories receiving low priority could include illnesses with a low incidence and rehabilitation rate, in which intervention is expensive.[44] These criteria could exclude at least some methods of treating infertility, given the relatively infrequent occurrence of particular conditions and the cost and the low success rates of their treatment. Another egalitarian, Robert Veatch, expressly named IVF as a biomedical technology that might justly be excluded from the universally available health care.[45]

Critics of egalitarian theory argue that it is unfair and unjust to inhibit the development and the availability of particular health-care services merely because they are too specialized, too expensive, or too often unsuccessful to be supplied to everyone: "Granted that individuals are allowed to spend their after-taxes income on more frivolous items, why shouldn't they be allowed to spend it on health?"[46]

Moral philosophers constructing theories of justice and applying them to health-care distribution tend to speak in general terms. Each theory is intended as a "rough guide" for assessing the importance of health-care needs, rather than as a "practical handbook for health care planners."[47] As a consequence, many theorists fail to designate the importance of specific forms of health care, such as the new reproductive techniques. A number of speakers, however, have addressed the question of what position these particular interventions should occupy in a just health-care delivery system. These commentators often combine principles of the general theories of justice set forth above and may rely on additional ethical considerations that they believe are important.

Some ethicists question whether interventions to correct infertility ought to be classified as medical care, as opposed to a social service analogous to traditional adoption. Many believe that if reproductive techniques fail to qualify as health care, then these interventions join a group of other social services having less urgent claims on societal resources. These analyses begin by scrutinizing concepts of health and disease, for the definitions of these terms are controversial. *Health* may be described in terms of appropriate species functioning,[48] or as a state of physical well-being.[49] The World Health Organization has adopted an expansive definition: "Health is a state of complete physical, mental, and social well-being and not merely the absence of disease or infirmity."[50] According to these definitions, the inability to reproduce constitutes a departure from the healthy state, and treatment enabling the otherwise infertile to reproduce is an appropriate component of the health-care system. [51]

A few individuals, however, take a conflicting view. Leon Kass asserted that "Infertility is not a disease in the usual sense. . . . It is not life threatening or crippling, nor does it lead to detectable body damage."[52] Kass believes that procedures such as IVF and ET fall outside the proper purview of medicine because, instead of eradicating the underlying physical condition of infertility, they merely fulfill an individual's psychological desire to procreate. [53]

Others who debate the medical status of the new reproductive techniques inquire whether the wish to experience pregnancy or to transmit one's genetic characteristics is overstated in our society. [54] Even if infertility qualifies as a disease, is the need to develop and provide treatment for this condition as critical as the need for programs of crisis and preventive medicine? These challengers ask, "With limited resources should our country be pouring money into life-creating technologies when basic health needs go unmet?"[55]

Their points, however, are contested by several commentators who note that much of traditional medicine is intended to ameliorate unpleasant symptoms, rather than to eradicate underlying disease. [56] Thus, procedures such as IVF come "within the realm of traditional medical motivation—to remove a limitation on normal healthy life."[57] Many physicians apparently support this view, for the American Fertility Society has declared that, in particular circumstances, IVF is "the acceptable treatment for achieving pregnancy."[58] Finally, advocates of the new techniques believe that it is unjust to limit reproduction to persons lucky enough to possess the physical equipment for it. [59] If society can remedy the effects of the undeserved burden of infertility, a condition inflicting extreme suffering on thousands of men and women, then it is only just to do so.

Yet, even those who label infertility an illness deserving of medical attention might exclude at least some forms of its treatment from the health care that society should make available to everyone. As asserted by the President's Commission for the Study of Ethical Problems in Medicine and Biomedical and Behavioral Research, "the level of care deemed adequate should reflect a reasoned judgment not only about the impact of the condition on the welfare and opportunity of the individual but also about the efficacy and cost of the care that is available for them."[60] The present expense and low success rates characterizing IVF and ET might then justify their exclusion from the care universally available to the infertile. These factors could, instead, support utilitarian decisions to allocate resources to those forms of infertility treatment that would assist the greatest number of persons at the least cost. Gonorrhea is the most common cause of fallopian tube blockage; intervention to correct this source of infertility might benefit more people than can the complicated and costly IVF and ET procedure.[61] Furthermore, because gonorrhea is most prevalent among the poor, allocating funds to IVF and ET may discriminate against the infertile in low-income groups. [62] Mark Lappé has noted as well that investing medical resources in methods of initiating and sustaining pregnancy in otherwise infertile women may drain the funds available to assist women whose pregnancies are jeopardized by social conditions of poverty. [63]

In sum, in our pluralistic democratic society, various forms of health care will be included in the "adequate" or "decent minimum" category as a function of changing cultural attitudes and resource availability.[64] At this point, IVF, ET, ovum transfer, and the other new reproductive techniques seem to many of us to be exotic health-care frills.[65] They lack the status of established medical services, and they may be defeated in the present-day battles over the allocation of health-care resources.[66] Yet, it is possible that, as the incidence and efficacy of these techniques increase, and as control over other aspects of procreation expands, the population will come to see them as standard medical treatment, rightfully accessible to all.[67] Conversely, if the future brings continued scarcity of resources and extreme social concern about overpopulation, the plight of the acute and chronically ill, and the morally troubling aspects of the new reproductive techniques, then the procedures could eventually be reserved for the wealthy or could even be prohibited.

CRITERIA FOR RATIONING REPRODUCTIVE TECHNIQUES

Whatever allocation approach policymakers choose, the new reproductive techniques will probably remain a scarce resource in the near future. Programs offering procedures such as IVF and ET will set criteria for distributing these services among numerous applicants. What are just criteria for such rationing, and who should apply them?

Medical characteristics predicting successful intervention are the least controversial criteria for selecting who should receive health care.[68] These factors tend to be objective and easy to measure. They also help ensure that scarce resources will be distributed to the persons most able to benefit from them. Yet, commentators point out that even these factors may be biased and unfair, especially if they incorporate psychosocial assessments.[69] Thus, when British physicians choose IVF candidates based on "the sincerity of their intention to accept the duties and obligations of parenthood,"[70] we may question the fairness of such an approach.

Even an apparently straightforward medical-selection requirement such as the diagnosis of infertility can mask the application of value judgments.[71] Some adults are physically unequipped to conceive or bear children; others have acquired their sterility as a result of contracting sexually transmitted disease or exposure to environmental toxins.[72] A number of infertile people belong to couples in which both members are physically able to reproduce, but one is the carrier of a disabling genetic condition.[73] Still others are infertile because they previously decided to be sterilized or because they chose to forgo conception until their later reproductive years.[74] Many individuals are infertile simply because they lack the partner necessary to the customary methods of reproduction.[75] Finally, some people seeking access to the new reproductive techniques do so only after traditional adoption has proved unsatisfactory.[76] Differing value judgments about these groups are likely to influence physicians' selection of candidates who fulfill the infertility criterion.[77]

Some moral philosophers endorse the explicit incorporation of value judgments into selection criteria. They believe that utilitarian considerations entitle society to distribute its scarce resources to the persons most likely to contribute to its needs.[78] Others argue, however, that systems of rationing health care according to applicants' social value and contributions or fitness for parenthood risk arbitrariness and bias, for we lack consensual definitions of and objective tests for these qualities.[79] The Seattle experience in rationing dialysis according to social worth criteria demonstrated that the persons administering such a system resort too readily to intuitive judgments reflecting their class and ethnic backgrounds.[80]

Despite these concerns, existing IVF programs consider social worth in making rationing decisions. They typically require applicants to be legally married and to demonstrate that they can provide a stable environment for child rearing.[81] The marriage requirement may be challenged as unfair, in light of the growing cultural acceptance of single-parent and "blended" families, the lack of empirical evidence demonstrating that the marriage environment is necessary to healthful child rearing, and the value that procreation holds for some unmarried individuals.[82] A related issue is the availability of IVF and ET to married couples who require an ovum, sperm, or womb donor to reproduce. IVF clinics have been reluctant to perform the procedure if such third-party participation would be necessary, apparently because of an unwillingness to disturb the traditional reproductive unit.[83] Again, some would debate the fairness of a rationing system that disqualifies these couples from enjoying the genetic or gestational parenthood that they desire.[84]

The difficulties inherent in rationing according to social worth criteria have stimulated some ethicists to advocate a selection scheme based on randomization, lottery, or first come, first served.[85] These writers argue that the subjectivity and discrimination inherent in alternative rationing procedures make chance the fairest method of determining eligibility for scarce medical resources. Opponents, however, label this system arbitrary and unjust, on grounds that it fails both to reward individuals for their contributions to society and to distribute resources to those who can use them most efficiently.[86] IVF clinics have partially implemented chance selection criteria by maintaining first come, first served waiting lists of candidates who meet the programs' other rationing criteria.[87]

Lastly, the clinics now offering the new reproductive techniques employ what Rosenblatt called "traditional rationing."[88] In this system, priority is given to the candidates with the ability to pay for the services. Private medical-insurance programs generally cover none or only a portion of the costs of IVF, and public medical-assistance programs rarely provide funds for any infertility treatment.[89] As a consequence, access to IVF today is reserved for those who can afford the $3,000–$4,000 charge for each attempt, together with the travel costs and the salary losses, and other forms of treatment for infertility are typically denied to persons who lack their own funds or private insurance to pay for such treatment.

THE GOVERNMENT'S ROLE

The task of removing monetary and other barriers to health-care access commonly falls to the state. What role should the government take in allocating and rationing the new reproductive technology? The range of potential government involvement is broad, for it could incorporate elements of any of the theories of justice discussed previously. Besides philosophical theory, the U.S. Constitution sets standards against which the justice of various state actions must be evaluated.

First, the government might completely prohibit the new reproductive techniques. Such a move would deny to many persons the opportunity to reproduce because they were unfortunate enough to lose out in the natural lottery. Opponents of the ban would view it as an unjust distribution of burdens to infertile people. At minimum, those contesting the policy would argue that the state bears a heavy burden to justify prohibiting highly desired, technologically feasible reproductive services that the private sector is willing to make available. A government prohibition of the new reproductive methods might be supported by a showing of serious risk to parents or offspring, but thus far, no such evidence has surfaced.[90] The remaining grounds for a prohibition would rest on moral objections to embryo and ovum destruction and to alterations in the traditional patterns of reproduction and child rearing.[91] Whether or not these objections outweigh the interests that infertile individuals have in procreation is a point of contention in our pluralistic society. Yet, constitutional law decisions have given special protection to married couples' procreative autonomy.[92] This judicial protection indicates that infertile married couples could successfully challenge a government ban as unjust interference with a fundamental right unless the state could demonstrate a compelling need for the ban.[93] Prior court decisions suggest that the new reproductive techniques could be constitutionally prohibited only if the prohibition were necessary to prevent serious harm to parents or offspring.[94] A government ban of private research on the new reproductive technology would face the added burden of justifying an infringement of First Amendment rights.[95]

Second, the government could attempt to discourage private entities from offering the new reproductive techniques by imposing burdensome regulatory requirements on the private sector. For example, the state could set exorbitant licensing fees for IVF clinics. Unreasonably burdensome regulation could again be attacked by married couples as an unjust infringement of procreative autonomy. To withstand the challenge, the state would have to demonstrate that its regulations were necessary to advance an important state interest. As in the case of a complete prohibition, constitutional law would probably demand a government showing that the regulations were essential to prevent serious harm to participants in the reproductive procedures.[96]

Some government regulation of private programs, however, could meet the requisite showing. For instance, unless the IVF medical-team members possess certain training and experience, success rates are much lower than 15%–20%.[97] Thus, licensing criteria demanding that health-care workers conducting IVF programs demonstrate specific skills and knowledge are not unreasonable obstacles to the exercise of procreative autonomy.[98] State certificate-of-need legislation and appropriateness reviewed by health systems agencies are in this category as well.[99] Because such regulation encourages health planning and quality care, all perspectives, save the libertarian, would deem such government involvement sufficiently justified.

Several states have enacted legislation banning the payment of fees for adoption.[100] This government regulation could interfere with the ability of certain couples to reproduce using the new techniques. Those who require third-party collaboration may want to offer monetary compensation to encourage ovum, embryo, and womb donation. The asserted reasons for outlawing such compensation are to protect the offspring of collaborative reproduction and to prevent the exploitation of potential donors in extreme financial need.[101] But the prohibition actually rests on other, less compelling moral objectives, for there is no evidence that permitting fees in itself would endanger offspring conceived through these arrangements;[102] moreover, the state permits individuals to sell other physical products, such as blood and sperm.[103] Some writers also claim that choosing to donate an ovum, an embryo, or a womb is less subject to exploitation than is choosing to surrender a child for adoption.[104] Opponents may argue, then, that the state has insufficient justification to disallow payments for the donations necessary to enable certain couples to exercise their right to procreate using the new techniques.

Federal and state governments have, for the most part, taken a third path with respect to IVF: neutrality. U.S. Department of Health, Education, and Welfare regulations issued in 1975 set a moratorium on the federal funding of research involving human IVF.[105] Despite the 1979 Ethics Advisory Board report concluding that federal support of human IVF research would be ethically acceptable,[106] the U.S. Department of Health and Human Services has taken no action on the board's recommendations and has failed to process a 1977 proposal requesting support for IVF research.[107] This position may be criticized on grounds that the government's failure to support laboratory and clinical research on the new reproductive techniques is an unfair omission, given its heavy support of experimentation in other health-care areas.[108] On the other hand, the federal government has failed to inhibit the growth of numerous privately operated IVF centers, and the states have generally followed suit. Only in Massachusetts and Illinois has state legislation delayed the establishment of IVF clinics.[109] The present government position would probably withstand constitutional attack because, as the abortion funding cases indicate, the state has no affirmative obligation to furnish individuals with the means to exercise a constitutionally protected right.[110]

But those who include access to the new reproductive techniques as part of the health care guaranteed by a just society are discontented with the government's stance. In their view, current U.S. policy fails to recognize the extreme suffering that infertility inflicts on thousands of Americans.[111] In response to this genuine public need, they believe that the state should actively support laboratory and clinical investigations of methods of overcoming infertility.[112]

Finally, some commentators advocate an even more enthusiastic government policy on applications of the new reproductive techniques. Spokespersons for this approach argue that, besides allocating funds for the technology's development and improvement, the state ought to cover the costs of infertility treatment as part of its medical assistance programs.[113] Otherwise, low-income groups are unjustly denied an important opportunity accessible to persons with greater financial means.[114] These arguments gain strength on examination of an existing exception to the government's "neutral" stance toward IVF and ET. The federal government currently subsidizes some infertility treatment by exempting employers' contributions to health insurance from employees' taxable income and by permitting individuals to deduct from taxable income medical expenses greater than a certain percentage in income.[115] As a consequence of this tax policy, infertile individuals whose private insurance covers even a portion of the medical procedures' costs, together with those who are sufficiently wealthy to purchase the services outright, can receive indirect financial assistance from the federal government. The justice of this policy is highly debatable in light of the government's present unwillingness to provide funds to increase general accessibility to the new reproductive technology.[116]

Government involvement in programs offering the new reproductive techniques would expose to legal attack any rationing criteria based on social worth.[117] Thus, unmarried couples and single adults denied reproductive services could challenge their exclusion as violating due process or equal protection.[118] Given that court decisions have failed to include unmarried individuals within the family autonomy given special constitutional protection, the success of such challenges is uncertain.[119] Although some might argue that these restrictions lack even a rational basis, the state probably could demonstrate that the criteria were legitimate on general social-welfare grounds.[120]

Resolution of the controversy over the government's position on the new reproductive techniques, again, will reflect cultural judgments of what comprises an adequate or decent minimum of health care, as well as the need for public contributions to make such care available and the extent to which government funds can be devoted to health-care services.[121] As one indication of the current national opinion of IVF, a Harris poll conducted during the late 1970s revealed that, although the majority of respondents believed that IVF should be a treatment option, half of the group surveyed opposed federal funding of IVF research.[122] Existing cost constraints, together with popular attitudes toward the new reproductive techniques, create a likelihood that the government will channel support to other forms of health care in the immediate future. Change may be forthcoming, however, as the new technology's benefits become clear and individuals grow to expect its assistance in their quest to reproduce. These events could produce societal condemnation of a government policy that allocates significant resources to competing forms of health care, yet withholds support from procedures that would enable many citizens to participate in the personally and socially valued experience of reproduction.

CONCLUSION

Moral philosophers express a diversity of views on just distribution of the new reproductive techniques. Most ethicists agree that total prohibition would be unfair, although a few strongly dissent because of threats that they perceive to the sanctity of life and to the family structure. The issue of accessibility, however, is more unsettled. The panoply of pressing health-care and other social needs confronting society has convinced several commentators to give access to the new reproductive techniques low priority for inclusion among universally available services. Yet, there is also clear discomfort over reserving these procedures for the wealthy, a discomfort stemming from the belief that this unequal treatment on the basis of income is unjust. As a consequence, we can expect continuing debate on the justice of social policies affecting the availability of the new reproductive techniques.

ACKNOWLEDGMENTS

I thank Baruch A. Brody and John A. Robertson for their helpful comments.

REFERENCES AND NOTES

1. Estimates of success rates for surgery to correct tubal blockage range from 20% to 50%. See, generally, Walters, L., Human in vitro fertilization: A review of the ethical literature, *Hastings Cent. Rep.* **9**(4):23, 26 (1979).
2. Kolata, G., In vitro fertilization goes commercial, *Science* **221**:1160 (1983). The waiting period is shorter in some treatment programs. Address by Dr. Martin Quigley, Insights into Infertility Symposium, Houston TX (March 10, 1984) (two- to four-month waiting period at University of Texas Medical School at Houston).
3. Grobstein, C., Flower, M., and Mendeloff, J., External human fertilization: An evaluation of policy, *Science* **222**:127–30 (1983) (hereinafter cited as Grobstein). The cost figure includes nonmedical costs, such as transportation, lodging, and lost wages. *Id.* at 130. "Clinical" pregnancy rates may be higher, but many such pregnancies fail to culminate in live births. See Edwards, R., and Steptoe, P., Current status of in-vitro fertilisation and implantation of human embryos, *Lancet* **2**:1265 (1983).
4. See Walters, L., Ethical aspects of surrogate embryo transfer, *JAMA* **250**:2183, 2184 (1983). See also n. 89 and accompanying text *infra*.
5. See British Medical Association, Interim report on human in vitro fertilisation and embryo replacement and transfer, *Brit. Med. J.* **286**:1594 (1983); Marsh, F., and Self, D., In vitro fertilization: Moving from theory to therapy, *Hastings Cent. Rep.* **10**(3):5 (1980).
6. Infertility Network, Houston TX (Information Sheet, March 1984).
7. Address by Dr. Patricia Mahlstedt, Insights into Infertility Symposium, *supra* note 2 (quoting from material prepared by Resolve of Central New York).
8. See Grobstein, *supra* note 3, at 130 (estimating yearly U.S. candidate pool for IVF at 70,000). It is estimated that one in six couples of childbearing age in the United States is infertile at any given time. Infertility Network, *supra* note 6.
9. See Aral, S., and Cates, W., The increasing concern with infertility, *JAMA* **250**:2327, 2330 (1983).
10. See Jones, H., Variations on a theme, *JAMA* **250**:2182 (1983); Grobstein, *supra* note 3, at 127, 129.
11. See Jones, *supra* note 10; Walters, *supra* note 4; Grobstein, *supra* note 3, at 129; Robertson, J., Procreative liberty and the control of conception, pregnancy, and childbirth, *Va. L. Rev.* **69**:405, 422 (1983). See also Bustillo, M., Buster, J., Cohen, S., Thorneycroft, I., Simon, J., Boyers, S., Marshall, J., Seed, R., Louw, J., and Seed, R., Nonsurgical ovum transfer as a treatment in infertile women, *JAMA* **251**:1171 (1984).
12. President's Commission for the Study of Ethical Problems in Medicine and Biomedical and Behavioral Research, *Securing Access to Health Care*, **1**:4 (1983).
13. See Evans, R., Health care technology and the inevitability of resource allocation and rationing decisions, Part 2, *JAMA* **249**:2208–9 (1983).
14. Branson, R., Theories of justice and health care, in *Encyclopedia of Bioethics* (W. Reich, ed.), 630 (1978).
15. Feinberg, J., Justice, in *Encyclopedia of Bioethics*, *supra* note 14, at 802, 803.
16. Buchanan, A., Justice: A philosophical review, in *Justice and Health Care* (E. Shelp, ed.), 3, 4–6 (1981); Branson, *supra* note 14, at 631.
17. Buchanan, *supra* note 16, at 14–16; Feinberg, *supra* note 15, at 805.
18. Feinberg, *supra* note 15, at 805.

19. Buchanan, *supra* note 16, at 14–15.
20. See Evans, *supra* note 13, at 2208–9. See also Smith, P., Ethics and in-vitro fertilisation, *Brit. Med. J.* **284**:1287 (1982) (analogizing resource allocation issues raised by these two interventions).
21. See, e.g., Daniels, N., Health-care needs and distributive justice, *Phil. & Pub. Affairs* **10**:146, 161–2 (1981).
22. E.g., Daniels, N., A reply to some stern criticisms and a remark on health care rights, *J. Med. & Phil.* **8**:363, 369 (1983).
23. See Branson, *supra* note 14, at 632.
24. Ibid. See also Buchanan, *supra* note 16, at 17.
25. Buchanan, *supra* note 16, at 17.
26. Ibid.
27. Fried, C., Equality and rights in medical care, *Hastings Cent. Rep.* **6**(1):29 (1976). See also Buchanan, A., The right to a decent minimum of health care, in 2 *Securing Access to Health Care*, *supra* note 12, at 207.
28. Fried, *supra* note 27, at 33.
29. See Branson, *supra* note 14, at 633.
30. See Buchanan, *supra* note 16, at 17–19; Branson, *supra* note 14, at 634–5.
31. Daniels, *supra* note 21, at 160–1.
32. Ibid. at 158.
33. Ibid. at 155.
34. Ibid. at 158.
35. Ibid. at 159.
36. Ibid. at 157.
37. See Stern, L., Opportunity and health care: Criticisms and suggestions, *J. Med. & Phil.* **8**:339, 340 (1983).
38. See generally Branson, *supra* note 14, at 635–6; Veatch, R., What is a "just" health care delivery?, in *Ethics and Health Policy* (R. Veatch and R. Branson, eds.), 127–9 (1976).
39. See Branson, *supra* note 14, at 635.
40. See Veatch, *supra* note 38, at 150–1.
41. Buchanan, *supra* note 27, at 212.
42. E.g., Veatch, *supra* note 38, at 141–2.
43. Outka, G., Social justice and equal access to health care, in *Ethics and Health Policy*, *supra* note 38, at 79, 92.
44. Ibid.
45. Veatch, *supra* note 38, at 141, 149.
46. Buchanan, *supra* note 27, at 212.
47. Daniels, *supra* note 22, at 363, 369.
48. E.g., Boorse, C., On the distinction between disease and illness, *Phil. & Pub. Affairs* **5**:49 (1975).
49. E.g., Callahan, D., The WHO definition of "health," *Hastings Cent. Studies* **1**(3):77 (1973).
50. Ibid.
51. See, generally, Singer, P., and Wells, D., *In vitro* fertilisation: The major issues, *J. Med. Ethics* **9**:192–3; Walters, *supra* note 1, at 26.
52. Kass, L., Babies by means of in vitro fertilization: Unethical experiments on the unborn?, *N. Engl. J. Med.* **285**:1174, 1176 (1971).
53. Ibid. at 1176–7. See also Kass, L., Making babies—The new biology and the "old" morality, *Public Int.* **26**:18, 26 (1972).
54. See Ethics Advisory Board, Report and Conclusions: HEW Support of Research Involving Human *In Vitro* Fertilization and Embryo Transfer, Department of Health, Education, and Welfare, 44 *Fed. Reg.* 35033 (June 18, 1979).
55. Hellegers, A., and McCormick, R., Unanswered questions on test tube life, *America* (August 19, 1978), 74, 77.
56. See, e.g., Gorovitz, S., *Doctors' Dilemmas*, pp. 176–7 (1982); Walters, *supra* note 1, at 26.
57. Grobstein, *supra* note 3, at 127.
58. Ibid. at 129.

59. See Robertson, *supra* note 11, at 428; Walters, *supra* note 1, at 39; Edwards, R., and Sharpe, D., Social values and research in human embryology, *Nature* **231**:87 (1971).
60. 1 *Securing Access to Health Care, supra* note 12, at 36.
61. Hellegers and McCormick, *supra* note 55, at 78.
62. Ibid.
63. Lappé, M., Justice and prenatal life, in *Justice and Health Care, supra* note 16, at 83, 92.
64. See Veatch, *supra* note 38, at 142 (adequate care defined by "human norms of healthiness").
65. Thus, some would say at this stage that we have no greater "right" to IVF than to an artificial heart or a heart transplant. Annas, G., and Elias, S., *In vitro* fertilization and embryo transfer: Medicolegal aspects of a new technique to create a family, *Fam. L. Q.* **17**:199, 212 (1983).
66. See Evans, *supra* note 13, Part 1, *JAMA* **249**:2047, 2051 (1983).
67. See Aral and Cates, *supra* note 9, at 2330–1, noting that the generation now entering its reproductive years is the first to be accustomed to having total control over fertility.
68. See Evans, *supra* note 13, at 2211; Childress, J., Rationing of medical treatment, in *Encyclopedia of Bioethics, supra* note 14, at 1414, 1415. The University of Texas IVF program, for example, requires female patients to be capable of regular ovulation and male patients to have sperm meeting certain criteria. Address by Dr. Quigley, *supra* note 2.
69. Childress, *supra* note 68, at 1414, 1415.
70. British Medical Association, *supra* note 5, at 1594.
71. See Robertson, *supra* note 11, at 430 n. 67 (noting social and economic influences on the condition of infertility); Comment, New reproductive technologies: The legal problem and a solution, *Tenn. L. Rev.* **49**:303, 310–11 (1982) (describing varieties of infertility).
72. Aral and Cates, *supra* note 9, at 2329.
73. Reilly, P., *Genetics, Law, and Social Policy*, Cambridge, Mass.: Harvard University Press (1977), 190–1.
74. Aral and Cates, *supra* note 9, at 2329–30.
75. See Hanscombe, G., The right to lesbian parenthood, *J. Med. Ethics* **9**:133 (1983); Bermel, J. The birth of a feminist sperm bank: New social agendas for AID, *Hastings Cent. Rep.* **13**(1):3–4 (1983).
76. See Ethics Advisory Board, *supra* note 54, at 35052. Adopting a "healthy white infant" through a Houston adoption agency entails a wait of from 18 to 45 months and costs of $4,000–$15,000. Private adoptions can cost $30,000 and more; in addition they lack the legal protection conferred on agency adoption. Adoption agencies generally place children with adoptive parents of the same racial and ethnic backgrounds, although international adoption agencies will arrange for transracial and transethnic adoptions. The waiting period is greatly reduced if the adoptive parents will accept children over 9 years old or children with permanent handicapping conditions. Agencies vary in the eligibility criteria that adoptive parents must meet. Some require working women to leave their jobs for a certain period, most require a legal marriage that has lasted from two to five years, many require "proof of infertility," and some require membership in a particular religion. Address by Lynn Waldman, M.S.W. and adoption agency employee, Insights into Infertility Symposium, *supra* note 2.
77. See, e.g., Ooms, T., and Steinfels, M., AID and the single welfare mother, *Hastings Cent. Rep.* **13**(1):22, 23 (1983).
78. See Childress, *supra* note 68, at 1415–7.
79. Ibid. See also Annas, G., Fathers anonymous: Beyond the best interests of the sperm donor, *Fam. L. Q.* **14**(1): 6–7 (criticizing procedures for the selection of sperm donors).
80. See Fox, R., and Swazey, J., *The Courage to Fail*, Chicago: University of Chicago Press (rev. ed. 1978), 226–65.
81. In a recent review, Grobstein and his colleagues found no IVF program in the United States that will perform the procedure for unmarried couples. Grobstein, *supra* note 3, at 132. See also Marsh and Self, *supra* note 5, at 5. A few physicians and clinics, however, will perform AID for single women. See Bermel, *supra* note 75; Curie-Cohen, M., Luttrell, L., and Shapiro, S., Current practice of artificial insemination by donor in the United States, *N. Eng. J. Med.* **300**:585 (1979).
82. See, generally, Robertson, *supra* note 11, at 418 and n. 36. As Samuel Gorovitz pointed out, one issue is whether the new reproductive techniques should be rationed on a model similar to the traditional adoption system, or whether its relationship to health care supports a less restrictive system. Gorovitz, *supra* note 56, at 100–06. Two authors have commented that IVF clinics have political reasons for

limiting services to married couples, for such a policy is more likely to encourage public acceptance of the procedure itself. Annas and Elias, *supra* note 65, at 211–12.

83. See Grobstein, *supra* note 3, at 131–2; Ethics Advisory Board, *supra* note 54, at 35057. But see Bustillo *et al.*, *supra* note 11 (reporting the birth of an infant to an infertile woman following the transfer of an *in vivo* fertilized donated ovum).

84. See Robertson, J., Surrogate mothers: Not so novel after all, *Hastings Cent. Rep.* **13**(5):28 (1983); Somerville, M., Birth technology, parenting and "deviance," *Int'l J. L. & Psychiatry* **5**:123 (1982).

85. See Childress, *supra* note 68, at 1417.

86. Ibid. at 1416.

87. See Kolata, *supra* note 2.

88. Rosenblatt, R., Rationing "normal" health care: The hidden legal issues, *Tex. L. Rev.* **59**:1401, 1403–04 (1981).

89. See Walters, *supra* note 4, at 2184; Kolata, *supra* note 2; Marsh and Self, *supra* note 5.

90. See Grobstein, *supra* note 3, at 128–9; Annas and Elias, *supra* note 65, at 206–07. But see Lorio, K., In vitro fertilization and embryo transfer: Fertile areas for litigation, *Southwest. L. J.* **35**:973, 981–2 (1982) (discussing the potential risks to offspring).

91. See Walters, *supra* note 1, at 24–5.

92. See Robertson, *supra* note 11, at 414–7.

93. Ibid. at 427–32; Lorio, *supra* note 90, at 1006–08.

94. Robertson, *supra* note 11, at 433–6; Lorio, *supra* note 90, at 1008.

95. See, generally, Robertson, J., The scientist's right to research: A constitutional analysis, *So. Calif. L. Rev.* **51**:1203 (1977).

96. See Robertson, *supra* note 11, at 433–6; Annas and Elias, *supra* note 65, at 208–210; Katz, B., Legal implications and regulation of *in vitro* fertilization, in *Genetics and the Law II* (A. Milunsky and G. Annas, eds.), pp. 351, 361–2.

97. See Grobstein, *supra* note 3, at 130; Kolata, *supra* note 2, at 1160–1.

98. See Robertson, *supra* note 11, at 433–4.

99. The Norfolk Clinic encountered opposition at its certificate-of-need hearing, but the state issued the certificate. See Marsh and Self, *supra* note 5.

100. See Note, Surrogate mothers: The legal issues, *Am. J. L. & Med.* **7**:323, 328–32.

101. See generally Robertson, *supra* note 84, at 32–3.

102. This risk could be addressed through careful screening procedures. See Robertson, *supra* note 11, at 460 n. 179; Walters, *supra* note 4, at 2184.

103. These practices have their critics, however. See, e.g., Annas, *supra* note 79, at 6–7 (criticizing current AID administration processes).

104. See Blumberg, Legal issues in nonsurgical human ovum transfer, *JAMA* **251**:1178, 1179–80 (1984); Robertson, *supra* note 84, at 33. But see Annas and Elias, *supra* note 65, at 221 (supporting a payment ban because it discourages the disturbing view of children as commodities).

105. See Grobstein, *supra* note 3, at 131.

106. Ethics Advisory Board, *supra* note 54, at 35056.

107. See Grobstein, *supra* note 3, at 131. Current federal regulations prohibit federal funding until IVF research proposals are reviewed by the Ethics Advisory Board. 45 C.F.R. §46.204(d) (1983). For a summary and critique of these events, see Abramowitz, S., A stalemate on test-tube baby research, *Hastings Cent. Rep.* **14**(1):5 (1984).

108. The federal government's inaction also limits public oversight of private research and practice in this area. See Brinkley, Uncertain present for in vitro fertilization, *N.Y. Times* (Feb. 5, 1984), §4 at 20, col. 1; Grobstein, *supra* note 3, at 132; Ethics Advisory Board, *supra* note 54, at 35052.

109. See Grobstein, *supra* note 3, at 131. But see Annas and Elias, *supra* note 65, at 208 n. 41 (Boston's district attorney has stated that, if all fertilized eggs are implanted in donor women, IVF would comply with the law).

110. See Blumstein, J., Rationing medical resources: A constitutional, legal, and policy analysis, *Tex. L. Rev.* **59**:1345, 1378–82 (1981).

111. See Walters, *supra* note 4, at 2184.

112. See Fox, M., Scientist quits NIH over fetal rules, *Science* **223**:916 (1984), Ethics Advisory Board, *supra* note 54, at 35045–6.

113. Ibid. at 35045–6, 35052.

114. But see Ooms and Steinfels, *supra* note 77.

115. See 1 *Securing Access to Health Care*, *supra* note 12, at 160–7.

116. Ibid. at 167.

117. See Blumstein, *supra* note 110, at 1357.

118. See Robertson, *supra* note 11, at 427–36.

119. Ibid. at 417–20, 432–3; Lorio, *supra* note 90, at 1009–11.

120. But see Shapiro, M., and Spece, R., *Bioethics and Law*, p. 530 (1981) (reporting a case settlement on the availability of AID to single women, in which a state university clinic agreed that marital status would no longer be used to determine eligibility).

121. See Ethics Advisory Board, *supra* note 54, at 35057 (the question of government funding must be settled in a larger context, in which political, scientific, economic, legal, and ethical material is considered).

122. See ibid. at 35053.

DISCUSSION

DR. LEE ROGERS: I was curious about the statement by Dr. Annas that the Seed brothers were seeking a patent for the process. Is that correct?

MR. GEORGE J. ANNAS: That's my understanding. I haven't seen a copy of the patent.

DR. LEE ROGERS: Do you know if this is the same process used for cattle-embryo transfers?

MR. GEORGE J. ANNAS: Substantially identical. I don't have any problem with the cattle process. I don't think that human reproduction should be patentable. That should be against public policy. If the patent is granted by the U.S. Patent Office, it should be challenged or ignored. It may be unconstitutional in any event, if a physician wanted to use these techniques to help an infertile couple.

MR. ROBERT GREENSTEIN: I've been a member of institutional review boards [IRB], and as a chairman in the past, I'm impressed with the apparent ease with which medical schools and universities accept *in vitro* fertilization in terms of its development within institutions. I'm also impressed with the parallel development of declining funds for research at the same time that there's the development of IVF. I have a similar concern about the development of chorion biopsy. Yesterday, we were talking about doing no harm at the same time as failing not to do good. I was impressed with Dr. Dresser's argument about the just allocation of resources, particularly because it represents the social pressure as opposed to the scientific one. I would like to ask whether or not IVF is human experimentation or research or both or neither?

MR. GEORGE J. ANNAS: My personal view is that we are still in the research phase, and my evidence is that the techniques are different in almost every center in the world, and in this country.

DR. JOSEPH M. HEALEY, JR.: At the very least, one is dealing with an experimental procedure. The question that was hinted at yesterday is one of the most difficult for an IRB: At what point is one dealing with an innovative therapy not subject to regulation, in contrast to an experimental procedure that is the subject of research? There is continued debate back and forth. At the very least, *in vitro* fertilization is an experimental procedure.

DR. AUBREY MILUNSKY: Where is the magic line at which experimental technologies become standard care? How does one draw that line?

DR. JOSEPH M. HEALEY, JR.: Again, it's among the most difficult questions presented to an institutional review board. I think the difficulty of the IRB's dealing with it reflects the absence of any clear line between the two. It's an issue of judgment, and very often, the IRB in evaluating a specific case takes into account the concrete risks and benefits that are involved in a particular situation rather than applying a preformed standard that somehow can provide a preformed answer.

DR. AUBREY MILUNSKY: In the real world, in doctors' offices, there are no IRBs. How do doctors know, in their own practices, when they can or cannot proceed with a new reproductive technology? What kinds of legal restraints are there? For example, I know of at least one operation in California that has already established a business for chorion villus biopsy.

A PARTICIPANT: I think the answer is that doctors don't know. This is part of the problem in regulating the whole area. What kind of regulation could respond to this ambiguity? The difficulty is that we do not know how best to avoid the problems, while simultaneously maintaining the vitality of science and the benefit of progress.

DR. AUBREY MILUNSKY: State departments of health in all states have the legal power to exercise constraint over the application of new technologies. No new laws are required. All the proper regulatory agencies are in place, though poorly funded. They regulate inadequately, and they certainly don't have the staff to do the job. They appear to be impotent. Do I have the wrong perspective?

MR. GEORGE J. ANNAS: The answer is yes and no. Certainly, the department of public health in most states has the authority to regulate clinics and hospitals, but most of them have no authority to regulate private doctor's offices, except in the most blatant circumstances. The same is true of the boards of registration in medicine. Even the U.S. Food and Drug Administration doesn't attempt to regulate the private relationships of one doctor with her or his patient, even in the experimental setting. So, probably, the answer is that it's only the medical malpractice system that the doctor has to fear if she or he is going to use these techniques in private practice.

DR. AUBREY MILUNSKY: So it is the threat of malpractice that is our most serious governing modality?

MR. GEORGE J. ANNAS: It's all we've got. And if you don't think the risks of liability are very high, it probably won't deter you.

DR. REBECCA DRESSER: One reason for this situation is that the federal government, which is the level most geared up to regulate research, has taken a "neutral" stance. We aren't able to regulate the IVF process as we are with other forms of research.

MR. R. ALTACHARO: You mention that you find embryo transfer capable of commercial uses even beyond those of artificial insemination. Given some of the similarities between the two, and the limited donor involvement, could you spell out in more detail the problems you see in commercializing the procedure? Do you think these problems are inherent in any kind of commercial arrangement, or are they simply a matter of allowing contractual arrangements to go on without limitations set by statute?

MR. GEORGE J. ANNAS: I'm not thrilled about the sale of any human tissue. If pressed, I would prefer the Australian system, which doesn't permit the sale of blood, sperm, or any other human tissue. Certainly, I'm not happy about the sale of kidneys or any other organ in the therapeutic context. Even if I thought that it was acceptable to sell sperm and blood—and many do; it hasn't resulted in the complete breakdown of our governmental system—I would still argue that it's not acceptable to sell embryos because I think they are special, and sales could have a tendency to cheapen our respect for the embryo, the child, and the family. Also, when you are engaged in embryo sales, you are creating a child that is going to have four parents. That's one problem that we haven't articulated in public policy as yet. We have a hard time defining the principle better than saying that we think that this may undermine our view of the value, the quality, and the sanctity of life or of the family. I don't think that, because we have a hard time articulating what we mean, we can conclude it's unimportant or doesn't exist. It's like love: I can't tell you what love is either, but I know this world would be a much poorer place without it. I think it would be a worse place with commercialized embryos.

MR. R. ALTACHARO: Would you feel the same if it was simply the sale of ova?

MR. GEORGE J. ANNAS: No, I think that if you accept the sale of sperm, the sale of ova is acceptable, too. I don't think you can distinguish them, except it's harder to get ova. If you want to price them, I would price them higher, because women have to take higher risks to "donate" them. If a system of surrogate ovum donors was set up, and an ovum instead of an embryo was flushed out, I'd feel different.

MS. MARTHA KNOPPERS: I have a question for Rebecca Dresser on the social worth judgments that pass as medical decisions. Suppose we have a couple who meet the age criteria (in other words, the woman is under 35) and who can make the proper financial arrangements and can prove a suitable relationship (all of which are questionable criteria in and of themselves). What interests me is the social worth aspect. Suppose this couple's infertility problem is due to either past abortion, sterilization, or venereal diseases. Can the physician selectively put such couples further down on the waiting list because of their voluntary assumption of risk, by having previously engaged in relationships that caused them to be ill or sterile? What kind of legal recourse would such couples have against the social criteria that pass as medical reasons for putting them lower down on the list?

DR. REBECCA DRESSER: I don't know of any IVF program that will accept people who are infertile because of a former sterilization. The criteria may become less stringent as more centers open. As far as legal recourse goes, I don't think that the person would have much of a chance. A private clinic has no obligation to meet any sort of constitutional requirements. The person would just have to engage in strong individual lobbying and face what may well be an unfair situation.

DR. JOSEPH M. HEALEY, JR.: There are analogous situations with artificial insemination. The question is whether a person who would be rejected as a recipient of sperm has any cause of action? There is also the question of the insemination of single women and the insemination of women in homosexual couples. If there is a contractual relationship or a voluntary relationship, the power of compelling the provider of services to respond to the request is just not currently legally recognized. As such, there's no viable strategy to compel the alteration of criteria with which one disagrees.

A PARTICIPANT: Shouldn't there be screening, as there is for sperm donors, and specified regulations imposed on physicians to ensure the just distribution of these techniques?

A PARTICIPANT: Yes, if we knew what we wanted to screen for before we enacted regulations.

DR. RUTH HUBBARD: Dr. Annas, in your rating of the appropriateness or inappropriateness of these different ways of reproduction, you left out the question of who controls. I wondered why you did that. Clearly, there's a real difference between artificial insemination by donor—sometimes obtained without any professional intervention or control—and IVF. With surrogate motherhood and IVF, as you pointed out, attorneys and physicians are pretty much in control. Why is that not one of your criteria?

MR. GEORGE J. ANNAS: I think it's reasonable to put the control issue in there. I was looking at legal and ethical components. I suppose you can make an argument that control is an ethical component. I think of it more as a societal one: The control issue is a sex issue. Most of the reproductive techniques are controlled by men; there's no question about that.

MS. BEVERLY FREEMAN: I was intrigued by some of the difficult issues that we are considering today. One is the ambivalence or difficulty of discussing these issues. Infertility is by itself very hard to talk about. I think that explains why it is very hard to give it the consideration that it deserves from an ethical standpoint. I do agree that that needs to be done before the legal issues are considered. I think that it's easy for physicians to relinquish the responsibility of considering these difficult issues to attorneys, who understand the directions in which we need to go. We all have a responsibility to look at those issues. The federal government will have a hard time because infertility is sexual and personal and it raises so many different feelings in the minds of the people when it's discussed. We need to confront those issues and be honest about them. I hope that the discussions about the ethical aspects of infertility will find a forum in the next few years, because they are terribly important at this juncture.

DR. LIVIA STRAUS: My question concerns the commercialization of sex and reproduction. Sex and reproduction have historically both been commercial for a very long time, through both prostitution and harem procedures, and in the United States, legally, through adoption procedures. One problem that I am having with some of the arguments is that I see a linkage between adoption and the use of certain procedures to stop people from being infertile. I wonder if we can really separate legislation on the two if we remove the emotional aspects.

MR. GEORGE J. ANNAS: Certainly, sex has been commercial. I like to think reproduction hasn't necessarily been commercial. One of the the things that all of these techniques do is to separate sex from reproduction. The techniques make that distinction, and we can make it, too. We don't have to be for or against prostitution to be for or against buying and selling gametes. The second question, the adoption issue, is very similar to the AID issue. The argument is that, because AID is acceptable, surrogate mothers and surrogate embryo transfers should also be acceptable. The other argument is that, if adoption is fine, all these other techniques for having a child should be available, too. The short answer, which may not be satisfactory, is that, just because obtaining a child one way is acceptable, another way is also acceptable. We all feel that infertile couples should have a right to a fair chance of having a child, but we don't think that they should be able to go out and kidnap children, and we don't think that they should be able to go out and buy children. So we recognize that some limits are appropriate.

DR. LIVIA STRAUS: I was addressing the issue of commercialism. In other words, we sell children through adoption agencies.

MR. GEORGE J. ANNAS: I don't think we do; at least, we don't admit that we do. Most states have laws against that. We do charge a fee for the adoption agency. But I would say that's not the same as baby selling. I certainly wouldn't want to use that as a precedent, to say that, because we buy children through public adoption agencies, therefore we should be able to buy them on the open market. I think that's wrong, and baby selling is wrong. Some argue quite vehemently that baby selling is acceptable. The rich find a child whom they really want and love. The child is better off and the poor family is better off because they get money instead of a child, who would be a financial drain on them. I think that this argument misses the point. It's the old story that the economist knows the price of everything and the value of nothing—selling children degrades and devalues human life, and that is the critical issue.

Having Other People's Babies

MODERATOR: RUTH MACKLIN

15

Surrogate Motherhood
Legal and Legislative Issues

Bernard M. Dickens, LL.M, Ph.D., LL.D.
Professor
Faculty of Law
University of Toronto
Toronto, Ontario, Canada M5S 2C5

Introduction: Types of Surrogate Motherhood

The biblical account of the Creation, in the first book of the Old Testament, includes details of arrangements by which women deliberately conceived children in order for them to be surrendered to the families of their natural fathers.[1] Although surrogate transactions by normal conception may thus be found at the genesis of Judeo-Christian culture, the emergence of the surrogate phenomenon in recent years has found the law unprepared. New reproductive technologies have added significantly to the potential for surrogacy and may make it more necessary for the law specifically to address an agreement, in written form and perhaps for payment, by which a woman bears a child for the purpose of surrendering it to be reared outside her own nuclear family.

Pressure to have resort to such arrangements is strong[2] and comes from a number of origins, a major source being female infertility. In response, many organizations are being formed to assist those seeking surrogate mothers of their children to meet and complete agreements with women willing to bear children for others.[3] It has been estimated that one in six and perhaps one in five couples of reproductive age experiences infertility.[4] The condition of infertility may be rather differently defined in medical, demographic, and popular usage and may include infecundity, pregnancy wastage, and, for instance, stillbirth. Further, primary infertility, where conception has never been achieved, may be distinguished from secondary infertility, where at least one conception has occurred but the couple is currently unable to achieve pregnancy.[5]

Causes of female infertility may include natural reproductive pathology and therapeutic removal of ovaries or the uterus. Other causes may be advanced age for childbearing, perhaps associated with late marriage or remarriage; effects of chemical or mechanical contraception, such as pelvic inflammatory disease associated with use of an intrauterine device, and effects of sexually transmitted diseases and spontaneous and induced abortion. Wider causes may include alcohol; tobacco; certain prescription, non-prescription, and illicit drugs; and some environmental and industrial pollutants. A more direct cause is voluntary sterilization and undertaken in an earlier marriage. Fertile couples may seek a second woman's services when the female partner cannot bear a pregnancy, such as when she is affected by a heart condition or chronic spontaneous abortion, or when she would transmit a harmful genetic or other congenital condition to a child she might conceive and bear.

A number of these conditions may be relieved by *in vitro* fertilization, perhaps employed in combination with ovum donation. A fertile woman who is unable to conceive because of deformity or disease of the fallopian tubes might thus have her ovum fertilized in the laboratory and replaced in her reproductive system for normal development. Further, a woman who is unable to ovulate or who decides, for genetic reasons, not to conceive her own child might acquire another woman's ovum for fertilization with her husband's sperm, so that the resulting product might be transplanted into her for normal gestation. The fertilization of a donated ovum might be *in vitro* but might also be *in vivo* followed by the recovery of the fertilized ovum by a lavage or flushing technique. The fertilization of the second woman would probably be by artificial insemination.

A simple division of the possible surrogate motherhood scenarios, which are distinguished by the feature that the woman who gestates and gives birth to a child does so in order to surrender it to another, covers instances in which

1. a woman is artifically inseminated *in vivo* by the sperm of a man, and on birth, the custody of her child is surrendered to the man's family;
2. a woman's extracted ovum is fertilized *in vitro*, the fertilized ovum is transplanted into the uterus of another woman who is able to bear a child, and on birth the child is surrendered to the woman whose ovum is fertilized;
3. a woman is fertilized *in vivo*, the fertilized ovum is flushed from her and transplanted into the uterus of another woman who is able to bear a child, and on birth the child is surrendered to the woman whose ovum is fertilized;
4. a woman's ovum is fertilized, either *in vitro* or *in vivo*, followed by recovery through flushing, and is transplanted into the uterus of a second woman; on birth, the child is surrendered to a third person, such as the wife of the man whose sperm are used for fertilization.

A variant may occur when a woman intends to be an ovum donor by submitting to artificial insemination with a view to yielding the *in vivo* fertilized ovum to flushing, but, because of unavoidable (or negligent) failure of retrieval of the fertilized ovum by this technique, she becomes pregnant and gestates the conceived child for surrender at birth to the intended social parents. Variants of fatherhood may be introduced by the engagement of perhaps anonymous sperm donors who are not the intended social fathers, and by considering fathers who are single or, for instance, in homosexual relationships.

An important semantic and genetic distinction, though perhaps of little legal significance,[6] may distinguish so-called surrogate mothers from true surrogate mothers. The former are fertilized *in vivo* and bear their own genetic children; in that sense, they are genuine mothers of their own progeny, although, in surrendering the children to their biological fathers' families, the women may act as surrogate wives. True surrogate mothers, on the other hand, receive the ova of other women, fertilized *in vitro* or *in vivo*, in order to gestate them for surrender on birth. If they receive such ova for the purpose of retaining custody of the children to whom they give birth, the genetic mothers may be considered the female equals of sperm donors for artificial insemination, who are not considered, in a social sense, true fathers.[7] The genetic link will be of secondary account, and the women who rear the children whom they bear may be considered true mothers. The proposition that the law regards as the mother the woman who bears and gives birth to a child has recently been expressed in the classical form *mater est quam gestatio demonstrat.*[8]

A simplified tabulation of the major means of legal parenthood is accordingly expressed in Table I. The table recognizes that, under the impact of reproductive technology, motherhood may be a collaborative enterprise involving genetic, uterine, and social functions, which may be discharged by different women. The law has come to recognize that a child may have separate genetic and social parents through adoption, including, for instance, stepparent adoption on the remarriage of a custodial natural parent, and equally that comparable distinctions may arise without formal legal procedures, such as when a mother's partner in a stable unmarried union assumes parental responsibilities toward her child conceived by another man. Accordingly, the prospect of surrogate motherhood may fit into existing patterns of legal analysis and adds only the separate dimension of uterine motherhood, which links genetic and social motherhood.

BACKGROUND MODELS

An initial difficulty in addressing surrogate motherhood arrangements is that they do not conform to known patterns of predictable behavior, and no language exists to describe the human and social relationships that they create. The relation of the surrogate mother to the biological father's wife is not simply expressed, particularly when the women know each other's identity and interact with each other before and during the pregnancy.[9] Further, it is unclear whether the surrogate mother's mother becomes a grandmother; whether her husband has a relationship to her child, which may be conceived with his prior consent and which may be her genetic child,[10] and whether her existing children have a sibling. We may easily describe such ties in biological terms, but this language may not do justice to the social and psychological perceptions that govern human and social interactions. Indeed, it has been seen that the popularly employed term *surrogate mother,*

TABLE I. Table of Reproductive Options

	Sperm	Ovum	Uterus	Means of conception	Intended child custody	Explanation
1.	H[a]	W	W	Natural	H & W	Normal conception
2.	H	W	W	AI	H & W	AI by husband
3.	H	W	W	IVF	H & W	IVF
4.	D	W	W	AI/IVF	H & W	Conception by sperm donor
5.	H	D	W	IVF or IV+F & ET[b]	H & W	Conception by ovum donor
6.	H	D1	D1	AI	H & W	"SM" & SPA by W
7.	H	W	D	Any & ET	H & W	SM & SPA by W
8.	H	D1	D2	Any & ET	H & W	Ovum donation, SM & SPA by W
9.	D	W	D	Any & ET	H & W	SM of W's ovum & adoption
10.	D	D	W	Any & ET	H & W	W bears (unrelated) child & SPA by H
11.	D	D1	D1	Any	H & W	Adoption
12.	D	D1	D2	Any & ET	H & W	Adoption
13.	F	M	M	Any	F & M	Child of the union
14.	F	D1	D1	Any	F	Father has child
15.	D	M	M	Any	M	Mother has child
16.	F	D1	D2	Any & ET	F	Father has true surrogate child
17.	D	M	D	Any & ET	M	Mother has true surrogate child
18.	D	D1	D2	Any & ET	D2	True surrogate has child
19.	D	D1	D1	Any	Third party	Adoption
20.	D	D1	D2	Any & ET	Third party	Adoption
21.	H	W	W	Posthumous AI/IVF	W	Widow has child
22.	H	W	D	Posthumous IVF/IV+F & ET	W	Widow has true surrogate child
23.	H	W	D	Posthumous IVF & ET	H	Widower has true surrogate child

[a]Husband and wife are used to describe those to whom the law attributes qualities of partners in a marriage, whether or not they have conformed to legal forms of celebration of marriage.

[b]The description of the conceptus as an embryo may be biologically inaccurate, as transplantation occurs before the embryonic stage of development, but the expression is employed in popular usage. Another, more accurate, word may nevertheless be desirable, as the word embryo may induce a distorting imagery.

Note. Abbreviations: H = husband (legal or common law); W = wife (legal or common law); D = donor of sperm, ovum, or uterine service; AI = artificial insemination; ET = embryo transplantation; "SM" = so-called surrogate motherhood; SM = surrogate motherhood; F = single father; M = single genetic mother; SPA = stepparent adoption; IVF = in vitro fertilization; IV+F = in vivo fertilization (by AI) and flushing; Any = natural conception, AI, IVF, or IV+F.

which is strictly a misnomer to describe the female role in the arrangements, has been widely publicized. The women in these early cases conceived, gestated, and gave birth to their own biological children. Further, gestating a child at its prenatal stage of life constitutes authentic motherhood, even if the child is genetically unrelated to its host. The expression has been fashioned by social purpose, however, to describe a woman who fulfills a motherhood function toward her own genetic child that the father's wife, the child's future social mother, cannot discharge. The biological authenticity of such motherhood is socially perceived to be secondary to its purpose in the anticipated social experience of the born child.

Present law reflects both the general uncertainty of society regarding the acceptability and the incidents of surrogate motherhood agreements, and ambivalence over the appropriate role and level of intervention of public authority embodied in law. It is questionable whether such agreements should be described as contracts, as they may lack the legal recognition and effect that such a description may imply. Legislatures are unclear about the approach that they should take, and courts, acting in default of adequate legislative direction, are uncertain of the models that they should apply. As the future jurisprudence is poised on the brink of its evolutionary surge, it may be appropriate to address background models in light of which surrogate motherhood may be assessed. None of these models fits adequately, but they expose principles from which some guidance may be taken. The available legal models are (1) natural reproduction (unregulated but recognized); (2) adoption (regulated and recognized); and (3) artificial insemination by donor (unregulated and, often, unrecognized).

Natural Reproduction

A basic legal postulate is of legislative nonintervention in competent adult reproductive choice, consistent with fundamental rights to privacy.[11] The constitutionality of involuntary sterilization laws regarding the mentally handicapped has been upheld[12] but is coming under mounting challenge.[13] The practice of sterilization is increasingly considered legitimate only when it is shown to be in the handicapped subject's best interests and to be an expression of the individual's privacy right.[14] Regarding competent adults, however, society tolerates the risk that "unsuitable" people may determine to conceive children by natural means, to be reared in a variety of social environments.[15] The law does not prescribe who may be a parent; by whom a woman may choose to become pregnant and in what circumstances; nor, in principle, who may rear his or her own child. If, at or after birth, children are found by the courts to be in need of care or protection, they may be placed under appropriate supervision, but administrative and judicial intervention must accord to the principles of due process and must involve clearly demonstrated contravention or prenotified standards of child guardians' conduct.[16] No prospective assessment justifies interference, however, with powers of natural conception and gestation.

Physicians undertaking hormone and comparable treatments to relieve patients' infertility and, for instance, repairing reproductive systems by such means as the microsurgical reconstruction of diseased or damaged fallopian tubes have no legal duty to inquire whether their patients are married or in stable relationships and would be genetically or otherwise suitable to act as parents. There are few indications that a child born into an adverse social setting could recover damages for dissatisfied life,[17] and an impaired child might have difficulty pursuing a wrongful life claim[18] against a physician who created or restored a parent's natural reproductive capacity.

Children born by natural conception are recognized in law as their parents' children without a requirement of judicial or other approval, and no more need be done to establish their parentage than is required by the normal process of birth registration. The practice of registration may focus on social appearances rather than genetic origins, and difficulty may be experienced in giving a child a desired surname, depending on the mother's married status and name. Subject to minor bureaucratic requirements, however, parents by natural conception normally face no obstacles or preconditions in achieving their mutual wish to have the child recognized as theirs.

Adoption

BY STRANGERS.   The model of taking an unrelated child into legal membership in one's family is almost a diametric reverse of the natural reproduction model. Applicants for adoptive parenthood are very carefully screened by public authorities and courts before orders finalizing adoption are made. Initial assessments may concern age, health, marital status and history, family structure and stability, and employment status and economic means. More refined assessments address the physical, material, emotional, and psychological environment in which a child might be placed, including scrutiny of the applicants' personalities, motives, tolerance, compatibility, and congeniality and their philosophical, religious, political, educational, and child-rearing convictions.

The criteria for approval may reflect a decreasing supply of adoptable children, and somewhat different standards may be applied regarding handicapped, older, mixed-race, and comparably hard-to-place children. The eligibility criteria for acceptance as potential adoptive parents of normally matched children may indeed be so demanding that couples may turn instead to surrogate motherhood transactions. The patterns of adoption preparation may vary between jurisdictions, but there is often a provisional placement of a child in a screened and approved home, and, after a given time, a report on the child's experience in the home is presented to a court. On adoption,[19] the child is legally integrated into the new family by judicial and related administrative measures, including the issuing of a new birth certificate.[20]

BY A STEPPARENT.   When a partner in a union wishes to regularize in law the relationship to the other partner's natural child, born perhaps in an earlier marriage or outside marriage, stepparent adoption may be appropriate. Because the child usually resides in the home by virtue of his or her link to the natural parent (and by virtue of that parent's responsibility to the child) and will remain there in any event, little screening of the applicant stepparent is usually undertaken. Faced with a *fait accompli*, the courts have little alternative but to grant the application. Indeed, obstructing a desired regularization of the relationship may prejudice the child's emotional and practical interests. Accordingly, although some level of administrative and judicial monitoring is undertaken, stepparent adoption is something of a legal formality intended to achieve, through a judicial process, legal recognition of a *de facto* relationship voluntarily assumed by the adult partner. On approval, the same consequences will result as follow normal adoption.

Artificial Insemination by Donor (AID)

AID may not present a true legal model of bringing a child into a family, as the legal results, as often as not, flow from default of a positive policy. The example illustrates the incidence, however, of an unregulated and therefore largely unrecognized but not prohibited procreative practice.

It is not clear that AID is any more the practice of medicine, which only approved health professionals may lawfully be able to undertake, than the natural conception it replaces.[21] Courts have experienced cases in which AID was undertaken in the absence of professional assistance.[22] Not only is AID often unregulated, but recognition of its use among married persons is frequently legally suppressed. In about half of the jurisdictions of the United States, legislation provides that a husband who gives consent before his wife's AID shall be deemed, for all legal purposes, to be the father of the resulting child.[23] Legislation legitimizing AID children reflects the disposition of the courts, in the absence of such legislation, to apply a tenacious presumption that the children born to a married woman living with her husband at conception or birth, or born within about 300 days of the husband's death, are the husband's children and accordingly legitimate. The general presumption of legitimacy may also be applied in less obvious cases,[24] in the children's perceived interests in enjoying legal status and known paternity.[25]

Participants in AID often have every incentive to maintain the legal appearance. Sperm donors have no intention of assuming, or becoming burdened with legal consequences of, paternity, and couples having resort to AID because of male infertility or risk of harmful genetic transmission are rarely keen to advertise or register the fact. Indeed, when women conceive children through specialized medical care, they may loosen contact with the medical specialists involved and present themselves to their general medical practitioners as women pregnant through their own husbands. Legislation or legal presumptions will permit birth registration in accordance with the social appearance of legitimacy. Whether the child is subsequently informed of its genetic origins is a private matter to be determined within the family.

Public disclosure of a child's AID origins may disruptively affect the child's status,[26] support entitlements, and, for instance, rights of legal inheritance. It may also lead to the identified donor's voluntarily or involuntarily becoming involved in the child's life. The child's health care may benefit, however, from tracing of the biological father and acquisition of knowledge of his genetic and medical record. Thus, the child's social interests and health interests may conflict. Private preservation of the donor's medical data may ease problems, but legal issues of access and confidentiality often remain unresolved where they are not governed by clear legislation.[27]

AID reflects the general liberty, disorder, and unpredictability of the unregulated free-enterprise system, with its strength of accommodating individual choices and its weakness of rendering the vulnerable self-reliant for protection of their interests. Suppression or disclosure of biological truths is largely a matter of individual choice and record-keeping practice, influenced by legislation (for instance, on birth registration), which advances a perception of children's stereotypical interests.

Discussion

These three models (natural reproduction, adoption composed of both stranger and stepparent adoption, and AID) relate to surrogate motherhood at a number of points. The privacy protection of natural reproduction may appear to be applicable to a woman's decision to serve as a surrogate mother (for instance, by the acceptance of artificial insemination), but the recipient couple may find that their privacy is limited by their decision to involve a third person in their reproductive choice.[28] The idea that sexual privacy is confined to two individuals is deeply ingrained in cultural standards, and sexual privacy appears to be protected in both its heterosexual and its homosexual forms only if it involves no more than two persons. The analogy with sexual activity may be inapposite, however, where asexual reproduction is involved.

The normal practice of AID is that an anonymous donor provides semen with no contact with or knowledge of the identity of the recipient woman, and her medical insemination is also undertaken in isolation. A surrogate transaction may involve a sperm donor and a recipient who know each other's identity, but often they do not. When aware of each other's identity, however, they often act apart from each other, even when fresh sperm are employed. Similarly, *in vitro* fertilization and AID for *in vivo* fertilization followed by flushing may involve solitary actors and medical professionals. It is irrational that the constitutional protection of asexual reproduction should be affected by the details of the style of the clinical management of its procedures.[29] In the absence of a socially shared and legally respected morality of asexual reproduction, however, it may be unavoidable to apply principles that are derived from the more traditional but functionally inapplicable model of natural reproduction.

The stranger adoption model arises to serve purposes that may be the reverse of those that inspire surrogate motherhood. Adoption involves an existing child seeking a family, whereas surrogate motherhood involves a family seeking a child. Nevertheless, experience derived from the management of adoption may affect official attitudes toward surrogate arrangements. Although infertility may lead couples toward the pursuit of this option, social work professionals and governmental welfare agencies may regard these arrangements as an alternative not to natural reproduction or to childlessness, but to adoption. It is indeed the case that one pressure toward surrogate motherhood comes from the scarcity, delays, and scrutiny involved in adoption. Social workers exercise a significant gatekeeping function regarding adoption, based on the best interests of the child available for placement. They may regard surrogate arrangements as a means of evading their role of screening potential parents, and of placing children in homes that would not necessarily qualify for the receipt of a child by adoption. Clearly, the standards required to be satisfied by adoptive parents tend to be demanding and would not be tolerated as a condition of natural reproduction. Surrogate arrangements offer a couple the additional satisfaction of a child to which at least one partner has made a genetic contribution. Public child-welfare officers may nevertheless be suspicious of an artificial means of conceiving children to be born into possibly undesirable homes over which such officers are denied a power of scrutiny and anticipatory prevention.

The stepparent adoption model relates more directly to surrogate agreements in which a woman surrenders to its biological father the child to which she has given birth. Because of his biological and legal paternity, the father does not have to adopt his child[30] nor seek the judicial or other approval for the discharge of his responsibilities toward the child. Further, the mother cannot be said to be abandoning her child in surrendering it to the care of its other legal parent and guardian. Once the child is in its father's care following a mutually approved surrogate birth, his wife will minister to the child's needs and assume the social and psychological role of mother. She may regularize her legal relationship to the child by initiating stepparent adoption proceedings. By an interplay of perhaps differently directed legislation, however, such proceedings may raise legal difficulties where the surrogate mother received payment.

Many jurisdictions attempt to foreclose on a potential market in babies[31] by legislating against the offer or receipt of money in return for a woman's consent necessary [32] for the adoption of her child. The aim is to prevent a woman from being induced by the offer of money to surrender a child (newly) born perhaps into circumstances of economic and social hardship. Equally, the legislation limits a woman's power to offer her child for sale. The legislation may be considered to go further, however, and to limit the power to conceive a child for sale. A surrogate motherhood arrangement may be viewed as the conception of a child for sale, notwithstanding that the child remains in the custody of its legal father. This interpretation rejects the view that the payment is for the service of gestation and focuses on the inclusion of consent to adoption. Although this reasoning and the related condemnation may be invoked against surrogate motherhood arrangements, it may be analytically dysfunctional. The key to condemnation exists in the adoption process, so that the arrangement cannot be condemned under such legislation where no adoption is intended. It may violate the best interests of the child, however, to be denied the regularization of its legal link to the woman who will continue to act as its social and psychological mother. Further, such condemnation would place single fathers and men in unmarried or homosexual unions at an advantage over those in regular marriages. It may accordingly be unsatisfactory to assess the legality of surrogate transactions solely by reference to legislation affecting the child's subsequent stepparent adoption, which is a relatively incidental aspect of the discharge of the surrogate agreement.

A middle ground may be identified between the close monitoring of stranger adoption and the almost automatic approval given to stepparent adoption because of the social *fait accompli* underlying it. A procedure of surrogate adoption may be developed,[33] based on the principle of preconception adoption, in which parties to a surrogate motherhood agreement present its terms to a court for approval of the transaction before any steps are taken to implement it. This procedure would respect the parties' privacy—and, in principle, their freedom of reproductive choice—compatibly with the model of natural reproduction, but the court could be more vigilant than in the approval of stepparent adoption because no child would exist at that stage. The function of the court would be primarily to satisfy itself that the parties were in true agreement,[34] that the surrogate mother was suitable for the discharge of her role, that the intended social parents were not unsuitable for theirs, and that the interests of the future child were adequately protected.

Prospective social parents would not be held to the high standards usually demanded of adoptive parents, and following judicial approval of the agreement, the birth of the child would be registered in their names, in accordance with the principles of amended birth recording following the making of routine adoption orders. Financial and other provisions of the agreement, including terms relating to enforceability and breach, would be subject to judicial scrutiny in order to ensure that nothing was agreed to that was injurious to the interests of the child or to public order; payment of the surrogate mother *per se* would not be a ground of disapproval.[35]

Legislation of this nature, providing for prior judicial approval of agreements as a condition of their recognition, may respect individual interests in participating in such agreements and social interests in due regulation. Comparably intended legislation on AID undertaken by physicians may ironically prove dysfunctional, however, where surrogate motherhood is concerned. Representative is the California Civil Code, which provides that

(a) If, under the supervision of a licensed physician and with the consent of her husband, a wife is inseminated artificially with semen donated by a man not her husband, the husband is treated in law as if he were the natural father of a child thereby conceived. . . .

(b) The donor of semen provided to a licensed physician for use in artificial insemination of a woman other than the donor's wife is treated in law as if he were not the natural father of a child thereby conceived.[36]

This provision permits parties to AID to achieve their mutual goals of the woman and her husband's having a child that is legally only theirs, and the donor's not becoming a legal parent. This result is clearly wise in light of a couple's wish to have their child through the use of donated sperm. It may be anticipated, however, that, despite the options of *in vitro* fertilization and *in vivo* fertilization followed by retrieval of the fertilized ovum by flushing, most surrogate motherhood agreements will rely on an application of the techniques of AID. If the surrogate mother is married, and her husband has consented to the artificial insemination with sperm donated by the intended social father, the legislation might operate with the effect that "the husband is treated in law as if he were the natural father," and the donor is denied any of the claims of a natural father.[37] Indeed, even in the absence of legislation, the legal presumption of the husband's paternity might have extraordinary strength.[38] It may be, however, that new blood tests, particularly HLA screening, could establish the child's paternity[39] in a way that courts would recognize and permit to rebut the normal presumption. Legislation would preclude this judicial option, however, and may obstruct surrogate motherhood agreements by compelling the biological father and his wife to initiate full stranger-adoption proceedings. Accordingly, unless artificial insemination for surrogate motherhood is distinguished from artificial insemination with simply donated sperm, legislation to regularize AID may be interpreted as obstructing an approach to surrogate motherhood that is equally respectful of the parties' intentions.

Approaches in Principle

Legislation aimed at addressing surrogate motherhood and other forms of artificial or nontraditional conception may be designed in accordance with a small number of broad conceptual approaches that may produce cohesive law with integrated refinements of detail. Based on the proposal of Walter Wadlington[40] these may be described as (1) the static approach; (2) the private ordering approach; and (3) state regulation approaches.

The Static Approach

This approach is socially and psychologically rather than legally static, and it is essentially conservative in orientation. It may center on principles of biology, of social form, or of both where they are not incompatible.

Biology dictates that children be governed by their genetic constitution, and that biological parenthood determine status and social role. A biologically static approach would not accommodate so-called surrogate motherhood in which the host mother serves also as the ovum donor, although it might be more sympathetic to ovum transfer from the woman intended to be the social mother to the child gestated and delivered by the true surrogate mother. Regarding biological confusion or infidelity, where a child does not share the biological lineage of both of its social parents, the biologically static approach might seek deterrence through penalties for and obstruction of the achievement of the participants' intentions. It might not feel compelled to moderate its hostility by fear of penalizing children by denying them the status and entitlements that they were conceived in order to enjoy. It might be unwilling, for instance, to accord genetically unrelated children rights of inheritance to the estates of the family members of their social parents, such as of the children's ostensible grandparents who left bequests not to them by name or precise description, but to the testators' own children's "children" or to their own children and, for instance, their "bodily heirs."

Social form centers on family solidarity and stability. It dictates that married women may properly bear children only of their husbands, that husbands may properly conceive children only through their wives, and that unmarried persons cannot be participants in legitimate reproduction. When children could be conceived only by sexual intercourse, these premises may have contributed to social stability. Their application to asexual reproduction is unsympathetic and, like the biologically static approach, might produce hardship not only for adult participants in surrogate transactions but also for children conceived by asexual means.

The Private Ordering Approach

This approach may lead to a libertarian extremity of the free-enterprise system of social ordering. It would recognize the sanctity of contracts; accommodate commercialism in the supply of sperm, ova, and surrogate services; and compel recognition in principle of whatever arrangements private persons may determine among themselves to govern the conception, prenatal carriage, birth, and custody of children. No contracts would be void as against public policy, as public policy would be to require and permit individuals to enter agreements reflecting individual preference and bargaining power.

In practice, where areas of private ordering are favored in principle by the law, such as areas concerning the sale of blood, sperm, and other body substances excluding organs, they tend to be moderated by legislation or by judicial constraints that hold certain agreements void on public policy grounds. Further, courts may be slow to interpret surrounding legislation sympathetically to a private purpose that they feel should be constrained.[41] The underlying emphasis of the approach is, however, that the state should restrain its restrictive interventions in private arrangements and should interpose its preferences only on demonstration of a legitimate interest and by due process of law. This might mean that paid surrogate arrangements would be free of control as part of individuals' freedom of reproductive choice, and that public intervention would be permitted only after the birth of children resulting from surrogate birth arrangements and according to judicially or legislatively determined criteria of the best interests of such existing children.

This approach may be compatible with emerging concepts of lowered governmental involvement in private affairs and with deregulation, in particular, of health services.[42] Influential advocates have come to urge that there should be reduced governmental, professional, and other paternalism,[43] reduced monitoring of private conduct and arrangements by public officers, and greater respect for individual choice. Not all who advance these concepts in the economic sphere would necessarily adhere to them in the domestic, moral, and reproductive spheres of human activity, however, and a clearly demonstrated need to protect the vulnerable by legislation may be accommodated. Children of surrogate transactions may seem to be vulnerable, but it is less clear whether women offering to act as ovum donors and/or surrogate mothers are equally vulnerable parties in need of protection. The contention that they may be induced by money to offer themselves to the burdens, risks, and pressures of pregnancy and the immediate postnatal surrender of the children they have borne, and should therefore be guarded by at least protective terms in agreements prescribed by legislation, may be countered by the contention that they should be free to agree to participate in such arrangements and to negotiate the most favorable terms they can. Ambivalence may be due to uncertainty whether surrogate motherhood is a moral covenant and responsibility, an industrial occupation, or a cottage industry. Whether or not legislative intervention is justifiable, however, the burden of argument would seem to fall heavily on those urging intervention to make the case for it.

State Regulation Approaches

THE PUNITIVE APPROACH.   Opposing the laissez-faire approach respectful of private ordering is an approach of strict state control by legal sanctions. It might aim at the total prohibition of surrogate transactions or at certain aspects of them, such as payment or, for instance, the recruitment of younger women having contractual capacity. The approach might be implemented through penalization of medical and health practitioners, other facilitators, gamete donors, and those seeking and offering children through surrogate agreements. Penalties might affect agencies advertising surrogate services, seeking services, or offering and contributing to services and those that conceal such services. Although public bodies such as the Law Reform Commission of Canada have urged restraint in the recourse to criminal law to achieve social consequences,[44] it remains a popular conviction among both the lay public and political officers that "there ought to be a law" to prohibit opposed conduct. It is a matter of judgment whether a legislative assembly considers it appropriate to make offenders of those who wish to have children; the prohibition under penalty against payment associated with consent to adoption has been upheld.[45]

Punitive models of legislation directed against surrogate motherhood could differ in ferocity and orientation. The more severe could apply harsh penalties to knowing participation in proscribed arrangements, holding professional and private persons and institutions to strict account for deployment of the genetic material and facilities under their control. Legislation could also be employed on the practice of medicine, on the conduct of counseling, and, primarily through civil law, on compensation payable to children born into disadvantaged social or psychological settings,[46] to deter surrogate arrangements. Less severe provisions might punish recourse to centers other than those approved according to demanding standards for the arrangement of surrogate agreements, on analogy with the licensed private adoption agencies that exist in some jurisdictions.

Punishment invites evasion by deceit, suppression or distortion of the truth, and, for instance, recourse to other jurisdictions where penalties do not apply. In the latter case, punitive laws might prove to be laws for the poor because persons of means might turn to services of which they may legitimately avail themselves in other than their normal jurisdictions of residence. Evidence shows that this is frequently the case regarding the management and execution of surrogate motherhood agreements.[47]

THE INDUCEMENT APPROACH. An alternative to the stick may be the carrot. Public regulation of surrogate motherhood transactions may be approached by encouraging resort to preferred practice by attaching advantages to it that do not naturally attach to, or which are expressly denied to, alternative practices. The promise of full or facilitated legal recognition of the birth of children born through the services of an appointed agency, for instance, or born under an agreement conforming to model terms and conditions, might induce prospective parents to turn to that agency or to employ that specified form of agreement. The inducement of legal approval of services rendered by or according to preferred means, as well as the disincentive of legal ineffectiveness or nonrecognition of alternative means, may operate to condition conscientious participants to conform to an acceptable model of surrogate motherhood. A limit of imposed ineffectiveness as a sanction for nonconformity may be, however, that harm would result to the legal, social, or psychological welfare of children born through the disfavored means.

An alternative may be to seek to induce resort to a particular procedure or agency by assuring the quality of its services. Without creating penalties for participants in agreements who resort to unapproved means, legislation might give special recognition and perhaps support to identified practitioners or agencies that demonstrate or conform to prenotified high standards. These might relate, for instance, to the recruitment of potential surrogate mothers, health and social checking of both the potential mothers and the social parents, scientific and related management of the insemination procedures, prenatal care and postpartum care of the mothers, and follow-up care of the social parents and the children. Particularly when the surrogate mother and the social parents remain anonymous, it may be a source of comfort to the latter to know that the surrogate mother is in good health and brings a quality of dedication to her role, and it may be reassuring to the surrogate mother to know that the child she has borne is going to conscientious parents and a good home life.

Whether government relies on independent accreditation of practitioners and agencies, prescribes standards of its own making that have to be observed as a condition of approval, or invites individuals and facilities to declare their professed standards and to request governmental approval is a matter of more refined specification. The inducement approach depends, however, on governmental assurance of the quality of services in order to encourage conscientious persons to pursue their surrogate motherhood intentions through arrangements that the government considers scientifically and socially adequate and ethically appropriate.

Approval patterns may include preconception recourse to the courts, to endorse the parties' intentions regarding conception and the future custody of children and to ensure that the birth registration will be in the names of the intended social parents.

Governmental identification of approved agencies might involve continuing the monitoring of standards through an inspection or a periodic review, perhaps on application for renewal of approval. Similarly, government may have to become involved in the control of financial charges for scientific and other services, lest the poor be unable to avail themselves of good quality practitioners and agencies on an equitable basis. Public protection and equity of access to services may therefore draw government into more intensive levels of regulation of approved services.

LEGAL ISSUES

Surrogate motherhood may be approached through AID techniques, *in vitro* fertilization and embryo transplantation, *in vivo* fertilization followed by recovery of the fertilized ovum by flushing and its transfer to another woman, and, indeed, through the fertilization of a woman by natural means, whether she continues her pregnancy for surrender of the child at birth or surrenders her fertilized ovum by submitting to flushing. The practice of surrogate motherhood therefore incorporates many of the legal problems raised by these separate reproductive processes and is accordingly burdened in principle by the weight of legal uncertainty attaching to these forms of reproductive conduct. The purpose of this part of the chapter is to state a number of legal issues of this nature, without undertaking to resolve them. Resolutions may be proposed in the wider literature, pitched either at a popular or general level,[48] at a more highly scholarly, legalistic level,[49] or at an interdisciplinary level integrating the perceptions and doctrines of related bodies of knowledge.[50] Further, resolutions may be left to the private ordering of the affected parties, be submitted for prior judicial approval (for instance, in surrogate adoption proceedings[51]), or be determined by legislation directed at surrogate motherhood transactions.

Some legal issues are of overarching concern because they affect the status of surrogate motherhood as an expression of, or as an affront to, basic legal values, especially regarding family recognition, structure, and functioning. Other legal issues are common to a number of artificial conception techniques, such as the parental status of mere gamete donors, and some issues are peculiar to a particular technology, such as whether the flushing of an ovum fertilized *in vivo* constitutes abortion. The following listings aim to identify a number of significant legal issues, and to place them within a relevant context.

(a) *Transcending Issues*

1. The right to surrogate motherhood as an aspect of legally protected privacy and freedom of reproductive choice.[52]
2. Surrogate motherhood for reward, as a violation of legislation against baby buying[53] and against payment for consent regarding adoption[54] or surrender of custody.[55]
3. Surrogate motherhood for reward, as a violation of legislation against slavery and trafficking in human beings.[56]
4. Transplantation of the ovum fertilized *in vitro* or *in vivo* into a surrogate mother as controlled embryonic or fetal research.[57]
5. Regulation of surrogate motherhood as a violation of international undertakings regarding rights to parenthood.[58]
6. Regulation of embryonic or fetal research and research on, for instance, *in vitro* fertilization, as a violation of international undertakings regarding scientific research and access to the benefits of science.[59]
7. Artificial insemination for the purpose of surrogate motherhood as an aspect of reproductive privacy,[60] or as the practice of medicine legally restricted to physicians and those acting under medical control.
8. Birth registration and genetic recording, determining whether legal policy on birth registration seeks genealogical accuracy or serves goals of social intentions and appearances.
9. Recognition of surrogate transactions made or executed in another jurisdiction or country, possibly according to principles offensive to the public policy of the social parents' jurisdiction of residence.
10. Maintenance of and access to (anonymous) medical records of genetic donors involved in surrogate births.
11. Maintenance of and access to details of genetic donors' personal identities.
12. Donors' access to information about the condition of children born of their donations.
13. Blood, tissue, and related testing of participants in and children born of surro-

gate transactions, to monitor that the pregnancy arose in accordance with their provisions and to determine the children's genetic parentage.

14. Wrongful conception and wrongful birth claims by women and social fathers, alleging, for instance, negligent disclosure by or screening of gamete donors leading to the conception, birth, or surrender of handicapped or inappropriate children.[61]

15. Wrongful life claims by children alleging, for instance, negligence in screening gamete donors or in handling the fertilized ovum *in vitro*, leading to birth with handicaps.[62]

16. "Dissatisfied life" claims by children alleging, for instance, their birth or surrender to inappropriately selected natural or social parents.[63]

17. Marital status requirements of participants in surrogate transactions, whether as gamete donors, surrogate mothers, or intended social parents, and formal requirements of spousal consent.

18. Public policy provisions on whether surrogate motherhood agreements may be recognized only when the intended social parents are medically unable to have their own child, or when they are socially unable to do so (for instance, when single or in homosexual unions), or when they wish to use the procedure primarily for convenience.

19. Public policy provisions on whether such agreements should be limited to childless couples or individuals.

20. Appeal rights of applicants for parenthood by surrogate arrangements who are denied access to services through public facilities.

(b) *Issues Related to Sperm and Ovum Donation*[64]

1. Genetic and related testing of donors and the legal standard of required care.[65]

2. Termination of parental responsibilities of the donors to their genetic offspring.

3. Termination of parental rights of the donors over their genetic offspring.

4. Status of donors' genetic offspring under intestacy law and general testamentary dispositions made by donors' relatives, such as their parents.

5. Status of children born of gamete donation under intestacy law and general testamentary dispositions made by the social parents' relatives, such as their parents, who are unaware of the children's origins in donation.

6. Retrospective operation of newly legislated provisions on access to medical and other records.

7. Payments to donors, for genetic materials or for the donation of services.[66]

8. Donors' negligent or other misrepresentation of medical histories, leading to unsuitable donor recruitment and births of impaired children.

9. Donors' negligent or other failure to disclose supervening unsuitability (for instance, because of venereal disease) contracted between screening approval and donation.

10. Donors' rights after donation to withdraw the donation or to prohibit its use for insemination.

11. Operation of (commercial) sperm and ovum banks.
12. Standards for the preservation of gametes in cryostorage.
13. Limits on the frequency of use of individual donors, or on the numbers of children born of their donations.
14. Reporting back to donors on handicaps attributable to them found in children born of their donations, for purposes of their own counseling.
15. Reporting back to inseminating physicians (and, for instance, sperm and ovum banks) any handicaps attributable to donors found in children born of their donations.
16. Reporting back to inseminating physicians (and, for instance, sperm and ovum banks) any handicaps attributable to donors found in children naturally conceived by the donors.
17. Legal minors as donors of sperm and ova, in general cases and in special cases, for instance, of matching unusual ethnic features.
18. Posthumous use of donated sperm and ova.
19. Consent of donors when, for instance, ova become available by means other than express donation for purposes of surrogate motherhood.[67]

(c) *Issues Related to* in Vitro *Fertilization and Embryo Transplantation*

1. Legal status of fertilized ova *ex utero*.[68]
2. Control of fertilized ova *ex utero*.[69]
3. Preservation of fertilized ova *ex utero* not destined for implantation.
4. Destruction and planned wastage of abnormal or surplus[70] fertilized ova *ex utero*: wrongful death liability.[71]
5. Intended surrogate mother's refusal or inability to receive fertilized *in vitro* ovum.
6. Research involving fertilized ova *ex utero* not destined for implantation.[72]
7. Implantation of ova fertilized *in vitro* dependent on gender.[73]
8. Transplantation of fertilized ova composed of donated sperm and donated ova.
9. Transplantation of multiple ova.[74]
10. Cryopreserved fertilized ova and the legal rule against perpetuities, affecting distribution of estates tied to "a life in being": the analogy of a child *en ventre sa mère*.[75]

(d) *Issues Related to* in Vivo *Fertilization, Flushing, and Transplantation*

1. Legal status of flushing procedures: contraception or abortion.[76]
2. Pregnancy of the intended donor of a fertilized ovum on failure of the flushing procedure: possible transition to surrogate motherhood agreements.
3. Relevant issues listed above under "Issues Related to *in Vitro* Fertilization and Embryo Transplantation."

(e) *Issues Related to Surrogate Motherhood*

1. Legal status, enforceability, and remedies or sanctions for breach of surrogate motherhood agreements.[77]

2. Professional misconduct of lawyers drafting agreements if clearly void as against public policy.[78]

3. Judicial or other compulsion of surrender of custody of children born to surrogate mothers under recognized agreements.

4. Time when intended social parents assume legal custody of children: birth or surrender of children, at blood or tissue testing confirming parenthood, or at some other time.

5. Change in material circumstances of intended social parents between surrogate mother's pregnancy and planned surrender of children (for instance, death or separation).

6. Standing of surrogate mothers to contest intended social parents' suitability to assume parental responsibilities, for instance, because of changed circumstances.

7. Exclusion of status of surrogate mothers' husbands and of related inheritance rights.

8. Status of intended social parents: for instance, married; unmarried but in a stable heterosexual union; married and in a stable union; single, or in a stable homosexual union.

9. Responsibility of medical or other professionals involved to screen prospective social parents by appropriate standards, in the best interests of the intended children.

10. Responsibility of medical or other professionals involved to screen prospective surrogate mothers.

11. Development of surrogate adoption[79] procedure for judicial approval of agreements before implementation.

12. Role of (anonymous) prospective surrogate mothers as coapplicants with intended social parents in surrogate adoption proceedings.

13. Standard of proof judicially required for approval of surrogate adoption applications.[80]

14. Payments in principle to surrogate mothers: legal status; control by legislation or, for instance, by judicially applied public policy.

15. Payments to surrogate mothers for services rendered, pain and suffering, medical and out-of-pocket expenses of selection screening and pregnancy, including childbirth, surrender of custody, loss of income and of earning opportunities, and so on.

16. Taxation of payments received,[81] and tax deductions for expenses incurred, in surrogate motherhood agreements.[82]

17. Provision for handicapped children born of surrogate motherhood agreements: confirmation of genetic parentage and the intended social parents' duty to receive surrender and accept responsibilities.

18. Determination of parental decision-makers on the birth of seriously impaired children eligible for life-sustaining medical care.

19. Provisions on the surrogate mother's spontaneous abortion or premature deliv-

ery of a nonviable fetus: minimization of risks, allocation of risks, financial and other effects on the parties.

20. Provisions on the surrogate mother's induced abortion: distinction between therapeutically indicated and not so indicated abortions, possibly equating the former with Item 19 above.

21. Separate legal representation for the parties to surrogate motherhood agreements; possibility of separate legal representation for the interests of the prospective children.

22. Life and health protection—for instance, through insurance policies—of surrogate mothers, including risks in pregnancy and delivery (for instance, of impairment of future childbearing capacity).

23. Arrangements should both intended social parents predecease the child's birth, for instance, in a common disaster. Compare Item 5 above.

24. Preservation of the surrogate mother's postsurrender interests in the child and its welfare.

25. Prenatal restrictions on the surrogate mother's activities, prenatal maintenance of nutritional standards, dietary prohibitions and supplements, and so on: enforceability and financial and other consequences of breach.

26. Provision for prenatal screening or diagnosis of children, and for their medical or other management in utero[83] indicated by the results of the screening or diagnosis.

27. Age restrictions on potential surrogate mothers, particularly lower age limits, and their capacity for free and informed consent.

28. Management of generational confusion, for instance, in a daughter's bearing her reproductively disabled mother's fertilized ovum for surrender on birth, and vice versa.

29. Provisions for the replacement of the surrogate mother where the intended woman becomes unsuitable or unwilling to serve between approval and the time for the transplantation of the fertilized ovum: preservation of fertilized ovum in cryostorage pending the finding and preparation of a replacement.

30. Control of agencies (private and/or public) arranging surrogate motherhood agreements; advertising, recruitment of prospective surrogate mothers, and so on.[84]

31. Provisions of the general law for the welfare of children born and surrendered under surrogate motherhood agreements complied with by the parties but made or executed in breach of law: minimizing the effects on such children's welfare of sanctions affecting the adult participants.

LEGISLATIVE APPROACHES

A perceptive observation was made some years ago regarding artificial insemination by donor that has proved to be true in that area, and may prove to be equally applicable to *in vitro* fertilization and surrogate motherhood agreements. In their 1966 study *Infertility in Women*, S. J. Kleegman and S. A. Kaufman noted that

> Any change in custom or practice in this emotionally charged area has always elicited a response from established custom and law of horrified negation at first; then negation without horror; then slow and gradual curiosity, study, evaluation, and finally a very slow but steady acceptance.[85]

A number of legislative bills have been introduced in the United States that together span the range from horrified negation to steady acceptance. These bills are based on an already-traditional perception of surrogate motherhood arrangements in which women conceive their own genetic children through artificial insemination in order to surrender custody, on the birth of the resulting children, to the sperm donors and their wives. Forms of true surrogate parenting and the use, for instance, of *in vitro* fertilization in surrogate transactions have not, to date, been addressed in express terms. Further, it is supposed that the intended social parents are infertile, rather than affected by genetic conditions that they wish not to transmit to children.

The first proposal to gain a favorable legislative vote was presented in the Senate of the State of Michigan[86] and was a penal measure. Sponsored by Senator Connie Binsfeld, Michigan Senate Bill No. 63 was passed on November 15, 1983, providing a new Section 45A and amending Section 69 of Chapter X of Act No. 288 of the Public Acts of 1939, being Section 710.69 of the Michigan Compiled Laws, reading:

> Sec. 45A.(1) A person shall not be a party to a contract or an agreement in which a female agrees to conceive a child through artificial insemination or otherwise and to voluntarily relinquish her parental rights to the child through the execution of a release or a consent. (2) A person shall not knowingly facilitate or aid other persons in entering into or carrying out a contract or an agreement of the type described in subsection (1).
> Sec. 69(2). A person who violates section 45A of this chapter shall, upon conviction, be guilty of a misdemeanor and shall be punished by imprisonment for 90 days or by a fine of $10,000, or both, and upon any subsequent conviction shall be guilty of a felony and shall be punished by imprisonment for 5 years or by a fine of $10,000, or both.

Similar was New Jersey Assembly Bill No. 3139, introduced on February 28, 1983, by Assemblyman S. M. Terry LaCorte, the essential provision of which was

> 2. No person, firm, partnership, corporation, association or agency shall participate in, agree to participate in, offer to participate in or materially assist in a surrogate mother arrangement in New Jersey.

upon sanction of punishment for a crime of the fourth degree.

In contrast, but with comparable directness, was Alaska's failed House Bill No. 498, introduced to the House of Representatives by Reps. Michael F. Beirne and Ray H. Metcalfe on April 14, 1981. Amending existing provisions on artificial insemination, its essential proposal was

> Section 1. A.S. 20.20 is amended by adding a new section to read:

Sec. 20.20.020. Conception by Agreement. A written agreement providing that a woman be impregnated by artificial insemination for the purpose of conceiving a child with sperm from a man other than her husband and providing compensation to the woman for bearing the child may be entered into and is enforceable according to its terms. A child born to a woman as a result of artificial insemination under an agreement entered into as provided in this section is considered for all purposes the natural and legitimate child of the man who furnished the sperm. The rights of a parent are relinquished by the woman and the relationship of parent and child as to the woman is terminated on birth of the child.

Sec. 2. This Act takes effect on the effective date of an Act[87] which requires reporting to the court any compensation or expenses paid to the mother of a child being adopted and which allows relinquishment of the parent and child relationship on payment to the mother of an agreed-on compensation for time and services in bearing the child.

Similar was House Bill No. 83H 6132, introduced in the Rhode Island General Assembly on March 10, 1983, by Rep. Harold D. Cutting, Jr. This bill proposed to amend Title 15 of the General Laws on Domestic Relations to add Chapter 16, providing that

15-16-2. Regulations and Guidelines. (A) All parties in a case involving a surrogate mother must agree to and sign a legal and binding contract. Parties include the surrogate mother and the adopting parents including the father of the child (if the adopting father is the donor). (B) This practice is to be viewed as a business venture. The surrogate mother shall receive compensation agreeable to all parties which is stated in the signed contract. The "rights of motherhood" do not apply to the surrogate mother. (C) All contracts must include a clause stating the rights and obligations of the adopting parents. This clause will include the guaranteed adoption of the child under any and all adverse conditions. These would include any abnormal birth or period of gestation resulting in an unhealthy child or a child born with birth defects.

15-16-3. Penalties. There are no penalties for violating these regulations. However, if a contract does not exist, the participating parties will follow the decision handed down by the court.

The support of private ordering evidenced in the Alaska and Rhode Island proposals stands in clear contrast to the punitive approach of the Michigan Senate and the New Jersey Assembly bill. Both these permissive and these prohibitive approaches leave many unanswered questions, however, and may suffer from a lack of necessary sophistication. The prohibitive approaches fail to address the welfare of and the consequences for children in fact born and surrendered in breach of the legislated prohibitions, apparently leaving the children to suffer for the wrongs of the parents. The permissive provisions, on the other hand, although not making criminals of those who wish to be parents, introduce no fine tuning of the conditions under which they may achieve their goals through surrogate motherhood agreements, and they offer the courts minimal guidance on the resolution of related legal issues.

Bills more adequate in this regard have been proposed in a number of States, including

1. California Assembly Bill No. 3771, introduced on April 6, 1982, by Assemblyman Michael Roos.[88]

2. Kansas Senate Bill No. 361, Session of 1983.
3. Michigan House (of Representatives) Bill No. 4114, introduced in February 1983 by Representative Richard Fitzpatrick.
4. Minnesota Legislature Bill No. H.F. 534, introduced on March 3, 1983, by Representative John Clawson *et al.*
5. New York Assembly Bills No. 5537/A proposed by Assemblymen Patrick Halpin and Alan Hevesi on March 1, 1983, and No. 6624 proposed by Assemblyman Hevesi on March 28, 1983.
6. Oregon House Bill 2693, and amendments suggested by Representative Nanette Farmer *et al.*
7. South Carolina House Bill No. H.3491 (later No. 2098), introduced by Representative Victor Rawl in January 1982.

Although too much significance should not be given to the specific provisions of such proposals—because most have already failed and survivors may further evolve within their own legislative assemblies, on the initiatives of the sponsors or of the committees that may be mandated to give them further attention—they are of interest in illustrating the types of provisions that have appeared in bills designed to regulate surrogate motherhood agreements in a more comprehensive fashion, and to address a number of the legal issues listed above. Particular proposals may be reviewed[89] in the context of the following issues.[90]

Definitions

Most bills deal with "natural fathers" whose semen is used for the artificial insemination of "surrogates." None addresses the use of donated sperm or ova, although separate legislation in some jurisdictions provides that a man whose wife is artificially inseminated with donated sperm with his consent shall be deemed the resulting child's natural father. This legislation does not govern a man whose wife is not inseminated, and it is not clear that a man consenting to the insemination of a surrogate mother with donated sperm can be regarded as approving the employment of "his" sperm. The link between the intended social father and the sperm used for a surrogate's insemination is defined in terms of genetics, not legal ownership or control of the sperm. Similarly, the underlying belief is that a surrogate will conceive her own genetic child, as the definitions speak of her being artificially "inseminated."

Age of Surrogate Mothers

The Kansas proposal requires prospective surrogates to be at least 21 years old when signing a contract, but the other proposals with an age limit require her to be at least 18 years old.

Other Limitations on Surrogate Mothers

The South Carolina proposal requires the parties to agreements to be state residents, and it requires that a surrogate have given birth to at least one child before entering an agreement. This second requirement may be intended not so much as a genetic check as an assurance that the surrogate's consent to bear a child is adequately informed by experience. Oregon proposals require medical screening for diseases or defects that are genetically transferable or that might otherwise affect the child, and the Kansas proposal eliminates, in addition, prospective surrogate mothers who are mentally ill or whose pregnancy would unreasonably endanger an unborn child or the life or health of the surrogate mother herself. It excludes a woman whose mental or physical health would be endangered in the opinion of a licensed social worker, a certified psychologist, or a board-certified psychiatrist. Most proposals bear no such limits, apparently leaving the issue to medical screening and the woman's self-care.

Age of Natural Fathers

Provisions addressing this issue require natural fathers to be at least 18 years old.

Other Limitations on Natural Fathers

The proposals of Kansas, South Carolina, and California expressly require the natural father to be married and to have his wife's consent to the transaction, but New York expressly precludes a construction of its proposal prohibiting unmarried males from entering into surrogate agreements. The Oregon and Minnesota proposals permit a single natural father, although in the latter state a physician aware that the inseminated person is a surrogate mother must be professionally satisfied that the father is mentally and physically suitable for the role. Other requirements in proposals more generally concern the father's mental health, free consent, medical health including venereal disease, and ability to care for a child. The California proposal also requires judicial review of any prospective parent's criminal record, and whether it may affect ability to function as a parent. The Michigan proposal requires prior counseling and evidence of the understanding of the fathers and their spouses regarding the consequences and responsibilities of parenthood through a surrogate.

Payments

Most proposals require payment provisions to be expressly included in contracts. The Kansas bill requires specification of the surrogate's service fee, of how it is to be paid, and of who is responsible for medical and other expenses. The Oregon, South Carolina, and California proposals require proportions of payments to be placed in trust accounts or escrow accounts, Oregon further specifying periodic releases for living and medical expenses. A New York proposal limits payments to medical and maternity expenses, reasonable attorney fees, and income actually lost, excluding any fee for acting as a surrogate, whereas Minnesota's bill requires that a maximum fee be set for the compensation of a surrogate, and that it not be less than $10,000. Michigan's proposal expressly allows payment for a surrogate's medical expenses and psychiatric and/or psychological expenses, including those for screening and counseling during pregnancy and after delivery, but precludes payment for the child itself and any reduction of payment on stillbirth or the live birth of an impaired child. The South Carolina bill requires terms in contracts that, if miscarriage occurs before the fifth month of pregnancy, no compensation other than medical expenses will be paid, and that later miscarriage will justify additional payment of 10% of the agreed-on compensation for a live birth.

The Michigan bill also requires that the natural father file a surety bond by a state-registered surety company to indemnify the state for any costs incurred for the care of the child born to a surrogate up to $100,000, and that no state programs or money shall be devoted to allowing parties to enter surrogate parenthood agreements.

Consents

Most proposals require the written consent of the natural father and his wife (see "Other Limitations on Natural Fathers" above) and of the surrogate mother and her husband (if any). The surrogate's consent is both to serve as such and to relinquish parental claims to the child born of the agreement. A number of bills expressly preclude a surrogate from acting as such if her husband declines signed consent. None addresses the consent of the legal but long separated husband, with whom the prospective surrogate has no or few dealings. California's bill precludes a surrogate's withdrawal of consent to an adoption made under a judicially approved surrogate agreement (see "Role of the Courts" below) unless extraordinary circumstances require it in the child's best interests. Michigan's bill permits a surrogate's revocation of consent and her initiation of child custody proceedings within 20 days of giving birth, although the natural father and his spouse will retain custody pending the action.

Paternity Testing

Few proposals address the issue of paternity testing. The bills proposed in New York and Michigan require blood- or tissue-typing tests, not later than 24 hours (3 days in the Minnesota bill) from the child's birth, of the natural father, the child, the surrogate, and her husband. Under New York's proposal, the natural father can demand testing in order to deny paternity, and under Minnesota's bill, the surrogate's husband may assert paternity.

Children's Status

Most proposals provide that children born of approved agreements shall be legally considered in all respects to be the children of the natural fathers and their spouses, who will each have from birth the full rights and responsibilities of natural parents. The South Carolina proposal initiates such rights and responsibilities on making a final decree of surrogate adoption.

Birth Registration

Most proposals provide for the birth registration under an approved surrogate agreement to be in the names of the natural father and his spouse, some requiring filing of the agreement, showing the surrogate's name, but the sealing of this document and its opening only under court order. The Kansas and Michigan proposals would allow surrogate children to demand opening when they are of legal age. The South Carolina bill would follow adoption practice after a final decree of surrogate adoption, and would require the filing of an original certificate of birth showing the natural father and his wife as the real parents.

Legal Representation

Proposals addressing the issue require separate legal representation, during the arrangement of agreements, of the prospective natural father and the surrogate mother. None requires separate representation between husbands and wives nor mentions representation of the legal interests of the future children.

Physicians' Responsibilities

See "Other Limitations on Surrogate Mothers" and "Other Limitations on Natural Fathers" above. The Kansas proposal expressly requires an assurance of the prospective surrogate mother's fertility. A number of proposals require medical certification of the undertaking of artificial insemination on surrogates with the natural father's sperm. South Carolina's bill requires physicians to file notice with the court, sending copies to all parties or their attorneys, on verification of pregnancy under surrogate motherhood agreements.

Contract Terms

Only Oregon's bill is silent about required terms of surrogate contracts. The other bills specify, in differing degrees of detail, the terms that must be included, usually providing that the required details not be exhaustive. Terms affect such issues as fees and payments, the consent of parties, the relinquishment of the surrogate's rights and acquisition of custody, and the rights and responsibilities of the natural father and his spouse. Terms may also address medical examinations and care, married and other surrogates' abstinence from sexual intercourse from specified times until positive pregnancy tests or termination of contracts, and provisions on blood- and tissue-typing tests. The Minnesota bill requires the surrogate's express assumption of risks, including of death, which are incident to conception, pregnancy, childbirth, and postpartum complications. South Carolina's bill requires the express assumption of such risks by the surrogate and her husband, as well as the surrogate's express undertaking not to abort unless she receives advice by the inseminating physician that an abortion is necessary for her physical health.

Prenatal Death of Natural Fathers

The bills addressing this issue provide for the spouse of the natural father to assume all rights and responsibilities for the child if the father dies before the child's birth, and vice versa if the spouse dies earlier than such a birth. The Minnesota and South Carolina bills further provide that if both the natural father and his spouse die, the surrogate may recover full compensation as agreed and elect to keep the child or consent to its adoption. The Oregon bill provides that, when the natural father predeceases the child's birth, the child shall share in his estate as if naturally and legitimately conceived.

Home Studies

The bills of Minnesota and South Carolina, based on a surrogate adoption concept, require favorable home studies as a condition of the approval of surrogate motherhood agreements. California's bill also requires court-approved agencies to recommend approval of the intended social parents following home studies.

Role of the Courts

Most bills require the filing of contracts or consents in the appropriate courts or registries as a condition of their recognition and enforceability, the documents being unavailable to the general public. The Michigan and New York proposals permit surrogates to initiate court proceedings within 20 or 21 days of giving birth in order to contest the intended social parents' custody under such agreements. California's bill requires the parties to agreements to petition for their approval, the proceedings being modeled on the natural father's spouse's seeking to adopt her husband's children, and being concluded by entry of decrees of adoption by the spouse and of paternity of the natural father, both entered within 45 days of the birth. Bills may require the father to file written notice with a court or other authority of the birth to the surrogate not later than a stated time afterward.

Minnesota's and South Carolina's proposals are more closely based on the traditional adoption model, although carefully distinguished from the law of the state relating to adoption. The courts are required to direct the developed procedures, which are entitled "surrogate adoption."[91] These procedures provide in general for the filing of petitions for surrogate adoption on the parties' agreement to contractual terms, for court-ordered investigations for approval of the implementation of such agreements, and for the parties' filing notice of the surrogate's pregnancy followed by judicial orders of filiation. After the courts' receipt of notices of pregnancy and the sixth month of gestation, interim orders will be issued by the courts granting custody, care, and control of the child to the natural father and his wife, with exclusive authority to consent to all medical, surgical, and comparable services for the child. These interim orders become effective immediately on the birth of the child, although the surrogate may see and hold the child within the first 24 hours following birth, if practicable. Fourteen days after receipt of the notices of birth, the courts terminate the parental rights of the surrogate and her husband, unless the child's paternity is challenged. If not, or if the challenges fail, final decrees of surrogate adoption are entered on judicial satisfaction that this is in the child's best interests. Before the entry of the final decree, the natural father and his wife must file a statement of all money or the like paid in the surrogate motherhood transaction and related proceedings.

Records: Access and Confidentiality

Most bills provide that official records of surrogate motherhood agreements shall be maintained in confidence, but they tend to permit access by court order and, in some cases, on demand by a person whose birth was involved, if of full age. A New York proposal permits surrogates at any time to deny release of their names, but Michigan's bill would favor children's rights of access over surrogate mothers' rights of confidentiality. Court proceedings—for instance, under South Carolina's surrogate adoption process— must be confidential and held in closed court, and all papers and records must be sealed. None shall have access to such records, except on order of judges for good cause shown. Nevertheless, nonidentifying medical and related information may be given to the adoptive parents, the biological parents, and the adoptees when it is in their best interests to receive it.

Duties of the Natural Father's Wife

Bills usually provide for a wife's assumption of duties consequent on her express consent to her husband's artificial insemination of an approved surrogate mother and the resultant birth of a child. The wife may also be required to offer evidence of her infertility, of her ability to care for a child, and of her willingness to act alone as a parent if her husband dies before the surrogate child is born. She must also generally submit to a required medical, mental health, and related examination. Under the bills of Minnesota and South Carolina, the wife must be willing to participate in the surrogate adoption proceedings and the associated evaluations.

Termination and Breach of Agreements

Natural fathers are, at times, afforded access to procedures to deny their paternity of children born to surrogates, and to abrogate contracts on the surrogates' refusal to comply with reasonable requests on matters agreed to in the contracts. Reciprocally, surrogates may be afforded procedures to withdraw from agreements on the expiration of time without pregnancy or on other grounds, for instance, on service of written notice. The South Carolina bill provides for termination of an agreement by a natural father if pregnancy does not occur within a "reasonable time," meaning a period not less than three months nor longer than six months. Bills may provide that, on breach of agreements, the courts shall make available legal and equitable remedies. Where at birth the surrogate and the natural father disagree over the custody of the child, bills may provide that express terms of approved agreements shall prevail over the general law on the matter. Bills in general tend not to address breaches of agreements, however, which occur between the occurrence of pregnancy and the birth of the child, appearing to leave the issue to the regular law.

Penalties

Bills often provide that surrogate motherhood agreements may lawfully be made and acted on in accordance with their provisions, but not otherwise. Some specify levels of offenses committed by violators and prescribe fine and/or imprisonment. Although criminal responses to violations may be determined, however, no bill addresses the effects on children born of unlawful agreements with which the parties have, in fact, complied by giving and receiving the factual custody of the children. The consequences for such children may be governed by the law preexisting and surviving the enactment of bills designed to accommodate only specified approved surrogate-motherhood agreements. Accordingly, where these bills are restrictively designed, they may leave the substantive legal issues facing these children unaddressed.[92]

REFERENCES AND NOTES

1. See Genesis 16:3, in which Abraham had a son through the handmaiden of his barren wife Sarah, and Genesis 30:1–6, in which the maid of Rachel bore her husband Jacob's child.
2. The President of the Surrogate Parent Foundation, a California nonprofit organization formed to provide information to the public, has testified that, from early 1981 to early 1982, the foundation received 20,000 requests for information; see Winborne, W. H. (ed.), *Handling Pregnancy and Birth Cases*, Shepard's/McGraw-Hill, Family Law Series, Colorado Springs (1983), 252.
3. In *Kentucky v. Surrogate Parenting Associates, Inc.* (Franklin Circuit Ct. No. 81-CI-0121, October 26, 1983), revocation of the defendant's corporate charter, on allegation of violation of law on adoption and termination of parental rights, was denied. An appeal has been filed: see *New York Times* (Feb. 27, 1984).
4. Speross, L., Glass, R., and Case, N., *Clinical Gynecologic Endocrinology and Infertility*, Williams & Wilkins, Baltimore (2nd ed., 1978), 317.
5. See, generally, *Population Reports*, Series L No. 4 Population Information Program, The Johns Hopkins University (1983).
6. See note 8 below.
7. They may similarly not be considered fathers in a legal sense. About half of the states in the United States in 1982 had statutes relating to artificial insemination, which typically regard the husband who gives consent before artificial insemination of his wife as the father for all legal purposes; see Winborne, note 2 above, at p. 219.
8. Mason, J. K., and McCall Smith, R. A., *Law and Medical Ethics*, Butterworths, London (1983), 46.
9. In the earliest cases, physicians were not involved, and the process of the insemination of the surrogate mothers was physically undertaken by the wives of the sperm donors/social fathers; see Keane, N. P., and Breo, D. L., *The Surrogate Mother*, Everest House, New York (1981).
10. In *People v. Sorenson* (1968), 43 P.2d 495 (Cal. S.C.), it was held that a husband who consents to his wife's artificial insemination is legally deemed to be the lawful father for support purposes; see also *Anonymous v. Anonymous* (1964), 246 N.Y.S. 2d 835 (N.Y.S.C.) and *Strnad v. Strnad* (1948), 78 N.Y.S. 2d 390 (N.Y.S.C.), where semiadoption was found.
11. See the series of U.S. Supreme Court cases *Griswold v. Connecticut*, 381 U.S. 479 (1965), *Eisenstadt v. Baird*, 405 U.S. 438 (1972), *Roe v. Wade*, 410 U.S. 113 (1973), *Carey v. Population Services International*, 431 U.S. 678 (1977).

12. *Buck v. Bell* (1926), 274 U.S. 200 (U.S. Sup. Ct.), applied in North Carolina in *In re Sterilization of Moore* (1976), 221 S.E. 2d 307 (N.C.S.C.).

13. See, for instance, Burgdorf, R., and Burgdorf, M., The wicked witch is almost dead: Buck v. Bell and the sterilization of handicapped persons, *Temple L.Q.* 50:995 (1977).

14. See Dickens, B. M., Retardation and sterilization, *Intl. J. Law and Psychiatry* 5:295 (1982), for a review of standards of judicial decision-making.

15. See Somerville, M. A., Birth technology, parenting and "deviance" *Intl. J. Law and Psychiatry* 5:123 (1982).

16. See Goldstein, J., Freud, A., and Solnit A., *Before the Best Interests of the Child*, Free Press, New York (1979), and the discussion in Dickens, B. M., The modern function and limits of parental rights, *Law Quarterly R.* 97:462 (1981).

17. See *Zepeda v. Zepeda* (1963), 190 N.E. 2d 849 (Ill. C.A.), and the discussion in Winborne, note 2 above: "The courts that have considered a cause of action in dissatisfied life cases have uniformly rejected it," at p. 419.

18. See Winborne, note 2 above, at p. 393 *et seq.* Only two California decisions and one in Washington State have prevailed in recognizing this action; see *Curlender v. Bio-Science Laboratories* (1980), 165 Cal. Rptr. 477 (Cal. C.A.); *Turpin v. Sortini* (1981), 174 Cal. Rptr. 128 (Cal. C.A.), and *Harbeson v. Parke-Davis* (1983), 656 P.2d 483 (Wash. S.C.).

19. The natural parents' consent is often a precondition to final adoption orders' being made, but this requirement can usually be waived by judges in appropriate circumstances.

20. Practice varies on the judicial sealing of the original birth registration and on who may subsequently be afforded access to its details. See Simanek, S. E., Adoption records reform: Impact on adoptees, *Marquette L.R.* 67:110 (1983).

21. States may prescribe who may perform artificial insemination; see California: Cal. Civ. Code § 7005 (West 1980), Georgia: Ga. Code Ann. § 74-101.1 (1973), and Oregon: Or. Rev. Stat. § 677.360 (1977).

22. See note 9 above and, for instance, *C.M. v. C.C.* (1977), 377 A.2d 821 (N.J. Juv. and D.R.Ct.), where a woman artificially inseminated herself with the sperm of a male friend, who was granted visitation rights in the best interests of the child.

23. See Winborne, note 2 above, at p. 219, and the Uniform Parentage Act § 5, at *ibid.* p. 220.

24. On the tenacity of the presumption of legitimacy, see the Quebec case of *Bolduc v. Lalancette-St.-Pierre*, [1976] C.S. 41 (Que. S.C.), where, although a birth certificate named as a child's father the married mother's lover, with whom she had lived for three years before birth, and he had cared for the child for a further six years, it was held that the estranged husband was the legal father. The marriage had not been dissolved, and the husband had not disavowed the child.

25. In the future, less significance is likely to attach to the distinction between the legitimacy and the illegitimacy of children, as the distinction is being progressively abandoned in family legislation.

26. Early judicial responses to claims of AID were to consider the act adulterous and the children illegitimate; see *Orford v. Orford* (1921), 58 D.L.R. 251 (Ont. S.C.), and *Gursky v. Gursky* (1963), 242 N.Y.S. 2d 406 (N.Y.S.C.); contrast *Strnad v. Strnad*, note 10 above.

27. For recent practice on AID, see Curie-Cohen, M., Luttrell, L., and Shapiro, S., Current practice of artificial insemination by donor in the United States, N. Eng. J. Med. 300:585 (1979).

28. See *Doe v. Commonwealth*, 403 F.Supp. 119 (U.S. Dist. Ct., E.D. Va., 1975), ruling that the right to privacy did not apply when a couple performed sexual acts in the presence of an invited stranger.

29. Even regarding sexual reproduction, it has been observed that "It would be rather anomalous if such a decision [whether or not to bear a child] could be constitutionally protected while the more fundamental decision as to whether to engage in the conduct which is a necessary prerequisite to childbearing could be constitutionally prohibited"; *State v. Saunders* (1977), 381 A.2d 333 (N.J. S.C.) at p. 340.

30. See note 53 below.

31. In 1977, it was noted that the tariff for a healthy white infant ran from $4,000 to $40,000, and a verified Jewish infant could bring up to $60,000; see Lovenheim, B., Innocents, Inc., *Student Lawyer* (December 1977):23.

32. In most jurisdictions, a judge may waive the requirement of the mother's consent in an appropriate case.

33. See text below at note 91.

34. Fears may exist, for instance, that an infertile wife, under pressure of guilt, may agree to her husband's wish for his own child when she is not truly willing to rear the child.

35. A procedure of surrogate adoption has been proposed by the Law Reform Commission of Ontario; see its report on *Human Artificial Reproduction and Related Matters* (1985), 218–272.

36. Cal. Civ. Code § 7005 (West 1980).

37. In *Syrkowski v. Appleyard*, 9 *Fam.L.Rep.* (BNA) 2260 (Mich.Ct.App. Jan. 19, 1983), the Michigan Court of Appeal strictly applied the state's Paternity Act to deny an application to exclude recognition of a woman's husband as father of her child, when she had been artificially inseminated with a donor's sperm under a surrogate motherhood agreement with the husband's consent. The Michigan Supreme Court subsequently reversed that approval and permitted the donor to be recognized as father under the Paternity Act, *Syrkowski v. Appleyard* (1985) 362 N.W. 2d 211.

38. See note 24 above.

39. See Terasaki, P. I., *et al.*, Twins by two different fathers identifed by HLA *N. Eng. J. Med.* 299:590 (1978).

40. See Artificial conception: The challenge for family law, *Virginia L.R.* 69:465 (1983).

41. See *Syrkowski v. Appleyard*, note 37 above.

42. See Gordon, R. S. (ed.), *Issues in Health Care Regulation*, McGraw-Hill, New York (1980).

43. See for instance, *Goldstein, J., Freud, A., and Solnit, A.*, note 16 above.

44. *Our Criminal Law*, Law Reform Commission of Canada, Ottawa (1976).

45. See *Doe v. Kelley* (1981), 307 N.W. 2d 438 (Mich. C.A.) at p. 441.

46. In the absence of legislation, the courts have been very hesitant to allow children's claims for wrongful life or dissatisfied life; see Winborne, note 2 above, at pp. 393, 419.

47. A feature of the practice of surrogate parenting agencies is that they often deal with residents of a number of states and may arrange out-of-state births.

48. See, for instance, Andrews, L., *New Conceptions: A Consumer's Guide to the Newest Infertility Treatments, Including In Vitro Fertilization, Artificial Insemination, and Surrogate Motherhood*, St. Martin's Press, New York (1984).

49. See, for instance, the well-referenced article by Rushevsky, C. A., Note: Legal recognition of surrogate gestation, *Women's Rights L.R.* 7:107 (1982).

50. See, for instance, the helpful article by Annas, G. J., and Elias, S., *In vitro* fertilization and embryo transfer: Medicolegal aspects of a new technique to create a family, *Family L.Q.* 17:199 (1983).

51. See text above at note 33 and proposals in text at note 91 below.

52. See Robertson, J., Procreative liberty and the control of conception, pregnancy, and childbirth, *Virginia L.R.* 69:405 (1983).

53. In *Kentucky v. Surrogate Parenting Associates, Inc.*, note 3 above, Judge Henry Meigs asked, "How can a natural father be characterized as either adopting or buying his own baby? . . . He does not (and cannot) buy the right to adopt a child with which he already has a legal and natural relationship." (Judgment p. 3)

54. In *Doe v. Kelley*, note 45 above, the Michigan Court of Appeal upheld a refusal to declare invalid legislation prohibiting payment in connection with adoption. The applicants were parties to a prospective surrogate-motherhood agreement.

55. An agreement by a person entitled to custody of a minor to transfer this custody to another is usually illegal unless authorized by legislation, except when the agreement is between the child's two parents. Even then, however, the courts may recognize such agreements only when they appear to be in the best interests of the children; see *Commonwealth ex rel. Teitelbaum v. Teitelbaum* (1974), 50 A.2d 713 (Pa. Superior Ct.).

56. The Oklahoma Attorney General has issued an opinion that surrogate motherhood agreements involving both compensation above medical expenses and adoption are illegal as being in violation of Oklahoma's Trafficking in Children Statute (Title 21, O.S. 1981, § 866); see *Attorney General of Oklahoma*, Opinion No. 83-162 (Sept. 29, 1983).

57. See generally Code of Federal Regulations Title 45 Part 46 Subpart B (45 CFR § 46.201-211) regarding research involving fetuses, pregnant women, and *in vitro* fertilization.

58. The International Covenant on Economic, Social and Cultural Rights, in force since January 1976, recognizes in Art. 10(1) that "The widest possible protection and assistance should be accorded to the family . . . particularly for its establishment." The International Covenant on Civil and Political Rights, operative since March 1976, provides in Art. 23(2) that "The right of men and women of marriageable age to marry and to found a family shall be recognized."

59. The International Covenant on Economic, Social and Cultural Rights recognizes in Art. 15(1) (b) the right of everyone "To enjoy the benefits of scientific progress and its applications." By Art. 15(3), States

that are parties to the Covenant "undertake to respect the freedom indispensable for scientific research and creative activity."

60. See notes 9 and 22 above.

61. See, generally, Winborne, note 2 above, at pp. 103 and 372.

62. See *ibid.*, at p. 393.

63. See *ibid.*, at p. 419.

64. The terms *donation* and *donor* are used here to refer to a genetic contributor to a child's procreation who is not intended to be a social parent to the child on birth.

65. The 1979 publication by M. Curie-Cohen *et al.*, see note 27 above, indicated some laxity of genetic screening.

66. Ovum donors may be expected to be considerably better paid than sperm donors where ovum recovery involves invasive procedures and, perhaps, prior preparation for superovulation.

67. See, generally, Dickens, B. M., The control of living body materials, *U. Toronto L.J.* **27**:142 (1977), at p. 187.

68. See Dickens, B. M., The ectogenetic human being: A problem child of our time, *U. Western Ontario L.R.* **18**:241 (1979–80).

69. See *Del Zio v. Presbyterian Hospital*, 74 Civ. 3588 (U.S. Dist. Ct., S.D.N.Y. April 12, 1978), in Winborne, note 2 above, at p. 230 *et seq.*

70. Surplus fertilized ova occur when a donor of ova is treated for inducement of superovulation and laparoscopic recovery of multiple ova for fertilization *in vitro*. Evidence indicates that pregnancy is most likely when three or four ova are implanted on a single occasion; see Lopata, A., Concepts in human in vitro fertilization and embryo transfer, *Fertility and Sterility* **40**:289 (1983), at p. 298.

71. Where this claim is recognized before birth, it is usually limited to independently viable fetuses; see Winborne, note 2 above, at p. 352 *et seq.*

72. See note 57 above.

73. Gender identification of the ovum fertilized *in vitro* may not be more than a distant though foreseeable possibility.

74. See note 70 above.

75. See Sappideen, C., Life after death—Sperm banks, wills and perpetuities, *Australian L. J.* **53**:311 (1979).

76. See the statement of the English Attorney-General, regarding the legality of postcoital contraception, that the definition of legal abortion "is not apt to describe a failure to implant—whether spontaneous or not;" Sir Michael Havers, Hansard, H.C. vol. 42 No. 112, Col. 238 (May 10, 1983).

77. For an example of a fully developed model agreement, see Brophy, K., A surrogate mother contract to bear a child, *J. Family Law* **20**:263 (1982).

78. See opinion of the New York City Bar Association's Committee on Judicial Ethics, 8 *Fam. L. Rep.* (BNA) 4069 (Sept. 28, 1982).

79. See text below at note 91.

80. Between the conventional civil standard of proof on a balance of probabilities and the criminal standard of proof beyond reasonable doubt, the courts have developed an intermediate standard of proof on clear and convincing evidence; see *Santosky v. Kramer* (1982) 102 S.Ct. 1388.

81. Taxation as earned income may have different implications from taxation as, for instance, a capital gain. The transaction may be considered a contract of employment or, for instance, a contract for independently rendered services.

82. See Maule, J., Federal tax consequences of surrogate motherhood, *Taxes* **60**:656 (1982).

83. In *Jefferson v. Griffin Spalding County Hospital Authority* (1981), 274 S.E. 2d 457, the Supreme Court of Georgia ordered a pregnant woman to submit to a cesarean section to save a viable fetus and transferred the legal custody of the fetus *in utero* to the state. See E. P. Finamore's discussion of the case in *American J. Law & Medicine* **9**:83 (1983).

84. Analogies may exist with the control of private adoption agencies.

85. Kleegman, S. J., and Kaufman, S. A., *Infertility in Women*, F. A. Davis Co., Philadelphia (1966), 178.

86. Michigan seems to have been the scene of intensive lobbying, perhaps associated with the Detroit lawyer Noel Keane's prominence in arranging surrogate motherhood arrangements. In the Michigan House of Representatives, Rep. Richard Fitzpatrick has come close to success in urging (a substitute for) his House Bill No. 4114.

87. Alaska House Bill 497, then pending passage.

88. This bill, as amended to May 18, 1982, is presented in Winborne, note 2 above, at p. 247 *et seq*. The bill died in the California Assembly Committee on Judiciary.
89. For simplicity, no references will be given to the numbers of the individual clauses of the proposed bills.
90. I am indebted to Larry Fox, of the Law Reform Commission of Ontario for the original digest on which this review is based.
91. See text above at note 33, and the detailed proposal of the Ontario Law Reform Commission, note 33 above.
92. In the United Kingdom, the Report of the Committee of Inquiry into Human Fertilization and Embryology (The Warnock Report), H.M.S.O. Cmnd. 9314, 1984, recognized that ". . . there will continue to be privately arranged surrogacy agreements;" para. 8.19, at 47. The Report recommended that criminal penalties for professional persons involved be imposed, and that agreements not be judicially enforceable, but made no provision for the welfare of the children; contrast the Ontario Law Reform Commission Report, *ibid*.

16

ETHICAL ISSUES IN HUMAN *IN VITRO* FERTILIZATION AND EMBRYO TRANSFER

LeRoy Walters, Ph.D.
Director, Center for Bioethics
Kennedy Institute of Ethics
Associate Professor, Department of Philosophy
Georgetown University
Washington, DC 20057

My goal in this chapter is to survey the major ethical issues in human *in vitro* fertilization (IVF) and/or embryo transfer (ET)—both in the clinic and in the laboratory. More specifically, the chapter seeks to analyze six major alternative ethical positions on IVF and ET and to display the presupposition and the internal logic of each of these positions.

The method employed in identifying the six major ethical positions, or paradigms, has been an inductive one. Fourteen major statements on IVF and ET by medical or religious bodies have been analyzed to determine what ethical issues are treated in the statements. Eighteen distinguishable ethical issues are treated in the fourteen statements; most issues are discussed by more than one statement, but a few are unique to particular statements. A summary of the eighteen issues in the fourteen statements is presented in the accompanying 252-cell matrix (Figure 1).

The fourteen major statements, in chronological order, are the following:

1. The report of the U.S. Department of Health, Education, and Welfare (HEW) Ethics Advisory Board (May 1979).[1]
2. The report of a working party to the Australian National Health and Medical Research Council (August 1982).[2]
3. The submission of the Catholic Bishops of Victoria, Australia, to the Waller Committee (August 1982).[3]
4. The interim report of the Waller Committee in Victoria, Australia (September 1982).[4]
5. The statement of the British Medical Research Council (November 1982).[5]

	(1) HEW	(2) (Austr.) NH & MRC	(3) Catholic Bishops (Austr.)	(4) Waller I (Austr.)	(5) (Brit.) MRC	(6) (Brit.) RCOG	(7) Catholic Committee (UK)	(8) Royal Society (UK)	(9) Brit. Med. Assn.	(10) Waller II (Austr.)	(11) European MRCs	(12) American Fertility Society	(13) Warnock (UK)	(14) Waller III (Austr.)
Therapy														
A. Acceptability in principle	Yes	Yes	No	Yes	Yes	Yes	Yes	Yes	Yes	Yes	Yes	Yes	Yes	Yes
B. Freezing of embryos	—	Yes	No	Yes	No	Yes	Yes	No	Yes	Yes	—	Yes	Yes	Yes
C. Donation of oocytes	No	Yes	No	NR	—	Yes	No	—	Yes	Yes	—	Yes	Yes	Yes
D. Donation of embryos (*in vitro fertilization*)	No	—	—	No	—	Yes	No	—	Yes	Yes	—	Yes	Yes	Yes
E. Donation of embryos (*in vivo fertilization*)	—	—	—	—	—	—	—	—	—	—	—	—	No	NR
Laboratory research														
F. Acceptability in principle	Yes	Yes	No	NR	Yes	Yes	Yes[1]	Yes	Yes	NR	Yes[2]	Yes	Yes[6]	Yes[8]
G. Donation of embryos for research	Yes	Yes	—	—	Yes	Yes	—	Yes	Yes	—	Yes[3]	Yes	Yes	Yes
H. Freezing of embryos	—	—	No	—	Yes	Yes	No	Yes	Yes	—	Yes	Yes	Yes	Yes
I. Interspecies fertilization	No	—	—	—	Yes	—	No	Yes	Yes	—	Yes[4]	—	Yes[7]	—
J. Division of embryos	—	—	—	—	—	Yes	—	—	Yes	—	—	—	NR	Yes
K. Nuclear transfer (actual cloning)	No	Yes	—	—	—	—	No	Yes	Yes	—	—	—	NR	—
L. Gene repair	—	—	—	—	—	Yes	—	Yes	Yes	—	—	—	—	NR
M. Harvesting of embryonic cells for transplant purposes	—	—	No	—	—	Yes	No	—	—	—	—	—	NR	—
N. Production of parthenogenones	—	—	—	—	—	—	No	—	—	—	—[5]	—	NR	—
O. Teratogenic studies	No	—	No	—	—	—	No	Yes	—	—	—	—	NR	—
P. Interspecies fusion of embryos	No	—	No	—	—	—	—	—	—	—	—	—	—	—
General issue														
Q. Disposal of embryos	—	Yes	No	Yes	Yes	No	No	—	Yes	NR	—	Yes	Yes	Yes
Related issue														
R. Surrogate motherhood	No	NR	No	No	—	No	No	—	No	NR	—	—	No	—

Figure 1. Contrasting viewpoints on the ethics of *in vitro* fertilization and/or embryo transfer. Key: — = Not Discussed; NR = Not Resolved. [1]If research is beneficial to embryo itself; [2]Irish MRC had strong reservations; [3]Norwegian MRC limited to embryos following IVF; [4]Norwegian MRC limited to infertility studies; [5]Norwegian MRC disapproved; [6]majority view; [7]for fertility testing, developmental limit: 2 cells; [8]majority view, acceptable only if spare embryos used.

6. The report of the British Royal College of Obstetricians and Gynaecologists (March 1983).[6]
7. The submission to the Warnock Committee of a joint committee established by the Catholic bishops of the United Kingdom (March 1983).[7]
8. The submission of the British Royal Society to the Warnock Committee (March 1983).[8]
9. The interim report of a working group to the British Medical Association (May 1983).[9]
10. A report on donor gametes by the Waller Committee (August 1983).[10]
11. The recommendations of an advisory subgroup to the European Medical Research Councils (November 1983).[11]
12. The statement of the American Fertility Society (January 1984).[12]
13. The Warnock Committee report in the United Kingdom (July 1984).[13]
14. The final report of the Waller Committee in Victoria, Australia (August 1984).[14]

Five of the six ethical positions analyzed in the pages that follow have already been adopted in one or more of the fourteen statements enumerated above. The sixth and final position is, for the most part, an extrapolation from currently adopted positions and seeks to anticipate future ethical quandaries.

Position 1: Natural Reproduction Only

This first position is most clearly represented by the Catholic Bishops of Victoria, Australia, in their submission to the Waller Committee in Victoria (Column 3 of the matrix in Figure 1). According to the Victoria bishops, the use of IVF to move an egg from the ovary around a tubal obstruction to the uterus via a petri dish is morally unacceptable. The bishops argued as follows:

> In pursuit of the admirable end of helping an infertile couple to conceive and have their baby, IVF intervenes in their supreme expression of mutual love. It separates "babymaking" from "lovemaking."[15]

The argument is couched strictly in means–ends terms, and IVF is identified as an illicit means of achieving a worthy end. The same logic would seem to entail a moral prohibition of artificial insemination with the husband's sperm and of most contraceptive methods, as well.

Note that this first ethical position need not make any judgment about the moral status of the early human embryo. The emphasis here is on the naturalness or the artificiality of the reproductive method. The fact that IVF and ET involve an unnatural mode of egg removal, insemination, early culture, and embryo transport is sufficient to disqualify this mode of reproduction, from a moral point of view.

Position 2: Clinical IVF Only and Only within the Family

A joint committee established by the Catholic Bishops of the United Kingdom is the clearest proponent of this second ethical position (Column 7 of the matrix in Figure 1). Reduced to its essentials, this position states that, as long as both gametes are from members of a married couple, and as long as every developing embryo is transferred for further development, IVF and ET are ethically acceptable procedures.

This position is actually a composite of views on two different issues: the moral status of the early embryo and the appropriate context for human reproduction. On the first issue, Position 2 argues that the early human embryo is a new human being from the time of fertilization forward. As a human being, the early embryo is entitled to all of the moral protections generally accorded to human infants, children, and adults. But a second issue is also raised by Position 2, namely, the appropriate context for reproduction. Here, the British bishops and their lay colleagues argued that it is unwise to go outside the marital unit for gametes, either sperm or eggs. Thus, Position 2 would find both artificial insemination with donor sperm and IVF with donated eggs to be ethically unacceptable. Also excluded would be the artificial insemination of a donor woman followed by uterine lavage and embryo transfer—a technique pioneered by a team of researchers at UCLA.[16]

Note that the position of the British bishops' commission allows for considerable latitude within the practice of clinical IVF. The freezing of embryos is permitted if there is a "genuine and definite prospect for transfer, unimpaired, to the proper mother."[17] Similarly, research on early human embryos is permitted, but only if the research is for the benefit of those particular embryos. Thus, if laboratory research with nonhuman mammalian embryos leads to safe and effective preimplantation gene therapy by the middle of the next century, there is no reason in principle that this position could not accept the application of gene therapy techniques to early human embryos.

The major practical difficulty of Position 2, given the current state of biological knowledge, is that it creates dilemmas at the stages of egg harvest and especially fertilization *in vitro*. Briefly stated, Position 2 prohibits the creation of surplus embryos—embryos that cannot be transferred to the uterus of the woman who has contributed to the embryonic genotype. If six embryos begin to develop *in vitro*, the clinician may be faced with the difficult choice whether to transfer all six—causing some additional risk to both the woman and the multiple fetuses that may develop—or to transfer only some of the six, perhaps three. If the clinician transferred only three embryos, the remaining three could, of course, be frozen, but according to Position 2, they would have to be thawed and transferred to the genetic mother at some future time.

An alternative policy that would also respect the moral limits set by Position 2 would be to fertilize only the number of eggs that one would be willing to transfer, should they successfully give rise to developing embryos. Most clinics would probably be unwilling to transfer more than three embryos at a time and thus would fertilize only three eggs at a time. The practical problems with this policy are, first, that it may reduce the couple's chances for a successful pregnancy if one or more of the three eggs is not successfully fertilized and if only one or two embryos can therefore be transferred. Second, this lower probability of success could lead to increased risk for the woman if she must then be exposed to future egg-harvesting procedures under general or regional anesthesia.

Position 2 would also presumably not allow for any kind of preimplantation screening of human embryos—whether on a gross morphological basis or, in the future, on a biochemical, genetic, or chromosomal basis. In addition, any attempt to select only embryos of a particular sex for transfer would be excluded on moral grounds.

POSITION 3: CLINICAL IVF ONLY

This third position is best represented by the *Report on Donor Gametes in IVF* of the Waller Committee in Victoria, Australia (Column 10 of the matrix in Figure 1).[10] This position differs from the second only by allowing for the donation of an egg or even an embryo in cases where the involuntary infertility of another couple cannot be overcome by any other means.

Position 3 accords significant moral status to the early human embryo. It assumes that all early embryos will eventually be transferred for further development, but not necessarily within the same family unit. The freezing of early embryos is accepted, presumably as a technique that is not disrespectful of human embryos. The freezing of embryos would also facilitate embryo donation, as it does not require synchronous ovulatory cycles for successful transfer.

A practical problem associated with Position 3 is that infertile couples are confronted with a decision whether to freeze and save untransferred embryos for their own future childbearing or whether to donate those embryos to other infertile couples. Many couples will probably decide to keep the surplus embryos as a kind of familial insurance policy until they have attained the desired number of children for themselves. The Waller Committee recognized these problems and recommended counseling and careful attention to informed consent in any situation where the donation of either human eggs or early human embryos is contemplated.

On the issue of laboratory research on early human embryos, the Waller Committee was deeply divided. In its August 1983 report, the committee was unable to resolve this question. Position 3, as presented in this chapter, excludes laboratory research but allows the donation of eggs or embryos within the context of clinical IVF.

POSITION 4: CLINICAL IVF PLUS LIMITED LABORATORY RESEARCH ON EARLY HUMAN EMBRYOS

There is a significant watershed between Position 3 and Position 4. Only with Position 4 does one encounter an acceptance, in principle, of laboratory research on early human embryos. The most conservative of the proresearch options is Position 4, represented by the report of the HEW Ethics Advisory Board in 1979 (Column 1 of the matrix in Figure 1).

The presupposition that allows Position 4 to accept some laboratory research on human embryos was formulated by the Ethics Advisory Board as follows:

> The human embryo is entitled to profound respect; but this respect does not necessarily encompass the full legal and moral rights attributed to persons.[18]

In short, Position 4 adopts a developmental view concerning the moral status of the human embryo. At the earliest stages of development, the *prima facie* moral obligation to protect human embryos can be overridden by other moral obligations that are even more compelling.

Position 4, as delineated by the Ethics Advisory Board, accepts laboratory research on early human embryos if the research is designed primarily to assess the safety and efficacy of clinical IVF. In the deliberations of the Ethics Advisory Board, the principal argument for accepting a limited amount of research on embryos was that it would be hypocritical to allow U.S. clinics to proceed without having better data from the laboratory, particularly on the safety of *in vitro* fertilization and *in vitro* embryo culture. As matters have, in fact, progressed in the United States since 1979, the clinics have forged ahead while the laboratories have done very little research—in part, because of a *de facto* moratorium on National Institutes of Health (NIH) funding for such research.

Position 4 clearly does not endorse general basic research on early human embryos. The Ethics Advisory Board also disapproved, on ethical grounds, any attempts to create human–nonhuman hybrid embryos and any efforts to perform nuclear transfer (cloning, in the strict sense of the term).

The primary conceptual problem for Position 4 is to define clearly what types of research are designed primarily to assess the safety and efficacy of clinical IVF. A strict construction of this limitation would seem to exclude general research on causes of infertility and on new approaches to contraception. On the other hand, the limitation would seem to allow for laboratory research on the incidence of genetic or chromosomal abnormalities in a series of, say, 100 *in vitro* fertilizations. Position 4 would also seem to permit experimental variation in the timing of, and the media employed with, the IVF procedure.

Position 5: Clinical IVF plus Virtually Unlimited Laboratory Research on Early Human Embryos

Position 5 adopts an intermediate approach to the question of research on human embryos. This position first draws a sharp distinction between embryos that are destined for implantation and those that are not. Most experimental procedures are permitted only if the embryo will not be transferred for further development. Second, Position 5 sets a clear limit on the amount of time that human embryos may be cultured in the laboratory—usually 14 or 17 days, the approximate point at which implantation is completed *in utero*. This fifth position is, in general, the one adopted by the Australian National Health and Medical Research Council, the British Medical Research Council, the British Medical Association, the American Fertility Society, the Warnock Committee, and the Waller Committee in its final report (Columns 2, 5, 6, 9, 12, 13, and 14 of the matrix in Figure 1).

On one further point, there is a measure of ambiguity in Position 5. Some groups subscribing to this position require that laboratory research on early human embryos should be relevant—or, more strongly, *directly* relevant—to clinical problems.[19,20] Other groups do not explicitly limit the range of acceptable laboratory research in this way.[21,22] However, the stipulation of clinical relevance may be more rhetorical than substantive, as no examples of nonrelevant and therefore impermissible research are cited. (Indeed, if one examines Columns 2, 5, 6, and 9 of the matrix in Figure 1, one finds that every experimental procedure mentioned by the four medical and research bodies is judged to be acceptable.)

What are some of the experimental procedures permitted by Position 5 when embryo transfer is not envisioned and when the duration of embryo culture does not exceed 14 or 17 days? One procedure is the *division of embryos* by teasing apart some of the cells, or blastomeres, in the early cleavage stage of development. Researchers can then study whether all parts of the divided embryo will continue to grow normally as if each part were a biological individual. In other words, the researchers would be attempting to determine whether they can create multiple human embryos from one human embryo. This technique would have obvious potential relevance for future attempts to perform preimplantation genetic diagnosis or preimplantation sex determination.

The only statement of the fourteen here under review that critically addresses the question of embryo division is the one prepared by the British bishops' committee. In the opinion of the commissioners, studies that divide early embryos and then perform research on some of the cells are morally prohibited. The rationale for this position is the view that, in dividing the embryo, the researcher has created new individuals, some of which are then killed for the sake of the remainder.[23]

A second experimental procedure is the attempt to perform *gene repair* in early human embryos. If these studies extrapolate from already-performed studies in mice,[24] new genetic material will be injected into the male pronucleus at the time of fertilization in an attempt to modify all cells of the developing organism—which, in this case, would not be allowed to develop more than 17 days. Attempts may also be made to repair the genes of human embryos at a later stage, for example, after preimplantation diagnosis had discovered a single-gene defect. Again, subsequent development of the embryo would be curtailed at 14 or 17 days. The potential clinical relevance of gene therapy in embryos is clear, although serious questions remain about both the technical feasibility and the desirability of repairing genetic defects in human embryos.[25]

A third technique that could be employed experimentally is *interspecies fertilization*. This technique is often used in infertility clinics with human sperm and specially treated hamster eggs, to assess the fertilizing capacity of the sperm. However, one researcher has proposed attempts at interspecies fertilization as a means of reconstructing the family tree of humans and other primates.[26] The British Medical Research Council, which is one of the two research groups that have discussed the interspecies fertilization issue, set a strict temporal limit on the duration of embryo culture following such interspecies fertilization: No culture should occur beyond the early cleavage stage[27]—a stage far earlier than the 14 or 17 days otherwise considered acceptable.

The clear presupposition of Position 5 is that human persons owe few if any moral obligations to human embryos before the stage at which implantation is normally completed. Proponents of Position 5 may accept a developmental view of our obligations to the human embryo that sees implantation as a significant dividing line in embryonic development. Alternatively, they may hold that, after 14 or 17 days of development, twinning is unlikely, and thus biological individuality is well established. In fact, little justification for the 14- or 17-day limitation on embryo culture is included in the major statements that support Position 5.

POSITION 6: CLINICAL IVF PLUS ANY KIND OF RESEARCH ON HUMAN EMBRYOS

The sixth and final position in IVF and ET is, in part, simply a theoretical construct. It shows us what kind of ethical options would be chosen if either the temporal or the geographical limitations of Position 5 were relaxed, or if the ambiguity about the rationale for research in Position 5 were removed. The existing policy statement that goes furthest toward Position 6 is the statement prepared by the British Royal Society (Column 8 of the matrix in Figure 1).

For Position 6, basic research on early human embryos—that is, research that does not aim for clinical application—is clearly acceptable. The Royal Society defined *basic research* in this context as "research related to the acquisition of basic knowledge of human development and its disorders."[28] The Royal Society statement continued: "Such basic research is essential; as has so often emerged in the past, it can lead in unanticipated ways to future benefits to society."[29]

The second kind of limitation removed by Position 6 is the 14- or 17-day limit for embryo culture. The Royal Society presented a biological rationale for going beyond this limit to at least the end of the third week following fertilization. In the words of the Royal Society statement:

> The first stage in the development of a human fertilized egg is concerned almost entirely with the formation of extra-embryonic tissues that initiate and maintain interactions with the mother. . . . During this stage of production of the extra-embryonic tissues, which lasts for approximately the first three weeks after fertilization, the whole growing entity is termed an "early embryo." It is not until the fourth week that, within the tissues constituting the "early embryo," the cells making up the "definitive embryo" (which will eventually become the fetus) begin to be organized and grow.[30]

The Royal Society statement explicitly criticizes the earlier Medical Research Council statement for having set the temporal limit for embryo culture at the end point of implantation. The Royal Society noted that "experiments such as those concerned with investigating the teratogenic effects of viruses or drugs . . . might depend on the use of embryos in which organization of the definitive embryo had begun."[31]

How long would Position 6 advocate that embryos be cultured and studied in the laboratory setting? There are both practical and theoretical limits. The practical limit is that mammalian embryos cannot be cultured *in vitro* much beyond the implantation stage because no artificial environment delivers nutrients to the embryo as efficiently as does the placenta *in utero*. A theoretical limit is that, at eight weeks after fertilization, the technical name of a developing human organism changes from *embryo* to *fetus*. Thus, any research conducted after eight weeks (if *in vitro* culture beyond eight weeks becomes possible) would be research on a human fetus rather than research on a human embryo.

However, if one ignores the name change that occurs at eight weeks, the outside limit would surely be set by advocates of Position 6 before the point of viability. In this view, no research should be conducted on a human embryo or fetus that would sustain it to the point at which it could survive to adulthood, given standard newborn care. Earlier stopping points would be the stage at which the fetal brain structure reaches particular levels of development, the stage of spontaneous movement (10 weeks), the stage of readable brain activity (8 weeks), the stage at which all major organs are present (6 weeks), or the stage at which the heartbeat begins (about 4 weeks).

One problem with the notion of stopping the laboratory development of an embryo or fetus before viability is that viability is a context-dependent concept. As the duration of embryo culture increases and the efficiency of neonatal intensive care extends to smaller infants, one may reach a point where the same machines are employed for life support in both the laboratory and the clinic. At that point, one would have to choose an end point other than "viability" as the outside limit for laboratory research on human embryos and fetuses. Ironically, some proponents of Positions 2 and 3 might applaud the disappearance of the viability watershed and argue for the generous use of the artificial placenta as a therapeutic device. There is, after all, no ethical inconsistency between ascribing significant moral status to the early embryo and accepting extracorporeal, machine-assisted gestation until the appropriate time for the "delivery" of a viable, laboratory-nurtured infant.

The remaining limitation, the geographical limitation, will probably not be relaxed with human embryos—at least, in the case of nontherapeutic research. With some nonhuman mammalian species, developing embryos or fetuses are "explanted" from the maternal uterus at the postimplantation stage and are subsequently cultured as long as possible in the laboratory setting.[32] However, in humans, it would be difficult to justify the creation and termination of a pregnancy solely for research purposes. Most people would find the maternal morbidity associated with the surgical removal of an intact human embryo or fetus for research purposes to be ethically objectionable. Depending on the age of the postimplantation embryo or fetus, some would also argue that such a procedure, when performed solely for the sake of research, violates our moral obligations to the developing embryo or fetus, as well. No currently existing policy statement on IVF and ET has advocated the transfer of human embryos for subsequent implantation in and removal from human volunteers.

In the longer term future, however, one can envision the possibility that new therapeutic procedures—for example, gene repair—will be performed on human embryos *in vitro* and that the repaired embryos will then be transferred for implantation, gestation, and term delivery. This kind of therapeutic research plus embryo transfer and implantation would again be acceptable to Positions 2 and 3—provided, of course, that the risk–benefit ratio for all concerned were appropriate and that the parents had consented to participate in such an innovative venture.

CONCLUSION

The major watershed in the ethical debate about human IVF and ET occurs between Position 3 and Position 4. It concerns the ethical acceptability of laboratory research on human embryos. Even among those who advocate laboratory research on human embryos, there are at least three distinguishable positions, which have been labeled Positions 4, 5, and 6 in this chapter. Since the HEW Ethics Advisory Board adopted Position 4 in 1979, there has been a clearly discernible trend in most British and some Australian policy statements toward a heavier concentration on laboratory research issues and toward the adoption of Positions 5 and 6. In the final analysis, one's decision about accepting Position 4, 5, or 6 will not depend primarily on learning new factual information about mammalian anatomy or physiology. Rather, one's decision will depend on a *judgment* about the *starting point* and the *relative strength* of our moral obligations to those primitive beings that we who can reason have learned to call *human embryos.*

REFERENCES AND NOTES

1. United States, Department of Health, Education, and Welfare, Ethics Advisory Board, *HEW support of research involving human in vitro fertilization and embryo transfer*, 2 vols., Washington, D.C., HEW (May 4, 1979).
2. Australia, National Health and Medical Research Council, Working Party on Ethics in Medical Research, *Ethics in medical research*, Canberra, Australian Government Publishing Service, 1983.
3. Catholic Bishops of Victoria [Australia], *Submission to the Committee to Examine In Vitro Fertilization*, unpublished document (August 6, 1982).
4. Victoria [Australia], Committee to Consider the Social, Ethical and Legal Issues Arising from In Vitro Fertilization (Chairman, Louis Waller), *Interim report*, unpublished document (September 1982).
5. Medical Research Council [Great Britain], Research related to human fertilisation and embryology, *British Medical Journal* 285:1480 (1982).
6. Royal College of Obstetricians and Gynaecologists [Great Britain], *Report of the RCOG Ethics Committee on In Vitro Fertilization and Embryo Replacement or Transfer*, London, Chameleon Press (March 1983).
7. Catholic Bishops' Joint Committee on Bio-Ethical Issues [Great Britain], *In vitro fertilisation: morality and public policy*, unpublished document (March 2, 1983).
8. Royal Society [Great Britain], *Human fertilization and embryology*, London, Royal Society (March 1983).
9. British Medical Association, Working Group on In-Vitro Fertilisation, Interim report on human in vitro fertilisation and embryo replacement and transfer, *British Medical Journal* 286:1594 (1983).
10. Victoria [Australia], Committee to Consider the Social, Ethical and Legal Issues Arising from In Vitro Fertilization (Chairman, Louis Waller), *Report on donor gametes in IVF*, unpublished document (August 1983).

11. European Medical Research Councils, Advisory Subgroup, Human in-vitro fertilisation and embryo transfer, *Lancet* **2**:1187 (1983).

12. American Fertility Society, Ethical statement on in vitro fertilization, *Fertility and Sterility* **41**:12 (1984).

13. United Kingdom, Department of Health and Social Security, *Report of the Committee of Inquiry into Human Fertilisation and Embryology* (Chairman, Mary Warnock), London, Her Majesty's Stationery Office (July 1984).

14. Victoria [Australia], Committee to Consider the Social, Ethical and Legal Issues Arising from In Vitro Fertilization, *Report on the disposition of embryos produced by in vitro fertilization* (Chairman, Louis Waller), Melbourne, F. D. Atkinson Government Printer (August 1984).

15. Catholic Bishops of Victoria (n. 3), p. 6.

16. Buster, J. E. *et al.*, Non-surgical transfer of an in-vivo fertilised donated ovum to an infertility patient. *Lancet* **1**:816 (1983).

17. Catholic Bishops' Joint Committee on Bio-Ethics (see n. 7), p. 10.

18. United States, Department of Health, Education, and Welfare, Ethics Advisory Board, *Report and conclusions* (n. 1), p. 101.

19. *Ibid.*, pp. 106–111.

20. Medical Research Council [Great Britain] (n. 5), p. 1480.

21. Royal Society [Great Britain] (n. 8), pp. 7–9, 11.

22. United Kingdom, Department of Health and Social Security (n. 13), pp. 60–61.

23. Catholic Bishops' Joint Committee on Bio-Ethics (n. 7), p. 16.

24. Gordon, J. W., and Ruddle, F. H., Integration and stable germ line transmission of genes injected into mouse pronuclei, *Science* **214**:1244 (1981).

25. Anderson, W. F., Prospects for human gene therapy, *Science* **226**:401 (1984).

26. Short, R. V., Human in vitro fertilization and embryo transfer, in United States, Department of Health, Education, and Welfare, Ethics Advisory Board (n. 1), *Appendix*, Essay 10, pp. 6–7.

27. Medical Research Council [Great Britain] (n. 5), p. 1480.

28. Royal Society [Great Britain] (n. 8), pp. 5–6.

29. *Ibid.*, p. 6.

30. *Ibid.*, p. 3.

31. *Ibid.*, p. 10.

32. New, D. A. J., Studies of mammalian fetuses *in vitro* during the period of organogenesis, in Austin, C. R. (ed.), *The mammalian fetus in vitro*, London, Chapman and Hall (1973), pp. 15–65.

17

EUGENIC STERILIZATION IN THE UNITED STATES

PHILIP R. REILLY, J.D., M.D.
Department of Medicine
Boston City Hospital
818 Harrison Avenue
Boston, MA 02118

The most important event in the rise of state-supported programs to sterilize the feeble-minded, the insane, and criminals was the rediscovery in about 1900 of Mendel's breeding experiments. The elegant laws of inheritance were seductive, and a few influential scientists, convinced that even conditions such as pauperism were caused by defective germ plasm, rationalized eugenic programs.[1] But by the close of the nineteenth century, the science of eugenics was already well established.

The founding father was Francis Galton, who, in 1864, began to study the heredity of talent. His investigations of the accomplishments of the children of eminent British judges first appeared in the popular press in 1865.[2] Four years later his book *Heredity Genius: An Inquiry into Its Laws and Consequences*[3] provided a cornerstone for eugenics. A man obsessed with measuring, Galton returned to the problem of heredity many times throughout his long life.[4]

In the United States, evolutionary theory was complicated by the race problem. Some scientists argued that human races had degenerated from a common type and that color was a rough index of departure from the original (white) type.[5] Such notions accommodated the Old Testament and reinforced the convictions of Europeans and North Americans that the Negro was inferior. Particularly important was Morton's 1839 study of the cranial volume of 256 skulls from the five major races. He reported that the average Caucasian skull was 7 cubic inches larger than the average Negro skull—a powerful finding to explain "obvious" cultural superiority.[6]

Another important progenitor of eugenical theory was Cesar Lombroso, an Italian criminologist. Lombroso argued that the behavior of many criminals was the ineluctable product of their germ plasm. During the postmortem on a famous brigand, Lombroso noted a median occipital fossa, rarely found in human skulls, but commonly seen in rodents. That and similar findings convinced him that the criminal was "an atavistic being who reproduces in his person the ferocious instincts of primitive humanity and the inferior animals."[7] Late-nineteenth-century American criminology felt his influence. For example, a Pennsylvania prison official wrote that "everyone who has visited prisons and observed large numbers of prisoners together has undoubtedly been impressed from the appearance of prisoners alone, that a large portion of them were born to be criminals."[8]

Perhaps the single most important event in the rise of eugenics was a report written by Richard Dugdale, a reform-minded New York prison inspector. At one upstate prison, he was struck by the large number of inmates who were relatives. He eventually amassed a pedigree spanning five generations that included 709 individuals, the collective offspring of an early Dutch settler, all with a propensity for almshouses, taverns, and brothels. His study of "the Jukes" had an immediate success with the general public.[9] The family entered American folklore and came to symbolize a new kind of sociological study, one that eugenicists would repeat and refine in the early years of the twentieth century.

During the 1870s, there was a marked increase in the number of state institutions dedicated to the care of the feebleminded. But by 1880, lawmakers were reassessing their relatively generous funding of these institutions. The U.S. Census of 1880 alarmed those who cared for defective persons; it reported that whereas the general population had grown by 30%, the apparent increase in "idiocy" was 200%.[10] By the 1880s, optimistic views on the educability of the feebleminded were fading, and there was a steady increase in the number of "custodial departments." The "Jukes" stimulated much interest in calculating the cost of providing for the nation's feebleminded, insane, or criminal.

The rediscovery of Mendel's laws was timed perfectly to reinforce the popular suspicion that the defective classes were the products of tainted germ plasm. It prompted a deluge of articles on eugenics in the pages of the popular press. Between 1905 and 1909, there were 27 articles on eugenics listed in The Reader's Guide to Periodical Literature. From 1910 to 1914, there were 122 additional entries, making it one of the most referenced subjects in the index. Not a few of them were alarmist in tone.

The popularity of this new subject owed much to Charles B. Davenport, the first director of the Station for Experimental Evolution at Cold Spring Harbor, New York. Trained in mathematics and biology (he took a Ph.D. from Harvard in 1892), young, and ambitious, Davenport was well placed to capture the dramatic implications of Mendelism.[11] After convincing the newly endowed Carnegie Institute to create a research facility, he embarked on genetic studies in domestic animals and plants. But the appeal of human studies was irresistible, and he was soon publishing papers on the inheritance of eye color and skin color.

In 1909, Davenport convinced Mrs. E. H. Harriman, the wealthy matron of a railroad fortune, to underwrite the creation of a Eugenic Record Office (ERO) for five years. His first task was to build a cadre of fieldworkers, young women trained to conduct family studies, to amass the raw data of eugenics. Progress was swift, and the ERO soon was publishing monographs arguing that degeneracy was highly heritable and that affected persons tended also to have large families.[12]

Significant as these works were, the major eugenics document of this century was probably Goddard's 1912 study of "the Kallikaks."[13] In 1907, Goddard, a psychologist doing research at the Vineland Training School, traveled to Europe. In Paris, he visited Simon and Binet and learned their new methods for testing intelligence. When he returned to New Jersey, Goddard, closely assisted by an ERO-trained fieldworker, used the methods to study the families of Vineland patients.

One family fascinated them. It was composed of two branches, both descendants of Martin Kallikak, a soldier in the Revolutionary War. While in tbe army, Martin had got a girl in the "Piney Woods" pregnant. After the war, he married a respectable Quaker maid and engendered a line of eminent New Jersey citizens. Goddard believed that this natural experiment proved the power of heredity. For generation after generation, the "Piney Woods" line produced paupers and feebleminded persons who, often unaware of their biological ties, sometimes worked as servants to their more eminent cousins.

The Kallikak Family was an immediate success. Written in clear language, embellished with many photographs of the moronic, sinister-looking family, and relatively short, the book hit home with the public. Reprinted in 1913, 1914, 1916, and 1919, it earned Goddard not a little celebrity. Only recently did Stephen Gould discover that the photographs had been altered, thus casting doubt on the integrity of the entire enterprise.[14] But in 1912 or 1919, one could hardly read The Kallikak Family without worrying about the consequences of childbearing by the weaker stock in the human family.

The climate of nativism made a large number of Americans particularly receptive to the argument that, if the wrong people had too many children, the nation's racial vigor would decline. No study of eugenic sterilization in the United States can ignore the impact of immigration. The history of the growth of nineteenth-century America is a history of immigration. The first of four great waves rolled across the land in the 1840s. During the 1890s, immigration exceeded the wildest predictions, rising from 225,000 in 1898 to 1,300,000 in 1907. Large-scale assimilation was painful, sometimes agonizing. Perhaps the most dramatic perturbation was competition for jobs. Despite their commitment to internationalism, even the great unions favored restrictive immigration laws. Several states passed laws excluding immigrants from the public works.[15]

Beginning about 1875 proposals to curtail the entry of aliens became a perennial topic before the U.S. Congress. The earliest laws were stimulated by fears in California that the importation of coolie labor had gone too far. Starting with the "Chinese Exclusion Acts," the federal government built the walls even higher. In 1882, a new law expressly excluded lunatics, idiots, and persons likely to become a public charge. During the late 1890s, the most ardent restrictionists sought to condition entry on a literacy test, but success in Congress was damped by President Cleveland's veto.

The early responses to fears of a rapidly growing number of defective persons were proposals that they be incarcerated. The first asylum dedicated to segregating feebleminded women during their reproductive years was opened in New York in 1878. But by the 1890s, it was obvious that only a tiny fraction of feebleminded women would ever be institutionalized. This harsh reality engendered a successful campaign to enact laws to prohibit marriage by the feebleminded, epileptics, and other "detective" types. Beginning with Connecticut in 1895, many states passed eugenic marriage laws, but this solution was unenforceable. Even the eugenicists dismissed it as ineffective.[16]

Perhaps the most lurid alternative to proposals for lifetime segregation was mass castration. Although never legally implemented, proposals to castrate criminals were seriously debated in a few state legislatures during the 1890s.[17] With the development of the vasectomy, a socially more acceptable operation, procastration arguments (usually aimed at male criminals) faded.

The Surgical Solution

The first American case report of a vasectomy was by Albert Ochsner, a young Chicago surgeon. He argued that the vasectomy could eliminate criminality inherited from the "father's side" and that it "could reasonably be suggested for chronic inebriates, imbeciles, perverts and paupers."[18] Three years later, H. C. Sharp, a surgeon at the Indiana Reformatory, reported the first large study on the effects of vasectomy. He claimed that his 42 patients felt stronger, slept better, performed more satisfactorily in the prison school, and felt less desire to masturbate! Sharp urged physicians to lobby for a law to empower directors of state institutions "to render every male sterile who passes its portals, whether it be almshouse, insane asylum, institute for the feebleminded, reformatory or prison."[19]

In 1907, the governor of Indiana signed the nation's first sterilization law. It initiated the involuntary sterilization of any habitual criminal, rapist, idiot, or imbecile committed to a state institution whom physicians diagnosed as "unimprovable." Having operated on 200 Indiana prisoners, Sharp quickly emerged as the national authority on eugenical sterilization. A tireless advocate, he even underwrote the publication of a pamphlet Vasectomy.[20] In it, he affixed tear-out post cards so that readers could mail a preprinted statement supporting compulsory sterilization laws to their legislative representatives.

Although the simplicity of the vasectomy attracted their attention to defective males, the eugenicists were also concerned with defective women. But the salpingectomy was not yet perfected, and the morbidity from intraabdominal operations was high. Eugenic theoreticians had little choice but to support the long-term segregation of feebleminded women. They were, however, comforted in their belief that most retarded women became prostitutes and were rendered sterile by pelvic inflammatory disease.[21]

Prosterilization arguments peaked in the medical literature in 1910, when roughly one half of the 40 articles published since 1900 appeared. The articles almost unanimously favored involuntary sterilization of the feebleminded. Appeals to colleagues that they lobby for enabling laws were commonly heard at meetings of state medical societies.[22] At the annual meeting of the American Medical Association, Sharp enthralled his listeners with reports on a series of 456 vasectomies performed on defective men in Indiana. After hearing him, a highly placed New Jersey official announced that he would seek a bill for the compulsory sterilization of habitual criminals in his state.[23] New Jersey enacted such a law 18 months later.

The most successful physician lobbyist was F. W. Hatch, Secretary of the State Lunacy Commission in California. In 1909, he drafted a sterilization law and helped convince the legislature (made highly sensitive to eugenic issues by the influx of "racially inferior" Chinese and Mexicans) to adopt it. After the law was enacted, Hatch was appointed General Superintendent of State Hospitals and was authorized to implement the new law. Until his death in 1924, Hatch directed eugenic sterilization programs in 10 state hospitals and approved 3,000 sterilizations, nearly half the nation's total.[24]

THE EARLY STERILIZATION LAWS

In studying the rapid rise of the early sterilization legislation, one is hampered by a paucity of state legislative historical materials.[25] Four small, but influential, groups lobbied hard for these laws: physicians (especially those working at state facilities), scientific eugenicists, lawyers and judges, and a striking number of the nation's richest families. There were, of course, opponents as well. But except for a handful of academic sociologists and social workers, they were less visible and less vocal.

The enthusiastic support that America's wealthiest families provided to the eugenics movement is a most curious feature of its history. First among many was Mrs. E. H. Harriman, who almost single-handedly supported the ERO in its first five years. The second largest financial supporter of the ERO was John D. Rockefeller, who gave it $400 each month. Other famous eugenic philanthropists included Dr. John Harvey Kellogg (brother to the cereal magnate), who organized the First Race Betterment Conference (1914), and Samuel Fels, the Philadelphia soap manufacturer. Theodore Roosevelt was an ardent eugenicist, who favored large families to avoid racial dilution by the weaker immigrant stocks.[26]

Of the few vocal opponents to the eugenics movement, Alexander Johnson and Franz Boas were the most important. Johnson, leader of the National Conference of Charities and Correction, thought that sterilization was less humane than institutional segregation. He dreamed of "orderly celibate communities segregated from the body politic," where the feebleminded and the insane would be safe and could be largely self-supporting.[27] Boas, a Columbia University anthropologist, conducted a special study for Congress to determine whether immigrants were being assimilated into American culture. His findings argued that Hebrews and Sicilians were easily assimiliable—a conclusion that was anathema to eugenicists.[28]

The extraordinary legislative success of proposals to sterilize defective persons suggests that there was substantial support among the general public for such a plan. Between 1905 and 1917, the legislatures of 17 states passed sterilization laws, usually by a large majority vote. Most were modeled after the "Indiana plan," which covered "confirmed criminals, idiots, imbeciles, and rapists." In Indiana, if two outside surgeons agreed with the institution's physician that there was no prognosis for "improvement" in such persons, they could be sterilized without their consent. In California, the focus was on sterilizing the insane. The statute permitted authorities to condition a patient's discharge from a state hospital on undergoing sterilization. California law was unique in requiring that the patient or the family consent to the operation, but as the hospitalization was of indeterminant length, people rarely refused sterilization; thus the consent was rendered nugatory.[29]

How vigorously were these laws implemented? From 1907 to 1921, 3,233 sterilizations were performed under state law. A total of 1,853 men (72 by castration) and 1,380 women (100 by castration) were sterilized. About 2,700 operations were performed on the insane, 400 on the feebleminded, and 130 on criminals. California's program was by far the largest.[30]

Sterilization programs ebbed and flowed according to the views of key state and institutional officials. For example, in 1909, the new governor of Indiana squashed that state's program. In New York, activity varied by institution. In the State Hospital at Buffalo, the superintendent, who believed that pregnancy exacerbated schizophrenia, authorized 12 salpingectomies, but in most other hospitals, no sterilizations were permitted despite the state law. Similar idiosyncratic patterns were documented in other states.[31]

The courts were unfriendly to eugenic policy. Between 1912 and 1921, eight laws were challenged, and seven were held unconstitutional. The first two cases were brought by convicted rapists who argued that sterilization violated the Eighth Amendment's prohibition of cruel and unusual punishment. The Supreme Court of the State of Washington, impressed by Dr. Sharp's reports that vasectomy was simple, quick, and painless, upheld its state law.[32] But a few years later, a federal court in Nevada ruled that the vasectomy was an "unusual" punishment and struck down a criminal sterilization law.[33] Peter Feilen, the appellant in the Washington case, was probably the only man ever forced to undergo a vasectomy pursuant to a law drafted expressly as a punitive rather than an eugenic measure.

In six states (New Jersey, Iowa, Michigan, New York, Indiana, and Oregon), constitutional attacks were leveled at laws that authorized the sterilization of feebleminded or insane persons who resided in state institutions. The plaintiffs argued that laws aimed only at institutionalized persons violated the Equal Protection Clause and that the procedural safeguards were so inadequate that they ran afoul of the Due Process Clause. All six courts invalidated the laws, but they were divided in their reasoning. The three that found a violation of the Equal Protection Clause did not clearly oppose eugenic sterilization; their concern was about uniform treatment of all feebleminded persons. The three that relied on due process arguments to reject the laws were more antagonistic to the underlying policy. An Iowa judge characterized sterilization as a degrading act that could cause "mental torture."[34]

From 1918 to 1921, the years during which these cases were decided, sterilization laws faded as quickly as they had appeared. One reason that the courts were less sympathetic to sterilization laws than the legislatures had been was that sterilization petitions (like commitment orders) touched the judiciary's historic role as protector of the weak. The judges demanded clear proof that the individual would benefit from being sterilized. Another important reason was that scientific challenges to eugenic theories about crime had appeared. For example, two physicians who studied 1,000 recidivists to determine whether inheritance was a factor in criminal behavior found "no proof of the existence of hereditary criminalistic traits."[35] But their voices were soon lost in the storm as another huge wave of immigrants swept across America.

THE RESURGENCE OF THE STERILIZATION MOVEMENT

Despite the judicial rejection of the earlier laws, after World War I arguments that mass eugenic sterilization was critical to the nation's "racial strength" resurfaced. Probably the major impetus was the sudden arrival of hundreds of thousands of southeastern European immigrants.[36] The xenophobia triggered by this massive influx had widespread repercussions. It reinforced concern about the dangers of miscegenation and helped to renew interest in biological theories of crime.

The concurrent concern about miscegenation reflected the weakening of southern white society's control over the lives of blacks. During the eighteenth and nineteenth centuries, the southern states forbade marriages between whites and Negroes. After the Civil War, the burgeoning "colored" population (largely a product of institutionalized rape before then) stimulated amendments that redefined as "Negro" persons with ever smaller fractions of black ancestry.[37] This trend culminated when Virginia enacted a marriage law that defined as white "one who has no trace whatsoever of any blood other than Caucasian." It forbade the issuance of marriage licenses until officials had "reasonable assurance" that statements about the color of both the man and the woman were correct, voided all existing interracial marriages (regardless of whether they had been contracted legally elsewhere), and made cohabitation by such couples a felony. Several other states enacted laws modeled on the Virginia plan. It was not until the 1940s that states began to repeal miscegenation laws, and only recently did the U.S. Supreme Court declare them to be unconstitutional.[38]

The early 1920s were also marked by an interest in biological theories of criminality somewhat akin to those legitimized by Lombroso. Orthodox criminologists were not responsible for this development.[39] The notion of biologically determined criminality was fostered largely by tabloid journalists and a few eugenically minded officials. For example, World's Work, a popular monthly, featured five articles on the biological basis of crime. One recounted the innovative efforts of Harry Olson, Chief Justice of the Chicago Municipal Court. Convinced that most criminals were mentally abnormal, Olson started a Psychopathic Laboratory and hired a psychometrician to develop screening tests to identify people with criminal minds.[40]

During the 1920s, many eugenics clubs and societies sprouted, but only two, the American Eugenics Society (AES) and the Human Betterment Foundation (HBF), exerted any significant influence on the course of eugenic sterilization. The AES was conceived at the Second International Congress of Eugenics in 1921. Dr. Henry Fairfield Osborn, President of the American Museum of Natural History, and a small group of patrician New Yorkers initiated the society. By 1923, it was sufficiently well organized to lobby against a bill to support special education for the handicapped, an idea that it considered dysgenic.

In 1925, the AES relocated to New Haven, Connecticutt. For the next few years, its major goal was public education. The Great Depression caused a great fall in donations, and when Ellsworth Huntington, a Yale geographer, became president in 1934, the society was moribund. With the aid of a wealthy relative of the founder, Huntington breathed new life into the organization and realized that politically the AES would fare better if it pushed "positive" eugenics policies, such as family planning and personal hygiene. By 1939, the AES had dissociated itself from hard-core sterilization advocates.

The wealthiest eugenics organization was the Human Betterment Foundation (HBF), started by California millionaire Ezra Gosney, who in 1926 convened a group of experts to study the efficacy of California's sterilization program. This group eventually published over 20 articles confirming the safety of being sterilized and concluded that the state had benefitted. Gosney was convinced that a massive sterilization program could reduce the number of mentally defective persons by one half in "three or four generations."[41]

For five years after sterilization statutes were struck down by the courts, there was little legislative activity. Then, in 1923, four states (Oregon, Montana, Delaware, and Ohio) enacted new laws, and by 1925, eight other states had followed suit. The new statutes were drafted with much greater regard for constitutional issues. Besides frequently requiring the assent of parents or guardians, the laws preserved the right to a jury trial of whether the patient was "the potential parent of socially inadequate offspring." Despite concern about the Equal Protection Clause, most laws were still aimed only at institutionalized persons.

Opponents of sterilization quickly attacked the new laws. Battle was joined in Michigan and Virginia. In June 1925, the highest Michigan court ruled that the state's sterilization statute was "justified by the findings of Biological Science."[42] But the crucial case involved a test of the Virginia law. Dr. A. S. Priddy, Superintendent of the State Colony for Epileptics and Feeble-Minded, filed a sterilization petition to test the judicial waters. Carefully amassing a wealth of proeugenic testimony, he shepherded the case through the courts. His strategy paid off. In May 1927, Oliver Wendell Holmes, writing for the majority of the U.S. Supreme Court, upheld involuntary sterilization of the feeble-minded, concluding:

> It is better for all the world, if instead of waiting to execute degenerative offspring for crime, or to let them starve for their imbecility, society can prevent those who are manifestly unfit from continuing their kind. The principle that sustains compulsory vaccination is broad enough to cover cutting the Fallopian tubes.[43]

YEARS OF TRIUMPH

The Supreme Court's decision to uphold the Virginia law accelerated the pace of legislation: in 1929, nine states adopted similar laws. As was the case before World War I, a small group of activists from influential quarters persuaded scientifically unsophisticated legislators that sterilization was necessary, humane, and just.

The lobbyists succeeded in part because of favorable views expressed in the medical profession. During 1927–1936, about 60 articles, the vast majority in favor of eugenic sterilization, appeared. In the general medical community, support was strong, but not uniform. Only 18 state medical societies officially backed sterilization programs. [44]

The legislative victories of the early 1930s were impressive, but the crucial measure of whether eugenic notions triumphed is to count the number of sterilizations. Data from surveys that were conducted by the Human Betterment Foundation and other groups permit minimal estimates of the extent of mass sterilization and compel some striking conclusions:

1. Between 1907 and 1963, there were eugenic sterilization programs in 30 states. More than 60,000 persons were sterilized pursuant to state laws.
2. Although sterilization reached its zenith during the 1930s, several states vigorously pursued this activity throughout the 1940s and 1950s.
3. At a given time, a few programs were more active than the rest. In the 1920s and 1930s, California and a few midwestern states were most active. After World War II, several southern states accounted for more than half of the involuntary sterilizations performed on institutionalized persons.
4. Beginning in about 1930, there was a dramatic rise in the percentage of women who were sterilized.
5. Revulsion with Nazi sterilization policy did not curtail American sterilization programs. Indeed, more than one half of all eugenic sterilizations occurred after the Nazi program was fully operational.

During 1929–1941, the Human Betterment Foundation conducted annual surveys of state institutions to chart the progress of sterilization. Letters from hospital officials indicate what factors influenced the programs. The most important determinants of the scope of a program's operation seems to have been the complexity of the due process requirements of the relevant laws, the level of funding, and the attitudes of the superintendents themselves. The HBF surveys strongly suggest that the total number of sterilizations performed on institutionalized persons was underreported. Respondents frequently indicated that eugenic operations were conducted outside the confines of state hospitals. [45]

Until 1918, there were only 1,422 eugenic sterilizations reportedly performed pursuant to state law. Ironically, the sterilization rate began to rise during the very period when the courts were rejecting the first round of statutes (1917–1918). From 1918 to 1920, there were 1,811 reported sterilizations, a fourfold increase over the annual rate during the prior decade. During the 1920s, annual sterilization figures were stable. But in 1929, there was a large increase in sterilizations. Throughout the 1930s, more than 2,000 institutionalized persons were sterilized each year, triple the rate of the early 1920s.

This rapid increase reflected changing concerns and changing policy. In the Great Depression years, the superintendents of many hospitals, strapped by tight budgets, decided to sterilize mildly retarded young women. Before 1929, about 53% of all eugenic sterilizations had been performed on men. Between 1929 and 1935, there were 14,651 reported operations, 9,327 on women and 5,324 on men. In several states, (e.g., Minnesota, and Wisconsin), virtually all the sterilized persons were women. This fact becomes even more impressive when one recognizes that salpingectomy incurred a relatively high morbidity and a much higher cost than did vasectomy. In California, at least five women died after undergoing eugenic sterilization.[46]

During the 1930s, institutionalized men were also being sterilized in unprecedented numbers, largely because of the great increase in the total number of state programs. Unlike the "menace of the feebleminded" that had haunted policy before World War I, the new concern was to cope with harsh economic realities. As the superintendents saw it, fewer babies born to incompetent parents might mean fewer state wards.

The triumph of eugenic sterilization programs in the United States during the 1930s influenced other nations. Canada, Germany, Sweden, Norway, Finland, France, and Japan enacted sterilization laws. The most important events took place in Germany, where the Nazis sterilized more than 50,000 "unfit" persons within one year of enacting a eugenics law.

The German interest in eugenics had roots that twined with nineteenth-century European racial thought, a topic beyond the scope of this chapter. In the early years of this century, there was a spate of books that preached the need to protect Nordic germ plasm. A German eugenics society was formed in 1905, and in 1907, the first (unsuccessful) sterilization bill was offered in the Reichstag. The devastation of World War I halted the German eugenic movement, but by 1921, groups were again actively lobbying for eugenics programs. Hitler advocated eugenic sterilization as early as 1923.

When the Nazis swept to power, they quickly implemented a program to encourage larger, healthier families. Tax laws were restructured to favor childbearing. In 1933, a companion law was enacted to prevent reproduction by defective persons. The work of Gosney and Popenoe was extremely influential on the Nazi planners.[47]

The law created a system of "hereditary health courts," which judged petitions brought by public health officials that certain citizens burdened with one of a long list of disorders (feeblemindedness, schizophrenia, manic-depressive insanity, epilepsy, Huntington's chorea, hereditary blindness, hereditary deafness, severe physical deformity, and habitual drunkenness) would be subjected to compulsory sterilization. In 1934, the courts heard 64,499 petitions and ordered 56,244 sterilizations, for a "eugenic conviction" rate of 87%.[48] In 1934, the German Supreme Court ruled that the law applied to non-Germans living in Germany, a decision that had special import for Gypsies. From 1935 through 1939, the annual number of eugenic sterilizations grew rapidly. Unfortunately, key records perished during World War II. But in 1951, the "Central Association of Sterilized People in West Germany" charged that, from 1934 to 1945, the Nazis sterilized 3,500,000 people, often on the flimsiest pretext.[49]

The Nazi program was eugenics run amok. In the United States, no program even approached it in scope or daring. But there is no evidence to support the argument, frequently heard, that stories of Nazi horrors halted American sterilization efforts.

The Quiet Years

With the onset of World War II, there was a sharp decline in the number of eugenic sterilizations in the United States. Although manpower shortages (surgeons were unavailable) directly contributed to the decline, other factors were also at work. In 1939, the Eugenics Record Office closed its doors; in 1942, the Human Betterment Foundation also ceased its activities. Later that year, the U.S. Supreme Court, considering its first sterilization case in 15 years, struck down an Oklahoma law that permitted certain thrice-convicted felons to be sterilized.[50] After the war, as the horror of the Nazi eugenics movement became more obvious, the goals of the lingering American programs became more suspect. Yet, despite these changes, many state-mandated sterilization programs continued, albeit at a reduced level of activity.

Between 1942 and 1946, the annual sterilization rate dropped to half that of the 1930s. Reports of institutional officials make it clear that this decline was largely due to a lack of surgeons and nurses.[51] There is little evidence to suggest that the Supreme Court decision had a major impact. Avoiding an opportunity to broadly condemn involuntary sterilization and overrule *Buck v. Bell*,[52] the justices demanded instead that such practices adhere to the precept of the Equal Protection Clause that like persons be treated in a similar fashion. The Oklahoma law was struck down because it spared certain "white-collar" criminals from a punitive measure aimed at other thrice-convicted persons, not simply because it involved sterilization.

During the late 1940s, there was no definite indication that sterilization programs were about decline. After hitting a low of 1,183 in 1944, there were 1,526 operations in 1950. Slight declines in many states were balanced by rapid increases in North Carolina and Georgia. By 1950, however, there were bellwether signs that sterilization was in disfavor even among institutional officials. For example, during the 1930s and 1940s, 100 persons in San Quentin prison had been sterilized each year. But in 1950, new officials at the California Department of Correction were "entirely averse" to the program.[53] During that year, sterilization bills were considered in only four states, and all were rejected.[54]

There were major changes in state sterilization programs in 1952. The California program, for years the nation's most active, was moribund, dropping from 275 sterilizations in 1950 to 39 in 1952. By that year, Georgia, North Carolina, and Virginia (having sterilized 673 persons) were responsible for 53% of the national total. General declines in most other states continued throughout the 1950s, and by 1958, these three states were responsible for 76% (574 persons) of the reported operations. The North Carolina program was unique in that it was directed largely at noninstitutionalized rural young women.[55] As recently as 1963, the state paid for the eugenic sterilization of 193 persons, of whom 183 were young women.[56] Despite their persistence, the southern programs must be seen as a local eddy in a tide of decline.

Involuntary Sterilization Today

During the 1960s, the practice of sterilizing retarded persons in state institutions virtually ceased. But the laws remained. In 1961, there were eugenic sterilization laws on the books of 28 states, and it was possible to perform involuntary sterilizations in 26.[57] Between 1961 and 1976, five laws were repealed, six were amended (to improve procedural safeguards), and one state (West Virginia in 1975) adopted its first sterilization statute. Currently, eugenic sterilization of institutionalized retarded persons is permissible in 19 states, but the laws are rarely invoked. A few states have enacted laws that expressly forbid the sterilization of any persons in state institutions.

If the mid-1930s saw the zenith of eugenic sterilization, the mid-1960s saw its nadir. But the pendulum of policy continues to swing. The late 1960s saw the first lawsuits brought by the parents of noninstitutionalized retarded females arguing that sterilization was both economically essential and psychologically beneficial to their efforts to maintain their adult daughters at home.[58]

In 1973, the debate over sterilzing institutionalized persons who officials had decided were unfit to be parents flared in the media. The mother of a young man whom physicians at the Partlow State School in Alabama wished to sterlize challenged the constitutionality of the enabling statute. When Alabama officials cleverly argued that they did not need statutory authority as long as consent was obtained from the retarded person, the federal judge not only overturned the law but decreed strict guidelines to control the process of performing "voluntary" sterilizations at Partlow. The key feature was the creation of an outside committee to review all the sterilization petitions.[59]

Also in 1973, the U.S. Department of Health, Education, and Welfare (HEW) became enmeshed in a highly publicized sterilization scandal. That summer, it was reported that an Alabama physician working at a family-planning clinic funded by HEW had sterilized several young, poor black women without their consent. The National Welfare Rights Organization joined with two of the women and sued to block the use of all federal funds to pay for sterilizations. This move prompted HEW to draft strict regulations governing the use of federal money for such purposes, but a federal judge struck them down and held that HEW could not provide sterilization services to legally incompetent persons.[60] Revamped several times, the HEW guidelines were the subject of continuous litigation for five years. Late in 1978, "final rules" were issued that prohibited the sterilization of some persons (those under 21, and all mentally incompetent persons) and demanded elaborate consent mechanisms when a competent person requested to undergo sterilization to be paid for by public funds.[61]

During the last few years, the debate over sterilizing the mentally retarded, although no longer cast in a eugenic context, reheated. The key issue was to resolve the tensions between the society's duty to protect the incompetent person and the *right* of that person to be sterilized. Of course, exercise of this right presupposes that a family member or guardian is, in fact, properly asserting a right that the subject is incapable of exercising on her own (almost all requests are filed on behalf of retarded young *women*), a matter to which judges devote most of their attention. The court must be convinced that the operation will benefit the patient.

More than 20 appellate courts have been asked to consider sterilization petitions. This spate of litigation has resulted because physicians are now extremely reluctant to run the risk of violating the civil rights of the retarded. The courts have split sharply. In the absence of express statutory authority, six high courts have refused to authorize sterilization orders.[62]

In the more recent decisions, most appellate courts have ruled that (even without statutory authorization) local courts of general jurisdiction do have the power to evaluate petitions to sterilize retarded persons. In a leading case, the highest court in New Jersey held that the parents of an adolescent girl with Down syndrome might obtain surgical sterilization for her if they could provide clear and convincing evidence that it was in "her best interests."[63] Since then, high courts in Colorado, Massachusetts, and Pennsylvania have ruled in a similar manner. These decisions promise that, in the future, the families of some retarded persons will be able to obtain sterilizations for them, regardless of their institutional status.

The great era of sterilization has passed. Yet, grim reminders of unsophisticated programs that once flourished linger. In Virginia, persons sterilized for eugenic reasons decades ago have sued the state, claiming a violation of their civil rights. Although they lost their argument that the operations were performed pursuant to an unconstitutional law, litigation over whether the state failed in its duty to inform them of the consequences of the operations continues. From pretrial discovery, it appears likely that not a few of the persons who were sterilized were not retarded.[64]

What of the future? Is the saga of involuntary sterilization over? Our knowledge of human genetics makes the return of mass eugenic sterilizations unlikely. However, it is more difficult to predict the future of sterilization programs founded on other arguments. During the 1960s, a number of state legislatures considered a bill to tie welfare payments to "voluntary" sterilization.[65] In 1980, a Texas official made a similar suggestion.[66] Unscientific opinion polls conducted by magazines and newspapers in Texas and Massachusetts found significant support for involuntary sterilization of the retarded.[67]

Although it is unlikely to happen in the United States, the pressing demands of population control in India and China have resulted in social policies that create strong incentives to be sterilized. Since launching the "one-child" program in 1979, China has rapidly altered the social fabric of 1 billion people.[68] As our resources continue to shrink and our earthly neighborhood becomes more crowded, compulsory sterilization may someday be as common as compulsory immunizations, but the eugenic vision will no longer provide its intellectual rationale.

REFERENCES AND NOTES

1. Estabrook, A., and Davenport, C. B., *The Nam Family: A Study of Cacogenics*, Eugenics Record Office, Cold Spring Harbor, NY, 1912.
2. Galton, F., Hereditary talent and character, *Macmillan's Magazine* 12:157–66 (1865).
3. Macmillan, London (1869).
4. Two other books by Galton, *English Men of Science: Their Nature and Nuture*, Macmillan, London (1874); and *Inquiries into Human Faculty and Its Development*, Macmillan, London, (1883), did much to legitimize eugenics.
5. Greene, J. C., Some early speculations on the origin of human races, *American Anthropologist* 56:31–41 (1954).

6. Morton, S. G., *Crania Americana*, John Pennington, Philadelphia (1839). After the Civil War, miscegenation took on new importance; the leading opponent of interracial marriages was a South Carolina physician: Nott, J. C., The mullatto a hybrid, *Am. J. Med. Sci.* 6:252–6 (1843).

7. Lombroso-Ferrerr, G., *Lombroso's Criminal Man*, Patterson-Smith, Montclair, NJ (1872).

8. Boies, H. M., *Prisoners and Paupers*, G. P. Putnam's Sons, NY (1893).

9. Dugdale, R. L., A record and study of the relations of crime, pauperism and disease, in *Appendix to the Thirty-first Report of the NY Prison Association*, NY Prison Assoc., Albany, NY (1875).

10. Kerlin, I., Report to the eleventh national conference on charters and reforms, *Proc. A.M.O.* (1884), 465.

11. Rosenberg, C. E., Charles Benedict Davenport and the beginning of human genetics, *Bull. Hist. Med.* 35:266–76 (1961).

12. See *supra* note 1; ERO workers also analyzed the inheritance of Huntington's chorea: Davenport, D. B., Huntington's Chorea in relation to heredity and eugenics, *Bull. No. 17*, Cold Spring Harbor, NY (1916); and early eugenic work was reported in a climate of scientific respectability.

13. Goddard, H. H., *The Kallikak Family*, Macmillan, New York (1912).

14. Gould, S. J., *The Mismeasure of Man*, Norton, New York (1981).

15. Higham, J., *Strangers in the Land*, Athenaeum, New York (1965).

16. Davenport, C. B., *State Laws Limiting Marriage Selection*, Eugenics Record Office, Cold Spring Harbor, NY (1913).

17. Daniel, F. E., Emasculation for criminal assaults and incest, *Texas Med. J.* 22:347 (1907).

18. Ochsner, A., Surgical treatment of habitual criminals, *JAMA* 53:867–8 (1899).

19. Sharp, H. C. The severing of the vasa defferentia and its relation to the neuropsychiatric constitution, *N.Y. Med. J* (1902), 411–14.

20. Sharp, H. C., *Vasectomy*, privately printed, Indianapolis (1909).

21. Ochsner, *supra* note 18.

22. Reilly, P. R., The surgical solution: The writings of activist physicians in the early days of eugenical sterilization, *Persp. Biol. Med.* 26:637–56 (1983).

23. Sharp, H. C., Vasectomy as a means of preventing procreation of defectives, *JAMA* 51:1897–1902 (1907).

24. Popenoe, P., The progress of eugenical sterilization, *J. of Heredity* 28:19–25 (1933).

25. But see Rhode Island State Library Legislative Research Bureau, *Sterilization of the Unfit*, Providence (1913); and Laughlin, H. H., *Eugenical Sterilization in the United States*, Chicago Psychopathic Laboratory of the Municipal Court, Chicago (1922).

26. Roosevelt, T., Twisted eugenics, *Outlook* 106:30–4, 1914; Eugene Smith, President of the National Prison Association, was a prominent lawyer pushing for sterilization laws—The cost of crime, *Medico-Legal J.* 27:140–9 (1908)—as was Judge Warren Foster, *Pearson's Magazine* (1909) 565–72.

27. Johnson, A., Race improvement by control of defectives, *Ann. Am. Acad. Penal Soc. Sci.* 34:22–29 (1909).

28. Report by the Immigration Commission, U.S. Government Printing Office, Washington, D.C. (1910).

29. See Laughlin *supra*, note 25.

30. *Id.*

31. *Id.*

32. *State v. Feilen*, 70 Wash. 65 (1912).

33. *Mickle v. Henrichs*, 262 F. 687 (1918).

34. *Davis v. Berry*, 216 F. 413 (1914).

35. Spaulding, E. R., and Healy, W., Inheritance as a factor in criminality, in *Physical Basis of Crime*, American Academy of Med. Press, Easton, PA (1914).

36. Ludmerer, K., *Genetics and American Society*, Johns Hopkins University Press, Baltimore (1972).

37. Mencke, J. G., *Mulattoes and Race Mixture: American Attitudes and Images, 1865–1918*, UMI Research Press, Ann Arbor, Mich. (1959).

38. *Loving v. Virginia*, 388 U.S. 1 (1967).

39. Parmelee, M., *Criminology*, Macmillan, New York (1918).

40. Strother, F., The cause of crime: Defective brain, *World's Work* 48:275–81 (1924).

41. Gosney, E. S., & Popenoe, P., *Sterilization for Human Betterment*, Macmillan, New York (1929). HBF was the leading source of prosterilization literature during the 1930s, sponsored a "social eugenics" column in the *Los Angeles Times*, aired radio programs, produced pamphlets, and underwrote lectures. It remained vigorous until Gosney's death in 1942.

42. *Smith v. Probate*, 231 Mich. 409 (1925).
43. *Buck v. Bell*, 274 U.S. 200 (1927).
44. Whitten, B. D., Sterilization, *J. Psycho-Asthenics* **40**:56–68 (1935). But in some states, like Indiana, support was very strong. Harshman, L. P., Medical and legal aspects of sterilization in Indiana, *J. Psycho-Asthenics* **39**:183–206 (1934).
45. See, e.g., Dunham, W. F., Letter to E. S. Gosney, *AVS Archive*, University of Minnesota (1936).
46. Gosney and Popenoe *supra*, note 41.
47. Kopp, M., The German sterilization program, *AVS Archive*, University of Minnesota (1935).
48. Cook, R., A year of German sterilization, *J. Heredity* **26**:485–9 (1935).
49. *New York Herald Tribune* (Jan. 14, 1951), 12.
50. *Skinner v. Oklahoma*, 316 U.S. 535 (1942).
51. Taromianz, M. A., Letter to NJ Sterilization League, *AVS Archive*, University of Minnesota (1944).
52. 274 U.S. 200 (1927).
53. Stanley, L. L., Letter to the NJ Sterilization League, *AVS Archive*, University of Minnesota (1950).
54. Butler, F. O., Report, *AVS Archive*, University of Minnesota (1950).
55. Woodside, M., *Sterilization in North Carolina*, University of North Carolina, Chapel Hill (1950).
56. Casebolt, S. L., Letters to Human Betterment Association of America, *AVS Archive*, University of Minnesota (1963).
57. Landman, F. T., and McIntyre, D. M., *The Mentally Disabled and the Law*, University of Chicago Press, Chicago (1961).
58. *Frazier v. Levi*, 440 S.W. 2d 579 (TX 1968).
59. *Wyatt v. Aderholt*, 368 F. Supp. 1382 (Ala. D.C. 1973).
60. *Relf v. Weinberger*, 372 F. Supp. 1196 (1974).
61. *Fed. Reg.* 52146-75 (1978).
62. *In the Matter of S.C.E.*, 378 A .2d 144 (1977).
63. *In re Grady*, 426 N.W. 2d 467 (NJ 1981).
64. *Poe v. Lynchburg*, 1981.
65. Paul, J., The return of punitive sterilization laws, *Law Soc. Rev.* **4**:77–110 (1968).
66. *New York Times* (Feb. 28, 1980), A16.
67. *The Texas Observer* (March 20, 1981), 7; *Boston Globe* (March 31, 1982), 1.
68. *Intercom* **9**(8):12–14, 1981.

Discussion

Mr. Norman Fost: As I'm sure you realize, what is going on today, in part, is a reaction against sterilization excesses, although excesses and eugenic ideas are alive in other ways than sterilization. We do have a reaction, and one of them involves the case Ruth Macklin just mentioned. As you know, in Wisconsin, a State Supreme Court Decision has made it impermissible to sterilize a retarded person involuntarily even when pregnancy is a significant risk and such pregnancy would offer little or no benefit and probably considerable harm, psychological and otherwise. The Wisconsin Supreme Court said that, in the absence of a statute, it would not be permissible to do that. Realizing the dangers of statutes and the excesses, I wonder if you could concisely tell us what sort of enabling statutes you would favor, if any, that would allow these therapeutic sterilizations.

Dr. Philip R. Reilly: I detect several trends in the current legal climate. One is for the courts to take a very conservative approach and to wait for enabling legislation. In other states, there's been a willingness for higher courts to say that courts of lower jurisdiction should have the right to act on such petitions without enabling legislation. I personally would not let "excesses in the past" take away rights from a family or a retarded individual. After all, a retarded individual, in my view, has as much right to be sterilized if he or she wishes, or if any appropriate proxy directs in his or her behalf, as anyone else. To be overly paternalistic is an ethical crime in the other direction. So I am opposed to states that take such an inflexible approach to the problem.

Ms. Sylvia Rubin (Columbia Presbyterian Medical Center): Professor Dickens, as a geneticist, I am specifically involved with genetic counseling, and I deal almost daily with issues that have been presented in this symposium. My question involves problems that will certainly come up with surrogate mothers but can involve any pregnancy. Can, for instance, a husband legally restrict a wife or a couple restrict a surrogate mother from smoking during pregnancy or drinking alcoholic beverages, and if so, how can the restriction be enforced? Both of these are harmful to a developing fetus. What

243

about the birth of an anomalous child? I'm sure everyone here knows there is a 2%–3% risk of any baby's being born with a severe defect. Is it genetic? Or can it be due to, or blamed on, the transplant process, whatever that process may be, and thereby, the physicians or anyone involved in the process would be to "blame." Or could the blame be put on an environmental factor in the womb and thereby be the "fault" of the surrogate mother? Are there precedents for lawsuits before or after delivery for any of these problems? As a scientist without any real legal knowledge, I feel that the potential problems haven't even begun to be recognized, and I wonder whether there's anything that individuals cannot be sued for regarding childbearing.

MR. BERNARD M. DICKENS: The problems certainly exists. I think you've located them in the right arena, in that they are inherent in childbearing. They're not special to surrogate motherhood. Where one has an adequately drafted agreement, one would expect the potential surrogate to give contractual guarantees about her conduct, such as not smoking, not drinking, and not having recourse to vigorous exercise. If a woman gives that guarantee, there would be no means of enforcement by specific restraints. On the other hand, a breach of contract could affect subsequent matters: it could affect her being entitled to payment, or to a bonus on the delivery of a healthy as opposed to an unhealthy child. In that sense, one could try to anticipate the problem and try to reduce it, but one couldn't eliminate it.

The question arises whether a woman who serves as a surrogate would have the right of recourse to nontherapeutic abortion if she chose to break the contract. The contract provisions could anticipate that right through a system either of sanctions or of proportionate rewards. There might also be a special obligation on those who screen potential surrogate mothers to eliminate those who would predictably pursue a wanton or inimical lifestyle. In a sense, one could try to deal with it.

Regarding the risk of anomalies (as you say, 2%–3% in "ordinary" pregnancies), one would have to rely on the doctrine of informed consent, so that both the social parents and the surrogate mother are aware of the inherent risk. It's fairly clear that the social parents would have obligations to accept the child even if it was born with anomalies. Some current contracts not only point out these risks but go so far as to require the payment of an insurance premium regarding the surrogate mother, her life, and perhaps her health. These are techniques of anticipation of problems and accommodation to them.

Regarding lawsuits, there is a so-called action for wrongful birth. The difficulty with surrogate motherhood is that one considers the action of the child, and that would be an action for a wrongful life (or sometimes for "dissatisfied life"). The courts fairly uniformly have rejected these claims. Indeed, only three decisions—two from California, and one from Washington State—have allowed children to sue for wrongful life. The philosophy underlying wrongful life actions is very complex and contentious. To that extent, I think that one could say that, if the alternative to the child's being born with the handicap is the child's not being conceived or, having been conceived, not being born, then all but two jurisdictions would conclude that wrongful life is not a legal cause of action. One normally sues for compensation: the measure of damages is the difference between the condition that one has and the position one would have been in had the wrong not occurred. The courts can accommodate the difference between normality and abnormality. They can't accommodate very easily the difference between abnormality and what the New Jersey Supreme Court calls the "utter void of non-existence."

Ms. TABITHA M. POWLEDGE (Bio/Technology Magazine): I'm a little troubled by the way in which we use the word *eugenics*, which has become a kind of umbrella term. Yesterday, we were talking about it mainly in the context of making changes in the gene pool. Today, Dr. Reilly used it in one context to mean either allowing the old or the handicapped to die or actually engaging in active killing, and this is a usage also honored by time. That is a preamble to my reiterating a suggestion I have made to Dr. Reilly before, that his extremely interesting data showing a change from sterilization of men to sterilization of women reveal a movement away from eugenic thinking, at least in the strict sense of alterations in the gene pool. The arguments for sterilizing men were very often couched in terms of not passing on criminal genes or genes for alcoholism and so forth, whereas the arguments for sterilizing women (beginning in the early 1930s) are couched in terms such as, "this woman is retarded," and she is therefore "not equipped to care for a child," or "This woman is retarded and therefore the state will have to bear the burden of caring for the child." I suppose you could say that that's eugenics once removed, but it seems to me to be quite a different sort of motivation from preserving the gene pool from harm. Would you comment?

Dr. PHILIP R. REILLY: I agree with you that where we diverge may depend on how precisely we use the term *eugenics*. My view is that the restatement of the rationale for sterilizing young retarded women came about because the purely genetic argument for sterilization was beginning to fade, that is, as more and more people said, "The simplified views of Davenport and Loughlin don't hold." People who still didn't want those retarded folks to have babies sought a new explanation and turned to the social cost argument. In fact, they still passionately believed that the retarded had bad genes and shouldn't be reproducing. I think that's part of it. I also do agree with you that there is still a eugenic argument implicit in what they did even if it is one step removed. But I think the original letters and the literature suggest that they were seeking a more palatable policy explanation to continue the same archaic eugenic goals.

Ms. TABITHA M. POWLEDGE: Was it a cover-up argument or was it a real argument? You made the case that the Great Depression provided all sorts of financial constraints.

Dr. PHILIP R. REILLY: I think it was a combination. I think there was definitely an impact of the Depression. One of the things that many of these state institutions did was to create a revolving door, where they admitted young women (there's some evidence that a significant number of them were not retarded by today's standards), sterilized them, and sent them out in a matter of weeks, so that they could not have children who would turn up in the institutions 20 years later. That suggests to me a financial argument to some degree. But when you become familiar with the people who were running these policies, you know they really thought that these women had bad genes, too. If you read their private letters, you see what they thought about.

Ms. TABITHA M. POWLEDGE: So it really was a mixture of motivations?

DR. PHILIP R. REILLY: That's my own feeling.

Ms. TABITHA M. POWLEDGE: To Bernard Dickens: I was absolutely fascinated to suddenly be faced with the notion that it is our tax laws that are going to solve all our regulatory problems. You may well be right. Are there any present examples where the taxing authorities in any country have made decisions on the questions you raised?

DR. BERNARD M. DICKENS: No, they remain very open. The difficulty is that a lump sum payment under an agreement could well be a payment under an unlawful agreement. That's not to say it's not taxable, but the tax authorities haven't made any systematic response.

Ms. BARBARA KATZ ROTHMAN (City University of New York): You called for an anthropologist to give us some language. As a sociologist, I would like to say that we don't have to look beyond our own culture and society. We have some language to use for the issue of surrogate parenthood, but we are very reluctant to use it. What we normally call a person who is a genetic parent is a *father*. What we are looking at in embryo transfer is the issue of women fathering children, and we are really reluctant simply to use that language. In all of our model building, there's been a real problem in the underlying assumptions. I think this is also the moment to respond to the issues that George Annas raised about surrogate motherhood: the issues of exploitation, the concern about the cheapening of embryonic and fetal life as they become purchasable commodities. I believe this issue builds on adoption, which has been largely and predominantly the purchase of babies. When we start building on models like that for the new technology, we are faced with the inherent problems of the exploitation of women.

What happens, for instance, when George Annas says that he's really uncomfortable about the sale of embryos (and I share that discomfort) is that as we focus on the problem that there really is something terribly wrong with selling embryos. But then, we go on to discuss the possibility of "renting wombs." One cannot rent a womb. One purchases a woman for the duration. Our wombs don't separate out that way. If we were really talking about taking a uterus out of one woman's body and putting it in another, it would be a very different issue. What we are talking about here, however, is something that is done either out of very, very great love (and it is the real contribution of one woman to another) or out of exploitation of one sort or another. And it's being purchased by what we are also calling one "couple" from a woman. So that the issues of exploitation are fundamental to the original models that we were building on: artificial insemination was based on the purchase of sperm, and adoption was based on the purchase of babies. As we start moving into new technologies, we are still looking at the same fundamental flaws. We are leaving out the meaning of the experience to the women involved, so that the meaning of the pregnancy can be eliminated as a significant moral factor in the surrogate motherhood issue. And this leaves out the exploitation that underlies all of this exploitation of some women for other women, often on a class basis.

DR. ELVING ANDERSON (Dight Institute, University of Minnesota): For Dr. Reilly: Do you think there are any acceptable or ethical concerns about the genetic constitution of future generations? If so, what label might be attached to them?

DR. PHILIP R. REILLY: If I understand you correctly, an ethical argument about a duty to the future that would justify some action in the present directed at an individual. Is that your concern?

DR. ELVING ANDERSON: It could be that, or it could be as simple as trying to find out what present policies may do. It could be either research along this line or something directed toward action. In other words, is it reasonable to have some concern about the genetics of the future, and then, because of the problem with the term *eugenics*, is there some other term that could be more acceptable?

DR. PHILIP R. REILLY: One of the bedrock documents in our society uses the term *posterity*, which is one I actually like very much. I would never attempt in this audience to engage in discussions of population genetics. I am ill equipped. However, having said that, I can imagine the development of policy arguments to shape reproductive behavior in gentle ways, because of proven concerns about the impact of failure to do that.

DR. BERNARD M. DICKENS: I think there is a cohesive link between Philip Reilly's observations and what we heard at the first session this morning. In discussing sterilization policy, one can assess the legislation that exists regarding screening for sperm donation, where certain particular traits have to be identified and eliminated. How far that can go is a speculative matter, but there seems to be some sense that one ought to undertake a form of positive eugenics in selecting gamete donors for artificial reproduction.

MR. JOHN L. COX, II (Chappaqua, New York): In connection with Dr. Reilly's discussion, I have a little information that might be interesting. I used to know the head of the Sonoma Home in California, and I know what his thinking was about the sterilizations that were being performed there. Well, I heard him, over and over again, say that he felt that the patients were being helped by what was being done. He felt that it was a mistake to keep them in institutions when they could live perfectly well on the outside, provided they didn't have things to take care of beyond their capability. He cited numbers of cases where a retarded person was brought to the institution and the people would say, "Don't ever let this person out. If you let them out, they are going to be in all kinds of trouble." He would respond, "It looks as though they could handle the situation if they didn't have any children." He cited any number of cases where people, who had been in the institution and had been sterilized, were released, got married, and lived perfectly happy lives. It was not a matter of eugenics primarily with him, but a matter of the social arrangement that would be more favorable for the patient.

DR. PHILIP R. REILLY: I don't think I said that the eugenicists were evil people. Indeed, I think many of them had the highest motivation for helping the persons whom they sterilized. However, when one looks closely, one begins to be concerned about the criteria used to decide who needed to be sterilized and how accurate they were. In fact, some of these people might have been able to raise children successfully. I'm not sure that intelligence is the *sine qua non* for being a parent. Indeed, it may sometimes be counterproductive.

MR. JOHN L. COX: The thing that made him saddest was when children would come to the institution to visit their defective parents. He said it was a tragedy.

A PARTICIPANT: I wonder whether Dr. Butler considered more reversible methods of contraception than surgical sterilization.

DR. PHILIP R. REILLY: The program in California had, among its prices, the death of five women from intra-abdominal procedures for involuntary sterilization conducted for their benefit. Those deaths would never have occurred if not for the well-meaning program, so there is a social cost in each direction.

A PARTICIPANT: We have a long history of paternalistic justifications for all kinds of behavior.

MS. PEGGY GLATNER (Albert Einstein College of Medicine, New York): I'd like to know how legally significant informed consent is in the eyes of the law as we use it in our institutions. A problem in obstetrics and gynecology arises when someone becomes impregnated in an institution and the person is of age to sign for consent for abortion but is unable to because of retardation, and there are no parents or next of kin responsible. Therefore, we can't have the consent signed, the pregnancy can't be terminated, and it goes to term. Would you comment on that, please?

MR. BERNARD M. DICKENS: The doctrine of informed consent can be analyzed in a number of ways. It is traditional to separate informed consent from free consent if one is dealing with a nonfree population. Then, it well could be that simply giving them data, even if the data are comprehensible, wouldn't resolve the legal problem. The issue may be that they are not in a position to exercise free choice, based on the data that they have.

MS. PEGGY BLATNER: How legally binding is informed consent when they understand the information conveyed?

MR. BERNARD M. DICKENS: Normally, if it's an exercise of their autonomy and is adequately informed and free, the courts would recognize it. If we are dealing with a dependent population, and if we are dealing with a legal guardian, then questions arise about whether the guardian can indulge his or her own wishes or whether the limitation of the power is to discharge the function of serving the best interests of the dependent individual.

PROTECTING THE VULNERABLE: AT WHAT COST?

Decisions about Seriously Ill Neonates

MODERATOR: ARNOLD S. RELMAN

18

"INFANT DOE"

Federal Regulations of the Newborn Nursery Are Born

I. DAVID TODRES, M.D.
Director, Neonatal and Pediatric
Intensive Care Units
Massachusetts General Hospital
Fruit Street
Boston, MA 02114
Associate Professor of Pediatrics
Harvard Medical School
25 Shattuck Street
Boston, MA 02115

The audience assembled represents a large cross section of individuals committed to health care: physicians, nurses, social workers, hospital administrators, lawyers, and the ministry. Most of you have read of the "Baby Doe" regulations and their implications for the care of severely handicapped newborns. It will be helpful to review the chronological events leading to these regulations and their present status. I should then like to consider why these are such difficult ethical dilemmas. As a physician practicing at the bedside, I shall be describing a perspective on these issues from the standpoint of the physician's role in the decision-making process.

BACKGROUND OF THE "BABY DOE" REGULATIONS

In February 1982, in Bloomington, Indiana, the Supreme Court for the State of Indiana upheld the wishes of the parents of a child with Down syndrome and tracheoesophageal fistula not to have the life-saving operative correction that would relieve the bowel obstruction and allow the infant to be fed. As a result of the nontreatment decision, the infant died.

Shortly after in April 1982, President Reagan instructed the Secretary of Health and Human Services (HHS) to notify health care providers of the applicability of Section 504 of the Rehabilitation Act of 1973 with regard to the treatment of handicapped patients. The following month, May 1982, the Department of Health and Human Services notified 7,000 hospitals, receiving federal funding, of the applicability of Section 504.

The following year, on March 7, 1983, HHS issued, with an effective date of March 22, 1983, an interim final rule requiring hospitals to post in conspicuous places a notice advising of the applicability of Section 504 and the availability of a telephone "hotline" to report suspected violations of the law.

This interim rule was successfully challenged by the American Academy of Pediatrics and other institutions in the courts. On April 14, 1983, Judge Gesell, U.S. District Judge of the District of Columbia, declared the interim final rule invalid on the grounds that it was "arbitrary and capricious" and that there was no justification for waiving the public comment period, an action that was a violation of the administration's Procedure Act. Thus, the rule was struck down on procedural but not substantive grounds.

On July 5, 1983, the HSS issued a revised notice and set up a 60-day comment period. While the rule was suspended, however, the "hotline" operation remained in effect.

HHS solicited and received approximately 17,000 comments relating to a variety of decisions involving severely handicapped infants. Following review, the final regulations were published on January 12, 1984, in the *Federal Register* with an effective date of February 13, 1984.

The new regulations required that life-sustaining treatment be provided for handicapped and seriously ill newborns, unless these medical procedures "are clearly futile and will only prolong the act of dying." The new regulations required institutions to post notices of their duty to provide care to the handicapped newborns. A "hotline" service for suspected violations was included in the notice.

In addition, the regulations advised the establishment of infant-care review committees to develop institutional policies and to review individual cases involving withholding life-sustaining treatment from handicapped or seriously ill infants. The new regulations also required state child-protective-service agencies to develop procedures for protecting handicapped infants.

The regulations also gave approval to a draft titled "Priniciples of Treatment of Disabled Infants" drawn up by the American Academy of Pediatrics, the National Association of Children's Hospitals, and the Associations for Handicapped (November 29, 1983). The principles stated:

> When medical care is beneficial it should always be provided. When appropriate medical care is not available, arrangements should be made to transfer the infant to an appropriate medical facility. Considerations such as anticipated or actual limited potential of an individual, and present or future lack of available community resources are irrelevant and must not determine the decisions concerning medical care. The individual's medical condition should be the sole focus of the decision. It is ethically and legally justified to withhold medical or surgical procedures which are clearly futile and will only prolong the act of dying. However, supportive care should be provided, including sustenance as medically indicated and relief of pain and suffering. In cases

where it is uncertain whether medical treatment will be beneficial, a person's disability must not be the basis for a decision to withhold treatment. When a doubt exists at any time about whether to treat, a presumption should always be made in favor of treatment.

As of this writing, the federal regulations arising out of the "Baby Doe" case have been suspended, pending further review.

The "Baby Jane Doe" case in New York State highlighted the problem again by bringing to our attention the ongoing agonizing dilemma confronting the parents of a severely handicapped infant. Infant "Jane Doe" is a severely impaired infant with multiple defects (including myelomeningocele, hydrocephalus, and microcephaly). It was anticipated that she would be so severely handicapped as not to be able to intereact with her environment or other people. After consultations with physicians, nurses, social workers, and clergy, the parents decided to forgo corrective surgery. HHS received a complaint from a private citizen and sought to investigate the records on the basis of Section 504 of the Rehabilitation Act. Federal District Courts and State Appeals Courts of New York have banned any investigation of the infant's records and, by so doing, have upheld the rigts of the family.

The Newborn Intensive-Care Unit

The birth of a seriously handicapped infant evokes powerful emotional responses in the parents. Instead of experiencing the joys of having delivered a healthy infant, feelings of numbness, grief, and disgust and waves of helplessness, rage and disbelief are experienced. Parents may at first wish to get rid of the infant. These feelings are quickly followed by intense guilt, self-blame, and anxiety. These reactions need to be recognized, as they can lead to hasty decision-making or paralyze it.

The sophisticated environment of the newborn intensive-care unit (NICU), in which these seriously ill newborns are cared for, has evolved relatively recently. These units are filled with advanced technological support systems that have significantly reduced morbidity and mortality in these infants. Follow-up of high-risk infants has attested to this reduction; however, at times, technological support preserves in life a child that biology's blueprint had not designed for human survival. We are, thus, presented with an ethical crisis that transcends our concepts of good and evil.

The physicians caring for the seriously ill and handicapped newborn may be faced with an agonizing dilemma. Although the physician has a duty to preserve life, she or he also has a duty to relieve pain and suffering—and sometimes these two aims are contradictory. Faced with decisions regarding the care of the infant, the physician should primarily perform what *is in the best interests of the infant*. The infant's well-being should not be contingent on the well-being of the parents, insurance companies, and taxpayers. Although these are concerns that we may have, they should not bias our decision making. The burdens that these groups will have are not ignored, but in considering burdens, we must consider the child and the burden that the illness places on the child for a future life.

In evaluating the mental and physical burdens of the handicapped, the physician requires a comprehensive understanding of the nature of the handicap, the possibilities for medical therapy, and the outcome.

The problem of uncertainty in our medical knowledge about these gravely handicapped infants makes prognostication difficult. In making predictions of future outcomes, statistical data are applied that may not necessarily reflect the most recent and evolving methods of treatment. The newborn is unique in that there has been no "previous life" to use as a measure of change from one state to another, as compared with a catastrophic illness that befalls an adult.

In recognizing and lessening the problem of uncertainty, it behooves the physician to consult appropriate colleagues for all the necessary information, and at the same time to recognize the limitations of present medical knowledge.

In the process of decision making, we need to consider the element of time as it relates to the urgency for medical intervention. For example, in infants with myelomeningocele, surgical intervention may be urgently required to prevent potentially lethal complications of infection. Under the pressure of urgent decision-making, difficulties may be encountered because of time constraints in getting additional medical opinions and thinking through the options to arrive at what is in the best interests of the infant.

For some of these ethical dilemmas, a single decision regarding treatment will determine the total management plan. However, what is often not appreciated is that the gravely ill and handicapped infant is experiencing a *changing* pathophysiological status from altered responses to therapy and further developing complications, thus necessitating frequent and difficult decisions in management.

Physicians, nurses, social workers, and families of severely handicapped infants have at times agreed that sustaining the infant's life was not beneficial, and that the technology applied only served to bombard and abuse the infant. Where one draws the line is extremely problematical. If doubts exist, then the infant should always be given the benefit of the doubt.

In the equation of decision making for severely handicapped infants, financial implications are usually not considered. The increasing high cost of intensive care for these infants is becoming an issue in these financially troubled times. I would not like to see the financial means of a family and our society be the determining factor in forgoing life support for these infants. However, financial restrictions may impose themselves in the future.

The Role of Infant-Care Review Committees

In difficult decision-making situations, an infant-care review committee might be helpful in an advisory capacity. The establishment of such committees has been proposed by the President's Commission for the Study of Ethical Problems in Medicine and Biomedical and Behavioral Research. It has also been suggested by the proposed federal regulations on management of the handicapped.

Such review committees may serve to establish guidelines for the institution by reviewing its practices and applying sound moral and ethical principles. The Academy of Pediatrics has supported the development of these committees and is advising on their constitution and function. For these committees to function in a practical way, substantive guidelines need to be drawn up so that individual situations are not dealt with arbitrarily.

SELECTED READINGS

Fletcher, J. C., Abortion, euthanasia and care of defective newborns, *N. Eng. J. Med.* **292**:76 (1975).

Fost, N., Ethical issues in the treatment of critically ill newborns, *Pediat. Ann.* **10**:17 (1981).

McCormick, R. A., To save or let die, *JAMA* **229**:172 (1974).

President's Commission for the Study of Ethical Problems in Medicine and Biomedical and Behavioral Research, *Deciding to Forgo Life-Sustaining Treatment*, U.S. Government Printing Office, Washington, DC (1983), 197–229.

Robertson, J. A., and Fost, N., Passive euthanasia of defective newborn infants—Legal considerations, *J. Pediat.* **58**:887 (1976).

Shaw, A., Randolph, J. G., and Manard, B., Ethical issues in pediatric surgery: A national survey of pediatricians and pediatric surgeons, *Pediatrics* **60**:588, Supp. 1977.

Sinclair, J. C., *et al.*, Evaluation of neonatal-intensive care programs, *N. Eng. J. Med.* **305**:489 (1981).

Todres, I. D., Krane, D., Howell, M. C., *et al.*, Pediatricians' attitudes affecting decision-making in defective newborns, *Pediatrics* **60**:197 (1977).

Wegman, M. E., Annual summary of vital statistics—1980, *Pediatrics* **68**:755 (1981).

Weir, R. F., *Selective Nontreatment of Handicapped Newborns: Moral Dilemmas in Neonatal Medicine*, New York, Oxford University Press, (1984).

19

AUTHORIZING DEATH FOR ANOMALOUS NEWBORNS

Ten Years Later

ROBERT A. BURT, J.D.
Southmayd Professor of Law
Yale University School of Law
New Haven, CT 06520

Ten years ago, at the first Symposium on Genetics and the Law, I participated in a panel discussion on withholding treatment from anomalous newborns. At that time, the issue had just come into public view, though it was common knowledge within the medical profession, and it was an open secret for anyone who chose to look at the question, that medical treatment was frequently withheld from some gravely ill newborns. The question we discussed when we met in 1974 was how public policy should respond to this practice. In my presentation, I considered three different solutions that were then (and still are today) the most common solutions advanced in public debate:

1. To stop the practice of withholding treatment altogether, so that every newborn no matter how gravely ill or impaired is provided with the most aggressive medical treatment technically available.
2. To enact a formal rule, by legislation or by judicial decision, recognizing that parents have a right to decide whether treatment should be provided for or withheld from some defined group of newborns (or, in a slight variation of this position, that parents have this right acting in consultation with physicians— much as the woman's right to choose abortion was formulated by the U.S. Supreme Court in *Roe v. Wade*).
3. To provide that parents (and physicians) who want to withhold treatment must go to court where it would be possible to obtain advance approval of this action from a judge.

In my presentation 10 years ago, I rejected each of these alternatives.[1] I found that each carried substantially undesirable likely consequences: that aggressive treatment of every newborn, no matter what the circumstances, could inflict terrible suffering on too many people (both the newborn and its family); that providing formal legal authority to parents (or to parents and physicians) to withhold treatment whenever they chose ignored the proper role of society generally in protecting vulnerable children against potentially abusive treatment from their caretakers; and that giving authority to a judge to decide beforehand whether treatment should be provided or withheld would provide only a hollow pretense of responsible, accountable public review of these decisions.

I opted for a different solution, a "least worst" choice among bad alternatives. I preferred to leave the law as it had been before the issue had been pressed into public attention. Physicians might withhold treatment, as they had in the past, without formal legal approval and without clear authority for this action. But physicians would act, and would know they were acting, with some risk of an adverse future judgment on this action. As a practical matter, I suggested, this might mean that most physicians would always provide aggressive treatment; but for some physicians, this course would seem so pointless and so cruel that they would be prepared to withhold treatment and take the risk that they would later be forced to justify this conduct in a public forum. Forcing physicians to face this unpleasant possibility was, I argued, the best way (or, more precisely, the least worst way) for the law to reflect the difficult conflicting concerns at stake in this issue.

I further suggested that no sensible physician would withhold treatment and take the risk of adverse future consequences unless he or she had consulted with and obtained approval from a wide range of others—typically, the newborn's parents, other professional colleagues in the hospital, perhaps members of ethics panels convened by the hospital, and so on. None of these people could decide to withhold treatment with the confidence that no one could later hold them all accountable and inflict some penalty on them. At the same time, because all of these people had participated in and had taken some responsibility for any decision to withhold treatment, I suggested that this risk of later penalty would most likely rarely materialize—that no sensible prosecutor would indict, no sensible jury would convict, no sensible judge would impose sanctions. Thus, I argued, this untidy resolution—this nonresolution, if you will—gave the best assurance that any nontreatment decision would be widely and intensely collaborative and would be reached only reluctantly and after agonizing self-scrutiny.[2]

This, in brief summary, was the best response I could offer 10 years ago. The question I want to explore in 1984 is whether this temporizing, avowedly "messy" solution has any current plausibility. One fact provides at least some support for the plausibility of my past position: the fact that this untidy situation has been the effective legal regime in almost every state during the entire past decade. Only recently, and in a few states, the courts have taken jurisdiction in these cases; and in a few of these cases, the courts have authorized the withholding of treatment (most notably in the Indiana *Baby Doe* case and the first *Phillip Becker* case in California—both of which I'll discuss later.) With these exceptions and a few others, the legal position has remained unresolved. But anyone involved in neonatal care knows that, during the past decade, the practice of withholding treatment has continued on a selective basis. Physicians have acted with knowledge of the legal uncertainties that they confront.

This practical experience does not, however, demonstrate the suitability of continuing this uncertain state of affairs; as a society, we have not reached a comfortable accommodation of the competing concerns in this matter. On the contrary, public concern about this issue is even more heated than 10 years ago. This greater intensity was particularly apparent during 1983 in the creation by the federal Department of Health and Human Services of the so-called Baby Doe squads, in response to the Indiana decision, and the litigation (and accompanying explosion of media attention) in the New York *Baby Jane Doe* case. Thus, it may be that the time has necessarily come for some definitive legal resolution of this issue: Who has the authority to withhold care from gravely ill newborns, and under what precise circumstances? It may be that the past decade of temporizing irresolution does not demonstrate what I had hoped—that this issue could remain formally unresolved indefinitely.

Many physicians are demanding some clear-cut resolution; they claim to find it intolerable to make difficult clinical and ethical decisions in the current politicized atmosphere, where they must expect squads of lawyers, federal bureaucrats, and media personnel pushing into the intensive care nurseries. Others are also demanding a definitive resolution, but one diametrically opposed to the regime demanded by the most vocal physicians involved in neonatal care. These others—most notably activists in the right-to-life movement—seek a definitive, aggressively enforced end to medical practices of withholding care from any newborn except (it would seem) on certification of death.

Ironically, this deep disagreement among the various disputants may in itself make any definitive resolution impossible, so that this untidy temporizing irresolution could remain, as a practical matter, the only attainable end. But for the purposes of this chapter, I want to assume that the position I have labeled the "right-to-life position" can be defeated before legislators or judges and that, as a practical matter, success is possible for physicians and others who are seeking the legitimation of, and the establishment of some clear procedures for, withholding treatment from some anomalous newborns. With this assumption, I want to explore whether substantial costs to our society, and to the medical profession in its customary social role, would accompany this kind of definitive resolution. I believe that there would be such costs.

Some might conclude that these costs are outweighed by other factors. That may be so. I will not propose any final tallying of the competing costs. My purpose is only to point to the substantial costs on one side of this argument because I think these costs have not been adequately understood or acknowledged by the proponents, particularly in the medical profession, of a legal regime legitimizing the withholding of care from anomalous newborns. We may, as a society, choose to run the risk of incurring these costs; but we should make this choice knowingly, if at all.

The first cost that I anticipate is related to the powerful tradition of the life-saving ethos in medical practice. That ethos itself has come under attack in recent decades. Physicians have been accused of deploying vast technological capabilities to prolong life without proper regard for the burdens imposed by that prolongation—without regard, that is, to the wishes of patients, without regard to the increased and ultimately pointless suffering that follows from life prolongation in many circumstances, and even without regard to the financial burdens on the patient's immediate family and on society generally imposed by this aggressive treatment ethos. I cite this criticism not to embrace or to reject it, but only to note how deep-rooted this ethos has been in medical practice. A legal rule specifying that physicians may legitimately decide to withhold life-saving treatment from some seriously ill infants would run against the grain of this entrenched ethos.

Twenty years ago, a similar kind of explicit, formalized, and legitimized acknowledgment of physicians' authority to withhold life-saving treatment was tried. But it was quickly abandoned; and I would draw a lesson from this abandonment. This all took place regarding access to life-saving kidney dialysis. When this treatment technique first became practicable, in the early 1960s, the cost was simply too great to provide dialysis for every patient in need. Formal mechanisms were accordingly created—most notably in Seattle, Washington, where the dialysis technology was pioneered—to make self-conscious allocative decisions.[3] These mechanisms became known, at least in the popular press, as "God committees." They were composed of a small group of clergymen, lawyers, and nonprofessional "citizens," with physicians serving as "advisers."[4] These God committees found themselves confronting impossible judgmental dilemmas in comparing the competing candidates for dialysis; and yet, the comparisons were somehow required because there were not enough resources to serve everyone.

In 1972, the U.S. Congress intervened in this dilemma to make it disappear, in effect, by promising an open-ended commitment of federal funds to provide dialysis (or some treatment) for all who needed it. The Congress thus made an extraordinary financial commitment, which soon (and predictably) involved a considerable annual expenditure (by 1977, some $600 million dollars) for a limited number (some 25,000 or so) of kidney patients throughout the country.[5] Many people have disputed the good sense of this extraordinary allocation of tax resources; the issue is surely debatable.[6] But the important point for our purposes here is to understand that this considerable, open-ended financial commitment was made in response to the social pressure—the moral pressure, if you will—created by the very existence of these so-called God committees. The fact that these committees were explicitly deciding who should live and who should die was simply intolerable in our society at that time.

Of course, it is a myth that everyone's life can and should be saved no matter what the cost. It is a myth that our society has sufficient resources for this purpose even if we wanted to commit such resources. As a society, we have not made this generalized commitment. But the myth nonetheless has a powerful hold on our collective moral imagination. The God committees were too explicit, too much a formal acknowledgment that we had fallen short of that mythic ideal. These committees, moreover, particularly offended the social ideal that the role of physicians was to save lives, that they should not decide who deserved to live and to provide treatment only on that basis. Current proposals for establishing regularized procedures for deciding which gravely ill infants should die and which should receive life-saving treatment explicitly run against this same social ideal.

Some people might argue that there is a significant difference in these proposals— that physicians would not decide, but that parents would decide to withhold treatment, or that judges would make this decision. But this is a disingenuous proposition; and even if true, it is an irrelevant proposition.

It is disingenuous because the underlying practical reality is that the physician will play the dominant role in these decisions no matter how they are formally structured. Parents of seriously anomalous newborns are typically overwhelmed and grief-stricken by the unexpected birth of this child, and they will inevitably rely heavily on guidance and support from physicians, particularly in the early days following birth when many crucial life-or-death decisions must be made.[7] Moreover, the medical prognosis for the infant will necessarily be a central determinant in decision making. Physicians will obviously dominate this aspect of the decision, even if the infant's prognosis is so much freighted with diagnostic uncertainties that the decision should not properly be characterized as medical and technical.

Even if judges are brought into these life-and-death decisions as a regularized matter, the physicians' role will remain predominant. All of our social experience with judicial involvement in these kinds of decisions points to this conclusion. The Indiana *Baby Doe* case—involving a Down syndrome infant with esophogeal atresia, where the judges approved the withholding of life-saving surgery—is a specific example of this general proposition.[8] The trial judge reportedly approved the withholding on the ground that the evidence established that both giving and withholding treatment were "medically acceptable alternatives" and that, therefore, the parents were entitled to choose between these alternatives. It was patent nonsense in this case to talk about "medically acceptable" alternatives. There was no medical issue, as such, at stake; the question was social and moral. But the judge in this case, as judges have done and will continue to do in such cases, was prepared to decide only if she could somehow hide her decision making behind the mask of medical expertise.[9] And thus, the ethos of medical caretaking will be unavoidably at issue in this kind of formalized, visible public decision making.

If this is so, the medical profession must confront the question of the true source of its cultural authority in our society. The profession must identify the basis for the extraordinary trust placed in it by the lay public. This trust, this once seemingly boundless faith, is important to physicians in a narrow, self-interested way, of course. But more fundamentally, this trust, this faith, is important both to physicians and to society generally because it is a crucial source of physicians' curative powers, because it leads patients to look to physicians for help, and because it bolsters physicians' confidence in their capacity to help. If this trust, this faith, comes from the basic conviction that physicians do not judge whether their patients deserve to live or to die—if it comes from the conviction that physicians work unquestioningly and unstintingly to save the life of every patient—then a public acknowledgment that sometimes physicians do not act in this way will have deeply unsettling implications for social confidence and for medical practice generally. This would be a heavy cost for the profession and for the society.

Even if physicians were not widely viewed as the dominant actors in withholding treatment from anomalous newborns—even if parents (or parents acting with the approval of judges) were viewed as the centrally responsible decision makers—the implications for our general social ethos of caretaking would still be profound and, I believe, profoundly transforming. For this reason, it is irrelevant whether physicians will be seen as the principal actors or merely as supporting players in this public drama. Parents who choose to withhold life-saving treatment from their child surely act against the force of the powerful social ethos that proper parents cherish and preserve their child's life no matter what sacrifice is involved (except, perhaps, the parent's own life). The proposition that parents have a right to decide otherwise is as much contrary to the dominant ideal of parenthood as the claimed right of a physician to withhold treatment contravenes our social ideal of medical practice. When parents and physicians act in concert to withhold life-saving treatment from a helpless, suffering child—even if the rationale is to avert further or greater suffering—then two conjunctive elements in our social ethos of caretaking have been radically redefined: the ideals that neither parents nor physicians ever withhold care from those dependent on them, that both parents and physicians give care without question.

The assumption that a true parent always gives and never withholds care can be seen at work in one of the legal cases I mentioned earlier. Phillip Becker's case in California involved a Down syndrome child, not an infant, but a boy of 10 when the litigation first began in 1977. Phillip had been placed in an institution by his parents soon after his birth; when he was 6 years old, physicians diagnosed a heart defect that, they said, could be surgically corrected but otherwise would lead to his early death. Phillip's parents refused permission for the surgery; after several years of desultory discussions, the physicians brought suit against the parents to compel surgery. The California courts decided, however, that Phillip's parents had a right to refuse this surgery.[10] That seemed the end of the matter (and, in due course, of Phillip).

But the case then took an extraordinary turn. Mr. and Mrs. Herbert Heath, who were volunteer workers in the retardation institution, had become emotionally attached to Phillip; they had spent considerable time with him both in the institution and on his numerous visits to their home. Now, they brought suit, alleging, in effect, that their involvement with Phillip, and the mutual emotional attachment between them and him, meant that they should be considered his parents, at least for purposes of authorizing the surgical treatment that could save his life. After extensive hearings and drawn-out appeals, the California courts, in effect, reversed their first decision and ruled that the Heaths could authorize this surgery for Phillip.[11] Thus, in this case, the very idea of parenthood was transformed from a biological to a psychological basis by the claim that Phillip's "original" parents had forfeited their parental status because they had decided against providing life-saving treatment for their retarded child.

Mr. and Mrs. Becker maintained throughout these proceedings—both in the courtroom and in the popular press, which extensively covered the case—that the Heaths were officious meddlers, interlopers who were stealing their child and their rights to control their child's fate.[12] It is, of course, possible that if the construct of the parents' rights to refuse treatment becomes more clearly established in our social mores, then this claim advanced by the Beckers will command firmer respect. But I suspect that, even if there is some formal legal acknowledgment of this claimed "parental right," nonetheless, for some considerable time, at least, a struggle will be waged in individual cases again and again between biological families (and their physicians) seeking to withhold treatment, on the one side, and intervenors ("interlopers," if one wants to call them that) who claim that they are the truer parents. I predict, moreover, that this claim will be increasingly advanced by people who offer to adopt the anomalous infant to provide it with medical treatment and with a new (and a nurturing) family. I expect, that is, the development of Baby Doe adoption squads composed of people committed to a "right-to-life" perspective and willing to act on that commitment by adopting such children.

Will many courts be moved to approve such adoptions, as the California courts were in effect moved in the *Becker* case? I don't know. But these adoption offers would find support in the underlying implication of our current social ideal of parenthood—that the "true" parent (like the "true" physician) always provides medical treatment for a needy child, no matter what. And if the courts are hostile to these intervenors, to these adoption squads, then we will have seen the transformation of this ideal of parenthood—a transformation that will, I believe, profoundly affect our general social definitions of what parenthood means, and what kind of caretaking ethos is dominant in our society.

In the New York *Baby Jane Doe* case, we have seen evidence of powerful judicial hostility to an analogous kind of intervenor: the attorney who repeatedly filed suits against the parents and physicians of this spina bifida baby. A Federal District Judge not only sharply criticized this attorney but imposed a $500 fine on him, purportedly to end his harassment, as the judge saw it, of the parents and the physicians.[13] There is, however, a different way to look at the conduct of this attorney.

As I was following various news accounts of the *Baby Jane Doe* case, I was somewhat startled to come across an account in the *New York Times* of a conference commemorating the twentieth anniversary of the Kitty Genovese case.[14] Miss Genovese, you might recall, was killed early one morning on a public street in a usually peaceful residential neighborhood in a borough of New York. Her killer had pursued her on this street for more than half an hour, and during this time she had frequently and loudly cried for help. Some 38 neighbors heard her cries, but none did anything to help her, not even by telephoning the police. Immediately after this event became widely known, many people were stunned by this evidence of the attenuation, even the disappearance, of a communal caretaking ethos in our urban, anonymous society; they were stunned that no one was prepared to acknowledge bonds of fellow feeling, of citizenship, with this helpless, suffering stranger.

Subsequent interviews with the witnesses to the event established that many of them thought Miss Genovese was being attacked by her husband or boyfriend, that this was a "family quarrel," and that, therefore, they should not "get involved."[15] But this rationale was itself disturbing to many people in retrospect, as if families in our society had become legitimate enclaves for the infliction of violence by one member on another. And at around this same time, in the mid-1960s, a strong social movement arose (as if in reponse to this feared implication) calling attention to the prevalence of child abuse in our society and pressing (with some success) for legislative action.

I was startled to read about the Kitty Genovese case, interspersed among news accounts of the *Baby Jane Doe* case, because none of the commentators (at least in the periodicals that I customarily read) saw any link between these cases. None saw the possibility that the intervening attorney was responding as good caretaking citizens should have responded when Kitty Genovese seemed to be under attack. Was this attorney an officious meddler? Or was he a good citizen prepared to seek protection for a fellow citizen who, though a stranger to him, appeared to be in need of help?

I raise these specific questions to point to the broader implication of the *Baby Jane Doe* case, and of these cases generally, regarding the withholding of medical care from anomalous newborns. These cases bring into question whether we live in a society where we can rely on mutual communal ties, on bonds of caretaking among strangers. I believe that if we, as a society, adopt formal rules demarking the nontreatment decisions by parents or physicians as legitimate and as "private," we will be ratifying and intensifying the general denial of communal caretaking obligations among "strangers" that seemed so inhumane and frightening in the Kitty Genovese case.

I further believe that the question of whether any communal caretaking bonds exist among strangers is raised with special symbolic and emotional force in social policy toward handicapped people generally and anomalous infants, who are mentally retarded or physically disabled, specifically. In 1975, American society made an extraordinary, and an extraordinarily expensive, commitment to these children specifically in the congressional enactment of Public Law 94-142, the Education for All Handicapped Children Act. In the same year, Congress made a comparable, though not as munificent, commitment to disabled people generally in the Developmental Disabilities Assistance and Bill of Rights Act. But the depth of these commitments and our social capacity to sustain them emotionally or financially remain open to question.[16] If we adopt an explicit social policy, by legislation or by judicial decision, that authorizes and legitimizes the withholding of medical care from anomalous infants, then we will have done more than signal a retreat from the commitments made in 1975. We will have significantly altered our currently accepted ideals of the caretaking obligations that accompany the status of citizen, parent, and physician in our society.

To be sure, these ideals are currently our public face, our Sunday best. In our private behavior, each of us, as citizen, parent, or professional, has frequently fallen short of these ideals. But when these shortfalls, these private lapses, become elevated into statements of public policy—become occasions for public social approbation as the exercise of "rights," albeit as "rights to privacy,"—then we transform the public ideals themselves. When a judge tells the anonymous Doe family in Indiana or in New York that they have a "privacy right" to withhold life-saving care from a Down syndrome or spina bifida child, this is a public and not a private act by the judge, the family, and the physicians. This act has more than private consequences. It sets a precedent. It invites others to act in the same way when they confront an anomalous child in their capacity as parent, physician, or citizen. It invites and legitimizes this conduct and thereby removes one source of constraint, one source of communal moral bond, that had joined the rest of us—however tentatively, however ambivalently—to these strangers among us. And by refusing any acknowledged communal bond with them, we turn our face more resolutely from other frightening strangers as well, from the Kitty Genoveses as well as from the Baby Does among us.

All of these, then, are costs that I anticipate if we, as a society, conclude that the time has now come to provide regularized, legitimized processes for withholding medical care from anomalous infants. There are, I know, countervailing costs in providing such care, and I have given no attention to them in this chapter.[17] It may still be possible to strike some untidy middle ground in this matter in order to avoid a definitive embrace of one set of costs or the other. I at least continue to nurture this hope as I examine recent judicial decisions.

The resolution of the *Baby Jane Doe* case in the New York courts suggests this possibility. The lower courts dictated conclusive resolutions; the trial court ordered treatment; and the appellate division reversed on the grounds that the parents had a right to deny treatment.[18] But the Court of Appeals took a temporizing route, ruling that the issue should not have been before any court but should instead have been considered, at least initially, by the state's child protective agency.[19] Because this agency is continuously responsible for the investigation of child abuse and neglect allegations generally, there is at least some prospect that a stable working relationship can evolve between the agency staff and the medical personnel in neonatal intensive-care units throughout the state. The agency might monitor the general conduct and policies of these units; it could conduct investigations in individual cases, where apparently necessary, that would be less intrusive than court proceedings and more respectful of confidentiality norms. And this agency would be in a position to demand treatment in "egregious" cases.

I have no clear-cut, generally applicable standard of "egregiousness" to propose. I would propose that, whatever the content of the standard that a particular state statute or child protective agency adopted, where the agency demanded treatment the courts should enforce that demand as a matter of course. I would also propose that where the agency refused to initiate this treatment demand, the courts should not override the agency's decision. In administrative law jargon, the courts would be deferring to the supposed expertise of the agency. From my perspective, the point of this judicial deference would be, on the one side, to avoid repeated public proceedings challenging nontreatment decisions that the agency was not also prepared to challenge. I would expect that the agency would develop a sufficiently close relation with neonatal intensive-care specialists throughout the state so that it would only rarely seek publicly to override nontreatment decisions. On the other side, the virtually automatic judicial enforcement of an agency demand for treatment would prevent any public legitimation of a decision by parents or physicians to withhold treatment—a legitimation that would necessarily be implied by a judicial refusal to enforce the child protective agency's demand.

A decision by the agency not to override a nontreatment decision should not, however, provide immunity for physicians and parents from the possibility of later criminal or civil liability. Thus, the agency refusal to intervene would not signify that nontreatment was necessarily legitimate (or that the agency had any authority to give formal legitimacy to a nontreatment decision). The parents and physicians who opted for nontreatment would be forced to accept the risk of later liability; no one could promise them immunity, even though the agency could have forced them to provide treatment.

This scheme is consistent with the decision of the New York Court of Appeals. But the court did not specify this arrangement in its decision; it left open the question of whether the courts might accept petitions even if the child protective agency failed to initiate them, and it did not address the possibility of subsequent criminal or civil liability for nontreatment. The scheme I have sketched is cumbersome, perhaps; but it is the best version that I can imagine in the current context that comes to my "least worst" preference for a continued regime of purposeful irresolution.

Finally, if the federal regulations for some form of Baby Doe squad are resurrected, after their demise at the hands of the Second Circuit Court of Appeals,[20] I would propose that federal intervention and investigation should not be permitted in individual cases, but that such intervention should instead be restricted to a general requirement that the states must establish an administrative regulatory regime of some sort to assure that the interests of anomalous newborns are being adequately protected. The state administrative regime that I have sketched should meet this kind of federal standard.[21]

Some have questioned whether there is any proper federal role in these matters. The image of an all-powerful, intrusive Big Brother is repeatedly invoked, with particular salience in this year 1984. But there is another image of Big Brother that seems at least equally plausible to me: the image popularly associated with Father Flanigan's Boys Town: one boy carrying a smaller boy on his back and saying, "He ain't heavy, Father; he's my brother." For all its heavy sentimentality, this invocation of the caretaking ethos that underlies brotherhood is an apt depiction of the Big Brother role that the federal government claimed in its efforts to undo the pernicious social implications of the Indiana Baby Doe decision that authorized the starvation death, by withholding treatment, of a child who suffered from Down syndrome.

In the current public posture toward these disputed issues, perhaps no temporizing resolution is possible. If that is so, then a hard choice must be made. As a result of this choice someone, some group, must suffer so that others can be protected from suffering. When we try to decide this question—Who should suffer on whose behalf?—I would urge that we give close attention to the possibility that public legitimation of withholding treatment from anomalous newborns may have substantial and ultimately excessive costs. These costs, moreover, may not fall solely on some infants who are wrongfully killed. These costs may also spread to undermine public trust in the medical profession and further to erode the caretaking ethos generally in this society.

REFERENCES AND NOTES

1. Authorizing death for anomalous newborns, *Genetics and the Law*, Plenum Press, New York (1975), 435–50.
2. The rationale for this position is developed at greater length in Burt, R., *Taking Care of Strangers: The Rule of Law in Doctor-Patient Relations*, Free Press, New York (1979).

3. Fox, R., and Swazey, J., *The Courage to Fail: A Social View of Organ Transplants and Dialysis*, University of Chicago Press, Chicago (1974), 240–79.

4. *Id.* at p. 244.

5. Rettig, R. The policy debate on patient care financing for victims of end-stage renal disease, *Law and Contemporary Problems* 40(4):196, 200–01 (1976).

6. Calabresi, G., and Bobbitt, P., *Tragic Choices*, W. W. Norton, New York (1978), 186–9.

7. See Guillemin, J. and Holmstrom, Legal cases, government regulations, and clinical realities in newborn intensive care, *A. J. Perinatol.* 1:89 (1983).

8. Neither the trial court nor the Indiana Supreme Court published opinions attempting to explain or justify their rulings in the case. The case and the judicial rulings are described in Pless, The Story of Baby Doe, *New Eng. J. Medicine* 309, no. 11:664 (September 15, 1983).

9. See Burt, *supra* note 2, at 155–8.

10. *In re Phillip B.*, 92 Cal.App.3d 796, 156 Cal.Rptr. 48 (Ct. of App., 1st Dist., 1979).

11. The unpublished court opinions are reproduced in Wadlington, W., Whitbread, C., and David, S., *Children in the Legal System*, Foundation Press, Mineola, NY, (1983), 921–23.

12. See the parents' article: Becker, W., and Becker, P., Mourning the loss of a son, *Newsweek* (May 30, 1983), 17.

13. See the report of this case in Steinbock, P., Baby Jane Doe in the courts, *Hastings Cent. Rep.* 14(1):13, 19 (Feb. 1984).

14. 20 years after Kitty Genovese's murder, experts study bad Samaritanism, *New York Times* (March 12, 1984), B1, col. 1.

15. *Id.* at B4, col. 3.

16. See the discussion of this legislation and judicial responses to it in Burt, R. A., Constitutional law and the teaching of the parables, *Yale Law J.* 93:455, 489–500 (1984).

17. For a thoughtful, balanced exploration of this question, see Arras, J., On the care of imperiled newborns— Toward an ethic of ambiguity, *Hastings Cent. Rep.* 14 (2):25 (Apr. 1984).

18. *Weber v. Stony Brook Hospital*, New York Law J. (Oct. 28, 1983), 3.

19. *Weber v. Stony Brook Hospital*, New York Law J. (Nov. 1, 1983), 5.

20. *United States v. University Hospital*, 729 F.2d 144 (2d Cir., 1984).

21. While this chapter was in press, the U.S. Congress enacted a new law that appears consistent with my proposal. The law requires state child-protective agencies, as a condition for receiving general federal funding support, to establish procedures that would "prevent the withholding of medically indicated treatment from disabled infants with life-threatening conditions." (Public Law 98–457 (Oct. 9, 1984); for the Conference Committee Report see *Congressional Record*, Sept. 19, 1984, at p. H9806.) The act, in effect, permits the withholding of treatment only for inevitably dying or "chronically and irreversibly comatose" infants (though the specific language gives some latitude for uncertainty about the inevitability of death; treatment must be "virtually futile" and "under such circumstances . . . inhumane"). As I read the legislative history, federal agencies could police the operations of state protective agencies regarding their general implementation of these standards; but federal intervention in specific, pending cases, as previously undertaken by the Baby Doe squads, would not be permitted under this act. (See the statement of six leading sponsors in the Senate, *Congressional Record*, Sept. 28, 1984, at p. S12392: "This legislation does not itself authorize direct federal involvement in individual cases.")

20

PROTECTING HANDICAPPED NEWBORNS
Who's in Charge and Who Pays?

JAMES F. CHILDRESS, PH.D.
*Commonwealth Professor of Religious Studies
and Professor of Medical Education
University of Virginia
Department of Religious Studies
Cocke Hall
Charlottesville, VA 22903*

Of the two questions assigned to me and indicated in the title of this chapter, I will concentrate on the first question ("Who's in charge?"), reserving the second question ("Who pays?") for brief discussion at the end. I shall construe both questions as normative rather than descriptive, as asking who should be in charge and who should pay.

The first question—Who should be in charge?—is one of the most important *procedural* questions about decisions regarding handicapped newborns. It is not the only procedural question; procedure involves more than *who* decides, and there may be procedures for the decision maker to follow in making the decision. Thus, under procedure, it is necessary to consider both *who* should make the decision and *how* the decision maker should decide. The question about *how* includes qualities that the decision maker should possess and display, such as competence and emotional stability. It is important to distinguish both of these procedural questions (who? and how?) from the main substantive question: *What* is the right decision? But even if it is important to distinguish these questions, it is impossible, or at least inappropriate, to try to separate them completely in decisions about handicapped newborns. There is what might be called an interactive or dialectical relation between procedural and substantive standards in decisions about handicapped newborns.

PROCEDURES AND OUTCOMES

According to John Rawls, there are at least three possible relations between procedures and the outcomes of those procedures. These three relations can be distinguished according to two questions: (1) Is there an independent standard of a just or right outcome, that is, a standard independent of the procedure for evaluating the outcome? And (2) can the procedure guarantee a just or right outcome, that is, one that satisfies the substantive standard?[1]

	Independent standard of just/right outcome	Procedure to guarantee just/right outcome
Perfect procedural justice	Yes	Yes
Imperfect procedural justice	Yes	No
Pure procedural justice	No	Yes

In Rawls's category of "perfect procedural justice," there is an independent standard of a just/right outcome, and it is possible to devise a procedure to guarantee this outcome. But it is difficult to find examples in the real world, and Rawls settled on an example of the distribution of a birthday cake at a children's party. The standard of a just/right outcome is equal shares, and there is a way to guarantee that this standard is met: tell the child who is going to cut the cake that he or she will have to take the last piece after all the other children have chosen theirs.

In "imperfect procedural justice," there is an independent standard of a right outcome, but the procedure is imperfect, flawed, or deficient in some respect and thus cannot ensure that outcome. For example, in criminal trials, there is an independent standard of a right verdict (conviction of the guilty and only the guilty), but society cannot design a procedure that guarantees a right verdict in every case. This relation between procedure and outcome is, of course, more common in social institutions than either perfect procedural justice or pure procedural justice.

In "pure procedural justice," any outcome of the procedure is just or right if the procedure has been followed, because there is no independent substantive standard of a just or right outcome. Justice or rightness inheres in the procedure, and whatever results is acceptable, as long as the procedure has been respected. Gambling is an example. It matters not who wins or loses as long as the game is fair.

At least one proposal about decision making regarding handicapped newborns approximates Rawls's conception of pure procedural justice. Raymond Duff, as shown in a series of articles, often in collaboration with A. G. M. Campbell, apparently believes that we do not have an independent standard for the evaluation of decisions about newborns and, thus, would allow familial discretion in these cases.[2] Whatever the parents decide is correct (within some vague and unspecified limits of child abuse). Society should almost always accept the results of the procedure of parental decision-making in consultation with physicians. And Duff emphasized the values embodied in the procedure, rather than a standard of a right or just outcome: letting parents make the decision reduces their helplessness and restores their sense of control.

Regardless of the values embodied in the procedure, Duff's approach may not be acceptable if there is an independent substantive standard of a just or right outcome and if the results of his procedure violate that standard. If there is such an independent standard, then we might seek "perfect procedural justice" in decisions about handicapped newborns, anticipating, however, that we will be able to realize only "imperfect procedural justice," in part because of unclear boundaries, indeterminate values in the standard, and the difficulties of making accurate prognoses.

This independent standard is, I would argue, the infant's *best interests*.[3] This standard establishes a presumption in favor of treatment to prolong life, itself a primary good and a precondition for other goods, but this presumption may be rebutted under some conditions, for example, when treatment can only prolong dying, when the accompanying pain and suffering outweigh the value of life to the infant, and when the resultant quality of life can be expected to be so low as to obviate the moral duty to prolong life.

This standard of the infant's best interests "excludes consideration of the negative effects of an impaired child's life on other persons, including parents, siblings, and society."[4] If the infant's interests provide a moral mandate for life-prolonging treatment, that treatment should be provided, even if other parties would suffer as a result. If, however, the infant's interests do not mandate life-prolonging treatment, the treatment is morally optional, and the impact on others may then be morally relevant and even decisive. But the threshold is the infant's interests.

Not only does this standard of the infant's best interests exclude the consideration of the interests of others, but it also provides one way of formulating the criteria of the traditional distinction between ordinary and extraordinary means of treatment. It is probably wise to replace the terms *ordinary* and *extraordinary* with *obligatory* and *optional*. The terms *ordinary* and *extraordinary* are misleading because they appear to focus our attention on such questions as whether the treatment in question is usual or unusual, customary or uncustomary, and so on. Then the criterion is whether a particular treatment is usual and customary medical practice in relation to a particular disease or illness. But morally, it is necessary to ask whether a particular treatment, even if it is customarily used for a certain disease, should be provided to this particular patient in view of his or her overall condition, for example, penicillin for pneumonia in a patient who is in the final stages of dying from a painful cancer. As this example suggests, the standard for decision making should be the patient's best interest considered as a whole. When this standard is employed, even usual treatment for a particular medical problem may be morally optional in view of the patient's overall condition, the negative and positive effects of the treatment, the chances of success, and so on.

Even though the best-interests standard establishes a presumption in favor of life-prolonging treatment, it also provides a way of rebutting that presumption: treatments are obligatory only when they are in accord with the patient's interests, optional when they are not required by those interests, and wrong when they violate those interests. There are thus at least three possible moral judgments about treatments for a patient: (a) obligatory; (b) optional; and (c) wrong (or obligatory not to do). If a treatment is obligatory to provide for a patient, failure to provide it is blameworthy. The treatment is obligatory if it offers a reasonable chance of success and a probable net balance of benefits over harms and other costs to the patient. If the treatment does not meet these conditions, it is optional. Treatment that is optional may be viewed in at least two different ways. On the one hand, it may be optional in the sense of morally indifferent. Thus, the appropriate agents would have total discretion about whether to provide the treatment. On the other hand, treatment may be optional in the sense of not being morally required, but it may still be considered heroic and perhaps even praiseworthy. Even though a treatment may not offer a patient a *reasonable* chance of success and may thus not be obligatory, providing it may offer the patient "a chance" and may merit praise as long as other duties are not violated.

Most ethical analyses in this area concentrate on obligatory and optional actions, rarely attending to the final category: wrong, or obligatory not to do. Perhaps the most common examples of this final category appear in the care of a competent or a previously competent patient who has clearly indicated his or her wishes; it would be wrong to treat against those wishes (except in very rare cases). Apart from those wishes, if a proxy decision maker believes that a treatment is mandatory or praiseworthy, he or she is acting in accord with the (rebuttable) presumption for life-prolonging treatment, and his or her decision is reversible, whereas the decision to withhold or to withdraw life-prolonging treatment may not be. Thus, observers are likely to accept this decision for the incompetent. But it is conceivable that observers could conclude that it is wrong to treat the incompetent patient, whose wishes are unknown, because of the pain involved for a limited benefit (e.g., a few additional days of life). Or the treatment could be viewed as wrong because it appears to offer no benefit to the patient and also violates the interests of other parties.

PROXY DECISION MAKERS

If the appropriate standard of a just/right decision regarding handicapped newborns is their best interests, what does this standard imply for the selection of proxy decision makers? In view of this standard, we might try to design a more perfect procedure to replace current procedures, or we might try to retain current procedures and reduce their imperfections. The latter is preferable for several reasons. As I have suggested, there is an independent standard of decisions regarding handicapped newborns, but this standard is obviously vague, value-laden, and difficult to apply, particularly in view of uncertain prognoses. There should be a *prima facie* or presumptive case for the parents as proxy decision makers for the handicapped newborn; they have made a series of decisions and have engaged in a series of actions that have resulted in the birth of their infant, and they will continue to make decisions regarding his or her care, unless they waive or forfeit their rights to do so. They should be permitted to make the decisions if they want to, unless it is necessary to disqualify them as decision makers.

Hence, I will focus on disqualifying rather than qualifying proxy decision makers in view of the presumption that parents will choose in accord with the newborn's welfare. What factors should be relevant to disqualification? In his valuable book, *Selective Non-treatment of Handicapped Newborns: Moral Dilemmas in Neonatal Medicine*, Robert F. Weir identified four major qualifications of acceptable proxies for newborns: (1) relevant knowledge and information; (2) impartiality; (3) emotional stability; and (4) consistency.[5] By contrast, I would propose the following list of qualifications, which overlaps with but is not identical with Weir's list: (1) ability to make reasoned judgments; (2) adequate knowledge and information; (3) emotional stability; and (4) commitment to the infant's interests.

I have added the first qualification because the ability to make reasoned judgments may be independent of adequate knowledge and information and emotional stability, both of which appear on both lists and both of which may be decisively affected by the actions of physicians and others, who may be able, for example, to impart adequate information. Perhaps more controversial is the fourth point on my list, commitment to the infant's interests, which replaced impartiality on Weir's list. As Weir interpreted this criterion of impartiality, it is close to my own criterion:

> For proxies of neonatal patients, the requirement of impartiality means that such persons should determine, as objectively as possible whether life-prolonging treatment would be in the best interests of the individual neonate in question.

He then suggested that objectivity is more likely if the proxies are "disinterested in the particular case at issue and dispassionate in weighing available alternatives."[6] I have substituted a form of partiality (the newborn's interests) because impartiality suggests neutrality in the consideration of the interests of various parties when the decision should be made in the infant's best interests.

My reasons for not including consistency are more complex. Weir used this term to highlight the moral requirement of treating similar cases in a similar way, and this moral requirement is certainly important. If life-prolonging treatment is held to be in the best interests of one newborn, it should also be held to be in the best interests of another newborn whose case is relevantly similar. But this criterion is not a matter of the qualification or the disqualification of particular proxies; it is a matter of the application of the standard of the infant's best interests in order to determine whether treatment is obligatory, optional, or wrong in a particular case. Furthermore, Weir's use of this criterion of consistency may obscure the point that, in cases where treatment is morally optional, different parents may choose in different ways. Consistency would then mean allowing discretion about relevantly similar cases even though the decisions might be very different.

The presumption in favor of parental decision making is a rebuttable presumption. It can be rebutted by appeal to the substantive standard of the infant's best interests. Procedurally, it is probably best to conceive of the relations between the parents and some other possible proxy decision makers as constituting a serial or lexical order: parents, physicians and other health-care professionals, hospital ethics committees, and the courts.[7] Nevertheless, I suggest that, in view of some evidence about the violation of the standard of the infant's best interests, it may be morally and politically advisable to require, at least temporarily, that parents and physicians *justify* their nontreatment decisions to an institutional ethics committee.

Parents have a presumed moral commitment to the infant because of pregnancy and nontermination of pregnancy; and they may be presumed to choose and act in the infant's best interests, unless there is evidence to the contrary. It has been deemed morally appropriate to grant parents a wide range of discretion in various decisions about their children, for example, decisions regarding education, religion, and lifestyles. This discretion is not, however, unlimited. Parents who refuse to consent to a medical treatment that offers a reasonable chance of significant net benefit to an infant can usually be disqualified as decision makers in that arena, especially if their refusal would probably result in the infant's death. An example is the refusal by Jehovah's Witness parents of a blood transfusion for an infant at serious risk of death. Apart from such clear exceptions, there will be considerable debate about where the limits should be set, in part because the standard of best interests presupposes values that identify and that weight harms (such as pain and suffering) and benefits (such as extension of life) and their probabilities.

In addition, most parents probably have the ability to make reasoned judgments, and some limitations that may be evident in a crisis, such as inadequate information and emotional instability, may be only temporary and correctable. If these limitations can be corrected (for example, by the provision of information and counseling), there is no excuse for disqualifying the parents as decision makers.

Physicians and other health-care professionals obviously play a critical role in decision making about the treatment of seriously ill newborns. Their diagnoses and prognoses determine the parameters of decision making by the parents, and what they say may be decisive. They may be able to correct the informational deficiencies and the emotional instability of parents who face a difficult decision. But their role is not simply to enable the parents to become better decision makers. They may sometimes have to try to disqualify the parents as decision makers, where, for example, they are convinced that the parents are acting against the infant's best interests or lack the capacities for decision making. In general, a patient's competence to consent to or to refuse treatment is rarely examined unless there is a conflict between the physician's recommendations and the patient's decision. The value dispute triggers an inquiry into competence. We can probably expect similar results in neonatal decision making, where the parents' qualifications for decision making will rarely be questioned unless there is a serious value dispute.[8]

In considering the role of physicians and other health-care professionals, it is important to examine some evidence about their *reasons* for their *willingness* to override parental decision making. First, there is evidence that physicians sometimes displace parents as decision makers in order to protect the parents rather than to protect the infant. One physician wrote, "At the end it is usually the doctor who has to decide the issue. It is . . . cruel to ask the parents whether they want their child to live or die."[9] This approach is paternalistic: paternalism is the refusal to acquiesce in a person's wishes, choices, and actions for that person's own benefit. It is a distinctive reason for nonacquiescence in that it focuses on the welfare of the one whose wishes, choices, or actions are overridden—in contrast to the welfare of some other party, such as the infant. Paternalism in relation to the parents of a seriously ill newborn usually involves nondisclosure of information rather than coercion. For example, the physician may not inform the parents that they have a decision to make or may not give them enough information to make the decision because allowing them to make the decision would overburden them, upset them, make them feel guilty, and so on.

Paternalism that is limited and constrained by the principle of respect for persons can be morally justified when certain conditions are met: (1) the beneficiary has some defect, encumbrance, or limitation in decision making; (2) he or she would suffer serious harm apart from intervention; (3) the benefits of intervention would outweigh the harms of nonintervention; and (4) the paternalistic agent chooses the least restrictive, humiliating, and insulting mode of intervention.[10] It is not clear how often, if ever, these conditions are met in relation to the parents of handicapped newborns, particularly because, as I have argued, the first condition can often be remedied by the provision of information or counseling. If the parents waive or relinquish their right to make the decision, assigning it to the physician, the physician's decision making is not paternalistic at all because it is in accord with, rather than opposed to, the parents' wishes, choices, and actions.

One difficult question about protecting the infant's (in contrast to the parents') interests is whether physicians are too ready to acquiesce in parental wishes and choices. In one survey of pediatric surgeons and pediatricians, the question was asked:

> Would you acquiesce in parents' decision to refuse consent for surgery in a newborn with intestinal atresia if the infant also had (a) Down's syndrome alone, (b) Down's syndrome plus congenital heart disease, (c) anencephaly, (d) cloacal exstrophy, (e) meningomyelocele, (f) multiple limb or craniofacial malformations, (g) 13–15 trisomy, or (h) no other anomalies, i.e., normal aside from atresia?[11]

The answers of 76.8% of the pediatric surgeons and 49.5% of the pediatricians indicated that they would acquiesce in parental decisions to refuse permission for surgery to correct intestinal atresia even if the infant's only other problem was Down syndrome. Of course, the term *acquiesce* does not imply approval, and it also fails to suggest the complexity of the physician's involvement in shaping the parents' understanding of the problem, the decision, and so on. But the term does indicate an unwillingness to override the decision. The Department of Health and Human Services appealed to this survey as evidence that some mechanism is needed to protect handicapped infants against discrimination, but critics have charged that the survey is not statistically valid and is outdated.[12] If pediatric surgeons and pediatricians are willing to acquiesce in parents' decisions to let a Down syndrome infant die rather than correct intestinal atresia, some procedure or mechanism is needed to protect the infant's interests, as there is no sound argument that the interests of an infant with Down syndrome are better served by nontreatment than by the surgical correction of intestinal atresia. Discretion is not appropriate in this type of case.

If parents sometimes refuse treatment against the interests of their infants, and if physicians sometimes, or frequently, acquiesce, then some mechanism or procedure is needed to break the closed, private circle of refusal and acquiescence. As an alternative to the proposed "hotline," with all of its adversarial features and moral costs, an ethics committee has been proposed. For example, the President's Commission for the Study of Ethical Problems in Medicine recommended "internal review whenever parents decide that life-sustaining therapy should be foregone."[13] In view of the (rebuttable) presumption in favor of life-sustaining therapy established by the standard of the infant's best interests, in view of the (frequent) irreversibility of the decision to withhold or to withdraw life-sustaining therapy, and in view of the uncertainty about current practices, it may not be sufficient simply to invoke an ethics committee when there is a conflict between parents and physicians. Evidence about physician acquiescence to parental wishes makes this approach unreliable. Nor is it sufficient to view such a committee as promoting a community of moral discourse in the hospital. Until there is greater clarity about the extent to which parents and physicians act or fail to act in accord with infants' best interests, it may be morally and politically appropriate for an ethics committee to review each decision for nontreatment. There is debate about whether such a committee is needed, would be effective, or would even be counterproductive. But if there is evidence that parents and physicians act against infants' interests in not providing treatment, then it may be appropriate to mandate review through an institutional ethics committee that can require the justification of nontreatment decisions. The composition of such a committee is obviously very important, but I will not discuss it here.

Finally, the courts should be invoked only as a last resort, when there are reasons to seek to disqualify other decision makers in order to protect the infant's interest or in order to adjudicate a conflict about those interests. At best, each decision maker in this serial or lexical order of proxy decision makers—and all of them together—can represent only imperfect procedural justice.

A Right to Medical Care?

Even if parents ought to authorize treatment for seriously ill newborns in most cases, and even if other agents ought to override the parents' refusals in some cases, there is still an important question about who pays or who should pay for such care.[14] Some have wondered whether we should not change the cliché "Whoever pays the piper calls the tune" in this setting: "Whoever calls the tune should pay the piper." The moral rationale for this shift is clear even though it may not be decisive. If treatment of a handicapped newborn is ordered against parental wishes, why should the parents have to cover the costs, which may include not only immediate care but also long-term institutional care?

There are, I believe, important moral reasons for providing and increasing support for the parents of handicapped newborns. Some of these reasons apply specifically to the situation of neonatal care; others apply more generally. First, the society should provide financial support in order to reduce some conflicts of interest between the newborn and his or her parents as primary decision makers. Other familial interests often masquerade as the infant's interests. The society should attempt to reduce and even to eliminate parents' worries about exhausting their financial resources in the care of a handicapped infant.

Second, there are solid moral arguments for a political-legal right to health care, when that care is in the recipient's best interests, and these arguments support societal funds for the care of handicapped infants. Apart from more general arguments for the equal distribution of all goods, including health care, most arguments for a political-legal right to health care rest on moral principles in conjunction with claims about the special nature and importance of both health needs and health care. As Tristram Engelhardt argued, one of the central issues in debates about the distribution of health care is one's view of the "natural lottery."[15] The metaphor of a lottery suggests that health needs, various diseases, and illnesses are largely the result of an impersonal lottery and are thus undeserved. But even if these needs are largely undeserved insofar as they result from chance, this does not determine why and how the society should respond to them, for, as Engelhardt noted, undeserved needs may be viewed as either *unfortunate* or *unfair*. If the needs are unfortunate, they may be the object of compassion. Other individuals, voluntary associations, and even the society ought to undertake efforts to try to meet those needs out of compassion and charity. But if those needs are unfair, there may be a duty of justice to try to meet them. If, of course, those needs result from the actions of others (e.g., assaults), or failures of institutions (e.g., environmental pollution), or actions on behalf of the society (e.g., military service), there may be special obligations of fairness to meet the needs. There is, however, less agreement about an obligation of fairness to blunt the effects of the natural lottery.

Whether a political-legal right to health care is based on charity or fairness, there is still room for debating the content and scope of that right and for making difficult allocation decisions. The question about who should pay for whatever care is available is not identical with the question about what level and kind of care should be made available. Policy decisons about the level and kind of care should involve answers to several questions: How much of society's resources (time, energy, and especially money) should go into health care (including critical care) versus other social goods? How much into preventive care versus critical care (and also chronic and rehabilitative care)? How much for various diseases? And how much for various technologies (such as NICUs)?[16] Although such questions have to be resolved politically (i.e., through the political process), they do involve several moral issues. Rather than trying to offer a comprehensive analysis of these issues, I will identify only a few points that merit consideration in determining our policies.

The costs of neonatal intensive care are staggering. In one study of patients with high-cost hospitalization ($4,000 or more in one year), the most expensive cases involved neonatal intensive care and averaged over $20,000 each. In 1978, the average expenditures for neonatal intensive care (hereinafter NIC) were estimated to be $8,000 per case, and the total costs of NIC throughout the United States were estimated to be $1.5 billion, similar to the costs of the end-stage renal disease program. Approximately 6% of all live births go to intensive care, and there are approximately 200,000 admissions each year. There is evidence that NIC has greatly reduced neonatal mortality, but there is more debate about the impact on neonatal morbidity.[17]

At the level of macroallocation—How much of a good such as neonatal intensive care should be made available?—it is impossible to avoid considerations of the value of life. Valuing lives is inevitable; it will be implicit or explicit. It occurs whenever we pursue or eschew policies that reduce the risk of death. But a policy that expresses an evaluation of life by refraining from reducing the risks of death is not as morally offensive as the comparative evaluation of individual lives that some propose at the level of microallocation. In part, the difference is between *statistical* and *identified* lives and between *impersonal* and *personal* approaches. To compare identified lives in order to determine their relative value to society for purposes of allocating scarce life-saving medical resources would infringe the principle of the equal and independent value of human life. Such an infringement does not occur when the society decides not to increase the number of emergency vehicles or ICUs or not to improve road barriers, even though such decisions statistically increase the risks of death.

If our society will spend X amount for the reduction of risks of death and morbidity to newborns, should it concentrate on NIC or on prevention (e.g., of low birth weight and anomalies)? Particular medical interventions in NIC have been validated as effective by randomized, controlled clinical trials, but NIC programs as a whole have not been evaluated for their effectiveness in reducing death and morbidity, particularly in comparison to other programs, such as various programs that might prevent low birth weight.[18] The best studies to date point to a significant role of NIC in the reduction of neonatal mortality among low-birth-weight infants. More controversial are studies of the morbidity, particularly the handicaps, of the survivors. As smaller and smaller newborns have been salvaged, *most* of them have been normal. Nevertheless, it appears that "the absolute number of seriously handicapped individuals may be increasing."[19] Even here, on balance, NIC appears to be effective.

However, it is probable that effective programs to prevent low birth weight could further reduce neonatal mortality and morbidity. Although noting that in California much of the decline in neonatal mortality has resulted from "the advent of neonatal intensive care and the increased rate of cesarean section," some analysts contend that "the prevention of low birth weight holds the greatest promise for improving the outcome of pregnancy and controlling the costs of perinatal care during the 1980s."[20] Such an argument, if sound, might lead to the conclusion that there should be a different mix of prevention and critical intervention. Such a mix might also be more cost-effective. But prevention might involve various activities ranging from education to prenatal care. In some other areas, such as the prevention of neural tube defects, screening might be involved, and abortion might be considered. But this is a different face of prevention: it might involve preventing the disease by preventing the offspring. Such prevention would encounter limits set by personal autonomy. Similarly, risks created for the prospective offspring by the mother's lifestyle would be difficult to reduce morally except through education. And as the debate about intrauterine interventions indicates, similar problems emerge when corrections might be made before birth.

All of these complications lead to the conclusion that we lack the data to offer cost-effectiveness analyses of NIC versus various preventive programs in the reduction of neonatal mortality and morbidity and that, even if we had the data, some possible preventive programs would encounter some moral constraints (not necessarily absolute ones). In addition, it has been argued that our society morally favors critical interventions over preventive programs because of a preference for identified over statistical lives and a conviction that critical interventions symbolize both the care and compassion of the rescuer and the value of the rescued. Although such a priority may not be defensible, it is at least understandable and may set political (if not moral) boundaries on allocation decisions and thus on the content and scope of a right to health care. At the very least, the weight of the financial burden should not fall on the family.

References and Notes

1. Rawls, J., A *Theory of Justice*, Harvard University Press, Cambridge, (1971), 85–86.
2. See Duff, R. N., and Campbell, A. G. M., Moral and ethical dilemmas in the special-care nursery, *N. Eng. J. Med.* **289**:890–4 (1973); On deciding the care of severely handicapped or dying persons: With particular reference to infants, *Pediatrics* **57**:487–93 (1976); Moral and ethical dilemmas: Seven years into the debate about human ambiguity, *Ann. Am. Acad. Political Social Sci.* **447**:19–28 (1980); Duff, R. S., On deciding the use of the family commons, in *Developmental Disabilities: Psychologic and Social Implications*, (D. Bergsma and A. E. Pulver, eds.), *Birth Defects: Original Article Series*, vol. 12, No. 4, Alan R. Liss, New York (1976), 73–84.
3. Martin Benjamin argued that we cannot use the language of "interests" except in relation to agents who have or have had wants, purposes, and so on. See Benjamin, M., The newborn's interest in continued life: A sentimental fiction, *The Bioethics Reporter* (Dec. 1983), Commentary, 5–7. By contrast I think it makes sense to talk about some interests in a more objective way and thus about harms (e.g., death) and benefits (e.g., life) even when we cannot identify conscious wants, purposes, and so on. At the very least, when an infant can be expected to survive with treatment, to be able to interact with his or her environment and others, and not to be overwhelmed by pain and suffering from handicaps or the treatment, prolongation of life is in his or her best interests and is a net benefit to him or her. Termination of treatment would be a harm—that is, a violation of his or her interests—even though he or she does not yet have conscious wants and purposes.
4. The President's Commission for the Study of Ethical Problems in Medicine and Biomedical and Behavioral Research, *Deciding to Forego Life-Sustaining Treatment*, U.S. Government Printing Office, Washington, DC. (March 1983), 219.
5. Weir, R. F., *Selective Nontreatment of Handicapped Newborns: Moral Dilemmas in Neonatal Medicine*, Oxford University Press, New York (1984), chap. 9.
6. *Ibid.*, 256.
7. For a discussion of the serial or lexical ordering of proxy decision-makers, see Childress, J. F., *Who Should Decide?* Oxford University Press, New York (1982), 172–4; and Beauchamp, T. L., and Childress J. F., *Principles of Biomedical Ethics* (2nd ed.), Oxford University Press, New York (1983), 141–3. This idea is developed further in Weir, *idem.*, chap. 9.
8. Carlton, W., *"In our professional opinion. . . ." The Primacy of Clinical Judgment over Moral Choice*, University of Notre Dame Press, Notre Dame, Ind. (1978), 5–6.
9. Rickham, P. P., The ethics of surgery on newborn infants, *Clin. Pediat.* **8**:251–3 (1969), quoted in Shaw, A., Dilemmas of "informed consent" in children, *N. Eng. J. Med.* **289**:886 (Oct. 25, 1973). See also The President's Commission, *idem.*, 210–11.
10. Childress, *idem.*, chap. 5.
11. Shaw, A., Randolph, J. G., and Manard, B., Ethical issues in pediatric surgery: A national survey of pediatricians and pediatric surgeons, *Pediatrics* **60**:588–99 (Oct. 1977).
12. *Federal Register* 49 (Jan. 12, 1984):1645.
13. The President's Commission, *idem.*, 227.
14. The Reagan administration has taken an active role in ensuring that newborns will receive treatment, while also reducing support for some programs, such as prenatal care, that statistically have an important impact on infant mortality and morbidity.
15. Engelhardt, H. T., Jr., Health care allocations: Responses to the unjust, the unfortunate, and the undesirable, in *Justice and Health Care*, (Earl E. Shelp, ed.), *Philosophy and Medicine*, vol. 8, D. Reidel, Dordrecht, Holland, and Boston, Mass. (1981), 121–37.
16. See Childress, J. F., Priorities in the allocation of health care resources, *Soundings* **62**:256–74 (Fall 1979).
17. See Office of Technology Assessment, *The Implications of Cost-Effectiveness Analysis of Medical Technology*, Background Paper #2: Case Studies of Medical Technologies, Case Study #10: The Costs and Effectiveness of Neonatal Intensive Care, August 1981 Office of Technology Assessment Washington, DC (1981).
18. Sinclair, J. C., *et al.*, Evaluation of neonatal-intensive-care programs, *N. Eng. J. Med.* **305**:489–94 (Aug. 27, 1981).
19. See note 17 *supra* at 38.
20. Williams, R. L., and Chen, P. M., Identifying the sources of the recent decline in perinatal mortality rates in California, *N. Eng. J. Med.* **306**:214 (Jan. 28, 1982).

Discussion

Dr. Arnold S. Relman (New England Journal of Medicine): I was particularly impressed by Dr. Todres's caution that you really have to be there in order to understand what we are talking about. Decision making for congenitally handicapped newborns, like all medical decision making, is not a one-time thing. It is not a kind of a theoretical argument: "Should we or should we not save this patient's or this infant's life?" That's not the way it is. The condition of the infant or the patient is changing all the time. There are multiple interventions that must continue with different consequences, which often change the picture. You start out doing one thing that you think is right or may help, and things end up being quite different from what you expected. Your decision making will be influenced by what happens as a result of the initial intervention. That's why I personally support the view that the less one formalizes, the less one institutionalizes, the less one has committees and courts involved, the better off one is. Committees can never take care of patients. Courts can never take care of patients. Decisions must be made all the time, and they must be made by people who are there on the spot, with the best interests of the infant always in mind. As far as Professor Burt's comments are concerned, he does make a powerful argument against institutionalizing or formalizing the withdrawal or the withholding of life-saving treatment. But it seems to me that it is just as bad to institutionalize the withholding of life-saving treatment as it is to institutionalized the requirement that life-prolonging treatment must always be given: institutionalization of any kind of treatment or decision formalizing and publicizing of any kind of management of desperately ill, incompetent patients is bad for the patient. It leads inevitably to injustice and damage. It seems to me that the people who are responsible for the care of the patient—the next of kin, the medical people, and any advisers that they wish to consult—must be the ones who make the decisions for these incompetent patients. I advocate avoidance of any kind of institutionalization. It seems to me that the law and society have an interest only after the event. If an injustice has been done, if somebody's rights have been violated, if somebody's been murdered in a hospital, that's when the law comes in. The law cannot and should not intervene in advance. There is no way it can do so helpfully. Finally, about

Professor Childress's comments, I found myself in agreement with almost everything he said, except that I think that review committees are very useful when there are very deep and irreconcilable differences between the family and the medical people who look after the patient. That sometimes happens, and there's no way to resolve it except by a committee. Also, it seems that, whenever a decision is made to withhold treatment, it's well to have that decision supported by more than one or two medical opinions. Committees can be very useful as medical consultants, saying, "Yes, there really is no medical reason, no medical justification to continue . . . to do any more." So, I think that committees can be very useful, and my personal view is that they ought to be used very frequently. Those are my personal views.

Ms. Barbara Katz Rothman (City University of New York): I'd like to address the issues of language that come up in the way that we think about these problems. One is the treatment; the word *treatment* is consistently used to mean "standard," "current," "this week's," "American medical practice." Treatment means different things to different people. So, when we talk about the giving and withholding of treatment, we're talking about the giving and withholding of what physicians define as appropriate treatment. This description casts the whole problem in a particular way. What happens (this is an issue that each of you approached and skirted) is that when there is a disagreement about whether treatment should be given or withheld, physicians are presumed actually to have the patient's best interest in mind. By virtue of being newborn, we all become patients. Every baby born is defined first as a patient, and then it is determined if it will continue in the patient role or leave that role. Physicians are defined as competent to define the patient status of the newborn, then further to define appropriate treatment. New persons come into the decision making only if someone disagrees with the physician. Physicians are always assumed to have their patients' best interests at heart. When the parents agree with what the physician wants, then the parents can make decisions. When the parents disagree, we call in the next level of arguer. Now, what was pointed out and then moved away from was that, certainly, when you bring in the state, the state turns to yet another physician to say, "Is this an appropriate medical treatment?", never questioning that there may be something else other than medical treatment. So, for those of us who are looking at this from the perspective of parents who are potentially in this situation, we might not choose to use the battleground analogies that you keep drawing of the frontline, and we might prefer to pull our babies out of that particular battleground and provide them with alternative treatments. Parents, for instance, can go back to some of the more interesting historical moments, such as parents who refused to have radiation treatment for their kids' tonsils and parents who refused to take DES to maintain pregnancies.

A Participant: The discussion is treatment of critically ill newborns.

Ms. Barbara Katz Rothman: I'm using other examples where medical intervention was not necessarily in the patient's best interests. Another is parents who disagreed about the routine use of incubators for premature infants and saved some of their babies from blindness. Medical decision making has not had a history of always being right. It is wrong to always assume that medical treatment is the only treatment and the correct treatment; this idea phrases the question in such a way that the parents' perspective is automatically discounted. I'd like you to examine the language you are using and see if this is exactly what you mean to say. Are you saying that the only treatment is always medical treatment? And that the only person ever qualified to determine the appropriateness of treatment is a physician?

DR. I. DAVID TODRES (Massachusetts General Hospital): I appreciate your comments because I think one of the things the medical profession is saying, and certainly I am saying, is "We need your help." We are not here to dictate that there is only one way treatment can be carried out. Your question is a well-thought-out one in terms of treatment. What is treatment? It's true that, when the infant comes to the intensive care unit, my focus is on that infant whose physiology is deranged. I'm hoping that I can step back and see the whole infant and not just the physiology of the heart or the lungs or the parts of the body. But initially, for life-saving, that's what's required, and I think that we have to concentrate on the physiology. That's why I said that, in some ways, the best way I could have presented my thoughts would be to ask you all to come with me to the intensive care unit and spend 20 minutes looking at these babies, to develop your own perceptions of what you think is treatment. I think we often are talking about different things when we talk about treatment or how we perceive the care of these very handicapped infants. If anything, from my perspective the infant is overtreated. I'm not saying that is wrong, that we shouldn't do that, but because we don't know the outcome, we're often going to the overtreatment point and then looking back and saying, "We gave this child every chance we could." We probably overtreated, and that hurts a great deal. At the same time, there are many infants lying in the newborn nursery who have tubes stuck into every orifice, are attached to monitors, and are difficult to recognize as human beings. And yet, it's necessary to do this to them because we know we can save these infants to live a healthy life in the future. Technology is applied where it can help the infant, but I think it may be better if we share this decision rather than dictate what's "treatment." I certainly have no intention of doing that.

DR. JAMES F. CHILDRESS (University of Virginia): I think you have made a very valuable contribution to our discussion by warning us about the kinds of language and metaphors employed in our interaction together. It is my contention about the relation between parents and physicians that there is an important range of discretion, in terms of both the definition of interests and what could be expected to meet those interests. It's hard to define that in an abstract way (as we've been reminded), but we have to recognize that it exists and work out ways to define it.

MR. ROBERT A. BURT (Yale University School of Law): I've been scanning my own remarks, and at least I was using the word *treatment* only where both physicians and parents agreed on the definition of treatment but decided that they wanted to withhold it. I think that my particular use avoided that general problem.

Ms. KAREN METZLER (Case Western University): I try to approach the problem intellectually, but I would like to bring a little bit of experience into it. I was born 33 years ago with spina bifida, among other birth defects, and it was at that time assumed that I could have been paralyzed, retarded, blind, and deaf. I am not. My concern is about handicapped infants who were born in the early 1950s, who are now young adults and have shown that they are intelligent and capable human beings, and who make up the bulk of the infants who were born with birth defects. The case of the anencephalic is really extreme in the context of the 2 million handicapped people in the United States who are not being given the opportunity to be productive because of social attitudes. I would like to remind people to consider how this debate plays into the development of social attitudes. I am particularly concerned about the upcoming generations who will be born into the midst of this debate who will survive and who will have the intelligence to ask their parents, as I know from my counseling experience, "If they had given you that option, would you have let me die?" What impact is this debate having on the quality of the lives of all handicapped persons? It's not a question; it's a reminder.

Mr. ROBERT A. BURT: I think it is a very apt reminder. In yet another context, the question of our social commitment to care for Down syndrome individuals, I agree with the implication that both this debate and the extent to which it becomes legitimized and authorized for somebody to withhold treatment from a Down syndrome child raises the question about all those Down syndrome individuals who have survived. It also raises a social question that never before was asked, directed at the handicapped individual, "How come you're still around?" You are right to remind us of that aspect of the cost of deciding formally to withhold treatment from some category of newborns.

Ms. KAREN METZLER: What will be the composition, the demographics, of institutional ethics committees? Studies show that, among individuals and parents who have children with birth defects, the higher their income and the higher their intelligence, the less likely they are to accept a person with a disability. So, if you have a professional group, is it going to be swayed toward not making a commitment to the best interests of a child, with some modification of the quality of life, compared to that of a person who is "boring" but ostensibly normal. I have a telling story. The last time I attended the Genetics and the Law conference, it was held at the Copley Plaza, and I was really frustrated because I didn't take the time to say my piece. I went out and crossed the street, and there was a bum who had probably been a rosy-cheeked, blossoming little kid because he didn't appear to have any anomalies. But he was a bum, and he wasn't struggling to get an advanced degree or a job, as I am, to be productive in society. And yet, he could stand there in front of a whole crowd of people and make a big scene, saying, "What's wrong with you? Why are you that way?" So there's no guarantee that we are all going to become presidents of the United States. We can't all do that. We each have a role to play, if we're given that role to play. You people hold the power, the keys. In terms of my education, in terms of my insurance, in terms of my employment, I have to turn to the medical community to define what I can and cannot do. If you have a limited view of what I can do because you've never seen me function outside the office or the surgical room, then society is going to persist in that as well.

DR. AUBREY MILUNSKY (Boston University School of Medicine): Karen, could we have you come back to the microphone. Karen knows how happy I am that she came again to our meetings. I've already told her that, and she represents a most important constituency in our country, that, indeed, is not well represented anywhere. I want to ask you if you'll take a few more minutes to address two questions from your perspective. The first is: Where, besides anencephaly, do you draw a line in the newborn nursery? How do you recommend that perinatalogists like Dr. Todres operate?

MS. KAREN METZLER: I'm not a doctor, not because I don't want to be one. I wanted to be one very badly. But my experience is that what is considered an impossible case today becomes possible tomorrow through research. My case was considered impossible in 1950; that's the way it was presented to my parents. My father said that, if doing what you can do will mean that, a generation from now, an infant will be born with a greater chance and a greater promise of living than my daughter, I'm willing to submit my daughter to this. And this was before they had my generation around to show them what those limitations were or were not. That was also at a time when the community was not making an effort to educate persons with disabilities. The government was not supporting the financial costs, so my parents did this all themselves. They were willing to do it as their contribution to society. In our family, people are judged by what they contribute, not by the power and money they have, or status, or whatever. We need education so that more people will see what the extremes are, so they will appreciate the whole spectrum. I don't have a definite answer. I don't feel qualified. I don't think you would accept my answer.

DR. ARNOLD S. RELMAN: I think Dr. Milunsky wants to know if the mental capacity is so severely impaired, does this justify allowing death to occur?

MS. KAREN METZLER: I think my IQ of 160 is a disability because people cannot accept a person with a disability who can function shoulder to shoulder in the job world with them.

DR. ARNOLD S. RELMAN: That's not the point, Karen.

MS. KAREN METZLER: I don't think that the money and that the human experience, the quality of it, should be the criteria.

DR. AUBREY MILUNSKY: Would you comment on society's continuing move toward perfection and on its lack of patience with imperfection.

MS. KAREN METZLER: Yes, I think it's a straightjacket for all of us because it teaches all of us not to accept ourselves. Striving to use the best of your capabilities is different from being perfect, from striving to be perfect. The point is, trying to be the best that you can be. I think the perfection model enhances the stigmatization of a person like me, not just because I'm not perfect, but because other people who do not accept themselves and their limitations, who are not comfortable with their own self-concept and are looking around society to see what their position is, are less likely to accept a person with a disability, too.

Ms. ALTA CHARO (Legislative Drafting Fund, Columbia Law School): Dr. Childress, I am rather puzzled by one thing that you said, and the previous speaker's comments just made my puzzlement more concrete. You spoke of using the best interests of the child as a definition of some sort of objective just outcome, which I'll shorten down to the "the right answer." The decisions are between disabilities (which can be very severe and can be overcome to differing degrees, based not only on the parents and the family, but on the motivation of the person with the disabilities) and what the courts call the "utter void of nonexistence." I find it difficult to say that there can be a "right answer" that is objective and just in any given situation, let alone as a generic answer. In fact, your attempts to describe a system of serial decision making struck me as coming much closer to an attempt to find a perfect procedure whose end would be the common wisdom of what's best for this child, which would become, by definition, the best-interests test. I wonder if you could explain to me any better how best interests can be an objective outcome.

DR. JAMES F. CHILDRESS: It seems to me very difficult to argue that survival is not in a particular infant's best interest. So it may well help us to establish some wrong answers that enable (or, perhaps, even require) later decision makers to override the primary decision maker, which would be the family or parents. I'm trying to hold onto both things: that there is a standard, and that we have a lot of difficulty in interpreting it in a variety of cases. This may well help us set some limits, and when those limits are violated, then perhaps we have to override the primary decision maker.

Ms. LYNDA MULHAUSER (Children's Hospital, Washington, DC.): I'm sorry, Dr. Childress, that you didn't further address the issue of cost and who pays, because within this whole argument, even though we have a set of parents who may make their decision based on the best interests of the child, and the physicians and everyone else in that process who may do the same thing, when an "objective third party" comes that issue is avoided totally. So from a legal standpoint—and Dr. Burt may want to address this—is there any current mechanism to require the people who are making the arguments to save the children to have some sort of responsibility for all the medical and social expenses, like leg braces at $2,000 each, that will help these people be independent and competitive?

DR. JAMES F. CHILDRESS: I think this is not different in principle from arguments we make about a right to health care in general, in the sense of setting limits on the scope and so forth. What I wanted to do is to insist that the question of decision making and the question of who pays should not be combined. The mere fact that we require treatment for someone, overriding the parents' wishes in this case, does not tell us who should pay the bill.

MR. ROBERT A. BURT: You knowingly pose the question. There are a lot of cheap shots in this area, and there are many advocates (the Reagan administration is particularly guilty of this) who take a rigid "right-to-life" position but are not willing to commit the kind of resources that are required by simple decency and humanity, as you indicate. At the same time, one has to acknowledge that 1975 was a banner year for this country in the social commitment of resources to these purposes because of the adoption of Public Law 94–142, the Education of All Handicapped Children Act and the Developmental Disabilities Assistance and Bill of Rights Act. When one looks from a 10-year perspective, when we first met to debate these issues, there was almost nothing by way of governmental funding, and now there is, in a certain sense, an unbelievable amount. There are still, however, nowhere near the kind of resources needed, and the Reagan administration is fighting those allocations tooth and claw at the same time that they are taking this rigid "right-to-life" position. The social position is not wholly bleak, but the inconsistency is an important point to make.

MS. LYNDA MULHAUSER: I find it ethically repugnant that the two are so divergent at this time.

MR. JIM WALTERS (Loma Linda University): As an illustration of the point, Paul Conrad in the *Los Angeles Times* a few weeks ago had a cartoon of President Reagan talking to this little needy handicapped person, saying, "Shut up, we got you here, didn't we?" Dr. Burt, I want to address the comments you made. I agree that there is a widespread myth in society that the individual has great sanctity and that this myth is valuable. Perhaps it's appropriate that we spend hundreds of thousands of dollars to try to rescue a coal miner, and we refuse to spend a similar amount to make railway crossings safe to save many lives. I am wondering, in this new medical economy and with the new medical technology, if physicians are going to be able to continue to have the sort of ethos of protecting life at all costs, and spending untold money for individuals regardless of other considerations. Given the new technology, and the new economy, aren't we going to have to expect the American public to be more mature than perhaps more paternalistic positions over the ages have assumed that they are? Then, a second question, Dr. Childress: I was surprised at your placing ethics committees in hospitals, and in the questionable way that you did. Given medical paternalism over the ages, given the need for a broader base for decision making, shouldn't the physician work in closer connection with those multidisciplined committees so that it's not just her or his values that are brought to bear on these sensitive judgments?

MR. ROBERT A. BURT: Your question is difficult to answer in a small compass. There was an implication that I heard in your question that this myth, this ethos of sanctity, is a symptom of social immaturity, and that we kind of grow up when we learn to be more bloodless and rational and cool about these matters. I don't find that implication compelling. We carry lots of emotive, symbolic, meaning-giving forces in our heads, and this is one in particular that I don't see why we should grow out of. But, of course, there are tensions and it's complex. Indeed, there may be occasions in the tightening of social resources that may force us back into the "God committees." The burden of my remarks was that I think we should genuinely be forced to that point before we accept it. In the context of treatment-withholding decisions about anomalous newborns, it is not yet clear to me that we have been forced to take those steps. There are great political pressures. Decision making in clinical settings is very difficult. There are pressures, particularly from the medical community, saying, "There's too much interference here. Regularize and formalize this in some kind of a way." I simply mean to be a Doubting Thomas on that score. It's not financial pressure that is primarily pressing in this area at this time as I read the current social debate.

MR. JIM WALTERS: I deal with a hospital that has spent, through a third-party payer, over $1 million for a neonate that no one thinks has any future. Is this sort of thing, in the name of the sanctity of life, to be accommodated in medicine today?

MR. ROBERT A. BURT: Well, you know it can be. Let me begin again with your example: a coal-mine disaster in which it is likely, though not a certainty, that most of the miners, or even all of the miners, are dead. Now, at the moment, we devote enormous amounts of resources, public attention, and focus to such a disaster. I am not sure that it is a sign of maturity or good social sense for us to say, "That's too expensive; to hell with the miners," rather than embracing the kind of social commitment that you were speaking of, which is "Now let's turn to saving people at railroad crossings." My prediction is—though who can know?—that we will be hard of heart in both contexts instead of in only one context, as we now are.

DR. JAMES F. CHILDRESS: Let me respond to your question and also to Dr. Relman's comments regarding hospital ethics committees. I serve on one that has the function of dealing with a kind of Infant Doe situation. I think that these committees have an important role to play. The question I was raising when I ran out of time was to what extent they're needed. Dr. Relman suggests that they serve a valuable function, although, interestingly, after he argued against institutionalization and the overcoming of distance, we got an argument for a central role for hospital ethics committees. What is the function of such a committee? If the committee is to recommend policy, as the one I serve on is in part designed to do, I think it has an important role. If it is educative, both for the staff and for the parents who want advice, that's fine, too. The big problem I have is whether a committee should have a primary role in the review of decision making day after day, or whether it should come into play only in certain limited settings. It was really more of a question than anything else. We need to ask how we are going to interpret the data that we have about decision making as to whether committees should have a role beyond educative and social policies.

DR. ARNOLD S. RELMAN: But the educative role is not to be minimized.

DR. JAMES F. CHILDRESS: No, I'd resign the committee if I didn't think it had an important educative role. I am agreeing with you. But then the question of the actual review of cases and how regularly it is done, and so forth, needs to be addressed.

DR. NORMAN FOST: Two comments on your comments, Dr. Relman. First, with regard to the importance of being there at the bedside, on the battlefield. My experience with institutional review boards and with our hospital ethics committee is that most of the most important information and pivotal arguments and facts come from people who aren't there. With regard to handicapped newborns, to cite one example, the very wide availability of adoption—say, for example, for Down syndrome children—is a very well-kept secret from many parents, as well as attending physicians. There are now many dead Down syndrome babies who, had their parents or doctors known about this adoption availability before the fact, would be alive today. That knowledge and access to information about it comes from people who sit on these committees who are not at the bedside. You suggested that we should wait for some murders to occur and then bring the troops in to punish the guilty. We've had, in the opinion of Professors Burt and John Robertson, homicides occurring for 10 years. Nothing has happened. There have been no prosecutions. And there won't be because it's too Draconian. No prosecutor wants to put a doctor in jail for doing something that is so complex and fraught with so many well-meaning intentions. It's because there are no prosecutions, and because child abuse and neglect laws have almost never been brought to bear, that we have the Baby Doe regulations and SWAT squads. Those regulations weren't written until laws were broken and not enforced. Waiting for prosecution after the fact is also small consolation to the dead children. The law hasn't changed behavior; it's too harsh. I think that's why we had something like the Baby Doe regulations, which I think were equally too harsh. We need something in between.

THE FETUS, THE MOTHER, AND THE STATE

MODERATOR: CHARLES H. BARON

21

ABORTION

A Decade of Decisions

LEONARD H. GLANTZ, J.D.
Associate Professor of Health Law
Boston University School of Public Health
80 East Concord Street
Boston, MA 02118

In 1973, the Supreme Court of the United States struck down all restrictive state abortion statutes in *Roe v. Wade*.[1] In doing so, it set forth a scheme by which the constitutionality of future statutes could be measured. In essence, the court ruled that, during the first trimester of pregnancy, the state could have essentially no role in the regulation of abortion; that in the second trimester, the state could regulate abortions in ways designed to further maternal health; and that after fetal viability (*not* the third trimester), in furtherance of the state's interest in protecting fetal life, the state could prohibit abortions except those that were necessary to protect the life or health of the pregnant woman. On the face of it, these are simple rules. However, over the last decade, many states have tried to pass the most restrictive abortion statutes possible under these rules, and indeed, some states have passed clearly unconstitutional abortion legislation. As a result of these state efforts, innumerable lawsuits have been brought in state and federal courts, and the U.S. Supreme Court has decided at least 14 abortion cases since *Roe v. Wade*. This activity indicates at least two things. First, the deceptively simple rules set forth in *Roe* are much more difficult to apply than they initially appeared to be. Second, those who are opposed to legalized abortion will work very diligently to have their voices heard and respected by state legislatures. It would also seem to indicate that the legal battles fought over abortion will not soon be settled.

This chapter will explore how the U.S. Supreme Court has dealt with various abortion issues presented to it since the last Genetics and the Law Conference in 1979, with the goal of ascertaining the constitutional boundaries regarding the regulation of abortion as the court sees them.

FUNDING

An important tactic that the "prolife" forces have adopted is withholding state or federal funding of abortions for poor women. The goal has been to reduce the total number of abortions performed. In 1977, the U.S. Supreme Court decided two cases that involved the public funding of "unnecessary" or "nontherapeutic" abortions. In the first case, *Beal v. Doe*,[2] the court decided that the Medicaid statute did not require states to pay for these abortions. In the second case, *Maher v. Roe*,[3] the court decided that a state policy that offered payment for the costs incident to childbirth, but not to abortion, did not violate the Equal Protection Clause of the U.S. Constitution.

At the time of the last Genetics and the Law Conference, I pointed out that these cases had been rather narrowly decided.[4] First, they dealt with "unnecessary" procedures that are usually not covered by Medicaid in any event. Second, the availability of funds was dependent on a determination of "medical necessity," which is left to the discretion of the women's physician. Finally, these cases allowed the withholding of funds in situations where the woman would not suffer any physical or mental harm from the continuation of the pregnancy. As it turns out, however, these factors were apparently not important to a majority of the court.

Harris v. McCrae[5] involved the constitutionality of the "Hyde amendment." The *Hyde amendment*, named after its congressional sponsor, is a term used to describe a member of federal restrictions on abortion funding. In 1980, the Hyde amendment forbade the use of federal funds to perform abortions except where

> the life of the mother would be endangered if the fetus were carried to term; or except for such medical procedures necessary for the victims of rape or incest when such rape or incest has been reported promptly to a law enforcement agency or public health service.[6]

However, there have been a variety of Hyde amendments over the years. In 1977, there was no rape or incest exception, and in 1979, there was an additional exception for instances where two physicians determined that a woman would suffer "severe and long-lasting physical health damage" if the pregnancy were carried to term. The court stated in footnote 4 that its opinion referred to all the versions of the Hyde amendment. This means that the court was rendering an opinion about the constitutionality of withholding funds for abortions except in life-threatening situations. Put another way, the issue was: Could the federal government deny funds to women who would suffer severe and long-lasting physical harm unless they had abortions, while providing funds for women who would undergo normal labor and deliver? The court, in a 5–4 decision, decided that the Hyde amendment was constitutional.

In rendering its decision, the court relied extensively on *Maher*, which involved nontherapeutic abortions, whereas this case involved therapeutic abortions. The court concluded that this distinction is without constitutional significance. In *Maher*, the court held that denying funding for nontherapeutic abortions did not impinge on a woman's right to privacy as described in *Roe*. Under *Roe*, the court explained, a woman must be free to decide whether or not to terminate her pregnancy, and the state must not place obstacles of its own making in front of a woman who wishes to act on her decision. However, by refusing to pay for abortions, the *state* has not placed any obstacles in front of her. As the court stated in *Maher*,

> The indigency that may make it difficult—and in some cases, perhaps, impossible— for some women to have abortions is neither created nor in any way affected by the [lack of state funding].[7]

In essence, the court was saying that one can have a right to make a choice but, if poor, is not entitled to have the state pay for the exercise of that choice. The court adopted this reasoning in *McCrae* and held that the state need not pay for therapeutic abortions.

There were vigorous, and even bitter dissents, in this case. Justice Stevens, who was a member of the majority in the nontherapeutic abortion cases, was a dissenter here. He felt that, once the government decided to alleviate some of the hardships of poverty by providing "necessary medical care," the government must use neutral criteria in distributing benefits. He was particularly concerned about the fact that, if the government decided to cut off funds for abortions that a woman needed to save her life, it would be constitutional to do so after *McCrae*. Indeed, the Solicitor General agreed with this proposition at the oral argument.[8]

This case stands for several propositions. The clearest is that neither states nor the federal government must pay for abortions for poor women. However, it also stands for the proposition that no government is required by the Constitution to pay for any medical care for the indigent no matter how necessary it may be, as long as the refusal to pay for such service is "rationally related to a legitimate government interest." Advocates for the poor see this case as an ominous foreshadowing of things to come. For example, anyone who ever believed that there is a "right to health care" will find that a constitutional basis for such a right has been undercut by *McCrae*.

Needless to say, both "prolife" and "prochoice" advocates tried to determine what *McCrae* meant in terms of the direction the Supreme Court was taking on abortion. Regardless of the fact that the court stated in *Maher* and *McCrae* that these cases did not lessen the right to privacy set forth in *Roe*, both sides of the abortion issue wondered if this was really the case. The vitality of *Roe* after *McCrae* is discussed in a later section.

ABORTION AND MINORS

Perhaps the most controversial issue that the U.S. Supreme Court has had to contend with in the abortion area is the access of minor women to abortion services. In *Planned Parenthood of Missouri v. Danforth*,[9] the court struck down a Missouri statute that required the written consent of a parent of a woman who was under the age of 18 and who was unmarried. The court noted that "constitutional rights do not mature and come into being magically only when one attains the state-defined age of majority."[10] Furthermore, the court argued that the "State does not have the constitutional authority to give a third party an absolute, and possibly arbitrary veto over the decision of the physician and his patient to terminate the patient's pregnancy."[11] The minor's right to consent to abortion on her own does not apply to every minor regardless of age or maturity; rather, it applies to a minor who is "sufficiently mature to understand the procedure and to make an intelligent assessment of her circumstances with the advice of her physician."[12] In effect, the court held that if, the state could not veto a woman's decision to have an abortion, it could not give anyone else veto power over a woman who could maturely and intelligently decide whether or not to have an abortion, regardless of the woman's age.

The Massachusetts legislature also passed a statute intended to limit a minor's access to abortion.[13] This statute provided that, if a woman was less than 18 years old, she had to obtain the consent of both parents in order to obtain an abortion. If one or both of the parents refused to consent, consent could be obtained from a judge of the superior court for "good cause shown." A three-judge federal district court struck down this statute,[14] and appeal was taken to the U.S. Supreme Court,[15] which, in essence, sent the case to the Massachusetts Supreme Judicial Court[16] for an interpretation of the statute. Five years after this tortuous litigation was commenced, the U.S. Supreme Court again heard the case and found the statute unconstitutional.[17]

In deciding this case, the court noted the interpretation of the statute by the Massachusetts Supreme Judicial Court. The Massachusetts court held, among other things, that (1) in most cases, a minor woman could not seek court approval until her parents refused to consent; (2) even if the judge decides that the minor woman is capable of making, and has made, an informed decision, she or he can still withhold consent to abortion if she or he deems that the best interests of the minor would not be served by an abortion; and (3) in most cases, the parents must be notified of any judicial proceedings brought by the minor. This holding means that, although the parents do not have unlimited veto power over the minor's decision to have an abortion, they are given a role every time a minor seeks an abortion.

Eight justices agreed that this statutory scheme was unconstitutional, and one would have upheld it. However, the eight Justices were split on how far the decision should go. Four of the Justices took it on themselves to set forth what they believed a constitutional statute would look like. They argued that a statute would be constitutional if a minor could go to court without first seeking a parent's approval. Moreover, the only role for the court would be to determine if the minor was mature enough and well informed enough to make an abortion decision in consultation with her physician. Once the judge decided that she was mature and well informed, the judge could not make an independent decision about the minor's best interests. Only if the court finds that the minor is not mature or well informed may it then make a determination of her best interests. Parental notification may not be required as matter of course. The proceeding must be conducted with anonymity and expeditiously enough to provide an "effective opportunity" for the abortion to be obtained. This scheme, four Justices held, would be constitutional.

The four other Justices who thought the Massachusetts law was unconstitutional felt that it was improper to discuss a hypothetical statute and so did not join in that part of the decision. As a result of this 4–4 split, it was not possible to determine how a majority of the court would view such a statute.

In *Akron v. Center for Reproductive Health*,[18] the court was asked to determine the constitutionality of a municipal ordinance that prohibited a minor from receiving an abortion without obtaining the "informed written consent" of one of her parents or "an order from a court having jurisdiction over her that the abortion be performed or induced." The court struck down this provision as unconstitutional because it did not limit the judge's discretion in making his or her decision in accordance with the *Baird* decision discussed above.

In a companion case, *Planned Parenthood Association of Kansas City, Missouri v. Ashcroft*,[19] the court upheld a statute regarding minors seeking court approval that the court believed was consistent with the guidelines promulgated in *Baird*. However, the fragility of this holding is demonstrated by how the Justices voted in this case. Only two Justices were satisfied with the constitutionality of the statute. Four Justices believed that a statute (including this one) that permits a "judicial veto" is unconstitutional. The three remaining Justices apparently believed that a statute providing parents with a veto is constitutional and therefore disagreed with the premise on which the two satisfied Justices based their opinions. There is, thus, a strange alliance between the first two Justices and the last three Justices, all of whom voted to uphold the constitutionality of the law, but for very different reasons. It was a 5–4 decision, with the Justices in the majority seriously split on the fundamental issue in the case. The four Justices in the minority were in solid agreement on the unconstitutionality of the statute. As a result of this odd voting distribution and the closeness of the decision, the constitutional dimensions of the right of a minor to obtain an abortion have still not been conclusively dealt with by the court.

In order to avoid the issue of parental veto, Utah passed a statute requiring parental *notification* before a minor undergoes an abortion.[20] The case was brought on behalf of an unmarried 15-year-old girl who was living at home. Additionally, no evidence was offered that she was either mature or emancipated. As a result, the court explicitly confined its decision to this category of minor women and upheld the statute.[21] The court based its holding on the finding that parents can provide an immature minor with suport, given the "medical, emotional, and psychological consequences of abortion," and further, that they could provide the adequate medical and psychological case history that is important to the physician.

Given the facts that this holding is explicitly limited to immature and unemancipated minors, and that it involves only parental notification and not parental veto power, the case is perfectly consistent with the *Baird* case discussed above.

The constitutional parameters of the state power to limit minors' access to abortion is still unsettled. This is not just a result of the difficult issues that abortion raises but is also a result of the court's continuing struggle to determine the nature of constitutional rights as they pertain to minors generally and the power of the state to abridge these rights.[22]

THE RESURRECTION OF *Roe v. Wade*

As we discussed earlier, following the court's decisions in the Medicaid cases, which held that neither the state nor the federal government was obliged to pay for abortions for poor women, there was a question concerning whether that decision signaled a retreat from *Roe*. This question was answered in June 1983, 10 years after *Roe*, when the court issued its opinions in *City of Akron v. Akron Center for Reproductive Health*[23] and *Planned Parenthood Association of Kansas City, Missouri v. Ascroft*.[24]

Akron concerned the constitutionality of a restrictive municipal ordinance that contained the following provisions:

1. All abortions performed after the first trimester of pregnancy had to be performed in a general hospital that was accredited by the Joint Commission on Accreditation of Hospitals (JCAH) or the American Osteopathic Association.

2. The woman's physician was required to inform her of the status of her pregnancy, the development of the fetus, the date of possible viability, the physical and emotional complications that might result from an abortion, and the availability of agencies that would provide her with assistance and information with respect to birth control, abortion, and childbirth. The physician was specifically required to state

> That abortion is a major surgical procedure which can result in serious complications, including hemorrhage, perforated uterus, infection, menstrual disturbances, sterility and miscarriage and prematurity in subsequent pregnancies and that abortion may leave essentially unaffected or may worsen any existing psychological problems she may have, and can result in severe emotional disturbances.[25]

The physician was also required by the ordinance to state that "the unborn child is a human life from the moment of conception," and to describe the anatomical and physiological characteristics of the fetus in some detail.

3. The attending physician was required to inform the woman of "the particular risks associated with her own pregnancy and the abortion technique to be employed" and other information that, in his or her medical judgment, he or she believed would be relevant to the woman's decision regarding the abortion.

4. At least a 24-hour waiting period was required between the time the woman signed the consent form and the performance of the abortion.

5. Physicians performing abortions were required to dispose of the fetal remains in a "humane and sanitary manner."

At the beginning of its opinion, the U.S. Supreme Court repeated the doctrines that it had set forth in *Roe*. Perhaps more significantly the court stated,

> arguments continue to be made . . . that we erred in interpreting the Constitution [in *Roe*]. Nonetheless, the doctine of *stare decisis*, while perhaps never entirely persuasive on a constitutional question, is a doctrine that demands respect in a society governed by the rule of law. We respect it today, and reaffirm *Roe* v. *Wade*[26]

Arguably, the court went even further than in *Roe*, as will be seen in the following analysis.

The court struck down the requirement that all abortions performed after the first trimester be performed in a general hospital. In *Roe*, the court had held that, subsequent to the first trimester, a state could regulate abortions to the extent that "the regulation reasonably relates to the preservation and protection of maternal health"[27] because the state's interest in maternal health becomes "compelling" at this point in the pregnancy. Needless to say, the city argued that the hospitalization requirement was designed to further its interest in maternal health.

In striking down this requirement, the court noted that a second-trimester abortion costs $850–$900 in a hospital, whereas it costs $350–$400 in a clinic. It also pointed out that hospitals in Akron only rarely performed second-trimester abortions, so that women who wished to obtain such an abortion were subjected to the additional financial burdens and health risks associated with travel. It concluded from these facts that the hospitalization requirement "may significantly limit a woman's ability to obtain an abortion."[27]

At the same time, the court noted that both the American Public Health Association (APHA) and the American College of Obstetrics and Gynecology (ACOG) had abandoned their recommendations that all second-trimester abortions be performed in hospitals, a standard that existed at the time of Roe. Instead, both organizations agreed that second-trimester abortions could be performed safely in adequately equipped clinics until 18 weeks of pregnancy. As a result, the court concluded that requiring all second-trimester abortions to be performed in a general hospital could not now be justified on the grounds of protecting maternal health, especially when the requirement placed a "heavy, and unnecessary, burden on women's access to a relatively inexpensive, otherwise accessible, and safe abortion procedure."

There are a number of important lessons in this part of the decision. First, a regulation that significantly increases the expense of an abortion, or that has the effect of requiring women to travel to obtain an abortion, can be seen as placing an "undue burden" on the women's abortion decision. Second, the court ruled that regulations designed to protect maternal health may not "depart from accepted medical practice."[28] Not only does this statement show tremendous deference to the medical profession, but it also indicates that, as medical standards evolve, the constitutionality of laws that restrict abortion practices may be affected. In this instance, a city ordinance that may have been constitutional in 1973 was unconstitutional in 1983 because the APHA and the ACOG had changed their standards as to the acceptability of performing abortions on an outpatient basis. This means that legislative bodies must pay close attention to standard medical practice when trying to restrict post-first-trimester abortions. It also means that those who wish to challenge such restrictive laws may be unsuccessful at one time but may succeed at a later data if accepted practice changes.

The court also struck down the detailed informed-consent requirement described in Point 2 above. The court's first opportunity to deal with the issue of informed consent occurred in Danforth.[29] In that case, the court upheld a Missouri statute that required a pregnant woman to verify in writing that her consent was "informed and freely given." In upholding this requirement, the court noted that the "right" set forth in Roe is to allow the woman to make a decision about whether or not to have an abortion. Therefore, by requiring a woman to give an informed consent, the state is enhancing her capacity to make an intelligent decision. As the court put it, "the decision to abort . . . is an important, and often a stressful one, and it is desirable and imperative that it be made with full knowledge of its nature and consequences."[30]

In *Danforth*, the challengers argued that the term *informed consent* was too vague. In a footnote, the court construed the term to mean

> the giving of information to the patient as to just what would be done and as to its consequences. To ascribe more meaning than this might well confine the attending physician in a undesired and uncomfortable straitjacket in the practice of his profession. [31]

The issue was whether Akron's informed consent requirements met this standard. The court struck down this portion of the ordinance for a number of reasons. First, the court said the purpose of the information required was designed not to inform the woman but rather "to pursuade her to withhold it altogether." Second, the court held that the requirement to inform the woman that "the unborn child is a human life from the moment of conception" was inconsistent with the court's holding in *Roe* that a state may not adopt one theory of when life begins to justify its abortion regulations. Third, the court stated that to require a detailed anatomical description would force a physician to speculate about the particular fetus. Fourth, the requirement that a woman be told that abortion is a major surgical procedure followed by numerous possible physical and psychological complications was described as a "parade of horribles" intended to make the woman believe that abortion is a particularly dangerous procedure. Fifth, the requirement was seen as an "intrusion upon the discretion of the pregnant woman's physician," forcing him or her to recite the same "litany" of "information" to every patient regardless of the physician's judgment about the relevance of the information to a particular patient.

Again, we see the court being very protective of physicians' prerogatives. Additionally, it is very clear that the court discerned Akron's motives for passing this ordinance and refused to allow the city to turn a physician into a "mouthpiece" for the expression of its unscientific and biased views to individual patients.

In the less burdensome informed-consent provision set out in Point 3 above, regarding the obligation of the woman's "attending physician" to inform the patient of the "particular risks associated with her own pregnancy and the abortion technique to be employed," the court found nothing objectionable in the substance of the requirement. The court, however, struck down this provision because it required the task of informing the woman to be performed only by her "attending physician." The court clearly recognized the state's interest in having the woman informed but found that nothing in the record indicated that a woman's consent would not be informed if a physician delegated the counseling task to another qualified individual. Thus, although the Court recognized that a state may mandate that only physicians can perform abortions, "there is not as vital a state need" for requiring that a physician do the counseling. This was the first time that the court even intimated that a standard for the review of an abortion regulation involved a finding of a "vital state need."

The Court did indicate that a physician could be required to verify that adequate counseling had been provided and that the woman's consent was informed. The state may also establish "reasonable" qualifications for counselors.

The court spent little time striking down the 24-hour waiting period. The district court had found that the 24-hour waiting period might increase the cost of abortions by requiring two trips, and that scheduling difficulties might increase the wait to more than 24 hours. Also, Akron was unable to demonstrate that any legitimate state interest was furthered by an "arbitrary and inflexible" waiting period. The court once again noted that this requirement interfered with the physician's discretion in the exercise of his or her "medical judgment."

If we read between the lines, the court viewed this provision as designed to make it more difficult for a woman to obtain an abortion and essentially as a form of state harassment. The judges on the court know that limbs are amputated and risky neurosurgery and heart transplants are performed without waiting periods: How could they possibly view this waiting period as anything less than arbitrary?

The court also struck down the provision requiring the "human and sanitary" disposal of the fetal remains. It was unclear what this requirement meant, and in a criminal statute, which is what this is, such vagueness is a fatal flaw.

The *Planned Parenthood*[32] case involved the constitutionality of a Missouri statute that required,

1. Abortions performed after 12 weeks of pregnancy be performed in a hospital.
2. A pathology report for each abortion performed.
3. The presence of a second physician during abortions performed after viability.[33]

The hospitalization requirement was struck down for the same reasons stated in *City of Akron.*

The court upheld the requirement that a second physician be present at postviability abortions. The court noted that, in *Roe,* it had recognized the state's compelling interest in the protection of potential human life after viability, and that a state could prohibit postviability abortions except where the abortion was necessary to preserve the life or health of the woman. Given this fact, and given the fact that in a postviability abortion the operating physician has to direct his or her attention and skills to the care of the woman, the court found that the presence of a second physician would serve to assure the state's interest in protecting the life of a live-born child.

The court also upheld the requirement of a pathologist's report. In Missouri, there is a statute requiring that most tissue surgically removed in a *hospital* be examined by a pathologist. The question in this case was: Can that requirement be constitutionally applied to tissue removed in a *clinic* during an abortion? The court found that the examination of tissue by a pathologist is a legitimate means of protecting maternal health, and that both medical testimony and the medical literature support the desirability of this practice. Additionally, the court found that a pathological examination of this tissue adds a "comparatively small additional cost" to the overall cost of an abortion, and that this small cost does "not significantly burden a pregnant woman's abortion decision." The estimated cost of compliance was $19.40. It is interesting that whether the cost is "unduly burdensome" or not was disputed by the dissenters, who argued that the cost of compliance might be as high as $40 in a first-trimester abortion. They sarcastically concluded,

> Although this increase may seem insignificant from the Court's comfortable perspective, I cannot say that it is equally insignificant to every woman seeking an abortion.

For the woman on welfare or the unemployed teenager, this additional cost may well put the price of an abortion beyond reach. [34]

There was a strong dissent in these cases against the court's actions striking down the various provisions in these laws, written by Justice O'Connor, joined by Justices White and Rehnquist, both of whom had been strong opponents of the court's prior decisions striking down restrictive abortions laws. The position that Justice O'Connor took was of particular interest because she is the first female Supreme Court Justice and because "prolife" advocates opposed her nomination because of their perception that she was too "prochoice." Justice O'Connor's opinion was essentially a dissent from *Roe v. Wade*. She argued that the trimester scheme is "completely unworkable" and was especially unhappy with the court's use of changing medical standards to determine the constitutionality of state laws. She was concerned that "without the necessary expertise or ability, courts must . . . pretend to act as science review boards." [35]

Justice O'Connor's opinion raises a serious generic question about the role that the courts should play when they are confronted with scientific evidence and scientific disputes. But it also indicates a lack of general awareness of the increasing role of scientific evidence in courts. More and more courts deal with public health regulations, the validity (or invalidity) of which is based on scientific evidence, whether one is talking about compulsory vaccination, using x-ray machines to determine if shoes fit, cotton dust standards, or nuclear-power-plant regulations.

Justice O'Connor did make the important point that the standards set down in *Roe* may be on a collision course with themselves because of advances in medical science. As she stated,

Just as improvements in medical technology inevitably will move *forward* the point at which the State may regulate for reasons of maternal health, different technological improvements will move *backward* the point of viability at which the State may prescribe abortions to preserve the life and health of the mother. [36] (Emphasis in the original.)

In her opinion, Justice O'Connor argued that, "even assuming there is a fundamental right to terminate pregnancy in some situations," [37] the state's interests in protecting maternal health and potential fetal life are compelling throughout the pregnancy. Thus, she asked if the Akron ordinance unduly burdened a woman's right to obtain an abortion and concluded that none of Akron's provisions did so. It would appear that, with the possible exception of outlawing abortions altogether, no state regulation would be deemed unduly burdensome by Justice O'Connor or the other dissenters.

In order to try to determine the direction that the court has taken on abortion generally, it is useful to see which regulations regarding abortion the court has upheld and which it has struck down over the last 10 years (see Table 1). We will put aside the cases regarding minors because that area is still unsettled, as discussed earlier.

What is striking about these lists is that, with one exception, the provisions that the court has struck down involve regulations that apply to the abortion procedure itself or to activities that occur prior to the abortion. On the list of provisions that are upheld, with

TABLE 1. Abortion Regulations Struck Down and Upheld by the Court

Struck down	Upheld
1. Recital of a "parade of horribles"	A. Pathological examination of tissue
2. Hospitalization in second trimester	B. Record keeping and reporting if not burdensome and confidentiality is assured
3. "Humane and sanitary" disposal of fetal remains	C. General informed-consent provisions
4. Twenty-four-hour waiting period	D. Presence of second doctor at postviability abortions
5. Legislative determinations of viability	
6. Spousal consent	
7. Ban on use of saline amniocentesis	
8. Requiring a *physician* to obtain informed consent	

one exception (C), they all apply to postabortion regulations. The general informed-consent regulation that was upheld does not single out abortion for special treatment, as informed consent is a requirement for all surgeries.

Based on this list and the recent and past U.S. Supreme Court cases, we can gleen the following tests to determine the validity of state regulations of abortions. These are not necessarily independent tests; they can be used in various combinations:

1. Has a state placed an obstacle in front of the woman or otherwise significantly burdened the pregnant woman's ability to choose or obtain an abortion?
2. Is abortion being treated differently from other similar medical or surgical procedures? This is a critical point in the early stages of pregnancy and is much less important after the fetus is viable.
3. Does the regulation interfere with the treating physician's exercise of professional judgment?
4. Does the regulation conflict with, or is it stricter than, accepted medical and scientific norms?
5. Is the regulation designed to protect maternal health?
6. If it is designed to protect maternal health, is there a less intrusive or less expensive alternative?

We can test this scheme against actions that the court has taken to see how it applies. In striking down the second-trimester hospitalization requirement, we can see that the requirement was determined to be "significantly burdensome" (raised costs several hundred dollars) and thus placed a significant obstacle in front of the woman, treated abortion differently from other procedures (state laws usually do not specify which procedures must be done in a hospital), interfered with a physician's professional judgment (usually it is left up to a physician to determine *where* she or he will perform a procedure), was stricter than accepted medical norms (see AGOG and APHA standards), and was only questionably designed to protect maternal health; there also existed less expensive means of protecting maternal health.

On the other hand, the pathological examinations placed no obstacles in front of the woman (it was after the fact), was not "significantly burdensome" (although how expensive it would have to be before it reached this point was unclear), did not interfere with the treating physician's professional judgment (it did not affect him or her at all), was consistent with medical norms of practice, did not treat abortion specially (applied, at least in hospitals, to most surgically removed tissue), and was designed to protect and in fact protected maternal health; also, there was no alternative method to obtain the same information.

The more "yes" answers (with the exception of Point 5) a given regulation induces, the more likely it is to be struck down. Again with the exception of Point 5, a "yes" answer to any of these questions does not automatically lead to invalidity; rather, it causes the state to meet a heavy burden of proof. In Point 5, the term *designed* is used because I believe that the court does look at the motive of the legislature in setting forth a regulatory scheme in regard to abortion. For example, in striking down the ban on the use of saline amniocentesis in *Danforth*, the court was well aware that, although there might be maternal health reasons for doing so, the Missouri legislature's *not* banning an even more dangerous procedure (hysterotomy) indicated an intent not to protect maternal health, but to mandate procedures that would protect fetal life.

Over the past decade, it is quite remarkable how consistent the court has been in protecting a woman's right to obtain an abortion and a physician's right to perform one. As to the latter point, what is striking about the *City of Akron* decision is just how zealously the majority of the court acted to protect the right of the physician to exercise individual medical judgment—it is an extremely prophysician case and will be of as much use in protecting "physicians' rights" in areas other than abortion, as it will be to argue for a woman's right to obtain an abortion. The problem with the "parade of horribles" was not so much that a woman had to listen to it as that a physician had to recite it.

As it turns out, the Medicaid cases really meant what they said: they were restricted to the issue of the governmental obligation to pay for abortions. These cases have not been cited by the Court as a means of regulating abortion, although dissenters have used them in this manner.

City of Akron is not the last abortion case that will ever be heard. There are still many ambiguities and questions, and the strong feelings and the political power that the members of the "right-to-life" movement have will continue to cause restrictive abortion legislation to be passed. What *City of Akron* does, however, is clarify the court's strong feelings about limiting the states' power to pass restrictive abortion laws, at least as the court is currently constituted.

References and Notes

1. 410 U.S. 113 (1973).
2. 432 U.S. 438 (1977).
3. 432 U.S. 464 (1977).
4. Glantz, L. H. Recent developments in abortion law, in *Genetics and the Law II* (A. Milunsky and G. J. Annas, eds.), Plenum Press, Boston (1979), 217.
5. 448 U.S. 297 (1980).
6. P.L. No. 96–123 Sec. 109, 93 Stat. 926.
7. 432 U.S. at 474.
8. *Supra* note 5 at page 354, n. 6.
9. 428 U.S. 52 (1976).
10. *Id.* at 74.
11. *Id.*
12. *Id.* at 73–74, citing the Dissenting Judge in District Court, 392 F. Supp. 1362, 1376 (E.D. Mo. 1975).
13. 1974 Mass. Acts, ch 706, Mass Gen. Laws, Ch. 112 Sec. 12S.
14. *Baird v. Bellotti*, 393 F. Supp. 847 (1975).
15. *Bellotti v. Baird*, 423 U.S. 982 (1975).
16. *Baird v. Attorney General*, 360 N.E.2d 288 (Mass. 1977).
17. *Bellotti v. Baird*, 443 U.S. 622 (1979).
18. 103 S.Ct. 2481 (1983).
19. 103 S.Ct. 2517 (1983).
20. Utah Code Ann Sec. 76–7–304 (2).
21. *H.L. v. Matheson*, 450 U.S. 398 (1981).
22. For a discussion of the effect of laws authorizing judicial intervention, see Donavan, P. Judging teenagers: How minors fare when they seek court-authorized abortions, *Family Planning Perspectives* **15**:259 (Nov./Dec. 1983).
23. Supra, note 18.
24. Supra, note 19.
25. Akron Codified Ordinances Ch. 1870.05 (5) as cited in 103 S.Ct. 2489 n.5.
26. 103 S.Ct. at 2487.
27. 410 U.S. at 163.
28. 103 S.Ct. at 2493.
29. 428 U.S. 52 (1976).
30. 428 U.S. at 67.
31. Id at 67 n.8.
32. 103 S.Ct. 2517 (1983).
33. Both the *Missouri* and *Akron* provisions dealing with the minors are above.
34. 103 S.Ct. at 2528 (Blackmun, dissenting).
35. 103 S.Ct. at 2507 (O'Connor, dissenting).
36. *Id.*
37. 103 S.Ct. at 2508.

22

SHOULD CHILD ABUSE LAWS BE EXTENDED TO INCLUDE FETAL ABUSE?

MARGERY W. SHAW, M.D., J.D.
Director, Health Law Program
University of Texas Health Science Center
Fanin Bank Building
1020 Holcombe, Suite 600
Houston, TX 77030

INTRODUCTION

Before we address the issue of fetal abuse, let us first ask whether the fetus deserves the protection of the state, and if the answer is in the affirmative, then we must delineate the legal duties of the mother not to harm her fetus and the legal remedies of the fetus if it is threatened or abused.

The law has spoken clearly on the rights of the state to protect a would-be child after viability. In *Roe v. Wade*, the court stated that after viability the state may, if it chooses, proscribe abortion except to save the life or health of the mother.[1] In addition, tort law may provide remedies that ripen at live birth for prenatal and preconception acts that result in harm to the child, and a few states have applied wrongful death statutes to fetal injuries that result in stillbirth.[2] Most of these tort cases involve third parties: doctors may be liable for medical malpractice and automobile drivers may be held negligent if the fetus is maimed or killed. But does the mother have a duty not to harm her fetus if she decides to carry it to term or if she waives her right to an abortion before viability? And if she does harm or threaten to harm her fetus, does the state have the right to place controls on her behavior on behalf of the fetus? Alternatively, does the fetus have a cause of action against the mother if she abuses it?

HISTORICAL ATTITUDES TOWARD CHILDREN

First, let us examine the history of child abuse laws in this country to determine societal attitudes toward the protection of infants already born. We would not expect the state to protect fetuses with any more vigor than that with which children are protected. The earliest cases of child abuse were intentional acts of assault and battery that were prosecuted under the criminal law. Curiously, they did not involve parents abusing their own children. Instead, these cases revolved around a master abusing his apprentice, a teacher whipping a student, or children in almshouses who were deprived of food and were falsely imprisoned. [3]

Under the common law, the parents had almost absolute control and custody of their children, who were regarded as their property, and the state practiced a hands-off policy in family affairs. Many children were disciplined severely and physically beaten for misbehavior. In an 1840 criminal case, the mother's conviction for repeatedly beating her child was reversed, in order to preserve the family unit. [4]

Early attempts to change this attitude that children were chattels were brought about by reform campaigns conducted by people connected with the American Society for the Prevention of Cruelty to Animals. Several commentators have referred to the case of Mary Ellen, an abused child, concluding that a child is a member of the animal kingdom that deserves the protection of the law. [5]

CHILD ABUSE

In 1953, an article written by a pediatric radiologist appeared in the *American Journal of Roentgenology*, calling attention to "unrecognized trauma" in children. [6] Such a diagnosis could be made only after the development and application of X rays. A decade later, the medical community began to recognize these injuries as having been caused by the intentional infliction of injury on children by their parents. The landmark article on the battered-child syndrome appeared in the *Journal of the American Medical Association* in 1962. [7] This article quickly led to child abuse legislation, and by 1965, 47 states had passed statutes under their criminal codes. [8] These are called *reporting statutes* because it was made a criminal offense for individuals who had knowledge of child abuse for failing to report it to welfare authorities.

As I reviewed the child abuse cases, they reminded me of the development of the wrongful birth and wrongful life cases that are well known to geneticists. These cases invoke the duties of a physician to provide parents with genetic testing and counseling, but they maintain a strict laissez-faire attitude toward the parents. A defective child may have a cause of action against the physician who fails to disclose risks or a laboratory that makes errors, but there is no legal duty of the parents to act to prevent a child's suffering if the proper medical standard of care has been met. In fact, after a California appellate court suggested, *in dictum*, that the parents might be liable for knowingly and intentionally bringing a child into the world to suffer and to die, [9] the legislature quickly responded by passing a statute disallowing children's suits aginst their parents based on a claim that the child should not have been conceived or, if conceived, should not have been allowed to be born alive. [10]

To return to an examination of child abuse, we can make some generalizations that have emerged from court opinions that interpret child abuse statutes as allowing state intervention in family affairs.

The Doctrine of Parens Patriae

Under the doctrine of *parens patriae,* the state assumes a responsibility for the welfare of children that is superior to that of the parents. The state may not intervene in family relations unless there is a compelling reason to do so because of the U.S. Supreme Court's holdings that family integrity, privacy, and reproductive freedom are fundamental interests that are protected by our constitution. The right to marry, to bear and beget children, and to raise them are examples of fundamental rights.[11] These rights, however, are not absolute.

Numerous state statutes have been upheld that speak to the state's interest in protecting abused and neglected children. What tests are applied by the courts to determine when a state may intervene in family affairs to subjugate parental rights and, in some cases, to terminate custody?

The Best Interests of the Child

The most widely used standard is called *the test of the best interests of the child.* This test elevates the child's interests to paramount value, subjugating the parents' interests to secondary importance. It has been criticized because it fails to take into account significant parental interests.

Parental Fitness

Under the parental fitness test, the parents' interests are balanced against their parenting capabilities. In child abuse and child custody cases, a significant showing of facts demonstrating parental unfitness is required before family intervention by the state is allowed. It is difficult to characterize an unfit parent, but certain categories of people, such as alcoholics, drug abusers, and mental incompetents, may be declared unfit *per se* by a court.

One of the issues raised by the parental fitness test is whether past parental behavior can be introduced in evidence when adjudicating the question of temporary or permanent termination of child custody. How one views this issue depends on whether the ultimate goal is preventing child abuse or merely removing the child after abuse has already taken place. Similarly, another factor to be determined is whether there is a threat of future harm even though no harm has yet occurred. In the Chad Green case, the court stated, "On a proper showing that parental conduct threatens a child's well-being, the interests of the state and of the individual child may mandate intervention."[12]

The Least Detrimental Alternative

When the state has demonstrated a compelling interest in the protection of a child, it is then required to apply the least detrimental alternative if there is an interference with parental constitutional rights. A termination-of-custody proceeding should not even be filed until other measures have been tried and have failed. These include parental supervision, parental counseling, and an offer to find solutions that the parents will find acceptable, such as temporary custody with a relative. The least detrimental alternative, from the parents' point of view, may not meet the standard of the best interests of the child but could be viewed as a compromise. It is believed that minimal state intervention is the most desirable approach and is in harmony with the stated policy of preserving the family.

Evidentiary Requirements

Traditionally, child custody cases were decided on the basis of the preponderance of evidence submitted to the judge by the parents, the guardian *ad litem* for the child, social workers, and other expert professionals such as physicians and psychologists. This preponderance of evidence standard was followed by a judicial trend toward requiring a stricter standard, such as a test of "clear and convincing evidence." In 1975, the American Bar Association's recommendations relating to abuse and neglect urged the use of this higher standard,[13] which has now been established by the U.S. Supreme Court for the termination of child custody proceedings.[14]

Legislative Mandates

The legislature is uniquely qualified to reflect society's goals. Some individuals feel that state intervention in family affairs should be nil unless a crime has already been committed. They would hold that no preventive measures should be imposed on a family and that the child should not be protected unless the parents have already produced a harm. Others feel that the state should intervene to prevent harm. A set of guidelines for the courts, with particular attention to the standards to be used in adjudicating family matters would be particularly helpful to judges who must make difficult decisions, balancing both parents' and children's rights.

FETAL ABUSE

Now let us turn to a discussion of fetal abuse and of court interventions meant to control a pregnant woman's behavior on behalf of her fetus. The preamble to the United Nations Declaration of the Rights of the Child states, "[T]he child, by reason of his physical and mental immaturity, needs special safeguards and care, including appropriate legal protection, before as well as after birth."[15]

In a California case, a criminal charge was brought against a pregnant heroin addict, and the prosecutor wanted to take custody of the fetus by incarcerating the mother. The court denied the request, holding that the California Penal Code did not include unborn children. The mother gave birth to twins, who suffered narcotics withdrawal at birth.[16]

In a Michigan case, a newborn infant's symptoms of narcotics withdrawal triggered a charge against the mother of prenatal abuse. The court held that there was sufficient evidence to uphold the charge but refused to decide that prenatal acts by the mother were sufficient to remove the child from the mother's custody unless her postnatal conduct also demonstrated neglect.[17]

In a Maryland case, a physician petitioned the court to enjoin a pregnant woman from using drugs. She was using Valium, Quäälude, morphine, and cocaine. A previous child had been born prematurely and was addicted at birth. The court ordered the woman to attend a drug rehabilitation clinic and to submit to laboratory tests for the last two months of her pregnancy.[18]

I could find no cases on maternal alcoholism; yet, it is known that fetal alcohol syndrome may be more detrimental than fetal drug addiction because alcohol can produce birth defects and mental retardation. It may be more difficult to order prenatal surveillance of an alcoholic than of a drug addict because the former behavior is not illegal. But does this make sense? There are strong sanctions against drunken drivers because they endanger others, and an alcoholic pregnant woman is certainly endangering her fetus.

Robertson has reviewed the rights of the state to intervene during pregnancy to provide the fetus with necessary medical and surgical care.[19] The most celebrated case is *Jefferson v. Spalding Memorial Hospital*, where the state took legal custody of the fetus and ordered the mother to submit to medical treatment, including cesarean section, if necessary, against her religious objections.[20] In a Colorado case, a hospital attorney petitioned the court for an order to require a woman in labor to undergo a cesarean section because of fetal distress. The court appointed attorneys for the mother and for the fetus and, after a hearing, ordered the operation.[21]

Another example of protection of the unborn is found in the increasingly frequent practice of placing brain-deceased pregnant women on respirators and circulatory pumps in order to continue the life of the fetus.[22] Such an intervention would probably be upheld, if ordered by the state, because there would be no maternal-fetal conflict to consider.

A Massachusetts case demonstrates the court's reluctance to intervene if the fetus is not yet viable. A lower court ordered a woman to undergo an operation to protect her against miscarriage because of an incompetent cervix, but an appellate court reversed.[23]

How would the courts consider a petition by a physician to require a PKU mother to maintain a low phenylalanine diet during pregnancy? Although it is impossible to predict a judicial decision, we can look at the arguments for and against state intervention on behalf of the fetus. First, it is clear that the fetus is under a threat of harm. Does this threat deserve protection? Under the test of the best interests of the fetus, the answer would be yes. Under the unfit parent test, one could argue that the mother is biologically unfit, although she may be a very fit parent emotionally. Under the least detrimental alternative test, one could argue that placing the mother on a diet is less intrusive than mandating the sterilization or the abortion of PKU women.

What is the evidence that the requested intervention would protect the fetus from harm? The answer is equivocal. There is insufficient medical evidence that proper dietary control would produce the desired objective. Is a mandatory maternal diet the least detrimental alternative? It is certainly less intrusive to require the mother to maintain a strict diet than to mandate an abortion.

A recent California court removed two children from a mother's custody because she kept them on a strict diet consisting only of grains and vegetables and they were found to be in a malnourished state. She followed the diet herself, based on her religious beliefs. The appellate court reversed a lower court's order that she use contraceptives to prevent future pregnancies but stated that, if she became pregnant, the state would have the authority to monitor her diet and subject her to blood tests to protect her fetus.[24] Thus, it would seem that dietary restrictions in a pregnant woman are within the purview of court-ordered supervision.

If it is known that a woman has PKU before she becomes pregnant, the parents could opt for fertilization with their own gametes, either *in vivo* or *in vitro*, with subsequent implantation of the blastocyst in the uterus of a surrogate mother. Clearly, the parents have no duty to reproduce at all, much less by artificial means. But if they choose to have children, they could be offered the surrogate mother alternative to the PKU diet. It would be necessary to impose the diet prior to the viability of the fetus. However, any state intervention on behalf of the father before viability is suspect under *Roe v. Wade*.[1] Yet, I would argue that, if the mother decides to carry a fetus to term, she incurs a conditional, prospective liability toward her fetus that ripens at live birth.[25] This liability would sound in tort and raises the need to overcome intrafamilial immunity to allow the child to sue the mother for wrongful prenatal care.

INTRAFAMILIAL IMMUNITY

I do not have time to review the history of the doctrine of parent–child immunity, but suffice it to say that it is being rapidly eroded. Only three states grant complete immunity to suits between parents and children. Four states have abolished the doctrine entirely. The remainder have modified the concept or have carved out many exceptions that allow a cause of action for intrafamilial torts. All states recognize that the exercise of parental authority and the use of parental discretion in the discipline of children are necessary to promote family harmony. It is significant that seven states have followed California's lead by using a "reasonable parent" standard.[26] Under this standard, a PKU woman might be held liable to her fetus for failing to maintain a diet to protect it if other PKU women, acting reasonably, maintained strict dietary control.

CONCLUSION

There is no doubt that, as genetic technology advances, the issue of fetal abuse and improper prenatal care will be heard about more often in the courts, just as wrongful birth and wrongful life are gradually becoming accepted as actionable torts. I would argue that, rather than addressing the issue of the rights of the fetus to be born alive, we should look to the duties and obligations of those who decide that a fetus shall be born. Before viability, it is the mother who decides, and she, therefore, carries the obligations; after viability, it is the state that incurs a duty to protect the fetus if it can do so without harm to the mother. Legal redress would sound in prenatal tort or wrongful life if the harm was done before viability, and fetal abuse charges could be brought by the state after viability. I am willing to predict that such cases will be discussed at our next conference: Genetics and the Law IV.

REFERENCES

1. *Roe v. Wade*, 410 U.S. 113 (1973).
2. For a discussion of cases, *see* Hartye, F. J., Tort recovery for the unborn child, *J. Fam. L.* **15**:276 (1976–77).
3. *Children and Youth in America: A Documentary History, 1600–1865* (R. Bremmer, ed. Harvard University Press, Cambridge, Massachusetts, (1970); Thomas, M. P., Jr., Child abuse and neglect. Part I: Historical overview, legal matrix, and social perspectives, 50 *N.C.L.* Rev. 293 (1972).
4. *Johnson v. State*, 21 Tenn. 282 (1840).
5. See Thomas, *supra* note 3 at 307–310.
6. Silverman, F. N. The Roentgen manifestations of unrecognized skeletal trauma in infants, *Am. J. Roentgenology* **69**:413 (1953).
7. Kempe, C. H., Silverman, F. N., Steele, B. F., Droegemueller, W., and Silver, H. K., The battered child syndrome, *JAMA* **181**:17 (1962).
8. Note, The federal and state response to the problem of child maltreatment in America: A survey of the reporting statutes, *Nova L.J.* **2**:13 (1978).
9. *Curlender v. Bioscience Laboratories*, 106 Cal. App.3d 811, 165 Cal. Rptr. 477 (1980).
10. Cal Civ. Code §43.6 (West 1982).
11. *Meyer v. Nebraska*, 262 U.S. 390 (1923); *Pierce v. Society of Sisters*, 268 U.S. 510 (1925); *Skinner v. Okla.*, 316 U.S. 535 (1942); *Prince v. Mass.*, 321 U.S. 158 (1944); *Loving v. Va.*, 388 U.S. 1 (1967); *Eisenstadt v. Baird*, 405 U.S. 438 (1972); *Wisconsin v. Yoder*, 406 U.S. 205 (1972).
12. *In re Custody of a Minor*, 375 Mass. 733, 379 N.E.2d 1053 (1978).
13. American Bar Association, Model Child Abuse and Neglect Reporting Law (1975).
14. *Santosky v. Kramer*, 455 U.S. 745 (1982).
15. U.N. Declaration of the Rights of the Child, preamble, G.A. Res. 1386, 14 U.N. GAOR Supp. (No. 16) at 19, U.N. Doc. A14249 (1959).
16. *Reyes v. State*, 75 Cal. App.3d 214, 141 Cal. Rptr. 912 (1977).
17. *In re Baby X*, 97 Mich. App. 111, 293 N.W.2d 736 (1980).
18. *New York Times* (Apr. 27, 1983) at 11, col. 4.
19. Robertson, J. A., Procreative liberty and the control of conception, pregnancy and childbirth, *Va. L. Rev.* **69**:405 (1983).
20. *Jefferson v. Griffin Spalding County Hospital Authority*, 247 Ga. 86, 274 S.E.2d 457 (1981).
21. Bowes, W. A., Jr., and Selgestad, B., Fetal vs. maternal rights: Medical and legal perspectives, 58 Obstet–Gynecol 209 (1981).
22. Dillon, W. P., Lee, R. V., Tronolone, M. J., Buckwald, K., and Foote, R. J., Life supoort and maternal brain death during pregnancy, *JAMA* **248**:1089 (1982); Siegler, M., and Wikler, D., Brain death and live birth, *JAMA* **248**:1101 (1982).
23. *Taft v. Taft*, 338 Mass. 331, 446 N.E.2d 395 (1983).
24. *State v. Pointer*, Calif. Ct. App. 1st Dist., *Family Law R.* 10:1270 (March 20, 1984).
25. Shaw, M. W., Conditional prospective rights of the fetus, *J. Legal Med.* **5**:63 (1984).
26. *Gibson v. Gibson*, 3 Cal.3d 914, 479 P.2d 648, 92 Cal. Rptr. 288 (1971).

23

THE FETUS AS PATIENT
A Philosophical and Ethical Perspective

ROGER L. SHINN, PH.D.
Reinhold Niebuhr Professor of Social Ethics
Union Theological Seminary
3041 Broadway
New York, NY 10027

LAW, ETHICS, AND SCIENCE

Our subject relates three social forces that influence the ethos, the structure, and the behavior of society: law, ethics, and science. The three constantly interact and influence one another.

Law is the fumbling and indispensable effort to enact those ethical standards that a society regards as obligatory on all and, at least to some degree, enforceable. Not all ethics is appropriately legislated: some matters are left to personal choice and commitment, and others concern inner attitudes that cannot be written into law. But the main content of law is ethics: the regulation of human behavior that helps and hurts people. I call law the "fumbling" effort to enact ethical standards because enactment involves political conflicts and power struggles that dim or subvert ethical intent. But I call it "indispensable" because it is the barrier against chaos and disintegration or, alternatively, unrestrained tyranny.

The third force, science, operates within an ethical and legal context, but it also functions to modify inherited ethics and law. It changes the understanding and the conditions of life, making some traditional practices obsolete and opening up new possibilities that require evaluation. It appears as threat and opportunity. Nowhere is the ambivalence of society about science more obvious than in the case of the biological and medical sciences. A public welcomes new possibilities of healing yet distrusts new powers of manipulating life.

There are many opinions on the relations between science and ethics. Consider, for example, three positions that have been influential in some times and places:

317

1. Many traditional philosophies have held that the general principles and values of ethics are eternal, but that they need to be applied deductively to particular situations, including those coming out of scientific change.

2. In sharp reaction to that position, John Dewey, a generation ago, urged that the experimental methods of science be transferred "from the technical field of physical experience to the wider field of human life," that "directive standards" of human behavior were destined to come not from tradition but "very largely from the findings of the natural sciences."[1]

3. Logical positivism, by contrast, separated sharply the verifiable knowledge coming from science and the emotive, noncognitive expressions of ethical discourse.

Contemporary discussions are likely to depart from all three of these patterns. A frequent assumption is that ethical analysis must be informed by science, which often makes possible radically new choices and realization of values; but that science is not the sole basis for evaluating its own achievements. Thus, a consultation on Genetics and the Quality of Life, convened by the World Council of Churches, came to this conclusion about the relation between science and ethics:

> Ethical decisons in uncharted areas require that scientific capabilities be understood and used by persons and communities sensitive to their own deepest convictions about human nature and destiny. There is no sound ethical judgment in these matters independent of scientific knowledge, but science does not itself prescribe the good. . . . Responsible ethical decision-making will require the most accurate knowledge of new scientific possibilities, but will still have to ask which possibilities are humanly desirable.[2]

In that context of ethical inquiry, I turn to the specific issue of the fetus as patient.

MOTHER AND FETUS AS PATIENTS

The expectant mother under medical care normally expects the physician to give advice and treatment for her own health and the health of the fetus. The physician usually recommends diet, possibly medicines, and habits of behavior that will foster the health of both woman and fetus. Increasing knowledge brings changes in medical advice. For example, physicians are likely today to prescribe kinds of exercise and avoidance of exercise different from those of a generation ago. Today's pregnant woman may be more careful than yesterday's about avoidance of tobacco and alcohol. In these and other ways, the health of the fetus has always been a concern. For most pregnant women and for their doctors, the health of the fetus has been so persuasive a concern that legislation on the subject may seem utterly superfluous. In some obvious nontechnical senses, the fetus has always been regarded as a patient.

On the other hand, there have always been some possible conflicts of interest between the woman and the fetus. The health of the two is not identical. Either may survive at the sacrifice of the life of the other. Maurice Mahoney put the issue this way:

> The existential duality of two individuals living very closely together and, simultaneously, of a single fetal-maternal unit, which thrives or suffers as a unity, creates complexities for ethical analysis. . . . In Western society, despite an emphasis on concomitant health of mother and fetus, most problems seem to arise from perceived conflicting interests of two separate individuals.[3]

In this characteristically human situation, the new element is innovations in fetal diagnosis and treatment of ailments. It is now possible, and will become increasingly so, to speak of the fetus as patient in far more specific terms than in the past.

Fetal diagnosis includes methods of amniocentesis, fetoscopy, ultrasonography, and various tests on the mother that may indicate a fetal disease. Recently, chorionic villus biopsy (a technique in which trophoblastic cells are removed via the cervix rather than the abdominal wall) has made some diagnoses possible as early as the sixth week of pregnancy—much earlier than amniocoentesis, usually done in the fifteenth or sixteenth week.[4] With remarkable speed, medical science has increased the number of ailments that may be diagnosed and the reliability of the diagnosis.

Progress in the treatment of fetal ailments is spectacular. Akin to traditional methods are the administration of medicines and vitamins to the mother for the benefit of the fetus. Far newer are blood transfusions to the fetus—not directly into the fetal blood vessels but into the peritoneal cavity. Nutrients, enzymes, and medicines are being transfused into the amniotic fluid or the fetus. Fetal surgery is going on for hydrocephalus, urinary tract malformations, and other ailments. In some cases, the surgery is performed within the uterus; in others, the fetus is removed (or partially removed) from the womb, subjected to surgery, and then restored to the womb.[5] Conjectures are frequent about possible—or impossible—genetic therapy through recombinant DNA.

In these procedures, actualized or projected, a new picture emerges of the fetus as patient. No longer is fetal treatment integrally related to treatment of the mother. The fetus becomes very distinctly a patient, possibly with major inconvenience or risk to the mother. The ethical and legal issues are complex.

THE PRESUMPTION IN FAVOR OF THERAPY

The starting point is a presumption in favor of therapy. Ill health jeopardizes many human values; healing is both a good and the prerequisite to many other goods.

If I may repeat my own statement to the U.S. House of Representatives Committee on Science and Technology, "Most religious communities have a basic commitment to health and to the arts of healing. The word salvation is derived from words for health and healing."[6]

Most secular ethics agrees. The burden of proof is not on therapy but on its rejection. On the specific issue of fetal therapy, John Fletcher wrote:

> The social promise of fetal medicine, at present, far outweighs any evident social costs that could be used to halt the new field in its tracks. Creative and ethical risk taking in

fetal medicine could result in great benefits for parents, children, and societies that support the enterprise.[7]

But that is only the beginning of the debates. There is no unanimity on what constitutes health and healing. As Alexander Capron has put it, "our definitions of 'disease' and 'health' are social as much as they are medical determinations."[8] In various times and places, some people have regarded skin color or certain facial profiles or even gender as liabilities. Recent American experience has been conspicuous changes in opinion about the value of electric shock treatment and lobotomies as valid therapies.

The perplexities increase when put in a global context. Different climates, cultures, economic situations, and religious beliefs mean different norms of health and therapy. Broadly, international discussions of medical issues usually have a tone notably variant from the dominant tone of discussions in a single nation or in a few culturally similar nations. Thus, a consultation called by the World Council of Churches, eight years after the consultation already quoted above, called for "protection for third world countries" in order to "ensure that therapies or products produced fit the local, cultural, economic and social needs," and to "protect against social impacts that tend to promote dependency rather than self-reliance."[9]

Granted the seriousness of all these difficulties, some ailments are so painful, so destructive of human life and potentiality, that few would argue against corrective therapies. The burden of proof is on the case against therapy. But there are times that call for acceptance of that burden of proof. The chief issue at stake is the risk of experimental therapies.

Assessing Risks

Because there is no life without risk, it is not strange that medical care involves some risks. The risks are especially associated with experimentation. But without experimentation, there is no medical progress. So it is not strange that the era of the greatest advances in medical science should be an era especially sensitive about risks. There is increasing discussion of iatrogenic (physician-induced or treatment-induced) illnesses, of unintended effects of drugs, and of the role of government in monitoring medical treatment and drug production.

In some forms of risk evaluation, there is considerable value in a risk–benefit calculation. The average person (often without conscious awareness) assumes such a calculation with every decision to get in an automobile, eat a meal, or take a bath. In view of the great benefits that have followed from some medical experiments, it is not surprising that some people are revising the ancient medical adage, "Do no harm," so that it reads, "Be willing to do some harm for the sake of greater good." The consequence is to exercise due caution in order to minimize risk, but to take some risks in order to gain some benefits.

But such a guideline of itself says nothing about the distribution of risks. The history of experimentation shows many cases where some people are subjected to risks for the benefit of other people. Those put at risk have often been the poor, the ignorant, prisoners, deprived racial groups, and institutionalized children. Sensitivity to that issue has led to the great emphasis on "informed consent" of the patient as an ethical prerequisite to experimental treatment.

But no fetus has ever given informed consent for medical treatment. The problem is not unique to the fetus. Similar issues arise in the treatment of infants, the senile, the mentally retarded, and patients in a coma. In all such cases, somebody gives consent in behalf of the experimental subject. There is no perfect answer to the question as it was put by André Hellegers: "By what reasoning can it be justified that one individual give such consent on behalf of another?"[10] The various answers usually involve the consent of somebody who is presumed to identify with the interests of the subject. But that is not enough. Such consent must often be supplemented by ethical boards of review—and the composition of such boards, including the representation of scientists and laypeople, is a subject of endless discussion.

The case for experimental therapy is strongest when such therapy offers the chance of relief from an ailment that is both severe and, apart from therapy, sure. Most of us, offered a choice of an overwhelming and certain evil or a possible but risky good, will choose the experimental risk. And we would probably make the same choice for a fetus under our responsibility. We would be slower to volunteer for a grave risk that offered us no benefit. And we would probably feel an overwhelming moral restraint on volunteering others, who cannot give informed consent, for risks that can bring them no benefit. Hence, the moral codes governing "nonbeneficial experimentation"—that is, experimentation of no direct benefit to the subject—are far more rigorous than the codes for "beneficial experimentation."

In the case of fetal therapy, the risk starts with diagnostic procedures. By this time, there has been sufficient experience with amniocentesis to determine that the minor risks to mother and fetus are very low and that the major risks are still lower. But a zero risk is extremely hard to assure for any procedure. For example, after 20 years of ultrasound techniques, regarded as harmless, a panel of the National Institutes of Health issued a warning of "hypothetical risks" and urged that ultrasound be used only when there is an "accepted medical reason" (not mere curiosity) for doing so.[11]

Risks mount when we move from diagnosis to treatment, especially to fetal surgery. Ruddick and Wilcox summarized the situation:

> There are risks to both mother and fetus; for example risks of uterine damage or hemorrhage and of premature contractions and delivery before fetal lungs are adequately developed to sustain extrauterine life. Without further laboratory investigation with the most exacting (primate) animal models, says [Michael R.] Harrison, "We should all maintain a healthy skepticism about fetal treatment."[12]

Researchers sometimes lament the public distrust that inhibits their experiments. They may point out that their only motives are the enhancement of knowledge and healing skills. And they may ask why moralists, journalists, and politicians have any right to deliver ethical warnings to scientists. One investigator, Allan J. Hamilton, research fellow at Massachusetts General Hospital, has given the answer with candid eloquence:

> I share in a common guilt to which all of us within academic medicine must admit, an ambitious hunger for new discoveries. While we do truly labor for the common good, we also strive for personal recognition; our own egos bob embarrassingly to the surface of swelling altruism.[13]

In quoting Hamilton, I am not in any sense implying that politicians and journalists—or clergy or academics—can claim superior virtue. The point is that nobody should be the sole ethical judge of an enterprise in which he or she has a major personal stake. In medical experimentation, there is need for the judgment of some whose loyalty, both professional and personal, is to the patient and not solely to the research project, admirable though it may be.

The ethical qualifications on fetal therapy, as I have been describing them, might be called prudential. They do not raise objections to therapy as such but try to surround it with appropriate safeguards. I have not yet mentioned a more general objection that is sometimes brought against new forms of therapy: the objection to unwarranted human interventions in nature or, as is often said, to "playing God." So often is this language used, even in our predominantly secular culture, that the President's Commission for the Study of Ethical Problems in Medicine and Biomedical and Behavioral Research used the heading "Concerns about 'Playing God'" for a section of its report on human genetic engineering.[14] (Fetal therapy, as of now, does not involve genetic engineering, but similar issues may be involved.)

The concern is not solely theological. Although traditional communities of faith may feel an awed restraint about intruding in a divine creation, many other people are concerned about brash interventions in the natural order. Thus, Barry Commoner announced one of the laws of ecology, "Nature knows best," and interpreted it to mean that "any major man-made change in a natural system is likely to be *detrimental* to that system."[15] Certainly, a kind of reverence before personality—whether it be regarded as a divine creation or the results of eons of evolution, or both—is ethically appropriate. But all medical treatment is a deliberate modification of the unsuperintended processes of nature.

A task force of the National Council of Churches, addressing this issue, stated its belief that God acts both through the processes of nature and through human actions:

> God acts through human freedom as humanity increases its knowledge, overcomes such ancient scourges as smallpox and malaria, modifies the natural environment by processes of civilization, expresses its joy and grief in the arts. The Christian doctrine of stewardship recognizes a human responsibility of trusteeship for the purposeful exercise of divine gifts. Nature's way of preserving species is to be prolific, allowing for many casualties. Most Christians accept as a divine gift the possibility of producing smaller families with fewer casualties. From this viewpoint "the natural" may be less moral than the purposefully human act.

The task force went on to warn against "the approach to nature as an object of plunder" but insisted that "the effort to improve on nature is not inherently wrong."[16]

The Changing Perception of the Fetus

A final issue concerns the changing perception of the fetus as fetal therapy becomes more common. I have already said that traditional medical practice in some vague sense perceives the fetus, along with the pregnant woman, as a subject of the physician's care and concern. But there is a difference between the mother and the fetus. It is the woman who seeks medical care, who enters into a contract (explicit or implied) with the physician, and who responds deliberately to medical advice. She is a patient in a far more definite sense than the fetus. But as fetal therapy increases, the fetus becomes more like other patients.

Ethical and legal questions will arise. For example, does the fetus have legal rights in any way analogous to the rights of other patients? The issue is already complicated. Aubrey Milunsky reported,

> The fetus has been seen to have property rights and estate rights as well as recourse to the courts in various ways such as to sue for damages. However, these civil rights do not vest until birth in those jurisdictions that recognize them.[17]

We can expect the issue to get more complicated. Will a person suffering a severe disease bring a lawsuit for damages, on the ground of past lack of fetal therapy? If so, will the lawsuit be directed against a physician for malpractice? Might it be directed against a mother who refused fetal therapy that would have been dangerous to her but possibly helpful to the fetus? There is little case law concerning such issues. We can expect more to come.

A different issue centers on the decision of the mother following a prenatal diagnosis showing a severe fetal anomaly. The present choices are most often between abortion and giving birth to a handicapped child. Fetal therapy may offer a third alternative in some cases, at first rare but later perhaps more common: treatment of the fetus with the hope of later giving birth to a healthy or more nearly healthy child.

In all these developments, it is conceivable that fetal therapy may, in the words of John Fletcher, "help to create a new stage of human life, prenatality, that will become as real to our descendants as childhood has become to us."[18] Fletcher reasoned, "The more living persons actually *see* the fetus, by ultrasound or in any future method to be developed, the more human and valuable will the fetus become."[19] He predicted that the present efforts of neonatal intensive-care units to protect newborn infants will be extended to comparable efforts of fetal therapy. And he conjectured that "abortion of a fetus treatable by a proven therapy with minimal risk to the mother will likely become progressively repugnant to physicians, most parents, and to society."[20] Whether that will happen—and whether it will have legal consequence—remains to be seen.

Our contemporary world has seen many revisions of ethical perception. Some of these have involved a dulling of sensitives, as in the massive destruction of civilian populations in war. Others have brought a heightening of sensitivities to the rights of women and oppressed ethnic groups. Biomedical achievements are changing other ethical perceptions and will continue to do so. The outcome is not predictable. But it is not too early to think about and talk about the ethical issues. Technical progress has a way of overtaking communities before they are ready.

REFERENCES AND NOTES

1. Dewey J., *The Quest for Certainty*, Minton, Balch, New York. (1929), 273.
2. Birch, C., and Abrecht, P., *Genetics and the Quality of Life*, Symposium Sponsored by World Council of Churches, Zurich, Switzerland, June 25–29, 1973, Pergamon Press, Elmsford, NY (1975), 203.
3. Mahoney, M. J., Fetal-maternal relationship, in *Encyclopedia of Bioethics*, Vol. 2 (Warren T. Reich, ed.), Macmillan, New York (1978), 487.
4. Schmeck, H. M., Jr., Fetal defects discovered early by new method, *New York Times* (Oct. 18, 1983), C1, C5. Yuet Wai Han, Genetic diagnosis by DNA analysis, *Advances in Gene Technology: Human Genetic Disorders*, Proceedings of the 16th Miami Winter Symposium (Fazal Ahmad *et al.*, eds.), International Council of Scientific Unions Press, Miami (1984), 79–81.
5. Ruddick, W., and Wilcox, W., Operating on the fetus, *Hastings Cent. Rep.*, **12**(5):10 (Aug. 1982), Fletcher, J., Emerging issues in fetal therapy, in *Research Ethics*: Proceedings of a Symposium Held in Oslo, Norway, August 23–25, 1982, Vol. 128 of *Progress in Clinical and Biological Research* (Kare Berg and Kunt Erik Trangøy, eds.) Alan R. Liss, New York (1983), 295. Since the initial presentation of this paper, the successful exchange of the blood of a fetus has been reported in France. See *New York Times*, January 14, 1985, p. A13.
6. Shinn, R. L., in *Hearings before the Subcommittee on Investigations and Oversight of the Committee on Science and Technology*, U.S. House of Representatives, Ninety-Seventh Congress, Second Session, Nov. 16, 17, 18, 1982, U.S. Government Printing Office, Washington, DC (1983), 301.
7. Fletcher, *idem.* at 298.
8. Capron, A., Genetic therapy: A lawyer's response, in *The New Genetics and the Future of Man* (Michael Hamilton, ed.), Eerdman, Grand Rapids Mich. (1972), 137.
9. *Manipulating Life: Ethical Issues in Genetic Engineering*, Report of a Consultation in Vogelenzang, Netherlands, June 15–19, 1981, World Council of Churches, Geneva, Switzerland (1982), 17.
10. Hellegers, A., Fetal research, in *Encyclopedia of Bioethics*, Vol. 2, p. 491.
11. Ultrasound: Unsound?, *Newsweek* (Feb. 20, 1984), 57.
12. Ruddick and Wilcox, *idem.*, 10. Michael Harrison is a pediatric surgeon at the University of San Francisco.
13. Hamilton, A. J., My turn: Who shall live and who shall die, *Newsweek* (March 26, 1984).
14. President's Commission for the Study of Ethical Problems in Medicine and Biomedical and Behavioral Research, *Splicing Life: The Social and Ethical Issues of Genetic Engineering with Human Beings*, U.S. Government Printing Office, Washington, DC (1982), 53–60.
15. Commoner, B., *The Closing Circle: Nature, Man and Technology*, Alfred A. Knopf, New York (1972), 41.
16. *Human Life and the New Genetics*, A Report of a Task Force Commissioned by the National Council of the Churches of Christ in the U.S.A., (Roger L. Shinn, ed.), NCC, New York, p. 42.
17. Milunsky, A., Prenatal diagnosis: Clincal aspects, *Enclyclopedia of Bioethics*, Vol. 3, p. 1335.
18. Fletcher, *idem.*, 298.
19. Fletcher, *idem.*, 307.
20. Fletcher, *idem.*, 308.

DISCUSSION

DR. SHEILA B. GOTTSCHALK (LSU School of Medicine): As neonatalogists keep smaller and smaller infants alive, and as the *in vitro* fertilization people may be able to keep more and more mature fetuses alive, somewhere along the line our technologies may meet. Then we will have to reexamine the whole issue of the continuity of the individual from the moment of the diploid cell to adulthood, and we will have to reexamine the right of other individuals to interrupt those individual lives. Second, I have no background at all in ethics, but I am very disturbed by the tendency of physicians to solve the problem of perceived imperfections by taking the lives of other individuals. We have traditionally been a profession of people who care for the living and the dying, and it disturbs me that we take the lives of some individuals. Third, I don't think it's been mentioned, but even infants with lethal congenital anomalies can, in a hospice environment, get care very similar to the type of care that we give to adults who are dying. The infants that I am thinking about are those with anencephaly, trisomy-13, and trisomy-18. We can care for those babies. We can give those babies the same types of medication and comfort that we give to dying adults. One of our big failures as pediatricians, neonatalogists, and physicians is that many of these babies are left to die in some corner of the well-baby nursery. We don't want to see them. We don't want to care for them. We don't want to know if they might be having pain. Most neonatalogists will agree that, even though we don't know if babies are having pain, they certainly appear at times to be in pain. So we just ignore that whole issue. I think the dying of newborn infants is very much an ethical issue. It can be addressed in the same caring way that the dying of adults can be addressed.

DR. AUBREY MILUNSKY (Boston University School of Medicine): Let me note that neonatalogists don't usually allow children to die but, much more often than ever before, save babies from dying. Only because of the technology are there these shady areas where opportunities arise for decision making. In the past, they all died.

DR. ROGER L. SHINN (Union Theological Seminary): I appreciate the ethical sensitivity in the comment. My own opinion about the nature of ethics is that it is more a matter of sensitivities than of rules that philosophers make up. On this point, I side with Carol Gilligan in her criticism of Kolberg and others who put so much emphasis on the intellectualizing side of things. I think it's because of that kind of sensitivity that has just been expressed that the presumption should be in favor of doing what we can do to promote survival. I share with Dr. Burt a desire for a bit of temporizing just the same. I am closer to the end of life than to the neonatal phase. My own mother, before her death, left very specific instructions with us that, if the time came when medical treatment was simply extending the dying process, she didn't want it. I don't either. And if at that point somebody—not kills me—but withdraws treatment—I think that is ethically sensitive. I think we must at least entertain the possibility of comparable situations for neonates but must be very reluctant to draw up rules, because this could become horrendous. The question, as Jim Childress put it, is "What is the benefit to the fetus or the neonate?", and with a kind of fear and trembling, we try to do the best we can.

DR. MARGERY W. SHAW (University of Texas Health Science Center): I'd like Leonard Glantz to comment on the new abortion laws when we have extrauterine development available.

DR. LEONARD H. GLANTZ (Boston University School of Public Health): It will be different at that time. I think that the whole nature of what it means to be pregnant and what it means to be in existence will change. As you know very well, a great deal of the law has to do with whether or not a child is *in utero*. Right now, all our laws are based on the fact that fetuses exist only *in utero*. When that fact changes, new laws will have to develop. All the rules will change at that point. We will have to deal with a very different set of issues. Once the fetus can exist separately from the mother, the interests of the various parties change, and then new rules will be needed and will be developed.

DR. BERTHA KNOPPERS (McGill Genetic Network of Quebec): We have two reported cases in Canada involving fetal abuse in the womb. Both of them used child protection laws and child welfare laws and extended them retroactively on the basis of anticipated deprivation. First, the fetal alcohol one involved an Indian woman, and there you can see, as in your Californian case—where there are cultural or other beliefs or lifestyles surrounding the pregnant woman—what effect those social or cultural factors can have on the determination of fetal abuse. In the second, a drug-addicted woman was involved in a mandatory, provincially imposed methadone treatment for heroin addicts. In that case, it was decided that it would be more harmful for the fetus to take the mother off the methadone than to allow her to continue. My two questions are: What kind of standards are we going to develop to measure the reasonable pregnant woman's standards under tort law? Or are we going to work backward into a coercive approach, by analogy with child protection laws and keep going further and further as viability moves earlier and earlier? Because if we do that, we have problems with contempt of court of pregnant women if they don't follow medical instructions. What kind of legal sanctions are we going to impose on these women? What kind of freedom would remain for pregnant women?

DR. MARGERY W. SHAW: I hope that the same freedom would remain for pregnant women that would remain for mothers of small children. Although a mother can drink herself, she should not give alcohol in large quantities, or drugs, to her child, and the state would have a right to intervene in that situation. It will start out at least with case-by-case analysis; each case will be different, and different courts will enunciate different standards. We may get a body of law building up. We will hear over and over again the standards that have been enunciated in child abuse laws: the unfit parent or the best interests of the fetus or the child. I don't see gross intervention into pregnancy and maternal lifestyle unless there is good evidence that it is harming the fetus. Again, the evidence may have to be clear and convincing, rather than just a preponderance of evidence. There will be some abuses, I am sure. I'm glad to get the Canadian cases.

MR. DANIEL AVILA (Massachusetts Citizens for Life): I really enjoyed the information that was given earlier on the status of abortion legislation and the legality of abortion in the United States. I attended a conference of Americans United for Life, which is the legal, public-interest group of the prolife movement. It was attended by over 500 lawyers, physicians, and other people concerned with the issue of *Roe v. Wade*. That decision is at a point now where it is teetering and could be reversed in several years. How do we even think of approaching changing the law in regard to abortion? The U.S. Supreme Court has become much more concerned with the factual aspects of abortion. The facts that were presented today about the development of the unborn child and its treatment as if it were one of us constitute a very important consideration in the legislative move to chip away at *Roe v. Wade*. The strategy is much like the strategy taken to chip away at and erode the separate-but-equal doctrine. For instance, can the state legislate to protect the child from undue pain? Currently, in Massachusetts, there is a bill sponsored by Massachusetts Citizens for Life (MCFL) that would require painkillers for abortion in the last 12 weeks of pregnancy so that the fetus would not go through the trauma of abortion. This bill could put before the Supreme Court the question: Does, at some point, the unborn child feel pain, and would this requirement be an undue burden on the woman?

Second, you ask how far the right to privacy and the right to choose abortion go to prevent state protection of the unborn child? Abortions cannot be interfered with throughout pregnancy if they are done in the interests of saving the woman's life or preserving her health. How broad is the health requirement? Can sex-selective abortion be protected from state interference? Can eugenic or race-related abortions, or abortions of defective children, be forbidden under the U.S. Constitution? And can we legislate to treat the fetus as any other person in the world? I would like to end with a question: By the time the next Genetics and Law conference comes around, do you foresee a change in the present legal situation?

DR. LEONARD H. GLANTZ: Do I see a change in the legal situation concerning something in particular or abortion law generally?

MR. DANIEL AVILA: Do you think that, in the next five years, you'll find states upheld by the U.S. Supreme Court if they ban sex-selection abortions or abortions done for eugenic or genetic reasons?

DR. LEONARD H. GLANTZ: I think that predicting what the Supreme Court will do is a dangerous undertaking. I would say that if the Supreme Court remained constituted the way it is today, you would not see them saying that states can outlaw abortions almost for any reason, whether for sex selection or racial selection or whatever. I don't see this court doing that. If the court changes, that may change. Right now, there are only three Justices who would review *Roe v. Wade*, In Justice Sandara Day O'Connor's dissent, she wrote that she would be willing to take another look at *Roe v. Wade*, and Justices White and Rehnquist would be willing to go along with her. If there were two new Justices, then conceivably there could be a switch. There are powerful ideological feelings on the court. How well *Roe v. Wade* and the other abortion cases will stand up as the court personnel change, I think is uncertain. The court has been remarkably stable during this period of time.

MS. BARBARA KATZ ROTHMAN (City University of New York): We come repeatedly to issues of definition, and then we come to the question of who has the power to define. There are definitions of fact and definitions of value. As Dr. Shinn said, people should have the right to decide about refusing treatment, and it's a value difference and there's not a single right answer on that. What happens then? Who has the power to decide, when we're dealing with newborns and fetuses, if similar issues come up and it's not just the value question but the very facts of the matter? Again, I remind you of a history of medical error that it seems to me is now going to be compounded. Would it have been fetal abuse if a woman rejected standard medical care that, within the last 15 years, required extreme calorie limitations in pregnancy? If a pregnant woman gained a lot of weight, physicians assumed that she was doing terrible things to her baby. The definition of what's appropriate behavior changes, and medicine does not have "final and right" answers at any given moment. This raises some real questions as our understanding of the facts changes, and as we recognize that reasonable people disagree about values. Who, then, do you see as having the power to define both the facts and the values?

DR. MARGERY W. SHAW: It's a big question, and I'd like to hear what your response to the same question would be, too. In terms of decision making, our title was "The Mother, the Fetus, and the State," and we have a kind of triangle. The state is ephermeral, and it is made up of people, too. I wonder whether the "reasonable parents standard" would meet your criteria of changing medical values. Dr. Shinn made the point at the very beginning that science does change ethics as new options are discovered by scientists. They are factored into the equation of the options, the benefits, and the risks. It is not a static thing. The rules do have to change as we live and learn, so I can't give you any kind of an absolutist answer.

DR. CHARLES H. BARON (Boston College Law School): It has always seemed to me that the courts are an appropriate place to have these things decided, in part because they have the ability to develop principles on the facts of specific cases that come before them. It doesn't make them a perfect vehicle. You're not going to find a perfect vehicle. But you can say of the courts what Winston Churchill said of democracy: "It's the worst of all systems, except for every other system." There is the possibility as time goes on of having the courts develop these principles out of the facts, leaving a great deal of discretion to parents and so forth, which the courts are capable of doing.

MR. PATRICK WALKER (Tulane Medical School): There doesn't seem to be much debate in this room that the current laws on abortion are the correct ones. And yet, I humbly offer the suggestion that, at the next Genetics and Law conference, we contact some of the right-to-lifers and invite them to come. I think it would provide some interesting discussion for a large segment of society who feel that the laws currently in practice are not correct.

TREATMENT OR AVOIDANCE OF GENETIC DISEASE

New Capabilities, New Issues

MODERATOR: MARGERY W. SHAW

24

PRENATAL DIAGNOSIS
New Tools, New Problems

AUBREY MILUNSKY, MB.B.CH., D.SC., F.R.C.P., D.C.H.
Professor of Pediatrics, Obstetrics, Gynecology and Pathology
Director, Center for Human Genetics
Boston University School of Medicine
80 East Concord Street
Boston, MA 02118

Prenatal genetic diagnosis provides reassurance to couples at risk that they may selectively have offspring without serious mental retardation and/or chronic or serious-to-fatal disease.[1] More babies are born *because* of the availability of prenatal diagnosis compared to the number of pregnancies terminated. Prenatal diagnosis is a life-giving, not a life-taking, technology. Amniocentesis for genetic diagnosis has been documented as a very low-risk procedure for almost a decade,[2] and less than 3% of women undergoing amniocentesis for genetic risks need to face a decision to terminate a pregnancy.[1] Abortions as a consequence of prenatal diagnosis account for a minute fraction of 1% of all abortions performed.

Despite the availability of prenatal genetic studies for over 15 years, it is still unusual for more than 50% of the women at risk in any given state to actually have these tests. Antipathy toward abortion accounts for some, but certainly not for all, of those not having such studies. Physician failure to counsel, to recognize disorders as of genetic origin, or to refer elsewhere for amniocentesis probably accounts for a significant proportion of those who are yet to benefit from this technology. Evidence of physician failure abounds in the rapidly escalating number of lawsuits originating after the birth of a child with a genetic defect that could otherwise have been avoided. Shaw has reviewed some of the cases involving physician or laboratory failure followed by the birth of a child with a genetic disorder.[3] Actions in the courts are replete with examples of physician failure to provide or to refer for genetic counseling on the basis of advanced maternal age, parental ethnic group, previous family history, erroneous or missed diagnosis, and laboratory errors.[4,5]

Recognition of wrongful life suits brought by children in states such as California[6] and Washington[7] may be the forerunners of like decisions in other jurisdictions. Shaw has pointed out the courts' view that obstetricians owe a duty to the fetus as well as to the mother and that the child, when born, both *exists* and *suffers*.[3] Moreover, these courts have maintained that there should be just compensation for legal wrongs.

Pari passu with the extensive use of a now well-established technology, new tools for prenatal diagnosis have been introduced. Ultrasound has become invaluable in the prenatal detection of many congenital malformations.[8] Superb technical improvements have sharpened the diagnostic potential and made the diagnosis of small lesions feasible and the detection of cardiac defects a reality. Nevertheless, even though obstetric ultrasound has been in use for about a quarter of a century, questions and concerns have again surfaced sufficiently through a consensus development report[9] to caution against simply routine ultrasound use in all pregnancies. There is, however, no compelling *human* evidence of problems in those exposed to ultrasound *in utero*.

Fetoscopy, which facilitates both fetal visualization and blood sampling, has enabled the prenatal detection of a number of disorders not approachable through amniotic fluid studies.[10] Even today, in Massachusetts, a fetal research statute[11] has effectively precluded the use of fetoscopy, thereby forcing citizens to leave the state to seek such studies. Those opposed to abortion and responsible for such developments have also thereby effectively blocked research avenues that will assist in the treatment and salvage of fetuses whose mothers desperately seek their own healthy child.

Three new major tools for prenatal diagnosis and one procedural innovation are in the process of emerging into the public arena: (1) chorion villus biopsy; (2) maternal serum alpha-fetoprotein screening; (3) molecular genetic analysis; and (4) selective feticide.

CHORION VILLUS BIOPSY

Notwithstanding the fact that amniocentesis represented the most significant advance ever in the early detection and prevention of serious mental retardation or fatal genetic disease, it still requires that women wait until the sixteenth week of pregnancy for the procedure and again some two to four weeks for a result of the analysis. Although less than 2% of the high-risk groups of women studied will need to consider the decision to terminate a pregnancy because of a diagnosis of a fetal defect, difficulty may be encountered after fetal movements have been perceived and after maternal-fetal bonding may have been initiated.

The most recent prenatal diagnostic tool to appear on the scene is in fact not so new. Attempts to biopsy the chorion were made during the late 1960s by Hahneman and Mohr in Denmark.[12] They used an endoscope to biopsy the chorion under direct vision and were only partially successful. Because of the various complications and the small percentage of cases in which they obtained diagnostically useful information, they were unable to establish this tool as a new diagnostic modality.

In 1975, the Chinese reported their experience with chorion villus biopsy, using a procedure in which they blindly introduced a catheter through the vagina and cervix.[13] They reported a 6% complication rate and a successful sex determination in 94% of sampling efforts. In the mid-1970s, we attempted to aspirate exfoliated trophoblast cells that had pooled at the external cervical os and succeeded with cell culture and chromosome analysis in 70% of the cases we attempted.[14] The early 1980s saw a rapid development utilizing various procedures, including biopsy forceps, blind aspiration, direct vision endoscopy, and ultrasound-guided catheter aspiration of chorionic villi.[15] A successful biopsy rate of 100% has now been achieved by Rodeck and colleagues in London, using combined ultrasound guidance and direct-vision endoscopic biopsy.[15]

Although the optimal timing has not yet been determined, most biopsy procedures have been successful between seven and nine weeks of gestation. The procedures require excellent ultrasound, careful eye–hand coordination, and adherence to aseptic technique.

The scope of first-trimester chorion villus biopsy is enormous. The tissue samples obtained can be processed directly to yield analyzable chromosome spreads with results within five hours of the procedure. Although this aspect of first-trimester biopsy is still to be fully refined and established, the growth of these tissues in cell culture is well established. Cells derived from the tissue culture process are usually available within two weeks for further chromosomal analysis, sex determination, biochemical enzymatic assays (for example, for Tay–Sachs disease), or DNA analyses (such as for sickle-cell anemia and thalassemia). It appears that virtually all disorders diagnosable through amniotic-fluid cell cultures will also be detectable by means of chorionic villi.

Chorion villus biopsy effectively represents a new diagnostic tool and not unexpectedly presents new problems, some of which are unique. Determination of the safety of the biopsy procedure requires careful and appropriately controlled studies, which have been initiated in the US and UK. These efforts, I hope, will provide vital answers about the safety, accuracy, and applicability of chorion villus biopsy, but unfortunately only in about five years. Meanwhile, it is judicious to exercise every caution in view of potential hazards to both mother and fetus. Infection and hemorrhage present the most significant complications to the mother. I am aware of one case in England in which septic endometritis followed the biopsy procedure, resulting in an emergency hysterectomy. Procedure-induced fetal death or abortion is a clearly recognized risk, whether it occurs as a consequence of immediate rupture of the amniotic sac, introduction of infection, or the causation of hemorrhage. Current risk figures suggest a fetal loss rate following biopsy of about 6%. Key to the analysis of such data is the realization that there is usually a spontaneous abortion rate during the first trimester ranging between 5% and 15%. The fetal loss (death) rate is considerably higher in the first few weeks than in the nine- to eleven-week period when biopsies are done. The available data would suggest that the spontaneous or natural fetal-loss rate during that period approximates 3% to 5%.

At first glance, accuracy of chorion villus biopsy analysis should not be difficult to achieve. One reason for desisting from our original studies still exists in the problem of maternal cell admixture. How frequent a problem this will be is still to be determined. However, one other and, hopefully, low-frequency aggravation is the occurrence of chromosomally aberrant cells derived from chorion. Such cells may indeed be the problem in causing the well-known difficulties with pseudomosaicism in amniotic-fluid cell cultures.[16] Another new problem requiring resolution hinges on the balance between nature's efficacy and our "unnecessary" diagnoses. The overall perspective is that about 97% of all trisomic fetuses are aborted spontaneously. Hence, from the cytogenetic viewpoint, we are focusing on the prenatal detection of some 3% of trisomies that escape the body's natural surveillance system. As a consequence, we will inevitably be diagnosing a significant number of chromosomally aberrant fetuses that would otherwise be spontaneously aborted. This, perhaps, creates no special burden other than a possible psychological one. Women who abort spontaneously in the first trimester may well be upset, but perhaps not as worried as when an actual chromosomal abnormality is reported, which would be the case in a significant number following chorion villus diagnoses. The effective response is that we already know that, in general, some 50% of first-trimester losses have chromosomal abnormalities.[17] Delineation of the specific abnormality may well yield important risk data for future pregnancies. Hence, if the chromosomal abnormality is found to be a translocation form of Down syndrome, further studies on both parents and possibly other family members would be recommended. This information may serve to explain previous recurrent abortions by the same couple as well as to alert both the couple and the particular relatives involved about further studies and specific risks, for example, of bearing a child with translocation Down syndrome.

Prodigious opportunities exist for the first-trimester diagnosis of many different genetic disorders as long as safety and accuracy are first assured. It is expected that all chromosomal abnormalities, biochemical genetic disorders whose enzymatic deficiencies have been characterized in cell culture, and all disorders in which the gene defect has been delineated will be detectable. The widest application of chorion villus biopsy is likely to occur for *all* pregnancies and not only those of women 35 years and over. The impact of amniocentesis and prenatal gentic diagnosis in the prevention of Down syndrome is quite unimpressive. Some 75%–80% of all babies with Down syndrome are delivered by women *under* 35 years of age. This new procedure may therefore, for the first time, present a significant opportunity for the very early detection and avoidance of births of those affected by this disorder. The ethical and value issues that some find in conflict will perhaps not be any different despite the diagnoses being made at a so much earlier stage of pregnancy. Current available insights suggest that amniocentesis will still not disappear, even if chorion villus biopsy is proved to be both safe and accurate. It is very likely, but not absolutely certain, that amniocentesis will be required for amniotic fluid alpha-fetoprotein studies for the prenatal detection of neural tube defects. The uncertainty, I suggest, may reflect developments in monoclonal antibodies to alpha-fetoprotein or neuronal tissues that may be demonstrable through cell-surface studies or maternal serum analyses.

Maternal Serum Alpha-Fetoprotein Screening

Since 1973, it has been possible to detect open neural-tube defects by the alpha-fetoprotein assay.[1] Some 11 years later (that is, a few months ago), the Food and Drug Administration (FDA) licensed the radioimmunoassay kits necessary for amniotic fluid diagnoses and serum screening. An approximate period of 8 years elapsed as a direct result of pressures by antiabortion groups aiming to prevent such licensing from occurring. During this period, about 50,000 children were born with neural tube defects, and their parents across the land were denied opportunities to prevent what, for many of them, subsequently became lifetime catastrophes. This licensing debacle has been further compounded by the final procedural decisions made by the FDA as they released the kits to the public. To explain the nature of the FDA's action, a summary of a typical maternal serum alpha-fetoprotein (AFP) screening program would be helpful. Our neural-tube defect-detection program utilizing both amniotic fluid[18] and serum[19] assays is the largest in this country, over 100,000 patients having been studied.

The serum alpha-fetoprotein screening program is initiated by a blood sample's being drawn during routine pregnancy at 16–18 weeks. Following the demonstration of an elevated maternal serum AFP value, a careful ultrasound study is recommended to determine whether fetal age has been estimated correctly, if multiple pregnancy is present, if fetal death has occurred, or if some congenital malformation, such as spina bifida or anencephaly, can be detected. If the fetal age is appropriate to the dates and no other explanation for the elevated AFP value has been found, amniocentesis for amniotic fluid AFP assay is recommended.

In our experience, extending over 40,000 women undergoing serum AFP screening, we find that 1.2% initially have a raised maternal serum AFP concentration. Following ultrasound, amniocenteses are recommended for only 1 in 400 (0.3%) screened patients. One in four women undergoing amniocentesis following screening in our hands is found to have a fetus with a congenital malformation/genetic disorder.[19] Hence, from the screening of a routine pregnancy population, we can extract a small group of women with risks approximating 25% for birth defects, equivalent to the risks of couples who are known carriers of an autosomal recessive disease (such as Tay-Sachs or sickle-cell diseases).

The efficacy of this serum-screening approach is all the more remarkable when contrasted with the results from genetic amniocentesis studies done mainly because of advanced maternal age. These latter studies yield diagnoses of chromosomal and other birth defects in about 1.3% of the women studied. The serum-AFP-screening program has about an eightfold greater efficiency.

Above and beyond the unquestioned value of a maternal serum AFP screening program have been the evolution of a variety of unexpected benefits.[1] Because of the need to utilize ultrasound in women thought to have elevated serum AFP values, a reduction in perinatal mortality has been achieved through more accurate gestational dating and the consequent reduction of unnecessary inductions of labor. In addition, a wider range of congenital malformations has been detected by ultrasound in such women—defects that would not otherwise have been found early enough in pregnancy. Routine screening has also identified women in whom fetomaternal hemorrhage has occurred early in pregnancy that has later been associated with intrauterine growth retardation, a five- or sixfold increased risk of subsequent fetal death or perinatal loss, and a group of women with about double the rate of low-birth-weight infants. For those women opposed to abortion, early detection of spina bifida has allowed carefully planned delivery in a tertiary-care center in which neurosurgical attention has been available immediately for that offspring. All of these benefits have been denied during the more than 26 million pregnancies in this country these past eight years.

What many of us regard as remarkable results from such serum screening programs have clearly been due to the closely linked and coordinated programs in which interdisciplinary connections between obstetrician. ultrasonographer, laboratory and geneticist are well established. The government's attitude and its actions aimed at deregulation now threaten the efficacy of serum-screening programs and could well destroy a valuable technology.

The FDA has licensed and released radioimmunoassay kits without the kind of restrictions advocated by professional societies, such as the American College of Obstetrics and Gynecology, the Amerian Academy of Pediatrics, and the American Society of Human Genetics. These and other groups have clearly delineated the need for the development of carefully monitored, coordinated, and linked programs. Failure by the FDA to impose such requirements on both pharmaceutical manufacturers and serum-screening programs is already having the expected results. Commercial laboratories have briskly added to their assay lists and provide results without further ado. Confronted by these results, physicians remain uncertain about the meaning of the assay figures and confused about the need for any further specific action. Although the commercial laboratories may measure alpha-fetoprotein accurately, they are not able to interpret the results and make recommendations to both obstetrician and patient. Nor are they able to provide the frequently necessary genetic counseling in situations of a truly suspected elevated serum alpha-fetoprotein value. Two consequences are predicted with relative certainty. The first is that many women will be rendered extremely anxious by such results and that some will undoubtedly seek pregnancy termination of what may be a normal fetus. The second certain consequence is that pregnancy terminations of normal fetuses will occur in the absence of informed counseling by an established team, including the geneticist. In our program of over 40,000 women screened, not a single pregnancy has been terminated with a normal fetus as a consequence of the program.

No requirement has been developed for quality-assurance programs for those undertaking serum AFP screening. From extensive experience overseas and early experience here, it is clear that serious variability in laboratory assay results is a reality. In the quality-assurance program established by the New England Regional Genetics Group, a sample mixup has occurred in one laboratory, and results in at least two others have been completely out of range and would have led to unnecessary amniocenteses, at the very least.

In addition to the abortion issue, the frequency of false-positive test results leading to the abortion of normal fetuses was raised as an objection. The initial FDA-proposed rules irritated some physicians, who argued that their imposition would lead to an unwarranted intrusion into medical practice. Allowing government inspection of patient records, they argued, would violate both the physician–patient relationship and the patient's privacy. The initial required record-keeping and reporting requirements by laboratories were regarded by many such facilities as extremely burdensome. The associated increases in costs for such efforts would translate into higher laboratory fees and would have the effect of reducing utilization by the public. Given these and other objections, the FDA concluded that their original proposed restrictions were not necessary and would not ensure the safety and the effectiveness of the AFP test kits. They therefore lifted their proposed restrictions and have established requirements for manufacturers to submit quarterly reports about their experience with these kits. The FDA apparently believes that these requirements should be sufficient to monitor future product performance.

There is a serious concern about the lack of requirements or regulation for maternal serum AFP screening.[20] The lessons from the newborn-screening programs for phenylketonuria in California provide sufficient evidence of the potential trouble that can be anticipated. Screening programs for phenylketonuria were initially allowed in a vast number of laboratories, which resulted in the diagnosis's being missed by the screening program and irreversible mental retardation developed in those children. After many years, states such as California have consolidated their testing into a few specific centers. Years elapsed, however, before the problem was sufficiently well documented for correction. A situation analogous to the phenylketonuria-screening problem is likely to evolve with the serum AFP program. Most laboratory testing may unwisely be performed at commercial sites and away from the direct scrutiny of state laboratories or university-affiliated institutions. Poorly functioning laboratories may be even harder to detect than those doing phenylketonuria screening, as the AFP-screening sensitivity is only between 70% and 90% for identifying open neural-tube defects. Hence, one poorly functioning laboratory may continue for many years without recognition of its inadequate standards.

Perhaps the very least is the expectation at this time that individual state governments and health departments institute the requirements that only programs that are interlinked and coordinated with obstetrician, ultrasonographer, geneticist, and laboratory be licensed. Only in this way can there be reasonable assurance that a most vital and valuable technology will not fall into disrepute.

Molecular Genetic Analysis

About 3,400 single-gene disorders have been cataloged, and over 300 human genes have been mapped. Current estimates suggest that the recognition of 10–15 common restriction-fragment-length polymorphisms regularly distributed along each chromosome at a distance of about 20×10^6 base pairs from one another would enable the construction of a total map of the human genome. If this expectation is anywhere near accurate, it will rapidly become possible to identify the location of the genes responsible not only for single-gene disorders but possibly the genes responsible for normal human inheritable variation. With these advances expected in the next few years, three direct potential applications of molecular genetic analysis can be anticipated:

1. Detection of single-gene disorders.
2. Recognition of oncogenes.
3. Gene therapy.

Detection of Single-Gene Disorders

Applications of recombinant DNA technology in these last few years have allowed for the prenatal detection of various types of thalassemia and of sickle-cell anemia.[21] Alpha-1, anti-trypsin deficiency[22] and, in some families, phenylketonuria[26] are also now diagnosable prenatally. Expectations are that Duchenne muscular dystrophy[23]—the most common known lethal X-linked disorder in childhood—and hemophilia[24] will undoubtedly be diagnosable prenatally within a short period. Proximate location of the gene for Huntington disease has been achieved,[25] and further refinement will facilitate detection of the mutant gene within a year or two. The search for the cystic fibrosis gene has been intensively and extensively joined and is ultimately likely to be successful. About one in five Caucasians carry the gene for cystic fibrosis.

The utilization of extracted DNA from cultivated or noncultivated amniotic-fluid cells has already facilitated the prenatal detection of the hemoglobinopathies. It is therefore certain that this same approach will facilitate the prenatal detection of a vastly increasing array of recognizable monogenic disorders. The conjoined developments of DNA technology and chorion villus biopsy (if proved safe) are likely to make prenatal diagnostic opportunities availabe for an increasingly larger percentage of all pregnancies. Hence, the day of the selected fetal gene profile-test is fast approaching.

Recognition of Oncogenes

Genes that cause or trigger cancer (oncogenes) are now known.[27] Genes transmitted in an autosomal dominant way may convert cells to malignant growth. The mechanism, however, may not be straightforward and may arise through several discrete events occurring within the emerging cancer cells. At least 18 different oncogenes have now been found in retroviruses, causing different tumors through a diversity of mechanisms. Although all cellular oncogenes are expressed during normal growth and development, it remains uncertain whether they are the root cause of every cancer. We do know that there is a common set of cellular genes that may mediate, if not cause, the genesis of all tumors. The complexity of the matter is exemplified, for example, by the discovery that about 30% of individuals with hereditary retinoblastoma die as a consequence of *another* cancer within 18 years after radiation treatment for their original tumor. Hence, a gene(s) causally related to retinoblastoma may confer cancer susceptibility leading to the development of other types of human cancers in the same patient.

SELECTED ISSUES. Considerable certainty attaches to the ultimate provision of a limited "gene profile" for individuals or for the embryo or fetus in early pregnancy. A host of issues arises, only some of which can be briefly addressed here.

Is Too Much Knowledge Hazardous to Your Health? Contemplate for a moment the unexpected knowledge culled from a gene profile study of the fetus that a high degree of certainty exists for the development of a specific malignancy sometime in the future. Decisions to continue such a pregnancy may not be difficult, but no psychologist is required to predict the mind set of a couple who bear a child with the full knowledge that such a catastrophe has to be anticipated. The surveillance and necessary monitoring against a background of chronic family anxiety can hardly be construed as advantageous. Would the contrary situation, in which no knowledge of the cancer genotype is provided, be a more rational approach? The issues, however, are likely to be more complex, and decisions might be necessary, for example, to avoid occupations with disadvantageous environmental effects.

Our new tools for prenatal diagnosis are likely to yield data about specific genetic disorders much sooner than about oncongenes. The first joyful trouble is already in the wings following the proximate location of the gene for Huntington disease on chromosome 4. It is a reasonable expectation that, within the next two years, at least those initially at risk for bearing progeny destined to develop Huntington disease will be faced with dilemmas about having such tests in pregnancy and/or about deciding whether to continue or terminate such pregnancies. This development will, for the first time, herald a situation in which a prenatal diagnosis is made of a fatal disorder that will generally manifest itself three to four decades later. Other examples are sure to follow and may eventually include disorders such as diabetes mellitus or coronary heart disease, representing conditions in which chronic illness but not necessarily early death can be predicted.

Other fundamental questions arise in the dissection of these technological consequences. Is the desire for perfection and excellence in health at all unnatural or inherently bad? What is the evidence that supports any contention that the "slippery slope" argument is more than theory? Are those individuals who seek prenatal diagnosis and selective abortion more likely to care poorly for their aged parents or for other handicapped people? Is it not equally likely that such individuals will be even more caring because of their acute sensitivity to defect and disability? Those opposed to abortion might be expected to care for their own defective offspring without burdening other taxpayers. My examination of this issue suggests that the religious affiliations in institutions for the mentally retarded closely represent what we find in society at large. There is no evidence that those opposed to abortion of the seriously defective fetus permanently care for their own retarded offspring in their own homes any more often than others with different views. Indeed, congressional politics has allowed us to observe that certain senators representing views in opposition to abortion work effectively to obstruct aid to women with dependent children, and to reduce care for the poor, among whom the disabled abound.

Do People Want the Right to Know Everything about Their Genotype?   At present, we all have the right to know the laboratory results on any tests we might have. The same would apply to "gene profiles" as these tests become available. With these rights come at least two responsibilities. The first is that we will have the responsibility of deciding not to have the tests, to have the tests for specific reasons but to request that no data be released about any other unexpected findings of ominous consequence, and, finally, to be prepared to deal with results with distant but difficult implications. The second responsibility devolves on our physicians, who, without permission, would be able to communicate selectively those results that might have a bearing on risks for future offspring while withholding other data that imply, for example, a future but still untreatable disease. The line between reckless negligence by the physician and a normal standard of care will be easily distinguished in such practice as it is now. Physicians will, however, need to pay close attention to this coming dimension in medical practice. More than 15 years after amniocentesis and prenatal genetic studies became available, we see an abundance of malpractice actions against physicians who fail to discuss these opportunities for prevention, or offer or refer appropriate patients for such studies.

SELECTIVE FETICIDE

Twins have a higher frequency of congenital malformations, and since the advent of prenatal genetic diagnosis, a steadily increasing number of pregnancies have come to light where one twin with a genetic defect has been detected. When such defects have involved disorders incompatible with life, such as anencephaly, the dilemmas have been less painful than with other disorders, such as a sex chromosome abnormality. I am aware of at least nine pregnancies worldwide in which the co-twin was affected by a serious disorder (included were Down syndrome, thalassemia, Hurler syndrome, and spina bifida) and in which the affected twin was terminated in order to sustain the pregnancy and save the normal twin.[28] Some of these dilemmas have evolved against a background family history of a previously severely affected child. Faced with the recurrence of the profound mental retardation in classical Hurler syndrome, for example, most would emphathize with a couple who elected to terminate the pregnancy or, given the chance, to at least save one of the twins. There are no easy answers to the obvious moral, theological, and philosophical questions posed by these difficult cases. Respect for and support of personal reproductive freedom within reasonable law and against a background of constitutional guarantees should remain as the principles guiding the delivery of care in such pregnancies.

At present, while we are still in Orwell's 1984, I predict that prenatal diagnosis in the twenty-first century will be different. Gene profile tests will be available *by law* to all couples prior to marriage. Although no compulsion will be exerted to obtain such profiles, societal pressure will influence couples to do all that they can to avoid having children with serious mental retardation or overwhelming physical defects. All pregnant women will automatically be offered prenatal genetic studies probably in the first trimester, and such studies will test for a large number of single-gene and possibly polygenic disorders. Chromosome analysis as we know it today will disappear, having been replaced by gene-specific and gene-dosage assays. Hopefully, these and other developments will occur with the retention of personal reproductive freedom and with the maintenance of respect and care for the handicapped.

REFERENCES AND NOTES

1. Milunsky, A. (ed.), *Genetic Disorders and the Fetus: Diagnosis, Prevention and Treatment.* Plenum Press, New York, 1979.
2. The NICHD National Registry for Amniocentesis Study Group, Midtrimester amniocentesis for prenatal diagnosis: Safety and accuracy, *J. Am. Med. Assoc.* **236**:1471 (1976).
3. Shaw, M., To be or not to be? That is the question, *Am. J. Hum. Genet.* **36**:1 (1984).
4. Milunsky, A., and Annas, G. J. (eds.), *Genetics and the Law I,* Plenum Press, New York (1976).
5. Milunsky, A., and Annas, G. J. (eds.), *Genetics and the Law II,* Plenum Press, New York (1980).
6. *Turpin v. Sortini,* 643 P.2d 954 (Cal., 1982).
7. *Harbeson v. Parke-Davis,* 656 P.2d 483 (Wash., 1983).
8. Campbell, S., Diagnosis of fetal abnormalities by ultrasound, in *Genetic Disorders and the Fetus: Diagnosis, Prevention and Treatment* (A. Milunsky, ed.), Plenum Press, New York (1979).
9. National Institutes of Health Consensus Development Conference, consensus statement, Diagnostic ultrasound in pregnancy, U.S. Government Printing Office, Washington, DC (1984).
10. Mahoney, M. J., and Hobbins, J. C., Fetoscopy and fetal blood sampling, in *Genetic Disorders and the Fetus: Diagnosis, Prevention and Treatment* (A. Milunsky, ed.), Plenum Press, New York (1979).
11. Mass General Laws chap 112, 12J.
12. Hahnemann, N., and Mohr, J., Antenatal fetal diagnosis in genetic disease, *Bull. Eur. Soc, Hum. Genet.* **3**:47 (1969).
13. Tietung Hospital Department of Obstetrics and Gynecology, Fetal sex prediction by sex chromatin of chorionic villi cells during early pregnancy, *Chinese Med. J.* **1**:117 (1975).
14. Rhine, S. A., and Milunsky, A., Utilization of trophoblast for early prenatal diagnosis, in *Genetic Disorders and the Fetus: Diagnosis, Prevention and Treatment* (A. Milunsky, ed.), Plenum Press, New York (1979).
15. Rodeck, C. H., and Morsman, J. M., First-trimester chorion biopsy, *Br. Med. Bull.* **39**(4):338 (1983).
16. Hsu, L. Y. F., and Perlis, T. E., United States survey on chromosome mosaicism and pseudomosaicism in prenatal diagnosis *Prenatal Diagnosis* **4**:97 (1984).
17. Boué, J., Boué, A., and Lazar, P., Retrospective and prospective epidemiological studies of 1500 karyotyped spontaneous human abortion, *Teratology* **12**:11 (1975).
18. Milunsky, A., Prenatal detection of neural tube defects. VI. Experience with 20,000 pregnancies, *JAMA* **244**:2731 (1980).
19. Milunsky, A., and Alpert, E., Results and benefits of maternal serum alpha-fetoprotein screening, *JAMA* **252**:1438 (1984).
20. Haddow, J. E., and Milunsky, A., Deregulation of screening for alpha-fetoprotein in pregnancy. *N. Eng. J. Med.* **310**:1669 (1984).
21. Little, P. F. R., DNA analysis and the antenatal diagnosis of hemoglobinopathies, in *Genetic Engineering I* (R. Williamson, ed.), Academic Press, London (1981).
22. Woo, S. L. C., Kidd, V. J., Pam, Z. K., *et al.* (eds.), *Banbury Conference on Recombinant DNA Applications to Human Disease,* Cold Spring Harbor Laboratory, Cold Spring Harbor, New York, 105 (1983).
23. Murray, J. M., Davies, K. E., Harper, P. S., *et al.,* Linkage relationship of a cloned DNA sequence on the short arm of the X chromosome to Duchenne muscular dystrophy, *Nature* **300**:69 (1982).
24. Choo, K. H., Gould, K. G., Rees, D. J. G., *et al.,* Molecular cloning of the gene for human antihaemophilia factor IX, *Nature* **299**:178 (1982).
25. Gusella, J. F., Wexler, N. S., Conneally, P. M., *et al.,* A polymorphic DNA marker genetically linked to Huntington's disease, *Nature* **306**:234 (1983).

26. Woo, S. L. C., Lidsky, A. S., Guttler, F., *et al.*, Cloned human phenylalanine hydroxylase gene allows prenatal diagnosis and carrier detection of classical phenylketonuria, *Nature* 306:5939:151 (1983).
27. Honey, N. K., and Shows, T. B., The tumor phenotype and the human gene map, *Cancer Genet. Cytogenet.* 10(3):287 (1983).
28. Rodeck, C. H., Mibashan, R. S., Abramowicz, J., and Campbell, S., Selective feticide of the affected twin by fetoscopic air embolism, *Prenatal Diagnosis* 2:189 (1982).

25

Perspectives on Fetal Surgery

On the Road from Experimentation to Therapy (and What to Do When We Arrive)

George J. Annas, J.D., M.P.H.
Edward Utley Professor of Health Law
Boston University Schools of Medicine and Public Health
80 East Concord Street
Boston, MA 02118

Sherman Elias
Director, Clinical Genetics Services
Prentice Women's Hospital and Maternity Center
Chicago, IL 60611
Associate Professor of Obstetrics and Gynecology
Northwestern University Medical School
Chicago, IL 60611

In 1982, we wrote: "Experimentation with fetal surgery has come of age, and its routine clinical application seems inevitable."[1] We still believe this statement, but the road from experimentation to therapy will be longer than most observers had originally predicted. The results to date have been disappointing, and although research continues, there is no longer a general expectation of immediate therapeutic application of these new surgical techniques. Nonetheless, the stakes remain high and the implications of successful fetal surgery for medicine, society, the pregnant woman, and the fetus are profound. In this chapter we review the current medical indications for fetal surgery, as well as the major ethical and legal issues that the use of this technology raises now and in the future.

MEDICAL ASPECTS

Ascertainment of Abnormal Fetuses

Only a small fraction of potential candidates for antenatal surgery are currently identified. Sometimes, a family history of a heritable condition will lead the obstetrician to monitor a fetus to determine if it is similarly affected. Some cases will be ascertained because of clinical suspicion (for example, oligohydramnios, which may be associated with urinary tract obstruction). And most important, with the current trend toward the liberal use of antenatal ultrasonographic monitoring for a variety of obstetric indications, the majority of cases in which fetuses are ascertained as candidates for antenatal surgery are likely to be diagnosed serendipitously.

Prerequisites for Fetal Surgery

In July 1982, a conference was hosted by the Kroc Foundation entitled "Unborn: Management of the fetus with a correctable congenital defect."[2] Perinatal obstetricians, surgeons, ultrasonographers, pediatricians, bioethicists, and physiologists intensively reviewed experimental and clinical experience with fetal surgical treatment to assess the potential benefits and liabilities of various interventions, the directions to be pursued, and the problems to be avoided.

Prior to considering a fetus for *in utero* surgery, a number of prerequisites must be met. First, the extent of the fetal malformation must be delineated, and a careful evaluation must be made for possible coexisting abnormalities through detailed ultrasonographic studies (so-called Level II ultrasound scanning) by an experienced ultrasonographer knowledgable in fetal anatomy and the natural history of fetal disease. Ancillary procedures should include amniocentesis for chromosomal analysis, determination of alpha-fetaprotein levels, and viral cultures; amniography or fetoscopy might also be considered. Second, the abnormality should be compatible with a reasonable expectation for a healthy infant as a result of the procedure. For example, surgery to repair a urinary tract obstruction would, in general, be contraindicated in a trisomy-18 fetus. Third, surgical intervention is indicated only when the fetus would be better off because of the performance of surgery before delivery, rather than after birth. In certain situations, the gestational age of the fetus will dictate whether or not preterm delivery followed by neonatal surgery offers an overall safer approach than *in utero* surgery. The primary rationale is that the fetal condition will progressively deteriorate to a point of irrevocable injury unless surgical intervention is undertaken. Lastly, the fetus should be a singleton, because of the risk to the other fetus. Fetal surgery requires a multidisciplinary team that includes an experienced obstetrician, ultrasonographer, pediatric surgeon, geneticist, and neonatologist, who will be required to manage the infant after delivery. Preferably, additional members would include a bioethicist, psychiatrist or psychologist, and social worker. Infants should be delivered at a tertiary medical center with a high-risk obstetrical unit and intensive-care nursery. Fetal surgery should also be performed only with the prior approval of an institutional review board and with informed consent.[3]

STATE OF THE ART

Erythroblastosis Fetalis

Surgical treatment of fetal disease is not in itself new. In 1963, Liley reported the first successful intrauterine transfusion for severe erythroblastosis fetalis.[4] This procedure involved the percutaneous insertion of a needle into the fetal peritoneal cavity under either roentgenographic or ultrasound guidance, followed by injection of group Rh-negative erythrocytes. Subsequently, intrauterine transfusion has become an integral part of modern obstetric therapy.[5]

Hydrocephalus

Current methods of ultrasonography permit the antenatal detection of at least some cases of fetal hydrocephalus during the second trimester; however, sensitivity and specificity have not be established. After 22 weeks' gestation, the outer border of the lateral ventricle should be extented no farther than half the distance of the midline to the skull wall.[6,7] In fetal hydrocephalus, the lateral ventricles become abnormally dilated prior to any changes in the biparietal diameter of the fetal skull. In addition, ultrasonographic studies of fetuses with hydrocephalus will detect association intracranial anomalies in 37% of cases and extracranial anomalies in 63% of cases.[8] Thus, a complete ultrasonographic evaluation of fetal anatomy is mandatory prior to any intrauterine surgical intervention.

The most widely used *in utero* treatment of fetal hydrocephalus has been the placement of a ventriculoamniotic shunt under ultrasound guidance. Clewell and associates first reported the placement of such a silicone rubber shunt with a one-way valve in a 24-week fetus with hydrocephalus caused by X-linked aqueductal stenosis.[9] The function of the shunt was confirmed by an increased cortical mantle thickness, a decreased ventricular-to-hemisphere ratio, and a normal biparietal diameter at 32 weeks' gestation. Shortly thereafter, this same group performed two other antenatal ventriculoamniotic-shunt procedures. Although initial evaluations suggested that all three infants benefited from this method of treatment, follow-up studies of at least one of these infants at 10.5 months of age showed considerable neurologic handicap (developmental quotient greater than 30), as well as physical abnormalities (e.g., flexion contractures and cutaneous syndactyly of the digits).[10] Other investigators have reported follow-up evaluation of infants with more encouraging results after ventriculoamniotic shunt placement.[11] In general, however, the outcomes following such shunt procedures have been disappointing. It is now clear that considerable screening is required to distinguish those fetuses that may benefit from such procedures (i.e., those with true obstructive hydrocephalus without associated malformations) from fetuses with nonobstructive ventriculomegaly associated with intrinsic brain malformations or extrinsic severe anomalies. In a retrospective review of 24 fetuses with ventriculomegaly at the University of California, San Francisco, it was shown that in the majority of the fetuses detected as having congenital hydrocephalus, prenatal intervention would not have improved the outcome.[12]

Urinary Tract Obstruction

Fetal urinary-tract obstruction may be ultrasonographically characterized by oligohydramnios, a massively enlarged bladder, and hydronephrotic kidneys.[13] Unrelieved complete urinary-tract obstruction as a result of posterior urethral valves or strictures leads to (1) hydronephrosis; (2) cystic dysplasia of the kidneys; (3) oligohydramnios with secondary facial deformities (hypertelorism, malformed low-set ears, depressed nasal tip, and micrognathia), flexion contractures in the extremeties, and pulmonary hypoplasis; and (4) abdominal-wall-muscle deficiency or "prune belly." In theory, drainage of urine from the bladder into the amniotic cavity prior to the time of irreversible damage may allow normal kidney development, restore normal amniotic-fluid dynamics, and thus prevent oligohydramnios and its sequelae.

Harris and co-workers reported a case of an 18-year-old primigravid patient who underwent ultrasonographic evaluation at 20 weeks' gestation because of an inappropriately small uterus.[14] There was oligohydramnios, and it was determined that the male fetus had bilateral hydronephrosis, dilated redundant ureters, and a large thick-walled bladder with a dilated bladder neck. The renal parenchyma did not appear to be cystic. Because of the fetal position and the oligohydramnios, the placement of a catheter shunt from the bladder to the amniotic cavity was deemed impossible. Therefore, it was believed that bilateral ureterostomies offered the only hope of saving the fetus. At 21 weeks' gestation, the lower part of the fetal body was lifted through a hysterotomy incision; the dilated ureters were exposed through bilateral flank incisions, opened in the midportion, and marsupialized to the skin. The fetus was then replaced and the incision closed. At 35 weeks' gestation, a 2,300-gm infant was delivered by cesarean section. The infant had mild facial deformities, limb contractures, a small chest, a slightly protuberant abdomen, and bilateral undescended testes. After 9 hours at maximum supportive measures, the infant was permitted to die. At autopsy, the lungs were found to be hypoplastic, and the kidneys showed Potter-type IV cystic dysplasia.

In a second case, Golbus and colleagues reported a 41-year-old woman who, by ultrasonography prior to genetic amniocentesis at 17 weeks' gestation, was found to have twins, one of which was a male with marked ascites.[15] At 23 weeks' gestation, this twin showed a marked increase in ascites, associated with a slight dilation of the left renal pelvis and ureter. At 30 weeks' gestation, the abnormal twin was found to have a significant decrease in ascites and to have oligohydramnios. An attempt to percutaneously place an indwelling catheter into the fetal bladder under the ultrasonographic guidance was unsuccessful. At 32 weeks' gestation, a polyethylene catheter was placed in the fetal bladder under ultrasonographic guidance so that the curled end was in the bladder and the other end drained into the amniotic cavity. At 34 weeks' gestation, the infants were spontaneously delivered vaginally. The affected infant had the features of the "prune-belly" syndrome. At 1 day of age, the infant underwent bilateral high-loop cutaneous ureterostomies, correction of an associate intestinal malrotation, and excision of a portion of the redundant abdominal wall. Renal biopsies showed mild dysplasia.

The largest experience in the management of fetuses with congenital hydronephrosis is that at the University of California, San Francisco.[12,16] Among their first 26 fetuses, 8 had unilateral hydronephrosis and were followed without intervention; all infants did well following postdelivery surgery. Three fetuses had bilateral hydronephrosis, which resolved spontaneously prior to delivery. Eight fetuses with bilateral hydronephroses were shown to have poor renal function: three were not treated and died after birth with dysplastic kidneys and pulmonary hypoplasis; three women elected to terminate their pregnancies based on diagnostic studies showing irreversible disease; in two cases, a drainage procedure was successfully performed, but the infants subsequently died of irreversible renal damage. Seven fetuses had bilateral hydronephrosis and "equivocal" function. Four were delivered prematurely and subsequently underwent surgical correction; three did well and one had renal failure. In three cases, shunts were percutaneously placed in the bladder and drained into the amniotic fluid; one infant died with multiple congenital anomalies, one developed severe renal failure, and one infant did well. These investigators have concluded that

> prenatal decompression should be reserved for the singleton fetus with bilateral hydro-
> nephrosis which has evidence of compromised renal function (oligohydramnios or
> documented diminution of amniotic fluid of serial sonograms) and is too immature to
> be delivered for postnatal decompression.[12]

Thus, from the very limited experience with surgery for fetal urinary-tract obstruction, as well as the natural history of such anomalies, it appears that the chances of fetal salvage are optimized by decompression of the bladder and the restoration of amniotic fluid dynamics as early in gestation as possible. However, the success rate measured by survival and ultimate prognosis remains to be established. Several additional approaches to the *in utero* surgical repair of fetal defects have been proposed.

FUTURE DIRECTIONS

Diaphragmatic Hernia

Many infants with congenital diaphragmatic hernia cannot survive because of pulmonary hypoplasia caused by a compression of the herniated viscera into the thoracic cavity. With the use of a fetal lamb model in which diaphragmatic hernias were created at at about 100 days' gestation, Harrison and associates[12,17] have developed a successful *in utero* surgical technique that involves reduction of the viscera from the thoracic cavity into the peritoneal cavity, repair of the diaphragmatic defect, and enlargement of the abdominal cavity by abdominoplasty by means of an oval silicone rubber patch sutured to the fascial edges followed by closure of the skin over this patch. They have concluded that the correction of congenital diaphragmatic hernia *in utero* appears physiologically sound and technically feasible. However, these investigators stress that the *in utero* surgical repair of human fetuses with diaphragmatic hernias should not be attempted prior to achieving a high degree of success in laboratory animal models.[12]

Spina Bifida

Using fetal rhesus monkeys induced to develop neural tube defects by the administration of synthetic corticosteroids and thalidomide between Day 18 and 28 or embryogenesis, Hodgen[18] has developed a technique in which an agar-based medium, containing crushed bone particles, is used as a "bone paste" for sculpturing antenatal enclosures to overlay and "correct" herniated nerve bundles. Although such patching techniques may seal the spina bifida lesion, the effects on neurological development and function are yet to be established.

Gastroschisis

The morbidity and mortality rate in neonates with gastroschisis has been significantly reduced since the mid-1960s by improved surgical techniques; however, serious complications are not infrequent and include respiratory distress, matted viscera, and peel formation. It is conceivable that early *in utero* repair of gastroschisis may ultimately prove to be the method of therapeutic choice. Fetal gastroschisis models have been created in rabbits and lambs, which would allow such investigation to be undertaken.[19,20]

Allogenic Bone Transplants

Michejda and co-workers have successfully performed intrauterine allogenic bone transplantations in the rhesus monkey at 120–135 days of gestation with the use of either fetus-to-fetus bone transplants or particles of crushed bone mixed with an agar-enriched culture medium.[9] They concluded that the immune surveillance system of fetal rhesus monkeys may be tolerant of such bone allografts, even when performed as late as the second trimester. Moreover, such transplants used in ablative long-bone surgery permit normal growth and development as compared with the contralateral unoperated extremity. Of particular interest was the fact that the "bone paste" had strong adhesive properties and could be sculptured into the desired conformation without forfeiting ultimate long-bone strength. Accordingly, these investigators suggest that this technique may offer potential in the human fetus for surgical repair of skeletal anomalies *in utero*.[21,22]

LEGAL AND ETHICAL ISSUES

Human Experimentation

Fetal research is one of the most controversial and complex areas in the entire field of human experimentation regulation. The National Commission for the Protection of Human Subjects of Biomedical and Behavioral Research, for example, spent the first year of its existence (1974–1975) working on fetal experimentation under a congressional mandate to make recommendations regarding fetal research before working on any other topic. This mandate itself was most influenced by the 1973 decision of the U.S. Supreme Court, which provided that the government could not interfere with the decision of a woman and her physician regarding abortion prior to fetal viability.[23] This decision invalidated criminal laws against abortion and increased the number of fetuses aborted and, therefore, the amount of fetal material available for research.

As adopted by the U.S. Department of Health and Human Services, federal regulations currently require that, prior to experimentation involving human fetuses, appropriate animal studies be done, and that researchers have no role in any decision to terminate a pregnancy. The purpose of any *in utero* experimentation must be to meet the health needs of the particular fetus and the fetus placed at risk only to the minimum extent necessary to meet such needs." In the case of nontherapeutic research, the risk to the fetus must be "minimal" and the knowledge to be gained "important" and not obtainable by other means. The consent of both the mother and the father is required, unless the father's identity is not known, he is not reasonably available, or the pregnancy resulted from rape.

In addition, the research protocol must be reviewed by an institutional review board (IRB), which, in addition to its normal duties, must take special care to review the subject selection process and the method by which informed consent is obtained. The consent process itself should probably be audited by a representative of the IRB as well. It has also been recommended by some that a special advocate for the fetus be appointed to help caution the parents against consenting to an experimental procedure on their fetus that they may not understand, or that they incorrectly may see as therapeutic. It appears, however, that, by the time parents reach the major medical centers involved in this research, they have already made up their minds to go ahead with what they consider the last hope that their fetus may have. Thus, the advocate notion may be too little too late if its purpose is seen as beneficially influencing the consent process.[24]

These federal human-experimentation regulations technically apply only to those researchers who receive federal funds or are affiliated with institutions that have signed an agreement with the Department of Health and Human Services that all research in their institutions and by their faculty and staff will be reviewed by their IRB. Nonetheless, these regulations are so fundamental to the protection of the integrity of the fetus, the potential parents, and the research enterprise itself, that they should be followed voluntarily in all institutions doing fetal research. In those cases in which surgeons are doing only one procedure, and it is contended that treatment is the primary goal, the IRB might consider expediting the review, but IRB protocol review should always be utilized.

State Statutes

The states that have legislated in this area have used a much more rigid and punitive approach; fetal research in many states is a criminal activity. Half the states now have statutes on fetal research; most of these (15) were passed soon after the U.S. Supreme Court's abortion decision and in direct response to it.[23] In fact, more state legislation has been enacted regarding fetal research than regarding any other type of research, and this legislative activity, together with its poor quality, indicates the emotional nature of this issue. Most state statutes prohibit or restrict both *in utero* and *ex utero* research, and the restrictions are generally more stringent than the federal regulations (only New Mexico's statute models itself on the federal regulations). In Massachusetts, for example, it is a crime to study the fetus *in utero* unless the study does not "substantially jeopardize" the life or health of the fetus and the fetus is not the subject of a planned abortion. Thus, therapeutic research, such as that on hydrocephalus, is permissible even in this restrictive state. Utah, the only state to deal exclusively with *in utero* fetuses, prohibits all research on "live unborn children." Eight states (Arkansas, California, Indiana, Kentucky, Montana, Nebraska, Ohio, and Wyoming) limit their prohibitions to the living abortus and so do not apply to fetal surgery at all. California, where much of the research to date has been done, restricts experimentation only on *ex utero* fetuses, outlawing "any type of scientific or laboratory research or any other kind of experimentation or study, except to protect or preserve the life and health of the fetus."

State regulation is a hodgepodge of restrictions and prohibitions, with little consistency over jurisdictions and no clear rationale. Nevertheless, researchers are bound by the law of the state in which they perform fetal experimentation, and knowledge of its provisions is obviously necessary in states that have such statutes. [23,25]

Therapeutic Interventions

The line between therapy and experimentation has never been a completely-clear one; some argue for delineation of a transitional state called *pretherapeutic* or *investigational*, and others contend that the distinction is usually intellectually pointless. [26] Therapy involves procedures done primarily for the benefit of the patient that are considered "good and accepted medical practice," whereas experimentation involves new or innovative procedures (not yet considered standard practice) for the primary purpose of testing a hypothesis or of gaining new knowledge. [27] The courts have not always been consistent in applying these criteria and have even rejected, for example, the argument that the first artificial heart implant was done for other than therapeutic purposes. [28] Nevertheless, it seems fair and accurate to conclude that all of the procedures described in this chapter must currently be considered experimental and subject to the rules already summarized. Specifically, IRB review, detailed consent, and a consent auditor are all morally and legally appropriate. An advocate for the fetus may also be appropriate in especially problematic cases.

Someday, however, it is likely that at least some types of fetal surgery will become accepted medical practice, and thus, the basic legal and ethical rules relating to therapy will apply. The most important issues will then be informed consent, resource allocation, and potential maternal-fetal conflicts.

Consent

It is a fundamental premise of Anglo-American law that no one can touch or treat a competent adult without the adult's informed consent. This doctrine is based primarily on the value we place on autonomy or self-determination and, secondarily, on rational decision making. The first requires that individuals have the ultimate say concerning whether or not their bodies will be "invaded"; the latter requires disclosure of certain material information (a description of the proposed procedure, risks of death and serious disability, alternatives, success rates, and problems of recuperation) before one is asked to consent to an "invasion."[29]

All of this is relatively straightforward when one is dealing with an adult, but how does it apply when the therapy is aimed at the fetus? In the experimental setting, federal regulations call for the consent of the mother and the father prior to any permissible experimentation. In the therapeutic setting, the consent of either one of the parents is generally sufficient consent for beneficial procedures on children. In the case of the fetus, however, if the proposed procedure will place the mother at any risk of death or serious disability, only she would have the right to consent (and the corresponding right to withhold consent). Even in the third trimester, the U.S. Constitution gives the woman and her physician the right to abort the fetus if the mother's life or health is endangered.[23] In an analogous case, the U.S. Supreme Court ruled that where conflict existed over the issue of an abortion between a potential father and mother, the mother's position should prevail because she has more at stake (that is, her own body and health) than the father.[30] The same logic applies here. The consent of the mother must be a necessary precondition for such surgery. Of course, her consent must be informed, and she should be told as clearly as possible about the proposed procedure and its risk to herself and her fetus, as well as about the alternatives, the success rates, and the likely problems of recuperation.

Resource Allocation

John Fletcher has raised resource allocation as one of the major ethical issues concerning fetal therapy.[31] Currently, the issue concerns how much funding the federal government and others should allocate to research in this area. This is fundamentally a political question, but it has ethical overtones. Is it acceptable, for example, to continue to place our most heavy emphasis on the extension of life for the elderly, rather than on providing fetuses and neonates with the best chance to live a healthy life? In an area in which early treatment can lead to the prevention of disease and misery and, perhaps, can reduce significantly the cost of a lifetime of care, both research and treatment warrant a high priority. When fetal surgery becomes accepted medical practice, issues of screening, selection, and indications will have to be addressed by insurance companies and other third-party payers. A liberal policy of reimbursement seems sensible.

MATERNAL-FETAL CONFLICTS

The emergence of fetal surgery brings the maternal-fetal conflict issue into sharp focus. This issue is, of course, at the heart of the continuing abortion debate, where the rights of the pregnant woman now take legal precedence. Putting the rights of the pregnant women first seems reasonable, but what if the woman "waives" her right to abortion, doesn't she then take on a new duty to the fetus that she has decided will become a child, a duty to ensure that it will be born as healthy as she can reasonably make it?[32] This is a complex issue, but we believe that no pregnant woman should ever be legally forced to undergo medical procedures that threaten her life or serious bodily harm for the sake of the life or health of her fetus. Much more difficult questions are raised when the intervention poses no physical threat to the woman (such as taking a vitamin pill), but she still objects to it on religious or personal grounds. Although this issue is not likely to arise very often, as most women will do almost anything to ensure the health of their fetuses, it is an issue of great symbolic importance because it determines what value and how much respect we accord to the autonomy of pregnant women. It has also been the most controversial issue touching fetal surgery. We, therefore, believe that it warrants careful review.

In 1979, four Israeli obstetricians suggested that when women in labor refuse surgical intervention recommended to save the life of their fetuses,

> It is probably that the patient hopes to be freed in this way of an undesired pregnancy . . . because it is an unplanned pregnancy, the woman is divorced or widowed, the pregnancy is an extramarital one, there are inheritance problems, etc.[33]

The view that women who refuse cesarean sections are in some way wilfully abusing their fetuses seems prevalent and deeply held, at least by some male obstetricians and judges. It is reflected in a number of cases in which judges have ordered women who were refusing surgical interventions during labor to undergo them.

Almost all of the cases decided to date are lower court decisions and so are of dubious precedential value. In the only state supreme court case (Georgia), this issue was decided under emergency conditions and the court misconstrued the law. Nonetheless, these cases represent the only judicial pronouncements on this subject to date and therefore must be addressed.

The Georgia Case

Jessie Mae Jefferson was due to deliver her child in about four days when the hospital in which she would be attended sought a court order authorizing it to perform a cesarean section and any necessary blood transfusions should she enter the hospital and refuse.[34] She had previously notified the hospital that it was her religious belief that the Lord had healed her body and that whatever happened to the child was the Lord's will. At an emergency hearing conducted at the hospital, her examining physician testified that she had complete placenta previa with a 99% certainty that her child would not survive vaginal delivery and a 50% chance that she herself would not survive it. On this basis, the court decided that the "unborn child" merited legal protection and authorized the administration of "all medical procedures deemed necessary by the attending physician to preserve the life of the defendant's unborn child."

The next day, a public agency petitioned for temporary custody in the same court, alleging that the unborn child was "a deprived child without proper parental care" and seeking an order requiring the mother to submit to a cesarean section. The odds that the unborn child would die if a vaginal birth was attempted were put at 99%–100% by the physician. The court granted the petition, on the basis that the

State has an interest in the life of this unborn, living human being [and] the intrusion involved . . . is outweighed by the duty of the state to protect a living, unborn human being from meeting his or her death before being given the opportunity to live.

The parents immediately petitioned the Georgia Supreme Court to stay the order; and on the evening of the same day as the hearing, the court denied their motion, with a two-sentence conclusory opinion, citing *Roe v. Wade*, *Raleigh Fitkin*, and *Strunk v. Strunk* as authority. A few days later, Mrs. Jefferson uneventfully delivered a healthy baby without surgical intervention.

Lower court decisions that were not appealed have been decided in courts in Colorado, Michigan, New York, and Illinois, and perhaps elsewhere as well. In the Illinois case, surgery was ordered and apparently thereafter consented to.[35] In the Michigan case, which involved a woman who refused a cesarean section on the basis of religious objections, surgery was also ordered, but the woman fled the jurisdiction and reportedly had a normal vaginal delivery without complication to herself or her child.[36] In the New York case, Judge Margaret Taylor refused to order a cesarean section on the basis of a prolapsed cord after talking with the pregnant woman, a 35-year-old black woman who had borne 10 children. The patient was competent and objected both on religious grounds and on the grounds that she had the right to control her own body. An hour after the judge's decision, the woman delivered a healthy baby without surgical intervention.[37] The best-documented lower court case is the Colorado one.

The Colorado Case

The pregnant woman in the Colorado case was unmarried, and had previously given birth to twins. She was described as obese, angry, and uncooperative. An internal fetal heart monitor suggested fetal hypoxia, and a cesarean section was recommended. Because of the patient's fear of surgery, she refused. Her mother, her sister, and the father of her child attempted unsuccessfully to change her mind. A psychiatric consultant concluded that she was neither delusional nor mentally incompetent.

The hospital administration was notified, and a decision was made to request court intervention. The hospital staff petitioned the juvenile court to find the unborn baby a dependent and a neglected child and to order a cesarean section to safeguard its life. An emergency hearing was convened in the patient's room, following which the court granted the petition and ordered the surgery. The cesarean section was performed, resulting in a healthy child and no complications for the mother. Because more than nine hours had elapsed between the external fetal heart-monitor tracings that indicated distress (and six hours from internal tracings) and the delivery, the physician was surprised that the outcome was not poor. He indicated that the case "simply underscores the limitations of continuous fetal heart monitoring as a means of predicting neonatal outcome."[38]

Three questions arise from a review of these cases: What is the state of the law? What should the role of the judiciary be in such disputes? And what position should physicians and hospitals take when confronted with a woman who refuses a cesarean section against medical advice?

The State of the Law

The cases all lack an analysis of the precedents and place heavy and primary reliance on *Raleigh Fitkin*[39] and *Roe v. Wade*.[23] The courts should at least have considered the severe limitations of these two cases. *Raleigh Fitkin* involved a woman who was approximately eight months pregnant. Physicians believed that, at some time before giving birth, she would hemorrhage severely and that both she and her unborn child would die if she did not submit to blood transfusions, which she refused because she was a Jehovah's Witness. The trial court upheld her refusal, and the hospital appealed to the New Jersey Supreme Court. In the meantime, the woman had left the hospital, against medical advice, and the case was moot. Nevertheless, the court proceeded to determine that the unborn child was "entitled to the law's protection" and that blood transfusions could be administered to the woman "if necessary to save her life or the life of her child, as the physician in charge at the time may determine."[39]

This opinion is of limited value. First, no one was forced to do anything as a result of the opinion; that is, no transfusion was actually performed, and no police were dispatched to apprehend the woman and return her to the hospital. Second, it was a one-page opinion, with little policy discussion. Third, the extent of bodily invasion involved in a blood transfusion is much less than that involved in a cesarean section, which is major abdominal surgery. And fourth, the case was decided eight years before the U.S. Supreme Court decision in *Roe v. Wade* and more than a decade before the same New Jersey court decided the case of Karen Ann Quinlan. One question posed (and not yet resolved), for example, is: Would the parents of Karen Ann Quinlan have been permitted to remove her from the respirator if she had been pregnant?

The second case, *Roe v. Wade*,[23] does stand for the proposition that the state has a compelling interest in preserving the life of viable fetuses. But it does not have such an interest if "the life or health of the mother" is endangered by carrying the child to term. The question that needs to be discussed is the relevance of the additional danger (physical or mental) to the mother of undergoing a cesarean section where its purpose is to protect the health of the fetus. In the Colorado case, for example, it was noted that excessively obese patients are "generally considered at increased risk of anesthetic and surgical complications."[38] When do such increased risk factors outweigh the child's right to be born via cesarean section? And what would happen if, despite a court order, the patient refused to submit to the cesarean section? The physician in the Colorado case cautioned that "had the patient steadfastly refused it might not have been either safe or possible to administer anesthesia to a struggling, resistant woman who weighed in excess of 157.5kg."[38] Surely, nothing in *Roe v. Wade*[23] gives either judges or physicians the right to favor the life or health of the fetus over that of the pregnant woman. No mother has ever been legally required to undergo surgery or general anesthesia (e.g., bone marrow aspiration or kidney transplant) to save the life of her dying child. It would be ironic if she could be forced to submit to more invasive surgical procedures for the sake of her fetus than for her child. For all these reasons, it is premature to label the conclusions of these quickly decided cases, which lack any meaningful analysis, "the law."

Judges in the Hospital

Judges are not terribly good at making emergency decisions. Perhaps the most famous example is the opinion of Judge Skelly Wright in the *Georgetown College* case.[40] The case involved an emergency petition to permit blood transfusions to a Jehovah's Witness to save her life. A lower court judge refused to issue such an order, but Judge Wright did, less than an hour-and-a-half after he was approached by counsel for the hospital. He went to the hospital and interviewed the woman and her husband. The woman, a 25-year-old with a 7-month-old child, was "not in a mental condition to make a decision." Her husband refused but said if the judge ordered it, it would not be his responsibility. Because the judge believed that the woman's reasoning would be similar, he ordered the transfusion.

The full bench of the U.S. Circuit Court of Appeals for the District of Columbia refused to review the case, but some of its members dissented from this refusal and noted their concerns. Judge Miller, for example, noted that Judge Wright was

> impelled, I am sure, by humanitarian impulses doubtless was, himself, under considerable strain. . . . In the interval of about an hour and twenty minutes between the appearance of the attorney at his chambers and the signing of the order at the hospital, the judge had no opportunity for research as to the substantive legal problems and procedural questions involved. He should not have been asked to act in these circumstances.[40]

Judge Warren Burger, now Chief Justice of the U.S. Supreme Court, quoted Justice Benjamin Cardozo on judicial restraint:

> The judge, even when he is free, is still not wholly free. He is not to innovate at pleasure. He is not a knight-errant, roaming at will in pursuit of his own ideal of beauty or of goodness. He is to draw his inspiration from consecrated principles. He is not to yield to spasmodic sentiment, to vague and unregulated benevolence.[40]

It is inappropriate for judges to act impulsively, without benefit of reflection on past precedent and the likely future impact of their opinions. The cesarean section cases discussed in this chapter suffer from a lack of reflection. Obviously, the delivery room is not conducive to such reflection, and judges probably do not belong there at all in such "emergency" circumstances.

What Should the Law Be?

The law can take one of two paths, neither completely satisfactory. The first is to follow the lead of most of the cases and require the woman to submit to a cesarean section when her physician deems it necessary to protect her fetus. The problems with this approach are illustrated by these cases. First, physician prediction of fetal harm may not be accurate. Indeed, in most of these cases, serious errors were made. In Georgia, a 99% certainty turned out to be wrong; the supposed 1% reality occurred. In New York and Michigan, intervention also turned out to be unnecessary. And in Colorado, the fetal heart monitor significantly overstated the amount of damage to the fetus from delayed delivery. So, permitting physicians to judge when fetuses are in danger may simply be giving them a license to perform cesarean sections or fetal surgery whenever they want to, without regard to the pregnant woman's desires.[41]

But suppose 100% accuracy. We should still permit pregnant women to refuse surgery, to protect their liberty as well as that of all competent adults. Practical considerations also support the woman over the fetus. Women may take matters into their own hands and not deliver in hospitals. Other interventions that they might consent to will be unavailable at home, and an opportunity to try to change their minds will be lost. The question of what to do with a woman who continues to refuse in the face of a court order remains. Do we really want to restrain, forcibly medicate, and operate on a competent, refusing adult? Such a procedure may be "legal," especially when viewed from the judicial perspective that the woman is irrational, hysterical, or evil-minded; but it is certainly brutish and not what one generally associates with medical care. It also encourages an adversarial relationship between the obstetrician and the patient, and it gives the obstetrician a weapon to bully into submission any pregnant women whom she or he views as irrational. Attempts at vaginal deliveries after one birth by cesarean section, for example, could fall victim to such a rule.

Could the case for forced cesarean sections be distinguished from fetal surgery when it becomes accepted medical procedure, or would pregnant women be forced to undergo fetal surgery as well? And if one can lawfully force surgery, one should certainly be able to restrain the liberty of a woman for the sake of her fetus, for example, by confining her during all or part of her pregnancy should she have an alcohol or drug problem that could adversely affect her fetus. It seems wrong to say that patients have the right to be wrong in all cases except pregnancy. In that case, why should only doctors have the right to be wrong?

The "waiver" argument that we opened this section with is not persuasive.[32] First, women never really do waive their right to an abortion; they retain it up to the moment of childbirth (although it should be termed *induction of premature labor* at some point) if their life or health is endangered by continuing the pregnancy. Second, this argument takes a right designed as a shield to protect pregnant women and turns it into a sword to be used against them by individuals who "know better." Finally, the argument ignores the fact that the woman and the fetus are biologically inextricable. As Ruth Hubbard noted: "To argue 'rights' of the fetus versus those of the mother ignores the organic unity and substitutes a false dichotomy [and] a false metaphor."[42]

Nor does the argument to provide children the right to sue their mothers for not properly taking care of them during pregnancy make policy sense. We may all agree that mothers should take care of themselves and their fetuses, but it is unlikely that the prospect of a damaged child suing its mother at some later date will be either an effective deterrent or a useful means of compensating the child. Indeed, it is more likely that this punitive approach will simply make it appear that we are doing something for fetuses when, in fact, we are not. Few children will ever find anyone to sue their mothers on their behalf, and even if they do, any funds gained would very likely be those that would be used for the child's benefit in any case.[43] More effective would be positive programs of education, the funding of maternal and child health programs, and medical research to help prevent the diseases that fetal surgery is designed to treat. Extending notions of child abuse to "fetal abuse" brings the state into pregnancy without any likelihood of benefit and great potential for invasions of privacy and massive deprivations of liberty. Treating women as incubators while they are pregnant represses them and deprives them of their human dignity and autonomy, and so dehumanizes us all.

The second alternative is to honor the unusual case of a woman's refusal. We assume that this is general practice at the vast majority of hospitals in the country regarding cesarean sections, and we believe that it should apply to fetal surgery as well; moreover, we believe that it is the proper practice ethically and legally. This view may seem callous to the rights of fetuses, as some fetuses that might be salvaged may die or may be born defective. This is tragic, but it is likely to be rare. It is the price that society pays for protecting the rights of all competent adults, and for preventing forcible physical violations of pregnant women by coercive obstetricians and judges. The choice between fetal health and maternal liberty is laced with moral and ethical dilemmas. The force of law will not make them go away.

We reach this conclusion primarily because fetal surgery entails serious risks to the mother and requires her body be "invaded" to reach and manipulate the fetus. If these considerations were not present (for example, if the fetus could be treated with a drug that the mother could take orally and that would not affect her own health), a much more difficult balancing test would be presented. In this latter case, we think that the woman would be morally wrong not to take the drug (assuming it was virtually 100% effective and had no adverse fetal or maternal effects). Nonetheless, we do not favor permitting police to forcibly administer such a drug under court order unless the woman has been determined to be mentally incompetent.[29] Education seems the more positive and beneficial route in the long run.

Conclusion

Fetal surgery is potentially a very positive development in medicine—one that enhances the status of the fetus and gives mother and child a better chance for a healthy life together. Done with informed consent and respect for the pregnant woman, it can reinforce our values of autonomy and respect for persons. Done forcibly, however, it threatens to return us to the day when pregnant women were considered incubators—a means to an end only, rather than ends in themselves. Preserving the requirement of maternal consent preserves the woman's dignity, and ultimately the dignity of us all.

References and Notes

1. Portions of this article are adapted from Elias, S. and Annas, G. J., Perspectives on fetal surgery, Am. J. Obstet. Gynecol. 145:807 (1983); and Annas, G. J., Forced Ceasarian sections: The most unkindest cut of all, Hastings Cent. Rep. 12:16–17 (June 1982).

2. Harrison, M. R., Golbus, M. S., Berkowitz, R. S., *et al.*, Occasional Notes, fetal treatment 1982, *N. Engl. J Med.* **307**:1651–2 (1982).
3. Council Report. In utero fetal surgery. Resolution 73 (I-81); Council on Scientific Affairs, *JAMA* **250**: 1443–4 (1983). See discussion, *infra*, notes 23–30 and accompanying text.
4. Liley, A. W., Intrauterine transfusions of fetus in haemolytic disease, *Br. Med. J.* **2**:1107 (1963).
5. Queenan, J. T., *Modern Management of the Rh Problem* (2nd ed.), Harper & Row, Hagerstown, MD (1977).
6. Campbell, S., Early prenatal diagnosis of neural tube defects by ultrasound, *Clin. Obstet. Gynecol.* **20**:351 (1977).
7. Denkhaus, H., and Winsberg, F., Ultrasound measurement of the fetal ventricular system, *Radiology* **131**:781 (1979).
8. Chervenak, F. A., Berdowitz, R. L., Romero, R., *et al.* The diagnosis of fetal hydrocephalus, *Am. J. Obstet. Gynecol.* **147**:703 (1983).
9. Clewell, W. H., Johnson, M. L., Meier, P. R., *et al.* Placement of ventriculoamniotic shunt for hydrocephalus in a fetus, *N. Eng. J. Med.* **305**:944 (1981).
10. Hecht, F., and Frix, Fr., A., Treatment of fetal hydrocephalus (letter), *N. Eng. J. Med.* **307**:1211 (1982).
11. Depp, R., Sabbagha, R. E., Brown, J. T., *et al.* Fetal surgery for hydrocephalus: Successful in utero ventriculoamniotic shunt for Dandy-Walker syndrome, *Obstit. Bynecil.* **61**:710 (1983).
12. Harrison, M. R., Bolbus, M. S., and Filly, R. A., *The Unborn Patient: Prenatal Diagnosis and Treatment*, Grune and Stratton, Orlando (1984).
13. Hobbins, H. C., Grannum, P. A. T., Berkowitz, R. L., *et al.*, Ultrasound in the diagnosis of congenital anomalies, *Am. J. Obstet. Gynecol.* **134**:331 (1979).
14. Harrison, M. R., Golbus, M. S., Filly, R. A., *et al.* Fetal surgery for congenital hydronephrosis, *N. Engl. J. Med.* **306**:591 (1982).
15. Golbus, M. S., Harrison, M. R., Filly, R. A., *et al.* In utero treatment of urinary tract obstruction, *Am. J. Obstet. Gynecol.* **142**:383 (1982).
16. Harrison, M. R., Golbus, M. S., Filly, R. A., *et al.* Management of the fetus with congenital hydronephrosis, *J. Pediatric Surg.* **17**:728 (1982).
17. Harrison, M. R., Ross, N. A., and de Lorimier, A. A., Correction of congenital diaphragmatic hernia in utero. III. Development of a successful surgical technique using abdominoplasty to avoid compromise of umbilical blood flow, *J. Pediatr. Surg.* **16**:934 (1981).
18. Hodgen, G. K., Antenatal diagnosis and treatment of fetal skeletal malformations with emphasis on in utero surgery for neural tube defects and limb bud regeneration, *JAMA* **246**:1079 (1981).
19. Haller, Fr., J. A., Kehrer, B. H., Shaker, I. J., *et al.* Studies of the pathophysiology of gastroschisis in fetal sheep, *J. Pediatr. Surg.* **9**:627 (1974).
20. Oshio, A. T., and Komi, N., An experimental study of gastroschisis using fetal surgery, *J. Pediatr. Surg.* **15**:252 (1980).
21. Michejda, M., Bacher, J., Kuwabara, T., and Hodge, G., In utero allogeneic bone transplantation in primates: Roentgenographic and histologic observations, *Transplantation* **32**:96 (1981).
22. Hodgen, G. D., Antenatal diagnosis and treatment of fetal skeletal malformations with emphasis on in utero surgery for neural tube defects and limb bud regeneration, *JAMA* **246**:1079 (1981).
23. *Roe v. Wade*, 410 U.S. 113 (1973). See Baron, C., Legislative regulation of fetal experimentation: On negotiating compromise in situations of ethical pluralism (this volume, pp. 435–437).
24. See, e.g., Jonsen, A., Fetal surgery (this volume, pp. 367–368).
25. Annas, G. J., Glantz, L. H., and Katz, B. F., *Informed Consent to Human Experimentation: The Subject's Dilemma*, Ballinger, Cambridge, MA (1977); Friedman, J. M., The federal fetal experimentation regulations: An establishment clause analysis, *Minn. Law Rev.* **61**:961 (1977); Brock, E. A., Fetal research: What price progress? *Detroit Coll. Law Rev.* **3**:403 (1979).
26. See, e.g., Fox, R., and Swazey, J., *The Courage to Fail*, U. Chicago Press, Chicago (1974).
27. Annas, G. J., Glantz, L. H., and Katz, B. F., *The Rights of Doctors, Nurses, and Allied Health Professionals*, Ballinger, Cambridge, MA (1981); Annas, G. J., Informed consent, *Ann. Rev. Med.* **29**:9 (1978).
28. *Karp v. Cooley*, 349 F. Supp. 827 (S.D. Tex. 1972), aff'd, 493 F.2d 408 (5th Cir. 1974), discussed in *Informed Consent, supra* note 25 at 11–7.

29. Annas, G. J., and Densberger, J. E., Competence to refuse medical treatment: Autonomy vs. paternalism, *Toledo L. Rev.* **15**:561 (1984).

30. *Danforth v. Planned Parenthood,* 428 U.S. 52 (1976).

31. Fletcher, J. C., The fetus as patient: Ethical issues, *JAMA* **246**:772 (1981).

32. See, e.g., Robertson, J., Procreative liberty, and the control of conception, pregnancy, and childbirth, *Virginia Law Rev.* **69**:405, 441–7 (1983); and Shaw, M., Conditional prospective rights of the fetus, *J. of Legal Medicine* **5**:63, 87–8 (1984).

33. Leiberman *et al.,* The fetal right to live, *Obstet. Gynec.* **53**:515 (1979).

34. *Jefferson v. Griffen Spalding Co. Hospital Authority,* 247 Ga. 86, 274 S.E. 2d 457 (1981). And see Note on this case, *W. New Eng. L. Rev.* **5**:125 (1982).

35. *American Medical News* (Feb. 19, 1982) at 11.

36. Goldman, E. B., Fetal versus maternal rights: Who is the patient? *Mich. Hospitals* (Apr. 1983), 23–25, in which the lawyer for the hospital in this case discusses it as a hypothetical.

37. Gallager, J., The fetus and the law—Whose life is it anyway? *MS.* (Sept. 1984), **62**:134–5.

38. Bowes, W. A., and Salgestad, B., Fetal v. maternal rights: Medical and legal perspectives, *Am. J. Obstet. Gynecol.* **58**:209 (1981).

39. *Raleigh Fitkin-Paul Morgan Memorial Hospital v. Anderson,* 201 A.2d 537, 538 (N.J. 1964).

40. *Application of the President and Directors of Georgetown College,* 331 F. 2d 1000 (1964).

41. It has also been noted that surgery will, of course, not always be successful and may lead to salvaging a fetus with a "dismal" prospect for whom the parents will be responsible. Ruddick, W., and Wilcox, W., Operating on the fetus, *Hastings Cent. Rep.* (Oct. 1982), at 10–14.

42. Hubbard, R., Legal and policy implications of recent advances in prenatal diagnosis and fetal therapy, *Women's Rights Law Reporter* **7**:201, 216 (1982).

43. Such suits may, however, make sense if confined to cases in which the mother has given the child up for adoption or has relinquished her parental rights.

26

THE ETHICS OF FETAL SURGERY

ALBERT R. JONSEN, PH.D.
Professor of Ethics in Medicine
Departments of Medicine and Pediatrics
University of California, San Francisco
1326 Third Avenue
San Francisco, CA 94143

Many thoughtful things have been said in this conference about the fetus as patient. I shall take them as prolegomena to my remarks, which are directed at the surgical treatment of the fetus *in utero* or *extra uterum*. At the present time, intervention for three serious threats to fetal life and well-being are considered feasible. The first is surgical relief of obstructive hydrocephalus secondary to stenosis of the aquaduct of Sylvius. In this procedure, a shunt is introduced into the ventricles of the brain of the fetus via a needle inserted into the uterus through the maternal abdomen, and cerebrospinal fluid is drawn into the amniotic fluid. The second procedure is correction of the blocked fetal urinary tract. This is done either by placing a catheter through the maternal abdomen into the fetal bladder or by removing the fetus partially from the uterus, decompressing the bladder, and creating a physical channel from the kidneys or the bladder into the amniotic fluid. This second procedure, which involves externalization of the fetus, has been done, to my knowledge, only twice. I was involved in both cases and was present at the second surgery. The third surgical treatment considered feasible is correction of congenital diaphragmatic hernia. This procedure has not yet been done.

The experience with these procedures is now being carefully collected and analyzed. In 1982, within a year of the first clinical efforts, an international conference was held to share experience, and a second conference followed in 1983. The status of these procedures is reported in Harrison, Golbus, and Filly.[1] John Fletcher and I authored the chapter on ethical issues in this volume.[2] The substance of that chapter is the basis of my remarks here, but the style is very different. In substance, we discussed the following points: whether fetal surgery is an innovative procedure or research; the problem of risks and benefits; and the problem of informed consent. These are the immediate issues. We also speculated on the long-term issues, such as the possibility of significant changes in the perceived moral and legal relationship between mother and fetus, the economic and eugenic implications, and the social consequences of prenatal therapeutic endeavors. The style of our essay is as straightforward as we could make it. We discussed the problems soberly and confined our speculation to the most likely scenarios for future problems. My style in this chapter is different. I shall abandon the straightforward and sober style in favor of the figurative. I shall employ simile and metaphor, allegory and parable, and, perhaps, even some hyperbole. I allow myself this departure from philosophical sobriety in order to convey to you vividly the impressions imprinted on me by my close association with our program in fetal surgery. It is my opinion that the ethical dimensions of this activity are, at this point, better conveyed by imagination than by rationality.

THE ADVENTURE OF FETAL SURGERY

Fletcher and I discussed at length the question of whether fetal surgery is an innovative procedure or research.[2] We try to define both alternatives and to draw the implication of each. Today, I want to confess that this rational distinction may not capture the reality of fetal surgery. It is better captured by the metaphor of adventure. In our scientific era, we disdain adventure. It is haphazard; it is clumsy; it is "uncautious." Adventures do not employ double blinds and randomnization. Yet, old-fashioned adventures can be described in ways that approximate what is actually going on in fetal surgery. Adventures have great and noble goals; they move through dark and mysterious places; the slightest misstep can mean disaster. After much effort, pain, and agony, the great and noble goal may be found to be an illusion. Disappointment darkens initial enthusiasm. Coadventurers are lost, and even then, something is learned and a chastened realism subdues the next venture.

This is what fetal surgery is like. Not many adventures have set off: less than 100 at last count. Out of these, some wonderful achievements, and many failures, have come. As in many adventures, the obstacle to success at first seems easy to vanquish. In fetal surgery, the physical barrier between fetal life and death, health or disease, is a simple mechanical obstruction. It can be cut or bypassed, and the threatening dam of cerebrospinal fluid or urine will flow. But, in fact, the simple barrier and the easy maneuvers that could overcome it are not simply a matter of inserting a needle and putting in a shunt or opening the uterus and cutting a ureter. The structure of the uterus, the life of the fetus, and the particular nature of its anomaly, even though open to view by ultrasonography and even though approached by the most skilled hands, present formidable dangers. (Could it be coincidence that the two medical centers where most of this work has been done are Denver and San Francisco, on either side of the Rockies: a barrier that a generation of adventurers believed they could vanquish easily?)

Not only is the surgery more difficult than might be theoretically thought, but also the vague map of the territory and the suitable time to set out pose great problems. It is not yet clear how the progress of the fetal malformations interacts with other organ development; not yet clear at what point in the pregnancy intervention is most appropriate; and not yet clear whether, in certain cases, a good outcome would result even without the intervention. Much more needs to be learned about the natural history of these malformations, much more about the diagnostic indications for interventions, and much more about the sequelae; and most of this can be learned only *in vivo* (*in utero*, we should say). The animal of choice is the human at this stage.

Some things have been learned, but the new information poses alternatives of daunting difficulty. For example, three years of placing catheters in brain and bladder have taught the surgeons that catheters are unreliable. They slip and clog even when designed with great care. The alternative, at least for the urinary tract malformations, is externalization of the fetus and marsupialization of the ureters. Percutaneus catheterization is clearly the less invasive procedure, creating much less risk of instigating premature labor, but it is much less efficacious. Hysterotomy and externalization of the fetus are much more risky but probably will be the most effective procedure, thus posing an experimental and therapeutic paradox. Fetal surgery is an adventure: risky, frightening, and exciting. Is it worthwhile? This is a question that adventurers seldom ask; they climb because "it's there." However, the pioneers in fetal surgery are not adventurers of this sort. They are carefully evaluating the effects of their work. Fletcher and Jonsen discussed at length the problem of risks and benefits.[2] Yet, behind that rational calculation burns something of the great and noble goal of adventure: the hope that, at its end, a live and well child will be born, a child who might have died *in utero* or, more likely, would have been born with severe problems pointing to an early death or lifetime deficits. The live, healthy, and wanted child is, in the eyes of most, worth the dangers. Adventure is literally, etymologically, *adventura*, "toward what is to come."

INFORMED FAITH

One is lead to a second figurative reflection about the ethics of fetal surgery. Fletcher and Jonsen wrote about the problem of informed consent,[2] as it is the parents, or the mother, who decide whether the goal, a live and healthy baby, makes the dangers and the adventure worthwhile. Our fetal treatment team are dedicated and ingenious about informed consent. They almost try to talk the parents out of surgery. We have had many of them decide against it, but the reality of consent is not captured by the sober rationality of "informed consent."

It has been my experience that, in this field of medicine, it is not informed consent, so much as informed faith, that directs parental choice. The New Testament has a definition of faith that catches the reality of this experience: the Epistle to the Hebrews describes faith as the "substance of things hoped for, the evidence of things unseen."[3] That thing hoped for, that thing unseen yet evident, is the baby in the womb who is to come into the world. It is not just a fetus viewed by ultrasound, but a baby dwelling within, beginning to move and communicate. The mothers who come to our program are not "carrying a fetus;" they are going to have a baby—a baby they desire to have and desire to be healthy. They come with a faith generated by that life in them. They believe, though they are not yet sure, that our services can help that baby. These parents have, in a profound sense, decided in faith before the "informed-consent process" begins. If they come as far as our program, they have come as pilgrims. Intense teaching efforts elicit simple responses: "We must do it for our baby;""We have prayed about it and know it's right. Even if it fails we've tried everything;" "It will turn out all right." They hear and understand our words about the uncertainties and the risks; but this is information given to the converted. It surrounds their faith but does not create it and does not change it, "just as the elucidations of theology broaden the faith of the religious believer, but do not initiate it." Some come without faith, and these leave. Most come with faith and, if they must leave, because surgery is contraindicated, leave with regret.

How does this faith—and my description is not hyperbole—force us to think about informed consent? Is this faith to be thought of as coercion? Are we ethically required to turn away the believers and only to accept the skeptics? Are we to mount a strong effort to undermine faith? Is there a way to dissipate the almost religious fervor of these parents and to convert them into rational calculators or, as the ethicists say, impartial observers?

I have tried to describe the ethics of fetal surgery, not with the cool eye of the philosopher, but with the poetry of a participant. Fetal surgery is, in fact, a serious scientific enterprise, a cautious therapeutic endeavor. It has weighty consequences for the fetus, for the parents, and for the providers of care. It has important implications for society. But beneath all this, it is an adventure in faith. Unfashionable as adventures and faith are these days in the world of scientific technology, that is how I have experienced this activity.

I am usually skeptical of this poetic approach: it turns ethical issues into ecstatic exclamations, in which rhetoric obscures the possibility of rationality. But in this case, I have permitted myself the liberty of poetry rather than philosophy because I believe that we can be misled by the rational conceptualization of problems of this sort. Only if we appreciate the profoundly emotional or symbolic roots of the issues of reproductive ethics can we begin to speak in rational categories of research and informed consent and to approach them with cautious reason and critical analysis. I am not denigrating such analysis; rather, I suggest that it can proceed on course only when we are vivdly aware of the prerational power that infuses our dealings with the fetus, in each one of whom lies, potentially, the future of our race.

REFERENCES

1. Harrison, M. R., Golbus, M. S., and Filly, R. A. (eds.), *The unborn patient*. Orlando, Florida, Grune & Stratton (1984).
2. Fletcher, J. C., and Jonsen, A. R., Ethical considerations, in M. R. Harrison, M. S. Golbus, and R. A. Filly (eds.), *The unborn patient*. Orlando, Florida, Grune & Stratton (1984).
3. Hebrews 11: 1.

Discussion

DR. MARGERY W. SHAW (University of Texas Health Science Center): As Dr. Todres told us yesterday, it helps to see the neonatal intensive-care unit before we discuss the decisions, and Dr. Jonsen's presentation shows us that it helps to be in the operating room watching the surgeons to really understand these issues that we are talking about on, as he says, a rational plane.

DR. FRANK CHERVENAK (Mount Sinai Hospital, New York City): I found Dr. Annas's comments most interesting. I don't necessarily disagree with the conclusion, but I would say, as a clinician, that certain points have to be emphasized that were not emphasized in the presentation. Let me begin by saying that there are times when coercion is indicated in intrapartum management decisions. I base this assertion on two ethical principles: With our current level of expertise in 1984, there are times when it can be predicted, with good probability, that the baby will die or suffer severe asphyxic brain damage under certain conditions, such as a scalp pH less than 7.20 or certain fetal-heart-rate tracings. There are other obstetrical times when there is an extremely high probability, almost a certainty, that the baby will either die or suffer severe asphyxic damage. This occurs when there is severe bradycardia that happens suddenly and inexplicably. In these situations, there are strong beneficent obligations to the fetus, and to the child it will become, to deliver the baby immediately and to avoid the often high probability of asphyxic brain damage or death. Now, the conflict, and what Dr. Annas has emphasized so strongly, is that this often presents a conflict with respect to maternal autonomy, that is, in those situations where the mother would refuse the cesarean section. The point that I would emphasize most strongly (not emphasized in Dr. Annas's presentation) is not to accept at face value a maternal refusal of cesarean section. A mother who has been cared for either by me or by one of my colleagues throughout her pregnancy has an implied understanding that the focus of obstetrical care will be the best for both her and her unborn child. For her at the last minute to make a decision not to do the cesarean section suggests that something isn't right. There is a need to explore with the woman exactly what is going on. Unfortunately, she may be paralyzed, either by fear, or by the anxiety or tension of the moment, in the same

369

way that a person would come to the emergency room with acute appendicitis and the surgeon would feel the high probability that immediate surgery is necessary.

I agree with Dr. Annas that perhaps the law is not the right way to go. In fact, from my experience in the labor and delivery room setting, I feel that the legal route is not an effective route. For those things with the highest probability of poor outcome for the fetus, there isn't time to go to court. There are times, however, for other forms of coercion. I would get the family involved immediately. I would get the father involved and say, "Look, there's a high probability that this baby is going to suffer. Immediate action is necessary." The tone that I would use to address the mother would not be the same tone that I would use in a more calm and relaxed setting, where I could explain all the advantages and disadvantages of the proposed intervention. So, in short, although I think that the points made are excellent, that legal intervention would not have any value, I think we need to explore the impingements of a truly autonomous decision, including the realization that the mother may be very regretful of a decision that was made on the basis of fear, anxiety, or pain. Respect for both autonomy and beneficence obligations to the fetus can sometimes best be served by using mild coercive measures, short of law.

MR. GEORGE J. ANNAS (Boston University Schools of Medicine and Public Health): I would like to respond, but probably not as vehemently as you might think. I don't think we have very much disagreement. The major point is that I want to keep judges and police officers out of the delivery room. I don't like the word *coercion*, but I have no problem with physicians' using persuasion. Physicians have a tremendous advantage. The pregnant woman in the middle of labor is at a significant disadvantage. A major point is that, if in that situation you cannot persuade her to change her mind, you should not be permitted to force her with the support of the state's police powers to change her mind. The only question you have is how far you can go to persuade her. That's a really difficult problem. You talked about caring for this woman during pregnancy and your implied agreement. I'd like to know about those implied agreements. In a number of the "forced-cesarean-section" cases, the women had religious objections to cesareans, and they had told the physicians about these objections well in advance. In those situations, I think you have to go with the woman. If you can't do that, you've got to refer the patient to another obstetrician, not when they're in active labor, but well before that. I think we want to preserve the situation where women and doctors can make agreements with each other. We don't want a situation where the law has proscribed and the police powers will dictate what the outcome is always going to be. I don't think we really have tremendous disagreement. If obstetricians stopped trying to do what they thought was best for women and trying to convince them of that they believed was the proper course, I think that would be very bizarre. I don't expect you to just stand back and say, "Well, whatever you want; if that's what you want, well, that's the end of it."

DR. FRANK CHERVENAK: The one thing that we find that's helpful is the use of the father or other family members in these situations.

MR. GEORGE J. ANNAS: It's a very strong woman who can stand up to that kind of pressure. But the point is that, if she can, there is something important going on.

DR. FRANK CHERVENAK: The thing I find most surprising about the situation is how uncommon it is.

MR. GEORGE J. ANNAS: That's the other thing. Do we really want to change the law and create this precedent that you can beat up pregnant women to save 3 or 4 fetuses when this applies to everybody—3.7 million fetuses a year? Because 3 or 4 of them might have problems, do we want to change the law to deal with those when you can persuade most of the mothers anyway?

MR. BERTIL WENNERGREN (Swedish Commission on Genetic Engineering): Just a short question about informed consent. According to Swedish law, we need informed consent from both parents with regard to the surgical treatment of a child. What about the surgical treatment of a fetus? Should there be informed consent from both parents, or just from the mother? You might say that the answer is easy to give: The fetus is not a person. Then, informed consent is not necessary from the father. But you might also reason by analogy and conclude that there should be informed consent from both parents.

DR. ALBERT R. JONSEN (University of California/San Francisco): In general, as far as the ethics of informed consent go, there is a stringent obligation to gain maternal consent. It's highly advisable to have the consent of both parents in any case of intervention on the fetus. I think the obligation is absolute relative to maternal consent and advisory relative to the consent of both parents. If a mother consented to surgery affecting her fetus and a father dissented, I would consider the consent to have been given, from the ethical point of view.

MR. GEORGE J. ANNAS: The law is similar.

DR. RUTH MACKLIN (Albert Einstein College of Medicine): My question is primarily for Dr. Jonsen. An article by one of your colleagues proposed that, while fetal surgery is still in either its experimental or its innovative stage, it would be a good idea to appoint an advocate for the fetus. I don't think that the author meant that in a legal sense that would have any standing in court, but an advocate in decision making about whether or not to go forward with a particular intervention. In support of that proposal, the author said that an independent advocate would be likely to be more objective than either the parents or the treating physicians and went so far as to suggest that, even when the parents and the physician are in agreement about *in utero* therapy, the advocate might have a different point of view and that that view might hold sway. I found this proposal bordering on incoherence primarily because, in the absence of the very knowledge that we seek about the risks and benefits, what is there to be objective about? I wonder if you think that proposal has any merit?

DR. ALBERT R. JONSEN: Dr. Macklin, it had merit, but not the merit we thought it was going to have. I guess I turned out to be the advocate. That proposal was in a fairly early book. Almost all the reports were fairly early. Those were 1981 articles. We thought that there might have to be some kind of presentation, in view of the great risks, and that somehow an outsider could be helpful. It turned out that that wasn't the case at all; because of the phenomenon that I described in my paper, it turned out you don't need an advocate for the fetus at all. What you really need is an advocate for the mother. You almost have to talk mothers out of it, in the sense that they've got to be very clear that they are going to undergo risks themselves. The whole process of attempting to talk to people who come to us for these sorts of procedures is to try to help the mother be aware that we may not have anything for her and for her baby. It's not been a fetus *versus* mother or a mother *versus* fetus thing. It's as incoherent as you suspected. We haven't gone ahead with anything of that sort. We've become very much aware that we have to make very ingenious efforts to educate and to enhance the persuasive approach (and I'm not using the term *persuasion* in the bad sense) and to diminish as much as possible the coercive elements of the situation. We've worked very hard to improve communication between the parties involved.

DR. BERNARD DAVIS (Harvard Medical School): I appreciated very much Dr. Annas's thoughtful analysis. But I would like to comment on one phrase toward the end that bothers me a little bit. When he expressed concern over the danger of society's taking steps on some societal idea of what constitutes normal or good health, it really didn't fit the rest of his talk, in which he was clearly drawing lines between healthy and unhealthy people. That phrase bothered me because it seems almost to trivialize or make arbitrary decisions about what individuals would be better off not being born. Those of us interested in ethics are constantly faced with having to draw lines because the world doesn't come to us in a nice map where all good is colored green and all bad is colored purple. You have to use judgments and draw lines. I'd like to make a prediction. This whole area is very new, and as time goes on and as this technology is equally available in parts of the world that don't have the democratic tradition and emphasis on autonomy that we all derive so much benefit from, we are going to see great pressure brought on people not to bring children into the world who are going to be terrible burdens to themselves, to their families, and to society. Even though I've mentioned the importance of judgment about what is healthy or desirable, and what is not, there's one line that is really very sharp: a person who can make a living versus a person who is a burden to society. We now accept even the idea of having to make people driving motorcycles wear helmets, although some people are very disturbed by that, because if the person doesn't wear the helmet and gets hurt, it affects our Blue Cross rates and our taxes. So society has an interest in the wearing of helmets. That kind of concept, I predict, will develop very rapidly and affect our attitude on these matters.

MR. GEORGE J. ANNAS: There's no doubt that it is going to develop rapidly and affect our attitudes. That's certainly true. The question is whether it's going to have the force of law behind it. Motorcycle helmet laws have been eliminated in most states— thankfully, not because we want to see people's brains splattered over the highways or not spend money in emergency rooms, but because we believe that people should have the freedom to make certain choices themselves. What this whole issue is about—and reproduction is more important than riding a motorcycle—is what decisions people are going to have the right to make for themselves. I don't remember the precise phrase I used—it may not have been apt—but the essential notion is that it's a dangerous society in which certain people cannot be born. What you can look at, for example, is mandatory chorionic villi biopsy when it works. If you can find 100% of all the Down syndrome fetuses, the question is: Are we going to pass a statute to require women to abort all Down syndrome fetuses? I would answer no. I don't think the law has any business in that area. With persuasion, we can probably convince most people, but if we can't, we should stop short of legal mandates.

DR. RUTH HUBBARD (Harvard University): My question is similar to that of the last speaker, although the viewpoint is different. I am very troubled by the facts that Dr. Milunsky has told us, and that we have heard for these three days, about all of these new technologies. And then Dr. Annas says, of course in a liberal society, in a democratic society, we have the choice to avail ourselves of them or not, we being pregnant women in this case. What troubles me is that the very existence of these technologies means that we have to relate to them positively or negatively just because they're there. And by virtue of their being there, they make it a personal responsibility for pregnant women to relate to a whole set of potential outcomes of their pregnancy for which we were not responsible before, that were acts of God, that just happened. That increasing responsibility is not accompanied by an increase in health or support services from the state. On the contrary, in line with what Dr. Davis was bringing up, insurance companies are already beginning to talk about whether they have an obligation to provide health insurance for a child that is born disabled when the woman knew enough, so to speak, to prevent its birth. The very existence of the technology raises issues that we can't really turn away from by saying that we're free to use them or not. One of the things that's really troubling me is that, in these three days of symposia, no one has addressed the question, "Is it really imperative to go ahead?" That's my question: Must we go ahead just because we can, and who should be the people who decide whether we go ahead and in what way?

DR. ALBERT R. JONSEN: That's an immense question. It is the constant question that has to be raised by every new technologic advance. One of the features of technology in a culture is that all technologies are ethically neutral. That is, they can become positive or negative, in terms of the values that we attach to them and the uses that we make of them. All of the new technologies that come into a culture have to have that question asked of them, but there is no simple, single answer to the question, "Must we go ahead?" For example, with regard to the particular issues of fetal surgery, must we go ahead? The *must*, in some sense, derives from the perception that, for certain cases, if we do not go ahead, what we are likely to end up with is a child who is very sick and whose sickness could have been prevented by some sort of intervention. That is different from many other possibilities that may eventuate, where the chance that we can save this life that would die *in utero* is a different sort of thing from correcting a defect of a child that's about to be born. With regard to the second sort, we might say, no, we ought not to go ahead because that has implications for a population and for eugenics. We ought to say no. We have to make those distinctions. How do we stop anything from happening in society? Well, we pass laws. We know that laws stop only a fragment of things, and not very well. We say that laws are morally inappropriate. That may just encourage people to go ahead anyway. We make unwanted acts financially unprofitable. Someone will find a way to make them profitable. There is no simple way of saying no. Nevertheless, the question has to be insistent and has to be attached to every new technology.

DR. AUBREY MILUNSKY (Boston University School of Medicine): Dr. Ruth Hubbard's question brings us back to the frontier again, asking why we exist, why life, and should there be babies and should we operate? It's the kind of question to which I will respond with a symposium question to you: When did we stop progress in our history? You are asking, "Should we progress?" Is there history to show that we stopped, took a tangential turn and said that fetal surgery, prenatal diagnosis, or the atomic bomb, for example, is not the way society should go?

DR. RUTH HUBBARD: May I ask a question in response to your question. It is a vocabulary question. I think it's the question we need to ask: Is all change progress?

DR. AUBREY MILUNSKY: It's clearly not. But my question is: What is there in history to show that we have the gumption to say that this is not going to be progress and let's stop it. Do you have a background to suggest that? Maybe the ethicist does.

DR. ALBERT R. JONSEN: Barbara Tuchman has published a book called *Paths of Folly*, which shows three great societies that went absolutely the wrong way in terms of their political and military adventures, leading to their own destruction. We ought to think more about how presumed progress can, in fact, be a route to destruction.

MR. GEORGE J. ANNAS: I find it interesting that you spoke about adventure and faith in your presentation and then gave a more intellectual response to this question. I think that's what progress is all about: faith and adventure. These values are ingrained in all of us.

GENETICS, FETAL MEDICINE, AND SOCIAL JUSTICE

MODERATOR: SEYMOUR LEDERBERG

27

Sociomedical and Ethical Dilemmas in Fetal Medicine

Charles L. Bosk, Ph.D.
Associate Professor
Department of Sociology
University of Pennsylvania
Philadelphia, PA 19104

Freud, in his despairing lament on progress and modernity, *Civilization and Its Discontents*, asked: Why should he be grateful for the advances in transportation and communication that enabled him to be in touch with loved ones at a distance when, without such technological advances, his loved ones would never have had either the capacity or the motivation to leave the family circle in the first place?[1] In the 50-plus years since the original publication of Freud's essay, our own awareness of the perils of progress has only deepened. The arena where our own ambivalence about technologic advance is the most apparent is the medical arena. At every turn, we are dazzled by new capacities and, at the same time, confused about how to apply them in ways that augment rather than shrink our humanity. To reask Freud's question in a slightly altered form: Why be grateful for the ability to prolong life, if, by so doing, we only increase suffering?

Perhaps nowhere is the advance of medical technology itself so mind-boggling and our collective uncertainty about how to use it so acute as in the area of applied human genetics. The reasons are not hard to locate. Advances in human genetics have generated public images of a brave new world that are a complex merger of fact and fear, of possibility and prophecy, and of desire and dread. Such images speak to the potential threat that genetic advances present to our normal taken-for-granted assumptions about what it means to be a person in modern American society. These attitudes are most baldly displayed in the recent "Theoretical Letter Concerning the Moral Arguments against Genetic Engineering of the Human Germline Cells." Two fears figure prominently in this letter, first, that genetic knowledge, when applied, will alter, in some fundamental way, the normal, natural methods of making babies, of being a parent, of belonging to a family, of being a member in the human community. With more than a little drama and within an indefinitely ambiguous but fast-approaching time frame, the letter's signatories fear, "It will soon be possible to engineer and produce human beings by the same technological design principles as we now employ in our industrial processes." Presumably, it is cold comfort for these clerics that the emphasis on standardization in the production phase gives way to an empasis on product differentiation in the marketing phase for most commodities. In fact, the second fear that the letter lays out is that genetic engineering will make possible increasingly subtle product differentiation and that this will lead to eugenic practices, to a greater and greater standardization in the design of acceptable human products:

> Once we decide to begin the process of genetic engineering, there really is no logical place to stop. If diabetes, sickle cell anemia, and cancer can be cured by altering the genetic make-up of an individual, why not proceed to other "disorders," myopia, color blindness, left handedness. Indeed what is to preclude a society from deciding a certain skin color is a disorder.[2]

The clerics' letter and the "Study Paper of Bioethical Concerns," prepared by the Panel on Bioethical Concerns of the National Council of Churches of Christ, present evidence that C. P. Snow's two cultures are as divided as ever. It is easy to dismiss the concerns of these groups (as the President's Commission for the Study of Ethical Problems in Medicine and Biomedical and Behavioral Research did) as "exaggerated."[3] Simply stated there is much to preclude this society from setting too high a floor on what constitutes genetic fitness. Not the least of these factors is the degree to which applied human genetics has developed in a public spotlight. Advances have been subject to appraisal by a broad spectrum of public opinion and by a wide-ranging array of experts: physicians, scientists, clerics, lawyers, ethicists, and social scientists in a variety of forms, from television talk shows to congressional committees. In addition, there is in place a structure of institutional review boards that would monitor any unconventional or experimental therapy. In theory, even dramatic and surprise advances in fetal medicine receive some scrutiny before they occur. Also, there are numerous proposals for establishing some type of regular, continuous oversight of genetic advances and their clinical application.[4] Finally, from Asilomar to this conference on Genetics and the Law, there is a rather well-established tradition of consultation over how to apply new technologies. So, the fears of the clerics notwithstanding, there are many forces at work in the society to preclude genetic adventurism. These same forces would also limit overly bold initiatives in the area of fetal medicine. By the same token, it is perhaps worthwhile to point out that none of this consultation has led to the shelving of any scientific advances. Once the genie is out of the bottle, we appear, as a society, utterly incapable of stuffing him or her back in.

In this chapter, I shall limit myself to those genies already out of the bottles. Although a purpose of symposia is to fret about the future. I find more than enough to worry about in our current practices. I will impose two further limitations on my subject matter. First, I shall not concern myself with the variety of ways that fetuses become fetuses. Artificial insemination by donor, surrogate motherhood, embryo transfer, *in vitro* fertilization—all of these have received much discussion elsewhere in this volume. By the division of labor in the obstetric subspecialties, they are part of reproductive rather than fetal medicine and it is as such that they receive attention.[5-7] Moreover, all of the problems of neonates and the social, medical, legal, and ethical questions raised by such things as the Baby Doe regulations are likewise outside the domain of this discussion.[8-10] What we now do to fetuses while they are fetuses is my concern.

WHAT WE CAN DO TO FETUSES

What we can do to fetuses is look at them, test them, treat them, and/or abort them. The primary modes of visualization are ultrasound and fetoscopy. Fletcher and Evans have suggested that "maternal viewing of the fetus by means of ultrasound examination results in an earlier initiation of parental bonding."[11] The current means of testing include alpha-fetaprotein screening (of which more shortly) and amniocentesis. There are hopes that, in the next few years, chorionic villus biopsy will permit first-trimester testing with results available virtually immediately.[12] This represents a dramatic technical advance (amniocentesis is not performed before the sixteenth week of gestation; there is generally a two to four week wait for results). To the extent that this new procedure makes the abortion of genetically abnormal fetuses psychologically easier, its adoption is not likely to occur without controversey. In fact, to the degree that all of this looking and testing is done with the explicit purpose of aborting the defective, such techniques meet with considerable moral and political resistance. For some, the question is to whom these techniques should be made available; for others, the question is whether they are ever permissible.

We can look at fetuses. We can test them. But perhaps even more astoudingly, we can correct a limited number of defects *in utero*.[13] A range of techniques are available for therapy: giving medication to the mother; injecting medication and nutrients into the amniotic fluid; transfusing the fetal peritoneal cavity directly; and, *mirabile dictu*, fetal surgery. Not surprisingly such techniques raise many ethical and social questions. These are questions that the leading innovators in the area have been attentive to; Ruddick and Wilcox reported that Harrison and de Lorimer have spelled out minimal requirements for fetal therapy.[14] These include (1) an obstetrician experienced in prenatal intervention; (2) a sonographer experienced and skilled in fetal diagnosis; (3) a surgeon experienced in operating on tiny preterm infants and in performing fetal procedures in the laboratory; (4) a perinatologist working in a high-risk obstetrical unit associated with a tertiary intensive-care nursery; (5) a reasonable and compassionate ethicist; and (6) uninvolved professional colleagues who both oversee and foster such innovative therapy (that is, a committee on human research). Leaving aside the question of whether there might not be a tension in the last item between "overseeing" and "fostering" innovative therapy, the list is quite impressive. It demonstrates that, as far as fetal therapy is concerned, commendable attention has been paid not only to developing techniques but to implementing them in a humane fashion. This fact alone provides some solace to those who fear adventurism in fetal medicine and genetics. Finally, we can abort fetuses, and I will return to this subject later.

THE RESOURCE ALLOCATION QUESTION

When asking what sociomedical and ethical dilemmas fetal medicine generates, we can focus on trees (individual procedures in the arena of fetal medicine)—or on the forest (the impact of the procedures on the total delivery of obstetrical services). Let us take the second question first. I have not been able to locate accurate data on the cost of the variety of therapeutic alternatives that might be performed on eligible fetuses. However, one need not be a wizard in accounting to recognize that interventions that occur under the conditions that Harrison and de Lorimer have identified as minimal are on a per unit basis quite costly. If we are limited by scarce resources, is fetal therapy one of those directions that it makes sense to pursue? John Fletcher, for one, answered this question in the affirmative:

> The final question is the social and economic priority that should be assigned to investigations of the risks and benefits of fetal therapy. In my view that priority should be high. The great appeal of fetal therapy is the promise of the earliest feasible treatment to correct diseases that result in a lifetime of physical suffering and economic burdens. The economic considerations should be secondary to the opportunity to relieve or prevent suffering, but the economic questions should not be passed over lightly. . . . Fetal therapy, in fact, may represent one example where treatment is indeed prevention. Early treatment could reduce some of the lifetime costs and there-by contribute to a future state of affairs when economic considerations would not be the overriding reason for medical decisions. [15]

At an individual patient level, Fletcher's argument has great cogency. But if we ask which patients are most likely to benefit, a different concern emerges. By and large, the most common indication for amniocentesis is "advanced maternal age." A great many of these older pregnant women are middle- or upper-middle-class women with careers who have deferred childbearing. To the degree that the kind of intensive prenatal care that results in fetal testing or therapy is a prerogative of class, the benefits of the advances in fetal medicine do not fall, like God's gentle rain, on the rich and poor alike. In effect, the field of fetal medicine may extend to the prenatal stage the types of advantages normally associated with birth into a good family.

If our interest as a society is in improving the overall health of all fetuses as a class, then we might ask if the kind of high-technology, low-yield approach exemplified by the kind of fetal interventions now possible is the best way to do this. There are certainly a number of underfunded low-technology, presumptively high-yield approaches available that would have a greater impact on the health of the entire class of fetuses. The kind of public health and educational efforts involved are not as dramatic, as newsworthy, or as professionally rewarding as the frontier efforts involved in fetal therapy. But they are not to be sneered at on that account.

Neither the dilemma posed by the choice between high-technology, low-yield strategies of intervention or low-technology, high-yield ones, nor the gap between the health services available to the comfortable and those available to the indigent, is peculiar to fetal medicine. Both issues run like an unbroken thread through all of American medicine.

What makes this question all the more insistent at present is how close to the ground the safety net for the poor has been moved lately. At the very least, we need to take care that, in discussing the social and ethical dilemmas brought on us by extraordinary advances in fetal medicine, we do not blind ourselves to the many inequities built into ordinary, everyday obstetrics. In my opinion, we need to develop mechanisms to distribute the benefits of progress equitably. From the viewpoint of a sociologist, the great social, medical, and ethical dilemmas of fetal medicine are those that surround everyday obstetric practice and that account for the difference in prenatal care that rich and poor receive. This difference, as well as the differential in infant mortality related to it, is much more vexing than the application of new technologies, however troublesome it might be. We are doing so poorly in managing some rather ancient problems of fetal medicine that there is something almost self-indulgent in worrying so much about the new ones.

If I feel from a demographic point of view that concern with the problems of fetal medicine is self-indulgent, I do not believe this is the case from a symbolic or cultural perspective. Much of the discourse in bioethics is a debate about the statistically improbable. The fact that so much intellectual energy is focused on such improbable events speaks to medicine's power to act as a symbolic filter through which many of our deepest human-condition concerns are expressed. To paraphrase Claude Lévi-Strauss, the technical advances of bioethics are good to think with; they allow us to ruminate collectively about who we are and what we are becoming. For example, at one level, the Baby Doe debate is a debate about how to care for handicapped infants. At another level, it is a discussion about the bonds of parenthood, the obligations of physicians, and the responsibility of the state. The debate is not heated because there are so many cases out there that the regulations fit. Rather, as moral tales, Baby Doe stories evoke a response in ways that a more abstract, philosophic engaging of the same issues could not.[16] I do not know what it means that the womb can now be invaded, but that that fact is culturally significant I have no doubt.

FETAL THERAPY AND ABORTION

Finally, I would like to outline some ethical and some pragmatic questions that our new capacities present. Ruddick and Wilcox asked whether the fact that a fetus can be treated changes its legal and social status. They presented—chiefly in order to refute it—the following propositional argument (which I am greatly condensing): (1) if someone is a patient, he or she is a person; (2) as a person, that patient has certain rights, including a right to life; (3) the capacity of fetuses to be patients entails status as persons; (4) as persons, fetuses have certain rights—including a right to life that they would not have if fetal therapy were not possible. Ruddick and Wilcox rejected this argument because they feel that its initial premise is mistaken. They stated, "The first premise is clearly false. Some patients are not persons—for example, patients who are brain-dead, anencephalic, or animal."[17] Through this argument, Ruddick and Wilcox dispensed with the allegation that fetal therapy enlarges the rights of fetuses as a class, entitles them all to personhood whatever the wishes of the mother, and makes abortion an ethically intolerable procedure. Ruddick and Wilcox were able to dispense with the personhood claims of the fetus because of the particular propositions that they employed and not on any universalistic grounds.

This disposal of fetal therapy as relevant in the abortion debate notwithstanding, the very potential of the procedure raises a number of issues. First, it magnifies the potential conflict of interest between mother and fetus. Although I find it a bit bizarre to think of mother and fetus as individual actors, each with its own inalienable set of rights and entitlements rather than as some community of common interests and shared risks, the current emphasis on individuality and autonomy found in the literature encourages the first approach. From this perspective, a number of questions, all flowing from the divergent interests of mother and fetus, arise. For example, can mothers be required to accept therapy on correctable fetuses rather than to abort them? How are the risks and benefits that therapeutic procedures represent to mothers balanced against those to fetuses? On the one hand, it is easy enough to agree with Ruddick and Wilcox that fetal therapy is unlikely to change any minds in the abortion debate. For those who oppose abortion, fetal therapy enhances personhood claims; for those who would permit abortion as a woman's right, the issue of fetal therapy is largely irrelevant. Perhaps fetal therapy will convince some that, as Charles Baron has suggested, personhood arguments only confuse our thinking about abortion.[18] However that might be, hospital staff might not be thrilled about aborting fetuses with correctable defects. This want of excitement might translate into care that is less than considerate to the woman.

SOME PRAGMATIC CONSIDERATIONS

If we move from ethical speculation to clinical concerns, another set of considerations emerges. Primary among these is the selection of eligible fetuses for treatment. According to a group of experts in fetal medicine, "The most difficult problem in prenatal management is how to select only the fetuses that might benefit from treatment." Selecting those that would most benefit is a fairly universal problem under conditions of scarce resources. However, it acquires an additional urgency in the area of fetal medicine. Some fetuses are so mildly affected with whatever their disorder is that they will do well with standard treatment after birth. In these cases, the risks of intervention far outweigh any benefits. By the same token, it is almost cruel to offer hope to those mothers whose fetuses are so severely affected that they are beyond the reach of even heroic therapy.

A concomitant of this medical problem is how these diagnostic uncertainties work themselves out in social settings.[19] The team of specialists involved in fetal diagnosis and therapy can include some or all of the following: perinatal obstetrician, surgeon, sonographer, bioethicist, psychologist, and neonatologist. This team needs to develop procedures for acknowledging its own differences of opinion internally; it needs to negotiate with the hospital's IRB over what is and what is not acceptable as a course of clinical action; and finally, it faces the difficult task of providing parents with clear expectations about the available technology and its limitations. Certain issues of uncertainty will resolve themselves with greater clinical experience. But fetal diagnosis has a large, irreducible component of uncertainty. This makes the procedural guidelines that have emerged very impressive.

The above discussion reads as if problems of uncertainty are approached in a rational way by rational actors. When we introduce the notion of false positives, false negatives, and inevitable error, the problem grows much more complex. Finally, when we consider the parents' emotional involvement in their own lives, it becomes clear that the solution to problems of uncertainty does not rest simply with finding a better slide rule. Here I would offer one caution. In our zeal to do the right thing in the right way, we need to install procedures for respecting both parental autonomy and parental privacy. Consulted by so many, talked to so thoughtfully and thoroughly, parents need permission not to feel coerced by medical kindness. The right to be squeamish, pessimistic, or afraid is not very well entrenched. Parents have a right to refuse fetal therapy without feeling criminally negligent for not doing the best thing for their baby.

CONCLUSION

Fetal medicine is expanding rapidly in the public spotlight. This chapter has given much more consideration to fetal therapy than to screening because it is the more recent development and the less discussed one. Experts in fetal medicine have devised commendable guidelines for therapy. The adequacy of these procedures requires that the diagnostic data evaluated be accurate. The limits of the technology, false positives, and uncertainty from inexperience pose a challenge to these procedures; nonetheless, considerable energy has been expended to provide an ethically responsible way of proceeding in a new area. Problems are posed by the ethics of resource allocation. Given our general obstetric problems, is this a way to help the greatest number in the most reasonable fashion? Question have also been raised about how fetal therapy affects the status of the fetus. The fact of fetal therapy is, however, not likely to change many minds in the abortion debate. Finally, fetal therapy is a complex team procedure; means for preserving teamwork in the face of conflicts that might erode it need development.

REFERENCES AND NOTES

1. Freud, S., *Civilization and Its Discontents*, W. W. Norton, New York (1961).
2. Both quotations are from Norman, C., Clerics urge ban on altering germline cells, *Science* 220:1360–1 (June 24, 1983).
3. For an analysis of the study paper and the commission's report, *Splicing Life: A Report on the Social and Ethical Issues of Genetic Engineering with Human Beings*, see Boone, C. K., Splicing life, with scalpel and scythe, *Hastings Cent. Rep.* (Apr. 1983), 8–10.
4. For a review see Moreno, J., Private genes and public ethics, *Hastings Cent. Rep.* (Oct. 1983), 5–6.
5. Grobstein, C., Flower, H., and Mendeloff, J., External human fertilization: An evaluation of policy, *Science* 222:127–32 (Oct. 14, 1983).
6. Krimmel, H. T., The case against surrogate parenting, *Hastings Cent. Rep.* (Oct. 1983), 35–9.

7. Robertson, J. A., Surrogate mothers: Not so novel after all, *Hastings Cent. Rep.* (Oct. 1983), 28–34.
8. Guillemin, J., and Holmstrom, L., Legal cases, government regulations, and clinical realities in newborn intensive care, *Am. J. Perinatol.* 1:89–97 (Oct. 1983).
9. Angell, M., Handicapped children: Baby Doe and Uncle Sam, *N. Eng. J. Med.* **309**(11):659–661 (Sept. 15, 1983).
10. Annas, G. J., Baby Doe redux: Doctors as child abusers, *Hasings Cent. Rep.* (Oct. 1983), 26–7.
11. Fletcher, J., and Evans, M., Maternal bonding in early fetal ultrasound examinations, *N. Eng. J. Med.* **308**(7):392–3 (Feb. 17, 1983).
12. Kolata, G., First trimester prenatal diagnosis, *Science* **221**:1031–2 (Sept. 9, 1983).
13. Harrison, M., Golbus, M., and Filly, R., Management of the fetus with a correctable congenital defect, *JAMA* **246**(7):774–7.(Aug. 14, 1981).
14. Ruddick, W., and Wilcox, W., Operating on the fetus, *Hastings Cent. Rep.* (Oct. 1982), 10–14.
15. Fletcher, J., The fetus as patient: Ethical issues, *JAMA* **246**(7):772–3 (Aug. 14, 1981).
16. Bosk, C., Pipers and tunes: Personhood in three clinical settings" (mimeo).
17. Ruddick and Wilcox. *idem.*, 13.
18. Baron, C., "If You prick us, do we not bleed?": Of Shylock, fetuses, and the concept of person in the law, *Law, Medicine and Health Care* (Apr. 1983). 52–61
19. Bosk, C., Occupational rituals in patient management, *N. Eng. J. Med.* **303**:71–6 (July 10, 1980).

28

Genetic Disease, Government, and Social Justice

Jessica G. Davis, M.D.
Associate Professor of Clinical Pediatrics
Cornell University College of Medicine
Chief of Genetics
North Shore University Hospital
300 Community Drive
Manhasset, NY 11030

A series of critical discoveries in biochemical, cellular, and molecular biology, coupled with an array of innovative technologies, inaugurated the "golden age of medical genetics" in the 1950s. A cascade of brand-new genetic information and techniques followed. Many of these discoveries had immediate and direct clinical application, leading to an expansion of diagnostic treatment and counseling capabilities. Comprehensive genetic service and screening programs began to be organized and implemented. These programs were designed to meet the needs of an ever-increasing number of individuals and their familes that had or were at risk for genetic disease or birth defects. Public interest and expectations grew, reinforced by the information media's unprecedented coverage of all aspects of medical genetics.

Despite the excitement surrounding medical genetics, there was a lack of large-scale financing for medical genetic services. The federal government greatly expanded its fiscal support of medicine in the 1960s, providing funds for medical genetic research and training programs, but few dollars for clinical genetic efforts. Third-party reimbursement was nonexistent. Fortunately, help did come from the private sector. Many medical schools allocated funds for medical geneticists and laboratory personnel. The March of Dimes Birth Defects Foundation supported a variety of medical-genetic research projects and provided funds to expand the clinical capabilities of a series of university-based genetic service programs. These service projects provided the basis for the present national genetics program.

Dedicated to Marjorie Guthrie

The first major federal sponsorship of clinical genetic services occurred in 1972 with the passage of the National Sickle Cell Anemia Control Act (Public Law 92-294). The act's goals were "to reduce the morbidity and mortality from sickle cell disease, to increase public awareness about the disease, and to develop and evaluate new modes of therapy for sickle cell disease."[1] This piece of legislation was followed in 1976 by the National Sickle Cell–Cooley's Anemia and Genetic Diseases Act (Public Law 94-278), which "unified and coordinated Federal Support for the provision of genetic services that had previously been fragmented."[2]

However, two years passed before funding was provided to implement the National Genetics Act, an amended version of P.L. 24-278. The 1978 appropriation enabled 22 states and Puerto Rico to obtain federal funds for medical genetic service and sickle-cell programs. Public and private third-party insurance groups began to underwrite limited reimbursement for medical genetic services. These decisions enhanced the fiscal stability of medical genetic services. Over the next four years, federal financial support increased, enabling additional statewide genetic service programs to receive federal funds and the already-established genetic programs to expand. During this period, federal directives encouraged statewide genetics programs to discard the former categorical or "disease-of-the-month" approach and to meld all existing resources into a united noncategorical plan.

By 1981, 42 statewide genetic service programs and sickle-cell projects had received federal support. Each of these programs basically fit into one of three models: (1) the state-health-agency grantee model, in which the state's department of health provided genetic services solely to its own citizens; (2) the university-based grantee model, in which all genetic services were university based; and (3) the regional-model state health agency, in which a consortium of state health departments and providers worked together.[3] The future of genetic services appeared secure.

This sense of well-being was short-lived. The federal government adopted a more conservative point of view in the 1980s. In its efforts to limit government spending and to reduce the role of the federal government, the Reagan administration cut back federal regulations, decreased public health services, and reduced federal financing for medicine, including genetic services and research. Congress repealed those laws authorizing funds for a variety of categorical health programs, including the then-underfunded National Genetics Act (P.L. 94-278).

Passage of the Omnibus Reconciliation Budget Act of 1981 followed. This act called for the consolidation of existing federal health programs in "block grants" and provided funds to the states to continue these categorical programs at their own discretion. The federal Genetic Diseases Program became part of the Maternal and Child Health Services (MCH) Block Grant. The MCH Block Grant combined genetic services with six other programs, including Title V Maternal Child Health (MCH) and Crippled Children's Services (CCS); Supplemental Security Insurance (SSI); hemophilia treatment centers; sudden infant death syndrome (SIDS); lead-based paint poisoning; and adolescent health services.

The Omnibus Reconciliation Act clearly states that the appropriation for the MCH Services Block Grant consists of two parts. One part of the appropriation (85%) is transferred directly to each state's coffers, and the remainder of the appropriation (15%) is set aside for disbursement by the Secretary of Health and Human Services. The 15% set-aside portion of the budget provides funds only for Special Projects of Regional and National Significance (SPRANS).

The creation of the MCH Services Block Grant led to major problems for the medical genetics community. First, although several programs were merged under the MCH Services Block Grant, the grant's overall 1982 budget was markedly reduced. The total appropriation was less than the sum of the 1981 budgets of its component parts. Second, the Omnibus Reconcilation Act clearly says that each state may use a portion of their MCH Services Block Grant to continue to fund their hemophilia centers and their genetics and sickle-cell testing and counseling projects. However, the Department of Health and Human Services (HHS) examined the limited funds appropriated for the MCH Services Block Grant and weighed the options. For reasons that remain unclear, HHS then decided to specifically exclude medical genetic service programs in their budget calculations for each state's block grant. This meant that funds for the medical genetic service programs had to come from the 15% set aside.

Unfortunately, the budget for the 15% set aside had also been drastically slashed by a 47% reduction. In 1981, $13.1 million had been allocated to the federal genetics program. The Omnibus Reconciliation Act's new budget awarded $7.25 million for medical genetic services in 1982. Furthermore "not all of this money was available to the state's genetic services programs, some went to the Center for Disease Control and to centralized education and information programs."[4]

In an effort to cope with the severely reduced budget for the 15% set-aside or SPRANS projects, HHS was forced to set new priorities. As a result, HHS adopted a new plan in an effort to allocate limited dollars. The plan's strategy was to declare those existing statewide genetic programs that had already been funded for four years ineligible for funds from the 15% set-aside or SPRANS dollars. Instead, HHS agreed to provide assistance to those "now ineligible statewide genetic programs to obtain funding from the consolidated 85% MCH Services Block Grants to the states, placing the funding hopefully under state authority."[5] The result was that 23 statewide genetics programs, including 17 sickle-cell projects, suddenly became ineligible for set-aside (SPRANS) funds. In addition, HHS decided to use the available 15% set-aside (SPRANS) funds to support only "those statewide genetics programs that had been funded for fewer than four years."[6] This meant that 19 statewide genetics programs, including 6 sickle-cell projects, were eligible for federal (SPRANS) support. Lastly, the HHS plan declared that funds would be available for new statewide genetic programs, but that, once a statewide genetic service program had completed its fourth years of federal support, it would be deemed ineligible.[7]

The reduced appropriation for the MCH Block Grant; the decision of HHS to declare 23 state-based genetics and sickle-cell programs ineligible; the inadequate reimbursement for genetic testing and counseling; and the limited university and local financing for these services—all precipitated a national fiscal crisis for genetic service programs.[8]

There was much anger and pain as model programs faced uncertainty. To quote Stephen Sondheim: "Success is swell/And success is sweet/But every height has a drop./The less achievement/The less defeat."[9] There was concern about issues of equity. Dr. Margery Shaw eloquently summarized the human consequences of the HHS decision:

> Diminished resources for providing genetic screening, prenatal diagnosis and counseling for high-risk parents with a resultant loss of reproduction choices to those who wish to avoid genetic tragedies and more importantly increased physical pain and suffering of affected offspring, increased emotional turmoil for the families, and increased economic burdens to individuals and to society in terms of health care costs.[10]

The staff of the Genetic Servies Branch, Division of Maternal and Child Health, then held a series of regional meetings to provide assistance in the transition period. These meetings brought together representatives of the now-ineligible programs, third-party insurance programs, private foundations, consumers, and key state-government personnel. Heated discussions occurred as genetic health-care providers tried to learn how to go about obtaining funds from their individual state's MCH Services Block Grant. The meeting participants expressed concerns about how to set priorities and how to allocate scarce resources, as well as how to seek alternate sources of funding and support. Medical geneticists worried about the disruptive effects of the budget cuts "on the partnerships that had been fostered, in some states, between academic geneticists, state health departments, and sickle cell screening and counseling programs."[11]

One general conclusion to emerge from these sessions was that third-party reimbursement for genetic services needed to change in order to ensure a radical turnabout in the economics of medical genetics. A cooperative study to review the status of third-party reimbursement was initiated by the March of Dimes Birth Defects Foundation, the Bureau of Health Care Delivery, and HHS.

The general outlook was grim. As talks progressed, genetic health-care providers finally understood there would be no magical restoration of the budget cuts and that the government's decision to declare some programs ineligible and others eligible would not be revoked. Representatives of each ineligible state's genetic services program began the herculean task of attempting to recoup all or a portion of their losses.

Many funded programs were well-coordinated efforts utilizing the resources of a network of tertiary-care medical centers and satellite centers working closely with a variety of state and local resources. Other programs were in the process of forging formal linkages. In some states, medical geneticists worked closely with their state health departments; in others, there was little or no cooperation. Geneticists in some areawide programs such as New York's had already established close working relationships with their state's sickle-cell projects and hemophilia centers. Other statewide programs lacked internal cohesiveness. Lastly, only a few state health departments were able to provide funds from their MCH Services Block Grants for statewide genetic programs. The majority had already committed their MCH Services Block Grant dollars to other existing programs.

It was clear that, in most states, funds for genetic services would have to come from other sources. This proved to be the major obstacle because most geneticists had little insight into the political process. Most had no experience in dealing with their state legislators and no knowledge of their state's budget process. For example, an article in the *New York Times* described the New York State budget as follows:

> In the grandest sense, it was said to be a "legislative budget," one written by the lawmakers themselves and imposed on the Governor. But in a far less visible sense, it was a legislative budget of a different sort, chock full of projects, constituent favors and just plain tidbits for each lawmaker. . . . It's a tradition with roots in clubhouse politics, days of pork barrels when politicians rewarded loyalty and perhaps themselves.[12]

Medical geneticists in each state had to devise their own strategies in accordance with their state's fiscal priorities and calendar. For example, in New York,

> Every year in June, the Budget Division issues a 'budget call letter' to all agency heads which provides guidelines for submitting their budget requests for the next state fiscal year which begins on April 1st; by September 15th, the agencies must submit their requests and then the Budget Division holds hearings to consider them. By late fall, the agency budgets are complete and the budget director prepares recommendations for the governor. The governor has until the third Tuesday in January to submit his budget to the legislature.[13]

This schedule meant that, by the time New York State's medical genetics community learned that the statewide genetics program was ineligible for federal funds, the budgets for programs now incorporated into the MCH Services Block Grant had already been determined. A careful review of the MCH Block Grant budget in January 1982 revealed that there were no extra dollars available for genetics services. It was clear that medical genetic services could be funded under the MCH Block Services Grant only if the other programs in the block grant experienced additional budget reductions.

New York geneticists quickly rejected this possibility, realizing that additional costs would cripple other existing maternal- and child-health programs. We began to search for other sources of funding. Time was short because New York State's laws stipulate that the state's annual budget must be approved by March 31 of each calendar year. With the assistance of Mr. James Couch (an educator and sickle-cell service provider), the late Mrs. Marjorie Guthrie (a consumer advocate for improved genetic services), and Mr. Thomas Parham (the New York State Genetics Program's chief fiscal officer), members of the New York State genetics community reviewed all available options. It was clear that we had only a slim chance of success because we would have to request new funds in order to maintain our statewide program. Our request was made at the same time that our state's administration had decided to hold over all budget growth below the level of inflation. We also faced one other enormous problem. No one in the New York State Legislature or Executive Branch knew about the medical genetics program.

With the help of consumers, we began to educate our state legislators about the benefits and accomplishments of our program. We learned that "the budget negotiation is the crux of the political process in that you are making political choices as to where to apply resources."[14] We learned that our governor's budget is sent to the Senate's Finance Committee and to our Assembly's Way's and Means Committee for analysis. Each of these committees then prepares an alternative budget based on constituent, regional, and party needs. The fiscal staffs of the committees then

> get together, compare notes, and assumptions and begin a series of technical negotiations, which are presumably matched by political negotiations between the legislative leaders and the governor.[15]

In order to become a line item on the budget, we learned that "you've gotta be a nudge. . . . If you miss one day, somebody else could take your money. There's a lot of legislators eyeing and vying for the same thing."[16] In the end, we New Yorkers were successful because many of our state legislators, particularly the Honorable James Tallon, Chairman of the Assembly's Committee on Health, and the Honorable Tarky Lombardy, Chairman of the Senate's Health Committee, as well as the Honorable Arthur Eve (Buffalo) and the Honorable Al Vann (Brooklyn) recognized our program's worth. They decided to sponsor a measure to fund our statewide genetics program, which, in turn, received the necessary gubernatorial support.

How did other statewide genetic programs fare? In a recent survey subtitled "The Impact of the Federal Cutback on Genetic Services,"[17] Neil Holtzman demonstrated the inability of most of the ineligible programs to make up the loss of federal support with funds from other sources. Ineligible states were less able than eligible states to maintain their current level of funding at or above their fiscal year (FY) 1982 level. There also was a significant discrepancy in per capita allocations to genetics and sickle-cell programs in FY 1983. The ineligible states fell well below the eligible states in allocations per capita and per child below the poverty level. A few ineligible states generated some revenue for genetic services from their block grants and/or from short-term federal supplemental appropriations. Some ineligible states instituted charges for services, including newborn screening tests. Most states did not rely on fee collections. Revenues obtained from third-party reimbursement varied greatly.[18]

What about the future? Of concern are the present federal administration's continued attempts to institute further budget cuts, to curb reimbursement, and to reduce the eligibility criteria for Medicaid. There is a cap on funds for medical genetic services. The federal budget for medical genetics for FY 1984 is $7.3 million. It also appears unlikely that the MCH Services Block Grant will receive an infusion of new dollars. Thus, no new federal dollars will be made available to states already declared ineligible. Furthermore, as the number of eligible states declines, the net result will be a nationwide decrease in allocations for genetic services per capita and per child below the poverty level.[19]

Because of their own internal financial problems, most states are not and will not be in a position to provide much relief. Medical genetics programs will continue to compete with a variety of other state programs for funds. There is a possibility of additional revenue from third-party insurers only if more consumers and employees demand insurance policies that include genetic services. Third-party insurers would then have to underwrite more insurance in order to meet the need. However, many individuals lack any financial protection. These include

> households with part-time or recently unemployed workers and the working poor who

> earned too little to afford assistance . . . along with the many poor people excluded
> from Medicaid because they failed to fit into eligibility categories.[20]

In addition, technological advances will not make genetic counseling more efficient. It is a labor-intensive activity.

Nance asked for "a re-examination of the justification for Federal funding of genetic services."[21] He recognized that "some health care programs such as neonatal metabolic screening can lay claim to Federal support because of their national relevance to public health measures,"[22] whereas "others such as transplantation programs may involve the distribution of limited or expensive resources."[23] Although he found it hard to justify the continued support of voluntary genetic screening and counseling programs, Nance made a strong case for continued support in order to ensure "the rapid dissemination and uniform application of important new research findings or technological advances . . . such as the use of restriction enzymes.[24] He emphasized that although "most genetic diseases are rare . . . they assume importance as a major public health problem only when considered in the aggregate."[25] Nance also pointed out that medical genetic diagnoses often involve other, healthy family members. Most medical geneticists encounter difficulty obtaining financial reimbursement for genetic studies involving healthy family members.

It is clear that the succession of laws that established and shaped the National Genetics Program were visionary and enormously beneficial. These congressional mandates were deftly handled by an elightened administration so that the prevention and treatment of genetic disease is now an important component of health care. However, recent events indicate that political and economic factors do have a direct bearing on the allocation of scarce resources. The resulting new priorities can and will

> severely restrict the medical geneticists' abilities to deliver a full range of medical
> genetic services to the citizens within our respective states. The values and priorities of
> those individuals who control the actual appropriations[26]

also play a key role in deciding whether expenditures for the diagnosis, treatment or other modes of management of relatively rare diseases can be justified. Yet, the present budget stringencies hold little promise of contributing to long-term solutions. Severe budget cuts can and will defeat the original purposes of the National Genetics Program.

There is an obvious need to develop new strategies to ensure adequate levels of support in order to preserve the program's momentum. The public, health professionals, and legislators must be made aware that genetic screening and counseling programs and medical genetic research can make major contributions to personal well-being and public health. This awareness can be accomplished through a well-organized, meticulous, ongoing educational effort aimed at all segments of our society.

In addition, I support the establishment of a permanent National Medical Genetic Advisory Council. This body should be composed of medical geneticists, genetic counselors, allied health-care providers, consumers, representatives of appropriate national bodies such as the American Society of Human Genetics, lay organizations and private foundations, educators and persons with legal and fiscal expertise. Working in close cooperation with our federal stewards, the council's members would provide current information about all aspects of medical genetic services, including new developments. The principal charge of this group would be to develop a bold, comprehensive, and flexible 10-year national genetic-service plan with well-defined goals and objectives. The program must be politically neutral and not subject to the vicissitudes of changing administrations. It should include an evaluation component with appropriate reporting mechanisms.

However, recent events indicate that the success of this program will rest on the abilities of its planners to secure stable and adequate financing to meet its goals. Public funds must be made available for genetic services in order to decrease inequalities in access to health care and to promote public planning and accountability. Medical geneticists must pay careful attention to the changing structure of medical care in the 1980s, particularly to "the rise of corporate enterprise to health services"[27] and "the growth of a kind of marketing mentality in health care."[28]

The corporate sector has already made major commitments to molecular genetic research. In some parts of the country, medical genetic and laboratory services are under the control of profit-making exterprises. Such trends are disturbing in that a health care system "in which corporate enterprises play a large part is likely to be more segmented and more stratified,"[29] with interests "determined by the rate of return on investments."[30]

Our task is clear. Our efforts must enable today's and tomorrow's citizens to have continued access to comprehensive genetic services. I am hopeful that our policymakers will recognize their duty to assist us in this process by allocating the resources to meet these needs. Such allocations, in turn, should lead to the renewal of a long-range commitment to excellence and accelerated progress in the field of medical genetics.

REFERENCES

1. Manley, A. F., *Legislation and Funding for Genetic Services, 1972–1982*. Proceedings of "Future Directions in Genetics Workshop" held on January 30–31, 1984. Sponsored by the Genetic Disease Service Branch, Division of Maternal and Child Health, U.S. Department of Health and Human Services, p. 6.

2. Nance, W. E., Rapid communication: Editorial comment on Dr. Holtzman's paper, *Am. J. Med. Gen.* **15**:375 (1983).

3. Fifth Annual Report, Genetic Diseases Program under Title XI. Part A, Public Health Service Act, Health Services Administratior Bureau of Community Health Services, J.S. Dept. of Health and Human Services. DHHS Publication No. (HSA) 81-5140 A, p. 14.

4. Holtzman, N. A., Rapid communication: The impact of the federal cutback on genetic services, *Am. J. Med. Gen.* **15**:353 (1983).

5. Manley, A. F., *Legislation and Funding for Genetic Services, 1972–1982*. Proceedings of "Future Directions in Genetics Workshop" held on January 30–31, 1984. Sponsored by the Genetic Disease Service Branch, Division of Maternal and Child Health, U.S. Department of Health and Human Services, p. 12.

6. *Ibid.*, 13.

7. *Ibid.*, 6.

8. Davis, J. G., Rapid communication: Invited editorial comment on Dr. Holtzman's paper, *Am. J. Med. Gen.* **15**:368 (1983).

9. Sondheim, S., Live, laugh, love. *Follies.* Copyright © the Herald Square Music Co., Rilting Music Inc., Burthen Music Co., Inc. All rights reserved.

10. Shaw, M. W., Rapid communication: Editorial comment on Dr. Holtzman's paper, *Am. J. Med. Gen.* **15**:375 (1983).

11. Nance, W. E., Rapid communication: Editorial comment on Dr. Holtzman's paper, *Am. J. Med. Gen.* **15**:375 (1983).

12. Gargan, E. A., The personal aspects of a public budget, *New York Times* (Apr. 1, 1984), 34.

13. Auletta, K., Profiles, Governor, I. *New Yorker* (Apr. 9, 1984), 96.

14. *Ibid.,* 99.

15. Auletta, K., Profiles, Governor, II. *New Yorker* (Apr. 16, 1984), 66.

16. Gargan, E. A. The personal aspects of a public budget, *New York Times* (Apr. 1, 1984), 34.

17. Holtzman, N. A., Rapid Communication: The impact of the federal cutback on genetic services, *Am. J. Med. Gen.* **15**:353–365 (1983).

18. Davis, J. G., Rapid communcation: Invited editorial comment on Dr. Holtzman's paper, *Am. J. Med. Gen.* **15**:369 (1983).

19. Holtzman, N. A., Rapid communication: The impact of the federal cutback on genetic services, *Am. J. Med. Gen.* **15**:363, (1983).

20. Starr, P., *The Social Transformation of American Medicine.* Basic Books, New York (1982), 374.

21. Nance, W. E., Rapid communication: Editorial comment on Dr. Holtzman's paper, *Am. J. Med. Gen.* **15**:376 (1983).

22. *Ibid.,* 376.

23. *Ibid.,* 376.

24. *Ibid.,* 377.

25. *Ibid.,* 377.

26. Davis, J. G., Rapid communication invited editorial comment on Dr. Holtzman's paper, *Am. J. Med. Gen.* **15**:369–370 (1983).

27. Starr, P., *The Social Transformation of American Medicine,* Basic books, New York, (1982), 421.

28. *Ibid.,* 448.

29. *Ibid.,* 448.

30. *Ibid.,* 499.

29

The Regulation of Alpha-Fetoprotein Test Kits by the Food and Drug Administration

Stuart L. Nightingale, M.D.
Associate Commissioner for Health Affairs
Food and Drug Administration
Room 1495 (HFY-1)
5600 Fisher Lane
Rockville, MD 20857

In this paper, I will describe the path that the Food and Drug Administration (FDA) has taken to arrive at a decision in one of the most complex and challenging regulatory episodes in recent memory: the approval for marketing of a diagnostic product—the alpha-fetoprotein (AFP) test kit—for the prenatal detection of neural tube defects (NTDs).

AFP Testing for NTDs

Between 1 and 2 out of every 1,000 infants born in the United States is affected by some degree of defect in the embryonic development of the neural tube, resulting in anencephaly or spina bifida. Approximately half of the NTDs are in each category. In anencephaly, the cranial vault fails to develop; affected infants who are not stillborn usually survive less than one month after delivery. Spina bifida is characterized by incomplete closure of the vertebral column and varying involvement of the spinal cord.

With surgery, about 40% of newborns with spina bifida survive five or more years. These patients can experience problems such as paralysis or weakness of the lower limbs, loss of sensation below the lesion, failure of bowel and bladder control, and hydrocephalus, which is present in about 75% of spina bifida patients and can cause mental retardation. Infants with closed (skin-covered) lesions, who comprise about 25% of spina bifida patients, may be less handicapped and have a more favorable prognosis than patients with open spina bifida.

More than 90% of NTDs occur in families with no previous history of the disease. Couples who have previously had a child with an NTD have a recurrence risk of approximately 2%.

The role of AFP testing for the detection of NTDs is based on the observations, reported more than a decade ago, that this fetospecific protein is detectable in maternal serum and amniotic fluid, and that, in the presence of an open neural-tube lesion, its concentration markedly exceeds normal limits. Hence, a finding of elevated AFP in maternal serum or amniotic fluid is suggestive, although not diagnostic, of a fetal NTD and warrants further tests to confirm or exclude the diagnosis. Other conditions that lead to elevated AFP in the serum include multiple pregnancy, omphalocele, congenital nephrosis, and fetal bowel obstruction.

APPLICATIONS TO MARKET AFP TEST KITS

The first application to market an AFP test kit for the detections of NTDs was submitted to the FDA in 1976. Although the radioimmunoassay technique employed in the test was not new and had been in general use for other indications, the application of this methodology to a test for the detection of NTDs did make the test materials, for this intended use, subject to FDA regulation under the 1976 Medical Device Amendments to the Food, Drug, and Cosmetic Act. AFP test kits had been used extensively in the United States as investigational products before 1976 in well-organized, highly sophisticated research programs. Experience gained in these programs served both to substantiate the safety and effectiveness of the test and to characterize the sequence of further testing that is required if an initial maternal serum is found to have an above-normal concentration of AFP.

The United Kingdom has been in the forefront of AFP testing and research. AFP testing has been used there since the early 1970s. A number of local health centers in the National Health Service provide maternal serum testing; an extensive quality-control program is in place; and test outcomes have been widely studied. The published results of a collaborative study of 19 centers conducting AFP testing in the United Kingdom, where the incidence of NTDs is higher than it is in the United States, document the effectiveness of the test.

As required by the medical device provisions of the Food, Drug, and Cosmetic Act, the FDA submitted the initial application to advisory panels of outside experts—in this case, in the fields of obstetrics and gynecology, radiology, and immunology. In addition to reviewing the data submitted in support of the marketing applications (the initial application was followed shortly by several others), the FDA held a public hearing on February 26, 1979, at which interested parties were given the opportunity to submit data and offer comments on the regulation of these devices. As a result of its review of the information provided at the hearing, as well as other communications, the FDA published in the *Federal Register* of August 3, 1979, a notice of intent to issue proposed regulations establishing restrictions on the sale, distribution, and use of AFP test kits as a condition of approval of any marketing application.

It should be emphasized that, unlike the regulatory authority governing drugs, the Medical Device Amendments of 1976 authorize the Secretary of Health and Human Services to grant restricted approval of a medical device if, in the secretary's judgment, such restrictions are necessary to ensure the safe and effective use of the device. Restrictions may limit those to whom the device may be sold or distributed, those who may use it, and those conditions (such as the availability of ancillary services and/or special competence) that may be required as a condition of receiving and using an approved, restricted device.

The FDA decided not to approve any AFP test-kit application until it had determined through the rule-making process what restrictions, if any, would be needed to ensure the safety and effectiveness of the kits in use. In fact, the Medical Device Amendments require that such public notice and comment rule-making be employed before any restrictions can be imposed. Such proposals for public comment are not required for the FDA to approve a device or a diagnostic product for marketing without restrictions.

On November 7, 1980, the agency published in the *Federal Register* a lengthy proposal to place restrictions on AFP test kits for use in detecting NTDs and announced a public hearing on the issue. That hearing, at which I was the presiding officer, was held on January 15 and 16, 1981.

Let me, at this point, interrupt this chronology of the regulatory actions surrounding AFP test kits to focus on the issues that relate to AFP testing in general and the FDA's regulatory stance in particular.

COMPETENCY

There is virtually unanimous agreement that the radioimmunoassay technique for the *in vitro* measurement of AFP in maternal serum and amniotic fluid is a reliable methodology in the hands of competent clinical laboratories. It is fair to say that the safety and effectiveness of the test itself and the reagents and other materials in the kits proposed for marketing have never been seriously challenged. The scientific—and, in a larger sense, the medical and ethical—issues that have prompted controversy have concerned the interpretation of the test results and the ability of the U.S. health-care system to ensure that AFP testing will take place only as part of a constellation of services (e.g., diagnostic and counseling) that must be available when suspicion of an NTD fetus is signaled by an initial positive AFP test result.

Concern was raised, notably by the American College of Obstetricians and Gynecologists, that physicians are unfamiliar with the test and unprepared to interpret the meaning of a serum AFP value. Further, it believed that the test should be performed only in specialized centers with formal programs for counseling and with sophisticated equipment. At public hearings and in other communications to the FDA, advocates of this viewpoint have argued that the marketing and promotion of the AFP test kit would rapidly propel this technology from availability in a comparatively few centers having highly developed comprehensive programs to general use in virtually every obstetrical practice in the country. It was suggested that rapid expansion in a health care system unprepared to utilize the technology responsibly would inevitably result in incorrect interpretations and failure to provide the necessary follow-up care. These, in turn, could cause needless anxiety on the part of pregnant women (or conversely, an unjustified confidence that the fetus was definitely not affected by an NTD). False positive results might lead to the termination of normal pregnancies; physicians could be exposed to charges of malpractice either for failing to offer AFP testing to their patients or for misjudging the meaning of the test results.

In addition to the concerns about the general unfamiliarity of physicians with the test and the correct interpretation of its results, concerns were also raised that many patients would not have access to competent counseling to aid them in making a decision. Some patients, frightened by an initial positive test result, might seek to terminate the pregnancy unnecessarily. Clinical laboratories might fail to maintain the high standards of performance required of AFP testing unless they were in a position to carry out many such tests on a regular basis. Some persons argued that any product or procedure that might lead to abortion was *ipso facto* unacceptable.

Others, notably the American Medical Association, were concerned that placing restrictions on the market availability of AFP test kits would tend to freeze technological development and would unnecessarily limit physicians' and patients' access to a valuable diagnostic procedure. The AMA also expressed concern that restrictions would represent an inappropriate and unnecessary intrusion by government into medical practice. Others with similar concerns emphasized that the health care system, including practicing physicians, radiologists, laboratories, and ancillary personnel, were sufficiently competent and had the technology available to adequately handle AFP testing for patients.

THE DIAGNOSTIC PROTOCOL

The concerns of some groups were predicated, in part, on the fact that the sequence of steps required to confirm the diagnosis of an open fetal NTD is critical as regards timing and laboratory technique, as well as demanding of a series of procedures, including patient counseling at each step, that require technical competence. The sequence set out in the 1980 proposal is generally as follows:

At 16–18 weeks' gestational age, a sample of maternal serum is tested for AFP. Blood drawn earlier than 15 weeks of gestation will yield a false low AFP value, whereas if the test cycle is started much later than the eighteenth week, the option to terminate the pregnancy is sharply reduced.

If the initial maternal serum AFP value is above the norm for the population group to which the patient belongs (AFP norms may vary both geographically and racially), a second serum AFP test is performed about one week after the first. If that value, too, is above the standardized norm, ultrasonography is indicated to establish fetal age. AFP values in maternal serum and amniotic fluid rise during the course of a normal pregnancy. Therefore, precise knowledge of gestational age, as determined by ultrasonography, is critical to the correct interpretation of AFP values. Moreover, factors such as twinning and fetal death also cause increased AFP levels. Sonography can rule out such non-NTD explanations of an elevated AFP value.

If sonography does not explain the reason for an above-normal AFP level, the patient is advised, following further, more sophisticated sonography (which may itself reveal an NTD), to have amniocentesis and a determination of amniotic fluid AFP. Elevated amniotic-fluid AFP levels can indicate an open NTD, although they can also result from other fetal abnormalities. Testing for acetylcholinesterase in the amniotic fluid, however, may confirm the presence of an open NTD and may rule out the potential for false positive results.

If this diagnostic sequence were followed in 1,000 pregnant women in the United States, the first serum AFP test would detect approximately 50 patients with elevated AFP. The second serum test would disclose repeat positive values in roughly 30–40 of those patients. Diagnostic ultrasound would designate approximately 17 patients who have a single, living fetus at the expected gestational age, without apparent anomaly, for whom amniocentesis is indicated. Measurement of amniotic fluid AFP levels would reveal 1 or 2 patients whose fetuses have a 50% chance of a serious abnormality, most of which will be open NTDs. An elevated acetylcholinesterase would make an NTD extremely likely, and a low or absent acetylcholinesterase result would point to a non-NTD fetal abnormality.

As amniocentesis is not without risk of fetal injury or loss, it should not be performed unless the earlier appropriate serum testing and sonography are carried out.

This diagnostic protocol was the one viewed as most appropriate, representing optimal medical care at the time of the FDA's deliberations in 1980.

THE PROPOSAL TO APPROVE THE AFP KITS WITH RESTRICTIONS

In seeking to reach a decision on whether to approve AFP test kits for marketing, the FDA obviously had to consider not only the ability of the kits to perform safely and effectively for their intended use, but also the issue of how safe and effective their use would be in obstetrical practice outside the investigational setting.

As stated above, on November 7, 1980, the FDA published in the *Federal Register* a proposed rule designating AFP test kits as restricted devices and describing the conditions under which such kits could be lawfully marketed. In essence, the proposal contained a set of proposed restrictions on clinical laboratories, physicians, manufacturers, and facilities at which sonography and amniocentesis are performed. The restrictions would have required written agreements, records, and reports.

Anyone offering AFP test kits for sale would have been required to designate a "program coordinator," an entity established by regulation to ensure compliance with the proposed restrictions. Among other things, the "coordinator" would see that all patients followed the diagnostic sequence outlined in the proposal. In addition to compiling and supplying detailed records on the use of the kits and the pregnancy outcome of each patient, the "coordinator" would have had to certify that the clinical laboratory was, in fact, maintaining proficiency in conducting the test by carrying out a certain minimal number of tests each week; that each patient was provided by her physician with a brochure explaining the meaning of the test; and that AFP testing would be carried out only on the order of a physician who had agreed to maintain and turn over to the FDA on request records of the patient's history, AFP testing and results, and signed patient acknowledgment that the implications of AFP testing had been explained and that the patient had consented to the testing.

In short, the restricted distribution scheme would have imposed a closed AFP-testing system constructed to guarantee that the test was offered only as part of a total spectrum of NTD detection procedures and services. Patients would have had ample opportunity to determine whether or not to accept such testing in order to make an informed decision to elect to terminate the pregnancy or to plan for the birth of an NTD child.

Also, the notice invited public comment on each of the specific aspects of the proposal, including the suggested language for a patient brochure, and on several broader issues, such as

1.   Should the FDA require that confirmatory procedures (following an initial positive maternal-serum test) be conducted or at least made available to the patient?
2.   How should a balance be struck between restriction on the use of the kits and the widest possible access to the technology?
3.   Is widespread access desirable?
4.   Would the proposed restrictions deny access to AFP testing to women in certain geographic areas and to women of limited economic means?
5.   Has the passage of time (since the FDA initially began consideration of the AFP test-kit applications) been accompanied by changes in the capacity of the health care system that reduce the need for restrictions on the distribution of AFP test kits?
6.   Should the FDA approve the kits without regard to resources, so that at least some women will have the benefit of AFP testing?

At the formal public hearing in January 1981, many of the concerns already mentioned were reiterated.

Numerous organizations opposed restrictions, including the American Medical Association, the College of American Pathologists, and organizations representing clinical laboratories and drug and medical-device manufacturers.

Obstetrical and pediatric societies, the Health Research Group, and the Spina Bifida Association supported restrictions for the reasons mentioned earlier, and academicians and others who were then involved in investigational AFP-testing programs expressed views ranging from disapproval of AFP testing, to permanent retention of the investigational status of AFP test kits with their restriction to certain genetic centers, and to approval without restriction. Also, many members of the public commented as individuals.

The above comments, together with more than 650 written comments from organizations and individuals on the proposal received by the FDA, presented an intriguing spectrum. Few comments supported the restrictions *per se*. Of the individuals who commented, 90% favored outright the banning or disapproval of AFP test kits on the grounds that the device would provide information that might lead to a decision to abort a pregnancy.

APPROVAL OF THE AFP TEST KITS WITHOUT THE PROPOSED RESTRICTIONS

The FDA withdrew its proposal to restrict the distribution of approved AFP test kits in a *Federal Register* notice dated June 17, 1983. What caused the agency to substantially reverse its earlier position? And what are the likely consequences of the decision to allow the marketing of AFP test kits without the restrictive scheme proposed in November of 1980?

The FDA's decision to withdraw the proposed restrictions reflected the fact that no data were presented to the agency to demonstrate that the health care system lacks the resources to make the full range of NTD detection and diagnostic services available if AFP tests kits were approved for marketing. On the contrary, information was submitted that showed that these services are and will be available and that the health care system will respond to the demand. Moreover, the acetylcholinesterase determination as an adjunct to the NTD detection and diagnosis process, not widely available earlier, greatly reduces the possibility of false positive results and their tragic consequences.

As explained in the *Federal Register* withdrawal notice of June 17, 1983, the safety and effectiveness of the test kits and the ancillary procedures had been thoroughly established by extensive laboratory and clinical investigations.

The notice stated that approval of the kits would be conditioned on the fact that manufacturers would be required to distribute FDA-approved physician, laboratory, and patient labeling to provide clear, thorough information for each intended recipient on the nature of the test, how to carry it out, how to interpret results, what is the significance of a positive test result, and what options exist for medical care and follow-up. On this last point, the June 17 notice states: "FDA expects that physicians will ensure that the proper diagnostic protocol is followed in a timely manner and that patients are adequately informed of the significance of test results."

FDA approval of AFP test kits would also establish certain conditions whereby manufacturers will be required to submit to the FDA quarterly and annual reports concerning postapproval experience with the products. These requirements will allow the FDA to monitor future product performance.

The notice also expressed the FDA's conclusion that existing controls on clinical laboratories—(including the rules of cognizant state and federal agencies), as well as voluntarily adopted proficiency testing standards, (such as those of the College of American Pathologists and the Joint Commission for the Accreditation of Hospitals) will ensure that clinical laboratories will maintain high standards of quality in performing the AFP *in vitro* tests.

On the issue of the capacity of the health care system to provide the array of services required for AFP testing for NTDs, the notice stated that there are no documented shortages of adequate facilities and qualified personnel for follow-up testing. The FDA estimates that only 30 out of 1,000 women who undergo a serum test will be referred for sonography, and that only 15 out of 1,000 will be referred for amniocentesis. Furthermore, the FDA believes that testing will not become universal on approval of the kits but will increase gradually over a five-year period following approval, allowing time for the establishment of the additional ancillary testing facilities that may be needed.

Parenthetically, some confusion arose about the role of FDA—an agency not involved in funding health care programs—in regulating how the test kits would be used. Much of the controversy centered on the use of the kit in mass screening programs. Whether or not and to what extent such programs materialize clearly depends on many factors not under the FDA's purview.

In summary, the FDA's decision not to restrict the sale, distribution, and use of AFP test kits, as well as the subsequent approval of the marketing of two such kits, is predicated on the conclusion that the devices are safe and effective for their intended use; that they are properly labeled for the guidance of physicians, laboratories, and patients; and that making this technology, along with the appropriate informational materials for laboratories, physicians, and patients, generally available under appropriate regulatory controls will benefit the public health.

Obviously, the FDA will closely monitor AFP testing. Of four test kits approved by FDA for marketing, two are now in commercial use—one approved in January 1984 and one approved in June 1984. The agency is reviewing the quarterly reports of experience with the kits that are required to be submitted by manufacturers.

The two manufacturers of approved kits and several others awaiting approval have provided to the FDA their plans for the distribution of patient and physician brochures and laboratory labeling. These plans specify how each manufacturer intends to ensure that physicians will receive supplies of both types of brochures before they offer AFP testing to a patient, and that laboratories will have detailed product information before they first receive a serum sample for analysis. All such plans are subject to prior approval by the FDA, and their effectiveness will also be monitored.

CONCLUSION

In the case of AFP testing and test products, has the regulatory process performed responsibly and in the public interest? In my opinion, the safety and effectiveness of AFP test kits have been thoroughly substantiated through extensive research; concerns about the propriety of allowing these kits to be generally marketed have been given ample opportunity for expression and have been thoroughly examined; the need for appropriate and timely ancillary and support services has been duly addressed; and a mechanism has been established that should facilitate the proper use of the AFP test without unnecessary and burdensome intrusion into medical practice or the delivery of clinical services.

The FDA, with its scientific advisers and through extensive public participation, reviewed the medical and scientific issues and then applied the criteria embodied in law and regulation. I believe that the FDA has reached an appropriate decision that is in keeping with evolving technology, the state of our health-care system, and, most important, the public interest.

DISCUSSION

DR. SEYMOUR LEDERBERG (Brown University): The theme of this particular session ranged from ethical dilemmas in fetal medicine to the FDA's position and also included, of course, governmental consent and funding for genetic programs.

MS. TABITHA M. POWLEDGE (Bio/Technology Magazine): I don't think the subjects of this session were as disparate as you say. In fact, I want to attract our attention back to the issues of commercialization that surfaced on the first day. Dr. Davis, it seems to me that one unavoidable implication of your presentation and Dr. Nightingale's is that genetic services are more and more going to be commercial services offered for profit to those who can pay. I invite your comment and anyone else's on whether you indeed think that is what is going to happen and, second, if it does, what are the implications for the ethical issues that we have been talking about for the last 2½ days?

DR. JESSICA G. DAVIS (Cornell University College of Medicine): I can't answer that question because it's so enormous. That's one that I and many of my colleagues have been grappling with. In a sense, I think this is a problem of all of medicine. I am personally quite dismayed by this direction, mostly because of some idealism and my own particular reasons for going into medicine and staying in academic medicine, and also because I feel that these technologies and developments really should be staying in the university and not be moving out into the marketplace, although I know this is the assault now on medicine and this is becoming increasingly so in all aspects of the work. As George Annas expressed a personal point of view, this is my own personal point of view. The President's Commission in its lengthy report on genetics and the bioethical aspects of screening, testing, and counseling identified many problems that we still have to wrestle with. Aubrey Milunsky talked this morning about new technology, and the whole panel yesterday morning was devoted to all this new research. I've heard many expressions of concern and anger about medicine and anger about men and a lot of anger that is a little dismaying to me. But I think it's good that these issues are being brought out in forums and discussed. I am afraid that they will not be discussed if the technologies become commercialized and go out into the "world."

Ms. ELAINE LOCKE (American College of Obstetricians and Gynecologists): I compliment Dr. Nightingale on the exceedingly difficult job of a comprehensive survey of the problem with AFP testing. I would like to emphasize that the opposition of the American College of Obstetricians and Gynecologists (ACOG) to the unrestricted release of the AFP kits has centered on the fact that this would imply the offering of the testing to all pregnant women throughout the country, which is something beyond what we have done at this point. Perhaps 1 person out of the 50 who are told that they have a positive result in the initial serum test would actually have an affected fetus. This means that a great number of people will be subject to further costly testing, or will be unable to pay for or to obtain access to further testing, or perhaps will have unnecessary abortions or worry because of misunderstandings. Dr. Nightingale touched on all of this. I guess that what's unusual is to find the College begging the FDA for restrictions and being on the side of Ralph Nader's Health Research Group. There was also support from the Spina Bifida Association. You could say that this has impressed us as a very scary situation. At the same time, we have been undertaking extensive efforts in physician education, which is no easy job. We have developed some patient education materials and intend to go forward with even more of these. Dr. Nightingale, we have been worried about the fact that physician labeling, in the usual sense, goes to the laboratory, not to the obstetrician/gynecologist who is drawing the blood sample. Hence, it is going to be even more difficult for that form of education, if it is usually effective, to be effective in this case. I believe you said that the manufacturers were going to be required to pass that education on to physicians in some specific way.

DR. STUART L. NIGHTINGALE (Food and Drug Administration): Yes, each company that gets the marketing approval has to present a plan to the FDA for distribution of the various materials. That includes how to get it into the hands of the physician and his or her patient. I've leafed through some of those myself to see how the distribution is being set up, and it appears to be mostly through the laboratories, then advertising directly to physicians through the various newsletters, journals, and so on that they would read. So, they would know about the availability of the tests and could write away, for example, for copies of the various physician leaflets and patient leaflets, and detail people would also be handing these out. The ACOG is doing an excellent job in terms of educating its members. There is a technical bulletin that the ACOG put out several years ago. I would hope that you'd update it, now that the test is commercially available. You have done a very good job on the patient brochure and leaflet. I recently spoke to a physician in one of these screening centers, and I said that each company has to develop its own patient brochure, which has to be approved by the FDA. I said, "How do you feel about that?" This individual knew about the ACOG leaflet and said, well, he'd never hand out something that was mandated or developed by the government but certainly would hand out the ACOG brochure. That's something that has to be looked at. The point is that the professional association is going to provide material that can be utilized by people in these various programs. I think the educational materials need to come from various sources.

Ms. ROBIN J. R. BLATT (Massachusetts Genetics Program): The screening process may subject parents to a high degree of anxiety and uncertainty. Before the first blood test, individuals need to be informed about the diagnostic protocol, which involves ultrasound and amniocentesis, that may be set in motion. In addition, the known and unknown risks of each procedure must be described. In my personal opinion, this has not been adequately done in the bulletins that have been put out by the different laboratories or the ACOG. Also, families need to be informed that open neural-tube defects may be detected and that in no way can the degree of severity or the degree of mildness be determined. The possibility of missing a neural tube defect or incorrectly identifying a healthy fetus as having a neural tube defect because of false positives and false negatives needs to be communicated. Families considering the test need to be provided with counseling during each phase. That's what everybody has been saying. This is directed to Dr. Nightingale and others who wish to comment. In the opinion of each of you, who's really responsible for communicating these facts to a pregnant woman, and in what way should they be communicated? Is a leaflet, a brochure, the most effective way? And if your answer is that it's the primary responsibility of the physician to tell these facts verbally to a pregnant woman, whose responsibility is it to make sure that the physician is aware of these issues and that the information is passed on?

DR. STUART L. NIGHTINGALE: I think it is indeed the physician's role and obligation to do this, to see that the patient is fully informed. The FDA, in this case, has gone so far as to say that there needs to be a brochure developed and approved by the FDA, which the manufacturer puts together, that needs to be in the patient's hands. It's not a regulation saying that is all that must be there. My view is that, following good medical practice, as this test expands, the leaflets will be made available initially to patients, and that a physician should begin by not only handing the patient one of these leaflets but also, obviously, explaining the whole situation. Written information is important, but what we are really talking about is an interaction that involves discussion about the various issues and the problems and options.

Ms. ROBIN J. R. BLATT: This will become the expected standard, then?

DR. STUART L. NIGHTINGALE: As far as the FDA is concerned, which is really what I can deal with best, the standard will be that the patient does receive this information prior to the time of the initial screen. It's not mandated in regulations that an FDA inspector will come into the doctor's office and observe to see that this is done, but it is what we— through our labeling approach and what we have done through manufacturers—feel is appropriate. My view personally is that it has to be done and will become standard practice, through the ACOG's efforts and through malpractice concerns.

DR. JESSICA G. DAVIS: I guess my own clinical experience leaves me rather skeptical that all this is going to happen overnight, and I must say that I do fear for my patients and their families and I fear for my associates in the medical field. Working in my own area, which is a rather sophisticated one in the Greater Metropolitan area, Nassau and

Suffolk Counties, particularly medically as well as genetically, I think that we have encountered grave problems in the past with this gray area. At least in my own area, my group of practitioners basically relay all these problems to our client. They do not really want to deal with this in their offices at this point because they understand the pitfalls. I also think you're being a little naive about what Dr. Lewis Thomas talks about, the nontechnological part of medicine, the "talk time." Busy obstetricians really don't have very much time to sit and explain at great length. That's why consortiums and working relationships with genetic units, genetic counselors, public health nurses who are trained in this field, and social workers is still going to be needed, and hopefully that will happen. My last comment is that I hope there is a monitoring system set up about what the experience is, not a lot of anecdotes about good work in Chicago or what's happening there or these six booklets. I'd like to know how many children are monitored and how many tests are performed, and I'd like record keeping on it.

DR. AUBREY MILUNSKY (Boston University School of Medicine): There is to me a greater concern even beyond what you've said. The history of screening for phenylketonuria—for example, in California—is abysmal. California, in its wisdom, allowed the screening for PKU in all laboratories, or in any laboratory, and for years this went on and laboratories would screen even a dozen cases a year. Of course, you can imagine that a laboratory that has very little experience in volume will err more often. It took years for them to realize that cases of PKU were being missed. Only in recent years have they coalesced laboratories into major centers and seen the error of their ways. With the alpha-fetoprotein going the same route (and we have already heard at this meeting how often we learn from history), all laboratories are offering alpha-fetoprotein screening. The same thing is going to happen, except worse. Now we know it's easy to detect over 90% of anencephaly and about 80% of open spina bifida. The problem is that, because it's only "a screening test," not a diagnostic test like PKU, it'll take years to detect the laboratory that's functioning poorly because, after all, if they miss a case, they'll say that only 80% can be detected. I don't know how anybody is going to identify a laboratory that is providing the most abysmal service. The consequence will be twofold. First, women will be having screening and they will end up aborting a normal fetus (something we haven't done in over 40,000 pregnancies that we have screened so far). The second consequence is that a most valuable technology may fall into complete disrepute, and that is my fear.

DR. PENELOPE ALDERDICE (Memorial University of Newfoundland): I appreciate very much being brought down into the mud by this talk about education and finance. I hope I speak for many people in this room who haven't had a chance to speak. I'd like to hear more about the cost. Dr. Davis, when you talk about the budget's being halved in one year, how much money should there be there? I also would like to say that I come from a place where half the children who start first grade never graduate from high school. Those young women are not going to gain from a pamphlet handed out to them. I'm sure that there are areas in the United States where the same thing happens. I think that we are very unrealistic in what is being voiced here.

Dr. Dorothy Helleman (Maryland): I'd like to focus on what I consider the true fetal abuse, and that is a rather dreadful international ranking in fetal and maternal morbidity and mortality. The low birth weight, the prematurity, and all the fetal surgery and neonatology could be avoided to a remarkable extent even without genetic testing.

The Role of Government

MODERATOR: WILLIAM SCHWARTZ

30

THE BIOTECHNOLOGY INDUSTRY
Impact of Federal Research and Regulatory Policies

JOSEPH G. PERPICH, M.D., J.D.
Vice President
Planning and Development
Meloy Laboratories
Revlon Health Care
6715 Electronic Drive
Springfield, VA 22151

The biological revolution underscores the success of the federal government's commitment to the support of basic research: the billions for health research through the National Institute of Health (NIH) in the 1950s and 1960s directly led to the discovery of recombinant DNA technology. As Dr. Donald Fredrickson, the former NIH director, has noted, there is a flood of basic discoveries in biochemistry, physiology, and medicine fueling today's revolution in biology. In a recent address, Dr. James Wyngaarden, the current NIH director, observed that the traditional biomedical research disciplines are becoming increasingly unified scientifically, in Dr. Arthur Kornberg's words, "by the common language of chemistry." For purposes of definition for this chapter, the focus is on biotechnology, a broad term that weds the fermentation industry and the new fermentation technologies with the genetic engineering industry, principally recombinant DNA technology and cell fusion, better known as *hybridomas* and *monoclonal antibodies*.

The impact of these discoveries will be very broad on government, universities, industry, and the public at large. I served during 1982–1984 as guest editor for a series of articles on the impact of biotechnology on society for the journal *Technology in Society*.[1] The purpose of the articles is to document and examine the new biology's present and future relationships with existing societal institutions. The first series of articles focuses on biotechnology from the perspective of research relationships and goals among government, university, and industry. Subsequent articles focus on the impact of biotechnology on government policy and its implementation; the specific problems posed to corporate, regulatory, and patent law; and the long-range public-policy and ethical questions posed by such a pervasive technology.

In the opening series of the *Technology in Society* articles, Dr. Richard Krause, the Director of the National Institute of Allergy and Infectious Diseases at the NIH, wrote how the cascade of information resulting from the biological revolution can deal with what he called "the trinity of despair": hunger, disease, and insufficient resources to support an expanding population.[2] The dimension of these problems, he noted, is worldwide, and yet, the application of these technologies gives hope to meet these challenges. In large part, it is through the industrial applications that we will meet those challenges.

The genetic engineering industry is a recent phenomenon, beginning in the mid-1970s. This industry combines the skills of academic research scientists, the fruits of federally funded basic research, and the venture capitalists' dollars. Companies like Cetus, Genentech, and Genex were formed initially with venture capital and equity investments by larger firms and refinanced through public offerings and research-and-development limited partnerships. The private markets responded rapidly and creatively to the promise of new biotechnology products. I would like to provide some data today based on the Office of Technology Assessment report on commercial biotechnology issued in early 1984.[3] There are approximately 220 biotechnology firms; 110 of them are the new firms commonly known as the genetic engineering companies, and 110 are from the established industries, principally pharmaceuticals, chemical energy, and agriculture. From 1976 to 1984, more than 100 of the newer firms were formed; in 1981 alone, 43 were formed. The equity investments in these companies by the larger companies during that period were approximately $350 million, and many of the bigger firms provided the operating revenues for the smaller firms through contract research, especially from the pharmaceutical industry. Virtually all of the newer companies were doing contract research for interferon production and other areas of pharmaceutical interest. One should also note the importance of the R&D limited partnership and the contribution of Bruce Merrifield of the U.S. Commerce Department, who vigorously promoted this mechanism as an effective method for the industrial R&D community to finance research. For biotechnology, $170 million of revenue was raised in 1983 via this mechanism, and $175 million is projected for 1984.

You can see the excitement in the 1984 business press. *Business Week*, on January 23, ran a cover story, "Biotech Comes of Age,"; February's *Venture Magazine* had a cover article entitled, "The Biotech Revolution Is Here—How the New Genetic Technologies Will Transform Industries and Our Lives"; and *Newsweek* had a cover article, "The Gene Doctors—Unlocking the Mysteries of Cancer, Heart Disease and Genetic Defects." For someone whose training and work experience has largely been in government and academic institutions, the plunge into this industrial and venture capital world has been exciting and bracing—it helps to be trained in psychiatry.

Government support for basic research and the dynamism of the private markets will bring biotechnology products into virtually every industrial sector. Thus, for product development in biotechnology, the genetic engineering companies join the major chemical, pharmaceutical, and energy companies that have significant internal biotechnology R&D operations. It should be noted that the larger companies are putting a good deal of money into their own biotechnology R&D centers. DuPont has committed $85 million for internal R&D, and Eli Lilly has committed an additional $50 million for internal R&D.

The objective of the biotechnology companies is to apply the emerging genetic-engineering techniques to the development of novel and profitable commercial applications. The R&D programs of these companies are set up to improve existing products, to increase the availability of rare products, and to create new products.

An example of how one can improve an existing product through genetic engineering is the work of several companies in producing rennin. Rennin is crucial to cheese making and currently is obtained by extracting rennin from a calf's stomach or producing it in bacteria, an inefficient process that simultaneously produces several undesirable by-products. The biotechnology companies hope to obtain the pure product with genetic engineering techniques. Scientists have isolated the gene for rennin and have cloned the gene in several bacterial systems to produce rennin. Several companies have filed applications with the Food and Drug Administration (FDA) for product approval. Through this technology, we can significantly improve the availability of an enzyme that, at present, is costly and is not a pure product. I should note that enzymes are an especially appropriate focus for biotechnology because they are the easiest to produce with genetic engineering techniques. Enzymes have wide applicability, particularly in food processing.

In the category of increasing the availability of rare products, a good example is human interferon. In 1977, the possibility of using recombinant DNA to produce insulin and interferon in bacteria was predicted to be 5 to 10 years away. Yet, these feats occurred far earlier, in 1978 and 1979, respectively. In early 1980, I was asked if I could obtain interferon for the use of a family friend who was diagnosed as having terminal cancer of the lungs. I called several drug companies, universities, and the American Cancer Society. None was available; the costs were prohibitive, and quantities were in micrograms. Today, virtually every genetic engineering and pharmaceutical company has produced liters of interferon—a dramatic example of the possible advances with this technology. In the health area, scores of industrial proposals have been approved by the Recombinant DNA Advisory Committee of the NIH for large-scale production of human insulin and proinsulin and animal and human growth hormones, to mention but a few, by such companies as Eli Lilly, Genentech, Hoffman-LaRoche, Cetus, and Molecular Genetics.

The third area, creating new products, often is synonymous with "protein engineering." One of biotechnology's major accomplishments will be the custom design of proteins and enzymes, a target that, when reached, will indicate that the new biotechnology has outgrown its infancy. This research focus is to understand the relationship between the structure and the function of proteins as the basis for their actions. The promise is great. Much work remains to be done. Many of the companies are actively involved in work in this area. Genex has a protein-engineering division funded in part through a contract with Allied. DuPont has an interest in the structure and function relationships of enzymes and the designing of genes in order to design better enzymes for agriculture. DuPont Laboratories has a number of projects under way here, and their research is a model for what should happen in the future.

FEDERAL RESEARCH POLICIES

The Office of Technology Assessment (OTA), in its biotechnology report, identified 10 factors responsible for the leadership of the United States in biotechnology and grouped them in the following terms: "most important," "moderately important," and "least important."[3] Two of the "most important" factors were government support for basic and applied research and support for training in the scientific disciplines, such as molecular biology. The OTA estimated that, in 1983, the government provided $511 million for basic research support in biotechnology and $6 million in applied technology. But these figures are very soft, because these are, after all, technologies that are used broadly in many of the research grants (which wouldn't be identified necessarily as recombinant-DNA research grants).

The genetic engineering companies and major companies with biotechnology divisions correspond to every major federal R&D program: health, chemicals, energy, agriculture, and environment.[4] The NIH has been a primary supporter of recombinant DNA research and related technologies for the past several decades. And many of the biotechnology companies are directly applying those research results in developing new drugs, vaccines, and diagnostic methods and treatments for cancer, heart disease, and genetic defects. Indeed, because of the enormous investment by the NIH in the basic research and because of the intensive research capacity of the pharmaceutical industry, with its enormous experience in fermentation, the wedding of the technologies occurred rapidly. Thus, according to the OTA, 62% of the biotechnology companies, or 135, are identified as being principally in, or at least involved in, pharmaceutical research. Several of the smaller biotechnology companies (Cetus, Genentech, Genetics Institute, Hybritech, and Biogen) and larger pharmaceutical companies (Eli Lilly, Upjohn, Schering-Plough, Merck, and Revlon, of which Meloy Laboratories is a subsidiary) are in the forefront of industrial applications here. In chemicals, the National Science Foundation (NSF) and the U.S. Department of Energy (DOE) have biological research programs to investigate the potential applications of biotechnology in the production of specialty chemicals. In the area of specialty chemicals (generally defined as costing more than a dollar a pound), 20% of the companies are involved. In addition, in the energy area, the DOE and the NSF have a number of research programs under way for refining biomass from trees or agricultural residues to produce fuel, feeds, and other useful chemicals. In the area of commodity chemicals and energy, 15% of the companies are involved. These areas are of special interest to smaller companies like Genex and Cetus and larger chemical companies like Dow, DuPont, Exxon, Monsanto, and Phillips.

In the agricultural area, the promise is especially great: animal production (growth hormones), vaccine development (hoof-and-mouth disease and chicken coccidiosis), and plant cell and tissue culture implants and nitrogen fixation, a whole host of applications to increase the food supply. In this area, approximately 28% of the companies are involved in animal health and 24% in plant biology. A number of smaller companies specialize in this area, including Agrigenetics, Cetus, and Molecular Genetics, as well as many of the big chemical companies with agricultural components, such as Dow, Monsanto, and DuPont. In the environmental area, the Environmental Protection Agency (EPA) is pursuing a number of promising opportunities to use biotechnology to deal with environmental wastes, the treatment of wastes, and the degradation of toxins. Companies like Genex, DuPont, and Dow have an obvious interest here. Approximately 11% of the companies are involved in the environmental area.

One should also note the broad interest of the U.S. Department of Defense in biotechnology research and development: the development of antiviral drugs and vaccines for our troops in Asia, Latin America, and Africa; the detection of, and defense against, chemical and biological weapons; and the development of biosensors and the production of new materials (biopolymers). With the president's commitment of building a space station, NASA will have an interest in the use of genetic engineering technologies for food production and the recycling of wastes in a space station. All of these agency programs are of interest as well to the Agency for International Development (AID). Biotechnology applications in health, agriculture, and energy are directly relevant to the needs of the less-developed countries. Here, the challenge for the AID is to harness the energies of the biotechnology industry for product development for the less developed countries.

In addition to federal research-and-development programs, a number of federal initiatives should be noted. For example, in 1981, the NIH changed its policy to permit companies to compete for grants. A major congressional initiative is the 1982 Small Business Innovation Development Act modeled on the NSF Small Business Innovation Research Grant Program. The act seeks to stimulate technological innovation, to use small businesses to meet federal research-and-development needs, and to increase the private sector commercialization of innovations derived from federal research and development. Another important law for small businesses is the Patent and Trademark Amendments Act of 1980, which gives universities, nonprofit organizations, and small businesses the first right of refusal to the title of inventions that they make while performing under government grants or contracts (subject to some limited exceptions). In creating this right to ownership, the act abolished approximately 26 conflicting statutory and administrative policies.

For the future, the OTA biotechnology report emphasizes the need for funding for general research in new fermentation and engineering technologies as well as relevant training, particularly in bioprocess engineering.[3] In this area, Japan is a leader based on its fermentation capacity. In addition, by "generic research," the OTA means, for example, research on developing better bioreactors, screening microorganisms for industrial products, and generally providing research support on the genetics and biochemistry of industrially important microorganisms. The OTA report also calls for enhanced support for molecular biology and related disciplines, especially in agriculture (plant molecular biology).

In addition to the OTA's identifying government support for basic research and training as "most important" factors, the other "most important" factor was financing and tax incentives, such as the R&D limited partnership, the low capital-gains tax rate, and R&D tax credits. Regarding the antitrust laws, the OTA noted this area as a "least important" factor, principally because U.S. biotechnology companies lack the requisite "concentration," and there is an absence of measurable markets. Thus, most joint biotechnology research arrangements would not be anticompetitive. Tax approaches such as the R&D limited partnership and joint R&D ventures will be necessary for such promising areas as protein engineering and bioelectronics, or "biochips," where there will need to be significant public and private investment for joint research ventures in the years ahead.

The OTA noted government and industry collaboration in biotechnology in the United States as a "moderately important" factor. University and industry collaboration is growing in biotechnology to enhance the rapid dissemination of basic science discoveries for potential product development. Mechanisms also need to be considered to promote the transfer of research discoveries in government laboratories to industrial application. Some of the university–industry arrangements might be applicable to the government laboratories.

I should also note the state and local initiatives to attract and invigorate the biotechnology industries. In the Washington, D.C., area, the National Bureau of Standards (NBS) has joined with the University of Maryland to plan a new Center for Advanced Research in Biotechnology. The NBS has issued a number of planning reports regarding needs associated with industrial biotechnology, particularly bioprocesses. The center will involve industrial firms with federal, state, and local government support. Several of the area's biotechnology companies are expected to affiliate with the center, including Genex, Litton, and Meloy Laboratories.

This center represents the efforts of many of us who have worked with the Montgomery County Economic Advisory Council in the development of a life sciences center. The life sciences center is a 298-acre industrial park, planned and developed by the county government to provide space for the growing biomedical and related industries. Recently, a Commission on Higher Education was established by the County Executive to seek the establishment of a high-level academic and research university presence in Montgomery County. In the State of Maryland, Governor Hughes has created a High Technology Roundtable with an agenda for increasing support for technical education in the public schools and in graduate and postgraduate education and for enhancing Maryland's financial climate for high-technology business. The Greater Washington Board of Trade has a Task Force on Technology aimed at bringing together a number of key players in the high-technology area in relating their work to governmental, industrial, and academic efforts in the Greater Washington community. Of particular interest to the Board of Trade is recruiting more venture capital funds in the area to serve the needs o the new companies. These efforts complement those occurring in virtually every other state in the nation.

Federal Regulatory Policies

The OTA identified as a "moderately important" factor health, safety, and environmental regulations in the United States, principally because the system has worked quite well with the NIH guidelines and voluntary industrial compliance, and federal regulations (FDA, OSHA, EPA) have not, to date, impeded product development.

Federal agency regulatory policies are a significant factor in the development of products by the biotechnology industry. The NIH Guidelines (developed in 1976–1978) have served as the standards to govern this research nationally.[5] Compliance by industry has been voluntary. The system of governance includes local institutional biosafety committees, whose responsibility for the oversight of this research has grown over the past five years. The NIH's Recombinant DNA Advisory Committee is a broadly based public advisory group that monitors the research and the initial industrial scale-up. The first products have come under the jurisdiction of the Food and Drug Administration (FDA). All of the FDA bureaus are involved; virtually all of the biotechnology companies are involved with the FDA as products come "on-line." From the industrial experience thus far, the FDA will be able to use its existing regulatory authority to deal with biotechnology products without major changes in FDA regulatory law. The leadership of individuals in the pharmaceutical industry, like Irving Johnson, Vice-President for Research of Eli Lilly, has ensured a smooth transition from the NIH's Recombinant Advisory Committee to the FDA regulatory processes.

A major biotechnology policy area for health is the application of gene-splicing techniques to human beings. The President's Commission for the Study of Ethical Problems in Medicine and Biomedical and Behavioral Research issued a report in 1982 entitled *Splicing Life—A Report on the Social and Ethical Issues of Genetic Engineering with Human Beings*. It recommended continuing oversight in this area. We have a system in place—the institutional biosafety committees and the institutional review boards—to ensure that this technology, as it is applied to humans in the experimental setting, will meet the requisite ethical and safety standards. However, because of the importance of the ethical issues raised, there are a number of proposals in Congress to reestablish a presidential commission devoted to oversight in these biotechnology applications.

In my series for *Technology in Society*, Alex Capron, Staff Director for the President's Commission, viewed the advances in the medical uses of gene splicing and addressed their consequences for (1) human genetic makeup; (2) intergenerational responsibilities; (3) the distribution of social benefits; and (4) the conception of what a person is.[6] He described the first two effects as posing new ethical uncertainties by being able to change the human gene pool and, with that change, to affect people's link to, and responsibilities for, their progeny. The latter two effects raise new questions of conceptual uncertainty concerning how these technologies will be distributed and to whom, as well as the resulting social and public consequences that will arise from the potentially profound genetic changes possible to the individual.

All of our companies must also meet occupational safety and health standards. The health and safety record of the fermentation industries has been excellent. Biotechnology firms have health surveillance programs, biological safety reviews, and waste disposal engineering, all currently performed under federal and state regulatory standards. Some have asked whether the small companies have health surveillance procedures, and they do, if only to answer the liability issues. Several of the smaller companies have instituted ongoing health surveillance and safety programs through outside contractors. In the Boston area, the biotechnology companies operate an excellent surveillance program in concert with Peter Bent Brigham Hospital. The program is monitored by the local Cambridge biosafety committee. The Boston model may be useful for the Washington area, possibly with Johns Hopkins University operating such a program for the bio-technology companies.

Another major policy area is the deliberate release into the environment of recombi-nant-DNA-containing organisms. The NIH Guidelines initially prohibited deliberate release into the environment in response to requests by environmental groups, which were most concerned about the potential effect of this technology on the environment. The prohibition was removed in April 1983 to permit case-by-case review by the NIH Recombinant Advisory Committee (RAC). Several proposals have come before the RAC and have been approved for field testing of genetically modified plants or organisms. These include the field testing of corn plants that have been transformed by corn DNA or corn sequences cloned in bacterial or yeast systems and field testing of tomato and tobacco plants transformed with bacterial and yeast DNA. One of the approved proposals involved the field testing of genetically modified bacteria for biologically controlling frost damage in plants. An environmental suit was filed in the district court in Washington to require environmental assessments of the proposed field testing, and the testing was held in abeyance pending the outcome of the litigation.

In May 1984, the District Court issued a preliminary injunction that temporarily enjoined NIH from approving the field testing of the genetically modified bacteria for controlling frost damage as well as any other deliberate release experiments. The order of the District Court was appealed by the NIH. In February 1985, the United States Court of Appeals for the District of Columbia Circuit vacated the District Court's injunction as it applied to future approvals of deliberate release experiments by NIH. However, the Appeals Court upheld the preliminary injunction as it applied to the field testing of the bacteria to control frost damage in plants. The Appeals Court concluded the injunction should remain in effect until NIH completed an appropriate environmental assessment of the proposed field testing. The NIH has completed the assessment, and the case is once again before the District Court for a rehearing.

There is a need for risk assessment in the deliberate release into the environment of genetically engineered microorganisms. A number of efforts are under way to bring together scientific leaders who know how to assess impacts on humans, animals, and plants. Martin Alexander of Cornell University noted that potential hazards associated with recombinant DNA technology will probably occur more quickly than with other technologies because of the speed with which this technology is advancing. He cited a number of examples of the harmful consequences of the introduction of organisms into the environment: chestnut blight, Dutch elm disease, and the flu epidemics.[7] He and others have focused on a recurrent theme: the need for a commitment from industry and government for research in this area. And, as John Donalds, Director of Biotechnology for Dow, has commented, industry has a responsibility for data gathering.[8] Industry must do the product development work and demonstrate the safety of its applications, and the EPA should map future action on the basis of these data.

In my biotechnology series in *Technology in Society*, former Senator Harrison Schmidt described his bill, which called for establishing risk-assessment demonstration projects for the federal government.[9] His proposal encouraged the government to tackle the multitude of statutes and regulations requiring different standards of risk assessment for purposes of regulation. He made a compelling case for this approach; EPA representatives have noted there are nine separate standards in nine statutes for the EPA's regulatory authority. Some of the regulatory standards are based on health effects and others on the best available technology. And EPA Administrator William Ruckleshaus has emphasized the need to distinguish risk assessment from risk management for the purposes of EPA regulation.

Because of the expanding industrial applications of biotechnology in health, agriculture, chemicals, and the environment, a Cabinet Council biotechnology working group was created in May 1984 with George A. Keyworth, the President's Science Advisor, as chairman. The working group reviewed all federal biotechnology research and regulatory policies and issued a report for public comment on December 31, 1984, recommending a number of administrative and regulatory changes to accommodate the accelerating pace of industrial R&D advances.

Noting the broad scope of applications beyond biomedical research of the NIH, the Cabinet Council working group recommended additional recombinant advisory committees be created for other federal agencies (Agriculture, National Science Foundation, Environmental Protection Agency, and Food and Drug Administration) with oversight by a government-wide Biotechnology Science Board reporting to the Assistant Secretary for Health of the Department of Health and Human Services. The report also provides policy statements by the Food and Drug Administration, Environmental Protection Agency, and Agriculture that address a number of the regulatory issues concerning health, agricultural, and chemical biotechnology applications. In its statement, EPA proposes regulations for genetically engineered products under the Toxic Substances Control Act and the Federal Insecticide, Fungicide and Rodenticide Act. Thus, mechanisms are coming into place to provide for product review by the EPA that complement those in place at the FDA.

The last area of regulatory oversight falls under the U.S. Department of Commerce's purview, namely, export controls. The OTA identified export controls as a "least important" factor, principally because there are few products from the industry, at present, that come under the purview of the Commerce Department's export controls. But the report noted that, as the products develop, export controls will become a very important area. Products are well under way, and actions must be taken now by the Commerce Department and the biotechnology industry to examine federal export policy for biotechnology products.

Action by the Department of Commerce to establish a technical advisory committee on export regulations for biotechnology is an important initiative. The Commerce Department is authorized to create advisory committees if there is sufficient industrial interest, and that interest has been documented in letters to the department from several biotechnology companies. Biotechnology representatives should also be given an opportunity to review and comment on drafts that include biotechnology and its products on the Military Critical Technologies List (MCTL). It should be noted that the application of genetic engineering to biological warfare was questioned at the Asilomar meeting in 1975, when scientists called for a temporary moratorium in the conduct of certain recombinant-DNA experiments pending the development of NIH guidelines. The U.S. government responded then and has reemphasized, most recently in 1983, that the Biological Weapons Convention prohibits such research for biological warfare purposes.

CONCLUSIONS

In biotechnology today, we have a vital and growing partnership among government, university, and industry, priming the flow of basic science discoveries and applications in virtually every industrial sector. Challenges by foreign competitors, like Japan, may loom on the horizon, but the biotechnology industry is healthy, vigorous, and well suited to meet those challenges. The OTA has noted that U.S. efforts to commercialize biotechnology are currently the strongest in the world. Japan's targeting of the biotechnology industry is regarded by the OTA as being a "least important" factor at present because of the strength of our national research capacity and industrial strength. However, Japan is, and will continue to be, our most serious competitor, principally because of its superb fermentation capacities. A key factor in our competitiveness is our patent system, which offers the best protection of biotechnology of any system in the world. But there are areas here as well, particularly in the plant area, where attention will need to be given to patent protection.

Our system for science support and industrial applications has served us well. As Dr. Lewis Thomas noted in the essay that concludes my *Technology in Society* series, "Today's biological revolution is unquestionably the greatest upheaval in the history of biology and medicine."[10] And as Dr. Thomas pointed out, the progress of science is not an orderly succession of logical steps but involves a cascade of surprises pursued by scientists who are generally curious as well as "nervous and jumpy" from ignorance. It is the recognition of this scientific process that has guided the NIH and the NSF in their support of investigator-initiated research grants through a rigorous peer-review system that fosters excellence in science, fueling advances such as today's biological revolution. We recognize the necessity of support for basic research from all major partners—government, academia, and industry—and, concomitantly, the indispensable need for circumspection and public oversight in the applications of this technology to humans and the environment.

REFERENCES AND NOTES

1. See generally Perpich, J. G., Guest Editor, "Biotechnology—The Impact on Societal Institutions," in *Technology in Society* 4(4) (1982), 5(1) and 5(3) (1983), and 6(1) (1984).
2. Krause, R., Is the biological revolution a match for the trinity of despair, *Technology in Society* 4(4): 267–282 (1982).
3. Commercial biotechnology: An international analysis, U.S. Congress, Office of Technology Assessment, Washington, DC (Jan. 1984).
4. See generally Perpich, J. G., Genetic engineering and related biotechnologies: Scientific progress and public policy, *Technology in Society* 5(1):27–49 (1983).
5. Perpich, J. G., Industrial involvement in the development of NIH recombinant DNA research guidelines and related federal policies, *Recombinant DNA Technical Bulletin* 5:59–79 (June 1982).
6. Capron, A. M., Human genetic engineering, *Technology in Society* 6(1):23–37 (1984).
7. Alexander, M., Spread of organisms with novel genotypes, *AAAS Advisory Committee, seminar series on bioengineering* (sponsored by the Environmental Protection Agency), May 17, 1983, Washington, D.C. (in press).
8. Donalds, J. E., Applications of Biotechnology in the Chemical Industry, *AAAS Advisory Committee, seminar series on bioengineering* (sponsored by the Environmental Protection Agency), February 9, 1983, Washington, D.C. (in press).
9. Schmitt, H., Biotechnology and the lawmakers, *Technology in Society* 5(1):5–14 (1983).
10. Thomas, L. S., Oswald Avery and the cascade of surprises, *Technology in Society* 6(1):37–41 (1984).

31

Governmental Responsibilities and Genetic Disease

Seymour Lederberg, Ph.D
Professor of Biology
Brown University
Box G
Providence, RI 02192

Governmental responsibility for dealing with genetic disorders is an old story that has expressed itself primarily through the knife, the law, and the purse. These past approaches are identified with the transmission of genetic handicaps, their detection by screening programs, and their understanding and treatment. In order to ask what government responsibilities should be, it may be instructive to review the contributions of these past efforts.

In the first quarter of this century, a number of states passed laws providing for the compulsory sterilization of mentally defective inmates of state hospitals.[1-4] Many of these statutes were judged unconstitutional for violation of the equal protection or due process clauses of the Fourteenth Amendment to the U.S. Constitution. However, these requirements were deemed to be met in the landmark case of *Buck v. Bell* in Virginia in 1925,[5] and shortly afterwards, Justice Holmes affirmed the constitutionality of the Virginia statute in a review by the U.S. Supreme Court.[6] The important elements accepted were the meeting of substantive and procedural due process and the existence of a minimal rational basis for the claimed interest of the state to promote the health of an individual and the welfare of the public.

In a later case, *Skinner v. Oklahoma*,[7] the Supreme Court approved of eugenic sterilization. It suggested that when due process is met, the primary question that remains is the uncertainty of the transmissibility of the socially injurious tendencies of an individual. Subsequently, in *Roe v. Wade*, the Court[8] drew on *Buck v. Bell* to affirm the right of the states to assert and protect important interests in safeguarding "health" late in pregnancy. A concurring opinion by Justice Douglas detailed compulsory vaccination in epidemics and compulsory sterilization of individuals with heritable forms of insanity or imbecility as examples of such important interest.[9] According to both liberal and conservative Justices of the Court, it would appear that, at present, the state has a far greater interest in preventing conception by certain individuals, than it has in preventing the use of contraception in general.

In the period 1907–1964, eugenic sterilizations were reported on about 64,000 persons, the actual number being probably significantly higher.[3] The practice is now less frequent. Compulsory sterilization laws have been repealed by many states or have been replaced by laws allowing voluntary sterilization. Reversible contraceptive measures have provided an alternative and less punitive protection to the institutionalized retarded female. A second pressure for voluntary action comes from the difficulty in determining the inheritability of mental deficiency and from the continuum in the empirical risk of the birth of retarded offspring to two retarded parents (as compared to nonsymptomatic or normal parents). Finally, a eugenic rationale for compulsory sterilization of the retarded could be levied against any serious genetic syndrome.

For example, cystic fibrosis is a life-limiting autosomal recessive genetic disorder. The frequency of heterozygote carriers in most Western populations is about 4%–5%.[10] The afflicted homozygotic person is rarely fertile, so most children with this disorder are born to parents who are asymptomatic heterozygote carriers. A family with a child diagnosed for cystic fibrosis has a 25% probability that another child will inherit this disease, a risk comparable to the estimates of inheritability of retardation in children of retarded parents.[11] Therefore, in order to reduce public health costs (or from a broader eugenic perspective), there is as much a state interest in sterilizing carriers of cystic fibrosis and other recessive genetic disorders as there is in sterilizing the institutionalized mentally retarded. Of the major governmental approaches to dealing with genetic handicaps, prevention of transmission by compulsory sterilization offers the gravest concerns and should find the fewest advocates.

Another major avenue of governmental involvement lies in the statutes and regulations concerned with screening people for genetic disorders. This theme was treated in the First Symposium on Law and Genetics, and only the broader issues are summarized here.

There are two major reasons for genetic screening. One is to identify a genetic condition presymptomatically in order to treat affected individuals before irreversible harm occurs. At present, only a few genetic handicaps are helped by this information. Phenylketonuria is the most frequently tested condition in neonatal screening programs, and even here a few states provide such screening as a recommended but voluntary, preventive medicine service.[12] The major requirement is not on family compliance but on the attending physician or the hospital to provide PKU screening as standard medical practice, and in most states, parents can object to neonatal screening. If early detection provides no therapeutic benefits, then a second reason for genetic screening should be to serve primarily as a family-planning aid available on a voluntary basis. Nondirective counseling and confidentiality are obligatory features of any mass counseling program where the intent is to be medically useful without doing harm to individuals in need. In practice, the populations at risk for sickle-cell anemia, thalassemia, and Tay–Sachs disease are large enough for practical mass programs that screen adults for heterozygous carrier status. These handicaps can also be detected prenatally if abortion is an option desired by the parents.

The third mode of governmental intervention is support for basic and applied biological medical research. Its precedents go back two centuries to the establishment of a Marine Hospital Service for sick and disabled seamen and of quarantine facilities for ships bringing contagious diseases from abroad.[13] The problem of contagion was aggravated by a yellow fever epidemic in 1793, followed by outbreaks of smallpox, and later of cholera. A Federal Quarantine Act in 1878 appropriated funds for research into epidemic diseases, especially yellow fever and cholera. For this purpose, a National Board of Health was established to prevent contagious diseases and was given $50,000 to sponsor the first federal grants to universities for medical research. Under President Theodore Roosevelt, the U.S. Marine Hospital Service added the title U.S. Public Health to its name and added divisions of chemistry, pharmacology, and zoology to those of bacteriology and pathology at its National Laboratory of Hygiene. In 1930, the Hygienic Laboratory was greatly expanded into the National Institute of Health in order to pursue public health problems other than infectious diseases.

Experience with federal support of basic research in World War II confirmed the arguments that such support was in the national interest. Following that war, extramural research and fellowship programs flourished in the National Institutes of Health (NIH). Based on the same perspective, a National Science Foundation (NSF) was created in 1950 to develop a national research policy and to support basic scientific research and training.

This same period marked the beginning of a revolution in genetics, funded by the NIH and the NSF. It resolved the structure of DNA, the genetic code relating protein structure to DNA, and mechanisms of gene mutation, DNA replication, and the regulation of gene expression. Human cells were cultivated and studied *in vitro*. Chromosome analysis was developed, from the level of chromosome number to the detail of nucleotide structure in specific chromosome regions. Improvement in biopsy methods allowed fetal cells from the amniotic fluid or the chorion to be sampled in addition to adult cells, so that DNA and enzyme studies could be made throughout a human life cycle. As a result of this swell in fundamental information, the molecular basis of a number of genetic disorders unfolded.

Current research on genetic disorders finds substantial support in different institutes of the NIH. The National Institute of Allergy and Infectious Diseases (NIAID) sponsors studies on the structure and function of microbial nucleic acids and on the manipulation of nucleic acids to make medically useful products, including hormones needed for the treatment of certain genetic disorders. The NIAID also supports work on the genetic control of the immune system and its disorders. Comparable work on nucleic acids is pursued by the National Cancer Institute.

The National Heart, Lung, and Blood Institute coordinates a National Sickle Cell Disease Program and also sponsors research on other genetic disorders of the blood, such as thalassemia and coagulation factor defects, as well as on genetic factors underlying hypertension. Its Division of Lung Diseases has helped studies on genetically determined emphysema and shares work on cystic fibrosis with the National Institute of Arthritis,

Metabolism, and Digestive Diseases. The latter is also important for its support of research on diabetes and endocrine and metabolic disorders. Studies on glycolipid metabolism in the National Institute of Neurological, Communicative Disorders, and Stroke are especially important for a number of genetic neurological disorders such as Tay–Sachs.

These categorical institutes deal with the development of an information base for the diagnosis and treatment of specific genetic deficiencies. By contrast, two institutes have more general missions. One, the National Institute of Environmental Health, conducts and supports research on the effects of environmental agents on human health. An area of special significance is genetic damage due to natural and manmade mutagens in our air, water, and food supply. A mutagen-testing program screens materials in tiers of experimental systems: microbes, mammalian cells *in vitro*, insects, and whole animals, where mutagenic, teratogenic, and carcinogenic data can be compared. A risk assessment program evaluates these experimental data to determine the significance of human exposure at levels of agents encountered in the environment.

Another institute, the National Institute for General Medical Sciences (NIGMS), has the charge of sponsoring research opportunities in basic medical sciences that may lead to generalizable concepts of significance. It shares with the National Science Foundation a goal of understanding fundamental biological processes. Its genetic program has been a major sponsor of research on gene structure, mechanisms of gene transmission and expression and the elucidation of genetic principles common to all genetic disorders. Toward this end, the NIGMS supports genetic research centers, favoring collaborative work between basic and clinical scientists and research training programs in the broad areas of basic and clinical genetics. It has been particularly helpful in mapping the chromosomal sites of human genes and in supporting a national repository for cells from patients with heritable disorders.

Since 1983, two broad lines of genetic research supported by federal and private foundation funds have become especially exciting. Restriction enzymes had previously been used to distinguish, at the DNA level, chromosomes bearing sickle-cell or thalassemia defects in hemoglobin.[14,15] A similar approach has now shown that a particular pattern of sensitivity to restriction enzymes is closely linked to the defective gene responsible for Huntington chorea.[16] The work is significant in that it should shortly lead to the isolation of the Huntington gene, from which its activity can be understood and possibly controlled. The restriction enzyme approach will allow the use of DNA probes for genetic screening, so that individuals at risk can be advised whether they have inherited the dominant gene for this disorder. However, unless a treatment is also found, this opportunity raises serious unresolved ethical problems.

A second major research direction has resulted in engineering defective retroviruses to carry particular genes that can be inserted into chromosomes and expressed in cells infected by these viruses.[17] The viruses are defective in their ability to make coats, and cannot mature to infect new cells. The target cells can be chosen with short lifetimes or with the ability to multiply and maintain inserted genes. The problem of gene therapy of deficient genes is now the regulation of the expression of the transferred ones. It is likely that the first success in humans will come for genetic deficiency disorders in which a small amount of the normal product made in a few cells will be adequate for an individual.

A century ago, the federal appropriation for medical research to the predecessors of the NIH and the NSF amounted to about $50,000. Now it is about $5 billion for fellowships, research and training grants, and intramural programs in the health sciences. This is an impressive amount, although we all feel that more is needed, especially for genetic health services. Only a portion of the medical research support can be identified primarily with genetic problems, yet a unifying view shows strong relationships among the mutational changes leading to genetic disorders, to oncogenes, to oncogene activation and cancer, and to the monoclonal origin of arteriosclerotic plaques in cardiovascular disease.

If we compare different governmental approaches to genetic problems, providing a generous purse for basic genetic and medical research and making this science available for noncompulsory use are effective roles. But the goal is to help people in need of medical care. When we wage wars on infectious disease, we envisage defeating hostile and alien forms of life. The idea of stamping out our own genes, when they do not work as well as they might, has led to concern that other improvements might be pursued. The best precaution against a self-directed genetic imperialism is to remind ourselves that our purpose in treating genetic handicaps should be to reduce illness and harm to the individual.

Finally, in response to earlier controversial remarks on progress, technology, and eugenics, I believe that we take ourselves too seriously. As with some strains of mutant mice, we are imperfect in genes that determine body hair. We correct this genetic defect by using appropriate clothing. Without this correction, we would at best have a very limited ecological niche. Comparable adaptive responses are available for other challenges. I don't know if we want to call these responses progress. We do call them civilization.

References

1. O'Hara, J. B., and Sanks, T. H., Eugenic sterilization, *Georgetown Law J.* **45**:20 (1956).
2. Haller, M. H., *Eugenics*, Rutgers University Press, New Brunswick, NJ (1963).
3. Robitscher, J., *Eugenic Sterilization*, Charles C Thomas, Springfield, IL (1973).
4. Ludmerer, K. M., *Genetics and American Society*, Johns Hopkins University Press, Baltimore (1972).
5. *Buck v. Bell*, 143 Va. 310 (1925).
6. *Buck v. Bell*, 274 U.S. 200 (1927).
7. *Skinner v. Oklahoma*, 316 U.S. 535 (1942).
8. *Roe v. Wade*, 410 U.S. 113 (1973).
9. See 8 supra and *Doe v. Bolton*, 410 U.S. 179 at 215.
10. Conneally, P. M., Merritt, A. D., and Yu, P-L., Cystic fibrosis: Population genetics, *Texas Reports on Biology and Medicine* **31**:639–50 (1973).
11. Reed, E. W., and Reed, S. C., *Mental Retardation: A Family Study*, W. B. Saunders, Philadelphia (1965), 56.

12. *State Laws and Regulations on Genetic Disorders, July 1980,* U.S. Dept. Health and Human Services, DHHS Publication No. (HSA) 81-5243 (1981).

13. Furman, B., *A Profile of the United States Public Health Service 1798–1948,* U.S. Dept. of Health, Education and Welfare, DHEW Publication No. (NIH) 73-369 (1973).

14. Chang, J. C., and Kan, Y. W. A sensitive new prenatal test for sickle cell anemia, N. *Eng. J. Med.* **307**:30–2 (1982).

15. Orkin, S. H., *et al.,* The molecular basis of α-thalassemias: Frequent occurrence of dysfunctional α loci among non-Asians with Hb H disease, *Cell* **17**:33–42 (1979).

16. Gusella, J. F., *et al.,* A polymorphic DNA marker genetically linked to Huntington's disease, *Nature* **306**:234–8 (1983).

17. Mann, R., Mulligan, R. C., and Baltimore, D., Construction of a retrovirus packaging mutant and its use to produce helper free defective retrovirus, *Cell* **33**:153–9 (1983).

32

LEGISLATIVE REGULATION OF FETAL EXPERIMENTATION

On Negotiating Compromise in Situations of Ethical Pluralism

CHARLES H. BARON, LL.B., PH.D.
Professor of Law
Boston College Law School
885 Centre Street
Newton, MA 02159

> *The general public must be heard on these debatable issues, and the medical profession has an obligation to assist lay people to understand the medical implications as well as to formulate its own collective thoughts.*
> Experiments on the Fetus, 2 Br. Med. J. 433, 434 (1970).

In 1977, the authors of a leading work on human experimentation stated, "Of all research discussed in this book, experimentation with fetuses is perhaps the most controversial."[1] It had not always been thus. Prior to 1973 and the decision in *Roe v. Wade*,[2] fetal experimentation had been conducted with little public concern.[3] This fact has led some to suggest that opposition to fetal experimentation is largely a rear-guard action being fought by opponents of the *Roe* decision who do not want burgeoning medical benefits from fetal research to impede their antiabortion efforts.[4] But the timing of the fetal experimentation controversy can be explained in other ways as well. Prior to *Roe*, most fetal research in the United States was claimed to be incidental to and consistent with therapeutic efforts.[5] Without widespread elective abortion, there were not widespread opportunities for *ex utero* experimentation on living abortuses or *in utero* experimentation on fetuses scheduled for abortion. After *Roe*, there was suddenly the prospect of millions of fetuses offered

I would like to dedicate this chapter to the memory of my former colleague and beloved adversary, James W. Smith.

as ideal subjects for such experimentation on the grounds that (1) they were of question-able status as human beings;[6] (2) they were scheduled to die; and (3) as experimental subjects, they could make important contributions to the power of medical science to save the lives or improve the health of others. To many observers, this scenario seemed frighteningly familiar. Just 30 years before, medical doctors had used the same grounds to justify human experimentation on the millions of inmates at the Nazi death camps.[7]

Three months after the *Roe* decision, the *Washington Post* published a series of articles that focused public attention on the ethical questions raised by fetal experimenta-tion.[8] One American physician was quoted as saying, "It is not possible to make this fetus into a child, therefore we can consider it as nothing more than a piece of tissue. It is the same principle as taking a beating heart from someone and making use of it in another person."[9] In what seemed a prediction of what could now be expected in the United States, the *Post* article reported disturbing experiments in other countries that had longer-standing liberal abortion policies. In Britain, a commission headed by Sir John Peel had had to lay down guidelines "to end what virtually everyone agreed was an abuse—obtaining months-old fetuses for research and keeping them alive for up to three or four days."[10] And the *Post* reported,

> some scientists have said that at least a few research programs involving the study of live aborted fetuses in the short time before they die have been supported with NIH funds, some of them performed by U.S. scientists abroad.[11]

In July of 1974, a congressional moratorium was imposed on federal funding of fetal research until the new National Commission for the Protection of Human Subjects of Biomedical and Behavioral Research promulgated guidelines governing it.[12] In the sum-mer of 1975, the commission issued, after months of hearings and deliberation, its final report.[13] Shortly thereafter, the commission's recommendations were partially codified as federal regulations.[14]

In the meantime, a great deal of legislative action was occurring at the state level. In 1973, statutes regulating some forms of fetal experimentation were passed in four states: California, Indiana, Minnesota, and South Dakota.[15] In 1974, five more states were added: Kentucky, Massachusetts, Montana, Ohio, and Utah.[16] In 1975, two: Arizona and North Dakota.[17] In 1976, California[18] and Massachusetts[19] amended their statutes. In 1977, Indiana amended its statute,[20] and three states passed new ones: Maine, Nebras-ka, and Wyoming.[21] In 1978, Louisiana and Oklahoma passed statutes.[22] A peak was reached in 1979, when Nebraska amended its statute[23] and new statutes were passed in five states: Florida, Illinois, Missouri, New Mexico, and Tennessee.[24] Since then, new statutes have been limited to one each year: Michigan in 1980, Rhode Island in 1981, Pennsylvania in 1982, and Arkansas in 1983.[25] However, there were also two amend-ments: Florida in 1980 and Louisiana in 1981.[26] At this writing (1984), the total of states with statutes explicitly regulating fetal experimentation is 25.

In some of these states, such statutes would seem to have only symbolic value. One would doubt that there were research facilities in states such as Wyoming or Montana set up for fetal research. On the other hand, the impact of such statutes in major research states such as California and Massachusetts is real. And there is a considerable potential price to be paid. Even those who take a cautious position regarding fetal research must admit that there is much medical benefit to be gained from certain sorts of fetal experimentation.[27] Studies on dead fetuses may be valuable for the same reasons as are autopsies on dead adults.[28] If recently deceased, the fetus may offer living organs to be transplanted[29] or living tissues that can aid "studies of developmental genetic problems, growth regulation, and discovery of the early antecedents of human disease."[30] Fetuses *in utero* that are scheduled for abortion provide opportunities for perfecting and practicing therapeutic techniques such as amniocentesis, fetoscopy, and chorionic villus biopsy without risk of inducing injury or abortion to a wanted fetus.[31] They also provide opportunities for research into other forms of fetal diagnosis and therapy, for research into methods of improved therapy, and for placental transfer studies that may improve medical care for expectant mothers and their wanted fetuses.[32] And research on nonviable but still living abortuses can produce data on fetal physiology and metabolism or develop new methods for neonate life-prolongation, which could improve techniques for saving the lives of prematurely born infants.[33]

Clearly, the great promise and the grave threat of fetal experimentation present our society with a painful dilemma. In many ways, the dilemma is the same as that presented by abortion: we are again weighing the life, dignity, and comfort of the fetus (or abortus) against the lives, dignity, and comfort of others. On the other hand, there are important ways in which the dilemmas differ. With rare exceptions, we are not faced in the case of fetal experimentation with the mother's claim to reproductive autonomy.[34] It does not seem to me to necessarily follow from the fact that the mother has a right to be free of an unwanted pregnancy that she has a right to determine what shall be done to the fetus before, during, or after its removal from her body.[35] Perhaps as a result, we are presented with another difference—a legal one. Thus far, there is no Supreme Court decision constitutionally restricting fetal experimentation laws in the way that *Roe* restricted abortion laws. Consequently, federal and state legislative bodies have felt free to engage in the development of substantive laws that reflect each jurisdiction's notion of the appropriate compromise of the competing values involved.

On the federal level, fetal experimentation is governed by the regulations that were promulgated on the recommendation of the National Commission.[36] Because federal substantive lawmaking powers are limited to those traceable to an explicit grant of power in the federal Constitution,[37] the federal regulations apply only to "all research involving human subjects conducted by the Department of Health and Human Services or funded in whole or in part by a Department grant, contract, cooperative agreement or fellowship."[38] On the one hand, these regulations go beyond the power of the states in that they regulate "research conducted or funded by the Department of Human Services outside the United States."[39] On the other hand, they do not regulate fetal experimentation in the various states that is not funded or conducted by the department.[40] Moreover, even as to fetal experimentation that is so conducted or funded, the regulations provide that "[N]othing in this subpart shall be construed as indicating that compliance with the procedures set forth herein will in any way render inapplicable pertinent State or local laws bearing upon activities covered by this subpart."[41]

The protections of the federal regulations are a function of three central concepts: (1) informed consent; (2) a weighing of the risks to the fetus against the benefits to be obtained by the research; and (3) the distinction between therapeutic and nontherapeutic research. Informed consent is required from both father and mother, except for certain instances where the father's consent is not required.[42] In addition, the risk to the fetus may not be higher than certain thresholds specified. Those thresholds fall into a small number of classes, which are a function of (1) whether the experimental procedure is therapeutic to either the mother or the fetus and (2) the status of the fetus, as either *in utero* or *ex utero*, living or dead, and viable or nonviable. Where the experiment is on a pregnant woman, it may proceed if it is for the purpose of providing therapy to the mother or if "the risk to the fetus is minimal."[43] Where it is on a fetus *in utero*, it may proceed if it is for the purpose of providing therapy to the fetus or if the risk is minimal *and* "the purpose of the activity is the development of important biomedical knowledge which cannot be obtained by other means."[44] If the fetus is *ex utero*, experimentation standards become a function of whether it is living and, if living, whether it is viable. If it is viable, it is considered a "premature infant" and is entitled to the protections of other portions of the regulations.[45] If it is not viable, experimentation may be done even if it is of more than minimal risk if "the purpose of the activity is the development of important biomedical knowledge which cannot be obtained by other means" and if the research will neither artificially maintain vital functions nor purposely terminate the fetus' heartbeat or respiration.[46] If it is not yet clear whether the fetus is viable or not, experimentation may proceed if it is for the purpose of providing therapy to the fetus or if "there will be no added risk to the fetus resulting from the activity and the purpose of the activity is the development of important biomedical knowledge which cannot be obtained by other means."[47] If the fetus is dead, regulation of experimentation on it is left entirely to applicable state law.[48]

The federal regulations also comprise a number of significant general provisions defining important terms, prescribing procedures, setting up institutions, and imposing broad substantive standards. Most important among the substantive standards specific to fetal experimentation are five that require (1) that animal and nonpregnant human studies be exhausted before fetal experimentation is resorted to;[49] (2) that "in all cases, . . . the least possible risk for achieving the objectives of the activity" should be the minimum standard;[50] (3) that participants in the research should have no part in decisions regarding the procedures used for abortion or regarding the viability of the fetus;[51] (4) that no changes in the abortion procedure solely in the interest of the research will be made if they create more than minimal risk;[52] and (5) that "no inducements, monetary or otherwise, may be offered to terminate the pregnancy solely in the interest of the activity."[53] Most important among the procedural and institutional provisions is the establishment, in addition to the institutional review boards,[54] of one of more ethical advisory boards to rule on questions regarding the applicability of the regulations to specific experimental projects and classes of projects.[55] With the Secretary of Health and Human Services, they also have the power to waive the provisions of the regulations in specific cases on the ground that the risks to the subject are so outweighed by the sum of the benefit to the subject and the importance of the knowledge to be gained as to warrant such modification or waiver and that such benefits cannot be gained except through a modification or waiver.[56]

Supplementing the federal regulations are the 25 state statutes mentioned earlier, which explicitly regulate fetal experimentation in one or another form. Supplementing these regulations as well is the Uniform Anatomical Gift Act (UAGA), which was passed in all of the 50 states in the five-year span from 1969 through 1973.[57] The UAGA governs experimentation on dead fetuses along with dead humans generally by dint of including within its definition of a "decedent" any "stillborn infant or a fetus."[58] As a result, it serves as a backdrop against which all the later-state statutes have been written. Its provisions allow for the gift of "all or part of the . . . body" of a dead fetus to be used for research or therapeutic purposes.[59] Such gift may be made by "either parent"[60] and must take the form of "a document signed by him or made by telegraphic, recorded telephonic, or other recorded message."[61] The act prescribes respectful treatment of the decedent's remains.[62] And it provides that

the time of death shall be determined by a physician who tends the donor at his death, or, if none, the physician who certifies the death. The physician shall not participate in the procedures for removing or transplanting a part.[63]

No sanctions are imposed for any violations of the terms of the act, and it provides that

a person who acts in good faith in accord with the terms of this Act or with the anatomical gift laws of another state or a foreign country is not liable for any damages in any civil action or subject to prosecution in any criminal proceeding for his act.[64]

When we move from the UAGA to look at the 25 statutes passed since 1973, we find anything but uniformity among the various provisions enacted. Indeed, 6 of these statutes undermine the uniformity provided by the provisions of the UAGA by placing serious restrictions or prohibitions on the use of dead fetuses for research,[65] and they range from the very strict to the very liberal. Perhaps the most strict statute is one passed in Arizona in 1975:

A person shall not knowingly use any fetus or embryo, living or dead, or any parts, organs or fluids of any such fetus or embryo resulting from an induced abortion in any manner for any medical experimentation or scientific or medical investigation purpose except as is strictly necessary to diagnose a disease or condition in the mother of the fetus or embryo and only where the abortion was perfomed because of such disease or condition.[66]

At the other extreme are a statute passed in South Dakota in 1973:

Experimentation with fetuses without written consent of the woman shall be prohibited.[67]

And one passed in Tennessee in 1979:

(a) It shall be unlawful for any person, agency, corporation, partnership or association to engage in medical experiments, research, or the taking of photographs upon an aborted fetus without the prior knowledge and consent of the mother.

(b) No person, agency, corporation, partnership or association shall offer money or anything of value for an aborted fetus; nor shall any person, agency, corporation, partnership or association accept any money or anything of value for an aborted fetus.

(c) It is the express intent of the general assembly that nothing in the provisions of this section shall be construed to grant to a fetus any legal right not possessed by such fetus prior to July 1, 1979.[68]

However, the vast majority of the statutes fall between these extremes, and despite their great variety, they are amenable to description in terms of a few helpful classifications.

Only New Mexico's 1979 statute models itself on the federal regulations, and even it differs from the federal model in many of its substantive provisions.[69] However, most of the criteria employed by the federal regulations have found their way into the state statutes as well. The difference is in the way that they are employed as combinations of necessary and sufficient conditions, the varying importance they are given, and the extent to which they are supplemented by additional criteria. Typically, the state statutes give lessened importance to maternal consent and a weighing of the costs to the fetus against the benefits to medical science.[70] Instead, they tend to ban all nontherapeutic research on the living product of conception. But there are two very common and interesting limitations. First, they most often prohibit such experimentation only on fetuses that are planned to be or that have been aborted.[71] Second, at least eight statutes do not explicitly prohibit research on the fetus *in utero*; they focus exclusively on use of the living abortus.[72] Presumably, one reason is the pragmatic and *ad hoc* nature of state legislation of this sort. In the wake of *Roe* and the revelation it generated of experiments on the living abortus, some legislatures concerned themselves solely with that acute problem. Where they did consider the problem of experiments on fetuses *in utero*, they again focused only on the plight of the fetus whose natural protector, its mother, had determined to have it aborted. Moreover, as some prochoice advocates have suggested, the legislators may also have focused on cheating medical science of any benefits that might flow from *Roe*.

Yet another difference from the federal regulations is a frequently found prohibition on trafficking in live abortuses. This may also be explained as a legislative *ad hoc* response—this time to post-*Roe* rumors that such trafficking had reached disturbing proportions in other countries. In two states, only trafficking in fetuses is prohibited.[73] There is no direct prohibition on experimentation.

Despite the lack of uniformity in the precise language of the various statutes, one finds, in reading them, a sense of development around certain issues and a repetition of concepts and terms of art. There is, however, only one instance of a statute's being taken as a form by other states and adopted by them in either unchanged or modified form. That one model is the statute adopted by Massachusetts in 1974.[74] In 1975, it was adopted in North Dakota with only one minor addition.[75] In 1980, the statute, this time with important improvements in language, was adopted by Michigan.[76] Finally, in 1981, Rhode Island adopted the statute in its original form.[77]

What do these state statutes add overall to the federal regulations by way of restrictions on fetal experimentation? In sum, their impact is as follows:

1. Twenty-five states have no restrictions. They have only the enabling provisions of the Uniform Anatomical Gift Act as to dead fetuses.

2. Two permit fetal experimentation of all sorts as long as maternal consent is obtained.[78]

3. Of the remaining twenty-three:

(A) Regarding dead fetuses. Nine permit experimentation on dead fetuses under the terms of the UAGA.[79] An additional eight permit experimentation on dead fetuses under the terms of the UAGA with very slight modifications.[80] The remaining six do not permit nontherapeutic research on even dead fetuses if they are the product of a therapeutic abortion.[81]

(B) Regarding live fetuses *in utero*. Eight place no restrictions on experimentation with fetuses *in utero*.[82] An additional two allow experimentation on fetuses *in utero* if "no significant risk to the fetus is imposed by the research activity"[83] or if "verifiable scientific evidence has shown [it] to be harmless to the conceptus."[84] The remaining thirteen will not allow nontherapeutic experimentation on the fetus *in utero* if it is the subject of a planned abortion.[85]

(C) Regarding live abortuses. Two states seem to place no restrictions on medical experimentation on live abortuses.[86] Two states allow experimentation on live abortuses if it poses no significant risk to the abortus[87] or if it is harmless to the abortus.[88] The remaining nineteen states allow no nontherapeutic experimentation on live abortuses.[89]

It might well be argued that this complicated patchwork quilt of legislation presents us with the worst of all possible worlds. It is a world in which no one seems to win. Defenders of the rights of the fetus have lost all protection for the fetus beyond those of the federal regulations in more than half of the American jurisdictions, and they have been cheated of many protections that they might want in many of the others. On the other hand, opportunities for important research are lost to the medical and scientific communities in those states that have restrictive statutes, and in all 50 states, medical researchers face the federal regulations that cover all federally funded research. And where is justice? If it is "right" to experiment on abortuses or fetuses under certain circumstances, then it should be permissible to experiment on them under those circumstances in every jursidiction. If it is "wrong," then it should be prohibited in every jurisdiction.

The problem is that there is no fast, easy, and satisfactory route to uniform "right" rules in a democratic society—especially one that is federated into 50 sovereign states. To whom shall we look for such rules? The medical community? As intelligent, well-educated, and expert in the field of medical science as its members may be, they are not experts in morals and statecraft. They are also, like all other mortals, capable of judging state questions from a viewpoint more narrow than that of the public good—more narrow even than their perception of the public good. As one Harvard researcher admitted in print:.

> I share in a common guilt to which all of us within academic medicine must admit, an ambitious hunger for new discoveries. While we do truly labor for the common good, we also strive for personal recognition; our own egos bob embarrassingly to the surface of swelling altruism.[90]

Shall we look then to religious leaders or philosophers to lay down uniform rules of right conduct here? Of course, even if we did, we would not find such leaders and thinkers speaking with one voice. And even if they did, we would still have to ask ourselves whether we agreed, after reflection, with the rules that they endorsed unless we were ready, for some reason, to delegate decision-making power to them. In a majoritarian democracy, the buck stops with us—the voters. And we, the voters, are still in the process of making up our minds about how we collectively feel about fetal experimentation. As one ethicist observed in his testimony before the National Commission for the Protection of Human Subjects of Biomedical and Behavioral Research:

> There are few published discussions of the ethical issues involved in live fetus research. The few documents which do exist reveal that the Commission is faced with a situation of ethical pluralism. So far as I am able to detect, there exists no national consensus on the question of fetal research.[91]

Of course, under our Constitution, there are methods for cutting short the slow democratic process of consensus building. These methods were employed in *Roe* to cut short the process as regards abortion. And there are those who would like to see these methods employed as well regarding fetal experimentation.[92] I have argued elsewhere[93] that the U.S. Supreme Court was mistaken in removing the abortion issue from the majoritarian democratic process. Prior to *Roe*, national and local efforts were afoot to develop a new national consensus in favor of liberalized abortion laws. By 1972, one author could report, "In the short span of years since 1966, the starting date of a definite trend toward liberalization of abortion laws, proponents of liberalized abortion have gained significant ground."[94] Some 13 states had adopted one form or another of the liberalizing provisions of the Model Penal Code.[95] Another 4 had adopted laws permitting "abortion on demand" in terms similar to those that would later be prescribed by *Roe*.[96] In legislatures across the country, prochoice advocates were at work arguing, lobbying, and negotiating for liberalization of laws that criminalized abortion. When *Roe* came down, that process ended. The Supreme Court's own legislative compromise was set in constitutional concrete.[97] Prochoice and prolife advocates were no longer forced to engage in dialogue with each other in an effort to win the hearts and minds of a majority or to negotiate compromise. Worst of all, the Supreme Court made its decision hinge simplistically on only one of many factors relevant to the value issue raised: the age of the fetus. By declaring the unborn human being a nonentity under the U.S. Constitution, the Supreme Court essentially told the prochoice advocates that there was no longer any need for them to argue and negotiate with the prolife movement. And the prolife advocates were told that they had lost and, worse yet, that they had been "wrong." For constitutional law purposes, at least, life did not begin at conception; it began at birth.

In my earlier article, I argued that more weighs in the balance when one is making an abortion decision than

> just the stage of development of the potential life involved. On the same side of the balance, there is the matter of how long a potential life is at stake. The anencephalic fetus can expect no future life outside its mother. The fetus with Tay-Sachs disease can expect only a few years. There is also the matter of what the potential life is likely to be

worth to the fetus. Is the short life of sickness and gradual decline of the Tay-Sachs child better than no life at all? On the other side of the balance are the interests of the mother, the other members of her family, the other fetuses she might conceive if this one were aborted, and society as a whole. Is the mother likely to die in childbirth or has she just decided that the child would be born at an inopportune time? Is the family threatened with being sapped of emotional, physical, and financial strength by the addition of a severely disabled child or have the parents just decided that they would prefer a child of a sex different from that of the fetus? Do the parents plan other children that they will not have if they are forced to devote all of their resources to raising a severely disabled child? And, perhaps most important, what stake do the rest of us in society have in the outcome of the particular decision? In most cases, the benefit or detriment to society of the particular birth will be insignificant. But patterns and principles that may be produced by many such decisions hold the potential for societal impact of great significance. . . .

If anything should be clear from all of this, it is that there is no one abortion problem. There are as many abortion problems as there are possible combinations of all of the elements that might make a difference in our thinking about whether an abortion would be justified.[98]

The same is, of course, true of fetal experimentation: " 'fetal research' is not one but many things."[99] The great merit of the federal regulations, in my opinion, is that they grant a great deal of recognition to this fact by making their operation a function not only of the stage of development and viability of the fetus, but also of a weighing of the risk to the fetus against the need for and the value of the medical benefits to be obtained through the proposed research. Moreover, they have built into them processes for a constant refining of the rules on the basis of the facts of individual research applications. Not only do institutional review boards, with variegated constituencies,[100] judge specific research applications for their compliance with the regulations as written, but the ethical advisory board, with its equally varied composition,[101] has the power to modify the regulations when a specific research application shows itself as warranting such a modification. As a result, the opportunity for rule making on the basis of all of the relevant factors presented by actual cases is maximized.[102]

In contrast, the vast majority of the state statutes are, in my opinion, defective in that they lay down blanket prohibitions largely based only on the status of the fetus or the abortus. However, unlike decisions based on the U.S. Constitution, they do not eliminate the opportunity for refining rules on the basis of argument, experience, and negotiation. Legislation is only as strong as the majority it commands in a current legislature. If the medical community in a given jurisdiction believes it has facts that demonstrate that extraordinarily valuable medical research is being stifled that can be performed at what should be acceptable risks to fetuses and cannot be performed in any other way, it may always present those facts to the legislature and the public in an effort to win a majority. And opponents of fetal research are always welcome to present their own opposing facts and arguments. Such debates may go on for many years in many jurisdictions before trends begin to develop into a societal consensus. In the process, not only may the opposing advocates educate and persuade legislators and their constituents, they may educate and persuade each other. At the very least, the opponents may learn to compromise for the good of the society as a whole. And through coming to know and work with each other in the negotiation process, opponents who begin the process in suspicion and antipathy may end it respecting and even liking each other.

But we need not talk about the potential virtues of the legislative process in this area entirely in the abstract. They are amply illustrated by the Massachusetts experience as that was reported in a two-part series in *Science* magazine.[103] There we are told that, following the decision in *Roe* and the *Washington Post* articles, Massachusetts State Representative William Delahunt decided to introduce legislation regulating fetal experimentation: "Delahunt knew he did not know much about biomedical experimentation, but he thought he knew all he needed to know about cruelty to the unborn."[104] Together with Professor James Smith of the Boston College Law School, he drafted legislation that would have banned all research on fetuses, living or dead, if they were the subject of planned abortions. Learning at the last minute of hearings to be held on the bill, Dean Jack Ewalt of the Harvard Medical School began a process of involving the Massachusetts medical community in an effort to kill or modify it. He arranged for Arthur Hertig, a scientist who had worked with John Enders on the discovery of the polio virus, to attend the hearings: "Hertig had obtained fetal tissues that were essential for Enders' studies and he testified at the hearing that research with human embryonic and fetal tissue is vital to medical advances."[105] Having been put on notice of medical opposition to the law, Delahunt, Smith, and others arranged to begin meeting with an expanding number of representatives of the medical research community. Among the new researchers brought into the process was David Nathan, Professor of Pediatrics at Harvard and Chief of Hematology and Oncology at Children's Hospital Medical Center.

Nathan began as one of the most intransigent of the advocates for fetal research. When other researchers seemed ready to settle for a compromise that would have pemitted experimentation on dead fetuses, studies on living fetal tissues, and amniocentesis on fetuses that were not scheduled for abortion, he objected: "In fact, he recalls, 'I was in a rage. I felt we were selling out.' "[106] Nathan was on the verge of a breakthrough with a method of antenatal diagnosis of beta-thalassemia and sickle-cell anemia that depended on sampling fetal blood by means of fetoscopy. Because use of the fetoscope was still sufficiently experimental so that it might pose a substantial risk to a fetus, it would be prohibited by the compromise legislation:

> Nathan recalls that he tried on his own to get through to Delahunt and Smith to effect a change in the bill. "I had to convince them," he said, "that if I could diagnose sickle cell anemia . . . and thalassemia and other disorders in utero, I'd be preventing more abortions than they ever could. We have women who have an abortion because they don't want to risk having an afflicted child. With antenatal diagnosis, I could tell them three times out of four, to go ahead and have the baby." They listened but they were not persuaded.[107]

But Delahunt, Smith, and members of the state legislature were persuaded to yield on other points. In a series of negotiating sessions covering several weeks, further compromises were worked out in the scope and the language of the legislation that was enacted in June of 1974. At the end, Delahunt was "the first to admit that his original version of the bill would have been disastrous for research."[108] He reported that his "experience with the fetal research law has been broadening, instructing him in the way of science and scientists."[109] In order to continue the relationship between the legislature and the scientific community, he established a state advisory committee on medical research of which David Nathan was made a member. And

> The confrontation between the scientists and the lawmakers [had] been equally illuminating for the scientists who, as Delahunt puts it, "have learned that we in the Statehouse do not have horns." In fact, the individuals involved in the struggle to save fetal research consistently say, still with surprise in their tone, that Delahunt is a very "reasonable, rational" fellow, as are the other public officials they got to know. But the process was a trying one.[110]

David Nathan never did get the permission he wanted to make the breakthrough that he was seeking in the antenatal diagnosis of thalassemia and sickle-cell anemia. However, he continued to work with James Smith, who had become a respected friend, on possible compromise legislation until Smith died in the fall of 1982. Together, they did get the legislature to enact in 1976 an amendment that added procedures for obtaining advance rulings on the legality of fetal research activities so that pioneering efforts would not be made at the risk of after-the-fact criminal prosecutions.[111] Nathan's research requiring fetoscopy was brought to fruition by researchers in London and in New Haven, Connecticut, where the law is more favorable to fetal experimentation. [112] He and his colleagues have developed alternative methods using amniocentesis and analysis of DNA to make the antenatal diagnosis that he was after in three out of four cases in his clinic. The other cases he refers to physicians in New Haven for blood sampling by means of fetoscopy. And he still speaks of his experience with Smith, Delahunt, and the legislative process with great enthusiasm. "In the end," he said recently, "I had enormous regard for Jim—we all did. He had a wonderful capacity for listening, for thinking things out, and then coming back at you at a higher level of thought on the issue. At one point when the fetal experimentation furor was at its height, I had him come to speak at a meeting of the Harvard Medical Society. They thought they would make mincemeat of him. When he was finished with their questions, he had just *destroyed* their arguments. They really learned something."[113]

Justice Holmes once observed:

> There is nothing that I more deprecate than the use of the Fourteenth Amendment beyond the absolute compulsion of its words to prevent the making of social experiments that an important part of the community desires in the insulated chambers afforded by the several States, even though the experiments may seem futile or even noxious to me and to those whose judgment I most respect.[114]

And Holmes's frequent partner in dissent, Justice Brandeis, added to that thought in one of his opinions:

> To stay experimentation in things social and economic is a grave responsibility. Denial of the right to experiment may be fraught with serious consequences to the Nation. It is one of the happy incidents of the federal system that a single courageous State may, if its citizens choose, serve as a laboratory; and try novel social and economic experiments without risk to the rest of the country.[115]

Such social experiments seem to me to be at least as important to the public good as fetal experiments. They are not at present conducted as scientifically as fetal experiments.[116] But when they affect medical science, it is in the power of medical scientists to attempt to make them more scientific. At one point during the negotiations over fetal research legislation in Massachusetts, an observer described a meeting between legislators and researchers with disgust: "There they were, some of the biggest names at the Harvard Medical School standing up like schoolboys to describe their work and ask, 'Please, Mr. Legislator, may I go on with what I am doing?' "[117] In the social experiment in majoritarian democracy that involves us all, it is sentiments such as the one expressed in that statement that present the gravest threat to success. Even the greatest medical researchers count as only one when it comes time to vote. If their influence is to be any greater than that, it will have to come through the power of the facts and thoughts that they have to share with the rest of society. And to share those facts and thoughts, there is no choice for them but to enter an arena in which one may not only inform but also be informed, not only persuade but also be persuaded, and not only gain way but also give it.

ACKNOWLEDGMENTS

I would like to thank my research assistants, Jennifer Parks and Frank Son, for their valuable assistance in the research for and the preparation of this chapter.

REFERENCES AND NOTES

1. Annas, G., Glantz, L., and Katz, B., *Informed Consent to Human Experimentation: The Subject's Dilemma*, Ballinger Publishing Company, Cambridge, MA (1977), 195.
2. 410 U.S. 113 (1973).
3. See Munson, J., Fetal research: A view from right to life to wrongful birth, *Chicago-Kent L. Rev.* 52:133 (1975); P. Lehman, The future of fetal research in California: A proposal for change, *San Diego L. Rev.* 15:859, 863 (1978); Reback, G., Fetal experimentation: Moral, legal, and medical implications, *Stanford L. Rev.* 26:1191 (1974); Holder, A., *Legal Issues in Pediatrics and Adolescent Medicine*, Wiley, NY (1977), 67.
4. Nathan, D., Fetal research: An investigator's view, *Villanova L. Rev.* 22:384, 386 (1976–1977).
5. Holder, *supra* note 3, at 67.
6. Indeed, the U.S. Supreme Court had held that they were not "persons" entitled to protection under the Fourteenth Amendment to the Constitution. *Roe v. Wade*, supra note 2, at 158–9.
7. See *Traials of War Criminals before the Nuremberg Military Tribunals*, vols. 1 and 2, *The Medical Case*, U.S. Government Printing Office, Washington, D.C. (1948). See also, Mant, A., The medical services in the concentration camp of Ravensbruck, *Medico-Legal J.* 17:99 (1950).
8. Cohn, V., Considering ethics—Live fetus research debated, *Washington Post* (Apr. 10, 1973), §A, at 1, col. 5; Cohn, V., NIH vows not to fund fetus work, *Washington Post* (Apr. 13, 1973), §A, at 1, col. 4.
9. Cohn, *supra* note 8 (Apr. 10), §A, at 9, col. 1.
10. *Id.*
11. Cohn, *supra* note 8 (Apr. 13), §A, at 1, col. 4. Most often cited to among these foreign experiments is one that used eight decapitated fetal heads to demonstrate complete cerebral oxidation of D-BOH-Butyrate to CO_2 in a physiological system. See Adam, P., Räihä, N., Rahiala, E., and Kekomaki, M., Cerebral oxidation of glucose and D-BOH-butyrate by the isolated perfused human fetal head, *Pediatric Research* 7:309 (1973).

12. National Research Act, Pub. L. No. 93-348, § 213, 88 Stat. 353 (1974); 42 U.S.C. § 2891-1.
13. The National Commission for the Protection of Human Subjects of Biomedical and Behavioral Research, Report and Recommendations, *Research on the Fetus* DHEW Publication, No. (05) 76–127, Bethesda, MD (1975).
14. 40 FR 33528, Aug. 8, 1975, as amended at 40 FR 51638, Nov. 6, 1975; 45 C.F.R. §§ 46.201–46.211.
15. West's Ann. Cal. Health & Safety Code § 25956; Ind. Code § 35-1-58.5–6 [10-112]; Minn. Stat. Ann. § 145.422; S.D. Compiled Laws Ann. § 34-23A-17.
16. Ky. Rev. Stat. Ann. § 436.026; Mass. Gen. Laws Ann. ch. 112, § 12j; Mont. Rev. Codes Ann. § 94-5-617; Ohio Rev. Code Ann. § 2919.14; Utah Code Ann. § 76-7-310.
17. Ariz. Rev. Stats. § 36-2302 A; N.D. Cent. Code §§ 14-02.2-01 and 02.
18. Cal. Stats. 1976, c.941, p. 1963, § 1.
19. Mass. St. 1976, c.551.
20. Ind. P.L. 335, § 3, p. 1513.
21. Me. Rev. Stat. tit. 22, § 1574; Neb. Rev. Stat. § 28-4, 161; Wyo. Stats. 1977 § 35-6-115.
22. La. Rev. Stat. Ann. § 14:87.2; 63 Okl. St. Ann. § 1-735.
23. Neb. Laws 1979, LB 316, § 8.
24. West's Fla. Stats. Ann. §§ 390.001(6) and (7); Smith Hurd Ill. Ann. Stats ch. 38, § 81-26(3); Vernon's Ann. Missouri Stats. § 188.037; New Mex. Stats. Ann. §§ 24-9A-1 to 7; Tenn. Code Ann. § 39-4-208.
25. Mich. Stats. Ann. §§ 14.15 (2685) to (2688); R.I. Gen. Laws §§ 11-54-1 and 2; 18 Pa. Cons. Stats. Ann. § 3216; Ark. Stats. § 82-437 to 441.
26. Fla. Laws. 1980, c.80-208, § 1; La. Acts 1981, No. 774, § 1.
27. See, for example, Walters, L., Ethical and Public Policy Issues in Fetal Research, in National Commission for the Protection of Human Subjects of Biomedical and Behavioral Research, *Appendix to Research on the Fetus*, (1975), 8-1.
28. Reback, *supra* note 3, at 1192–3.
29. *Id.*
30. Lehman, *supra* note 3, at 861.
31. Walters, *supra* note 27, at 8-4.
32. *Id.* at 8-5.
33. *Id.* at 8-6.
34. Two exceptions may be (1) those cases where fetal experimentation may be indicated for the purpose of diagnosing problems in the mother that implicate future childbearing and (2) those cases where fetal experimentation may enable an unwanted abortus to become an unwanted child.
35. See, on the subject, Somerville, M., Reflections on Canadian abortion law: Evacuation and destruction—Two separate issues, *Univ. Toronto. L. J.* **31**:1 (1981).
36. *Supra* note 14.
37. In this case, the "spending power" under U.S. Const. art I, § 8, cl. 1. See Oklahoma v. United States Civil Service Comm'n., 330 U.S. 127 (1947).
38. 45 C.F.R. § 46.101(a).
39. *Id.* § 46.101(a)(2).
40. Except to the extent that a funded research institution must gain approval of "A statement of principles governing the institution in discharge of its responsibilities for protecting the rights and welfare of human subjects of research conducted at or sponsored by the institution, regardless of source of funding." *Id.* § 46.103 (b)(1).
41. *Id.* § 46.201(b).
42. His consent is not needed where "(1) the purpose of the activity is to meet the health needs of the mother; (2) his identity or whereabouts cannot reasonably be ascertained; (3) he is not reasonably available; or (4) the pregnancy resulted from rape." *Id.* § 46.207(b). See also §§ 46.208(b) and 46.209(d).
43. *Id.* § 46.207(a).
44. *Id.* § 46.208(a).
45. *Id.* § 46.209(c).
46. *Id.* § 46.209(b).
47. *Id.* § 46.209(a).
48. *Id.* § 46.210.
49. *Id.* § 46.206(a)(1).

50. *Id.* § 46.206(a)(2).
51. *Id.* § 46.206(a)(3).
52. *Id.* § 46.206(a)(4).
53. *Id.* § 46.206(a)(5).
54. *Id.* §§ 46.102(h) to 46.115.
55. *Id.* § 46.204.
56. *Id.* § 46.211.
57. See Uniform Anatomical Gift Act, Table of jurisdictions wherein act has been adopted, 8A *Unif. Laws Annot.* 8A:15–6 (1983).
58. Uniform Anatomical Gift Act § 1(b).
59. *Id.* § 2(b).
60. *Id.*
61. *Id.* § 4(e).
62. *Id.* § 7(a).
63. *Id.* § 7(b).
64. *Id.* § 7(c).
65. The statutes are those passed in Arizona, Illinois, Indiana, Louisiana, Ohio, and Oklahoma.
66. Ariz. Rev. Stats. § 36-2302 A.
67. S.D. Compiled Laws Ann. § 34-23A-17.
68. Tenn. Code Ann. § 39-4-208.
69. New Mex. Stats. Ann. §§ 24-9A-1 to 7.
70. Exceptions are the statutes in Minnesota, New Mexico, South Dakota, and Tennessee.
71. Exceptions are the statutes in Louisiana, Maine, Massachusetts, Michigan, Minnesota, Montana, New Mexico, North Dakota, Pennsylvania, Rhode Island, South Dakota, Tennessee, and Utah.
72. The statutes are those passed in Arkansas, California, Indiana, Kentucky, Montana, Nebraska, Ohio, and Wyoming.
73. Kentucky and Wyoming.
74. Mass. Gen. Laws Ann. ch. 112, § 12j.
75. N.D. Cent. Code §§ 14-02.2-01 and 02.
76. Mich. Stats. Ann. §§ 14.15 (2685) to (2688).
77. R.I. Gen. Laws. §§ 11-54-1 and 2.
78. South Dakota and Tennessee.
79. Kentucky, Maine, Minnesota, Missouri, Montana, Nebraska, New Mexico, Utah, and Wyoming.
80. Arkansas, California, Florida, Massachusetts, Michigan, North Dakota, Pennsylvania, and Rhode Island.
81. Arizona, Illinois, Indiana, Louisiana, Ohio, and Oklahoma.
82. Arkansas, California, Indiana, Kentucky, Montana, Nebraska, Ohio, and Wyoming.
83. New Mexico.
84. Minnesota.
85. Arizona, Florida, Illinois, Louisiana, Massachusetts, Michigan, North Dakota, Oklahoma, Pennsylvania, Rhode Island, Utah, Maine, and Missouri.
86. Arkansas and Utah.
87. New Mexico.
88. Minnesota.
89. Arizona, California, Florida, Illinois, Indiana, Kentucky, Louisiana, Maine, Massachusetts, Michigan, Missouri, Montana, Nebraska, North Dakota, Ohio, Oklahoma, Pennsylvania, Rhode Island, and Wyoming.
90. Hamilton, A., My turn: Who shall live and who shall die? *Newsweek* (March 26, 1984), 15.
91. Walters, *supra* note 27, at 8-7.
92. On the prolife side are those who are pressing the Human Life Amendment. See Westfall, D., Beyond abortion: The potential reach of a human life amendment, *Am. J. L. Med.* 8:97, 120 (1982). On the prochoice side, see Holder, *supra* note 3, at 82–87.
93. Baron, C., The concept of person in the law, in *Defining Human Life: Medical, Legal, and Ethical Implications* (Shaw, M., and Doudera, E., eds.), AUPHIA Press ASLM, Ann Arbor, MI (1983), 121,

previewed *sub nom* "If you prick us do we not bleed?": Of Shylock, fetuses, and the concept of person, *Law, Medicine, and Health Care* 11:52 (1983). (Citations hereinafter are to Shaw and Doudera.)

94. George, J., The evolving law of abortion, *Case Western L. Rev.* 23:708 (1972).

95. *Id.* at 740–1.

96. *Id.* at 742.

97. On the status of the court's ruling as a legislative compromise, see, for example, Ely, J., The wages of crying wolf: A comment on *Roe v. Wade*, *Yale L. J.* 82:920 (1973).

98. Baron, *supra* note 93, at 134–5.

99. Walters, *supra* note 27, at 8–6.

100. For membership requirements, see 45 C.F.R. 46.107.

101. "Members of these board(s) shall be so selected that the board(s) will be competent to deal with medical, legal, social, ethical, and related issues and may include, for example, research scientists, physicians, psychologists, sociologists, educators, lawyers, and ethicists, as well as representatives of the general public." *Id.* § 46. 204(a).

102. As regards my own preference for consensus development through rule making which is incident to decision making—especially decision making in courts of general jurisdiction—see Baron, C. , Medical paternalism and the rule of law: A reply to Dr. Relman, *Am. J. L. Med.* 4:337 (1979).

103. Culliton, B., Fetal research: The case history of a Massachusetts law, *Science* 187:237 (1975); Culliton, B., Fetal research (II): The nature of a Massachusetts law, *Science* 187:411 (1975).

104. *Id.* at 237.

105. *Id.*

106. *Id.*

107. *Id.* at 238.

108. *Id.* at 241.

109. *Id.*

110. *Id.*

111. Mass. St. 1976, c. 551.

112. Interview with Professor David G. Nathan, Chief, Hematology and Oncology, Children's Hospital Medical Center and Sydney Farber Cancer Institute, Boston, in Boston, March 27, 1984.

113. *Id.*

114. *Truax v. Corrigan*, 257 U.S. 312, 344 (1921) (dissenting opinion).

115. *New State Ice Co. v. Liebmann*, 285 U.S. 262, 311 (1931) (dissenting opinion).

116. See generally, Caplan, N., What do we know about knowledge utilization? *New Directions for Program Evaluation* 5:1 (1980); Saks, M., The utilization of evaluation research in litigation, *New Directions for Program Evaluations* 5:57 (1980); Koretz, D., Developing useful evaluations: A case history and some practical guidelines, *New Directions for Program Evaluation* 14:25 (1982).

117. Culliton, *supra* note 103, at 411.

DISCUSSION

DEAN WILLIAM SCHWARTZ (Boston University School of Law): I would like Dr. Perpich to comment on a point raised by Mr. Baron. He referred to the issue of compliance with the NIH standards and guidelines. I think the real development may come not from the government regulators, but from the instigation of private individuals who, when injured, bring a private lawsuit for damages. Will compliance with the federal standards be a defense to that private common-law action?

DR. JOSEPH G. PERPICH (Genex Corporation): My response is that we have a system that has worked thus far. The federal regulators are coming in, are accepting some standards, and are developing their own. When the tort suits come, if they come, I think we have a corpus of regulatory law and standards that will be helpful in terms of the suit before the court.

DEAN WILLIAM SCHWARTZ: I think by analogy to other areas, it should be noted that compliance with the government standard would be evidence of due care, but not necessarily conclusive. It won't be a complete bar to the suit.

DR. AUBREY MILUNSKY (Boston University School of Medicine): I would like to ask Dr. Albert Jonsen, what are the controlling ethical imperatives that govern corporate efforts in biotechnology?

DR. ALBERT R. JONSEN (University of California at San Francisco): You threw me a curve. I think there are three controlling imperatives relative to corporate developments in this area. The first one may sound odd, but I think it is perfectly ethical and reasonable. The first controlling imperative is making a profit. I put that as an ethical imperative, which people usually don't do, because I think that is the corporate way of stating a legitimate self-interest in making a living. I think that there is a legitimate principle of ethics called *self-interest*, but it's only one. I think they have a right—and, in fact, in some sense a duty—to make a profit in doing what they are doing.

But there are two important additional ethical principles that pose limitations. The second one is not very surprising. It's "Do no harm." That is, corporate enterprises have an ethical obligation to guarantee that what they do is safe in a variety of dimensions. There is the imperative of being a safe corporate body or producer, and of course, much of the effort of exercising oversight and control has to do with the safety. The third ethical imperative is probably the most difficult to express and even to think about. I can, on the spot, think of only one way of describing it, and that is to say that there must be appropriate development. I mean appropriate also in the etymological sense of fitting and what it is supposed to fit. The development has to fit genuine needs. I recognize, in saying that, that I open up a lot of questions. What are genuine needs? I only mention this third principle in order to note that, frequently, corporate endeavors do not meet needs but create needs. It's a marvelous ability of medicine to create its own needs. Often, major abuses come in creating a new disease that didn't exist before because you've got a medicine that can treat it. It seems to me that the underlying ethical question for the corporate developments in biotechnology has to do with the perception of what are, in fact, genuine needs. That would open up a great deal of debate about what constitutes a genuine need in society or individuals. I think that's the way I would start thinking about the problem.

DR. JACQUES LORRAIN (Sacred Heart Hospital, Montreal): It's fine to screen for genetic disease or to treat genetic disease. But I would like to come back to the matter of prevention. I would like to give you an example of what's going on in the Province of Quebec as far as law is concerned. We have legislation that enables a physician to withdraw pregnant women from work who would be exposed to mutagens or teratogens. This law makes it possible for women to be paid 50% of their full salary for the total length of pregnancy, and also for the breast-feeding period. I would like to ask Dr. Lederberg, Is it possible to have such a legislation here in the United States? I think that we have to take care of the woman who wants to bear children, and we owe this to the future generation. It is very important for the government to take care of nutrition and the environment. It is also very important for geneticists to be involved whenever genetic damage is possible.

DR. SEYMOUR LEDERBERG (Brown University): My initial response is to applaud this policy and to lament the lag in this country's support of family services. But this policy also has drawbacks. The removal of one vulnerable class from working-place hazards reduces the pressure to correct the problem for others left at risk, although they may be intrinsically less sensitive. It also leaves uncorrected the possibility of contaminants' being brought home on the clothing of workers, as occurred with asbestosis. A more satisfactory solution would be to require health standards in the working environment that protect the more sensitive fetus and the pregnant woman, and therefore all of us.

DEAN WILLIAM SCHWARTZ: Actually, Dr. Baram will be touching on this subject in his talk in the next panel. He has a project going right now at the Boston University School of Public Health with the National Science Foundation on biological monitoring in the workplace.

DR. JACQUES LORRAIN: Half of the salaries are given by the government, half come from the industry.

DEAN WILLIAM SCHWARTZ: You assume that we remember Joan of Arc because she had an inspired earning capacity. There are other factors. We remember Joan of Arc because of the pain and suffering she endured, and there are other legitimate human interests at stake in biological monitoring, including the right to privacy and confidentiality, and if a person is identified as someone who should be removed from the workplace, there may be countervailing considerations.

MR. GEORGE J. ANNAS (Boston University Schools of Medicine and Public Health): When I was listening when you said that you were involved in abortion rights before *Roe v. Wade*, that you were invested in that activity and enjoyed the process, and that you thought the Supreme Court was spoiling your fun solving the problem. You couldn't stay involved in the political process of trying to change state laws. You almost seemed to me to be saying, with regard to fetal research statutes, that the process should go on almost for the process's sake. You liked the 50 states struggling through a process, and you argued that there are never any answers anyway, so that the best we can do is keep going on with the process. But why can't we just come up with the best answer that we can come up with and live with that, at least for a time? We have to do something in these situations. When women are pregnant, you can't tell them there's no answer. You can't say, "We can't tell you whether you can have an abortion or not." You have to tell them whether they can have an abortion or not. When a scientist wants to research with a fetus, she or he has to know whether it will be possible to do it or not. Why can't we have the best answer we can have and then have people argue that it's not the right answer and try to change it later on?

MR. CHARLES H. BARON (Boston College Law School): You raise a good point. I think, once again, the medium is the message. I value that criticism of me. I think you have to suspect somebody whose business is dialogue, dialectic, and argumentation, just as you have to suspect somebody whose business is experimenting for the purpose of producing truth and new means of therapy for other people. I am to be suspected. There's no question about it. I love to argue. It's my life's work. One of the reasons that I teach instead of practicing law is that I didn't have enough opportunity to argue in the practice of law. I didn't get into court often enough.

DEAN WILLIAM SCHWARTZ: The courts are still congested, despite your absence.

MR. CHARLES H. BARON: And despite my best efforts to try to get some of these issues into the courts. I'm half lawyer, half philosopher. One of the things to avoid is committing the genetic fallacy. What could be more appropriate for this meeting? The genetic fallacy is to think that just because you can see where this argument is coming from means that it's wrong. Sure, where it's coming from is the fact that I love this dialectic process, among other things. But I see it at work, and what is the alternative when you can't get people to agree on something? The Massachusetts fetal research statute was a much better statute than Jim Smith would have wanted initially, because of the involvement of David Nathan, who favored no statute. What came out of the legislative process was something better, and more important, what came out of it was that the ideas of both of them were changed as a result of their arguing with each other. Why do people come to these conferences? You all had answers before you came.

I found, when I first started dealing with the question of abortion in my classes in law school, that everybody knew the answer. I'd take a poll at the beginning of the class, and everybody knew what the answer was. The problem was that it wasn't the same answer. Some people thought absolutely that there is a right to life on the part of the fetus. Other people thought absolutely that it's just a lump of tissue. It's like removing a skin tag, to have an abortion. But the more we talked about it, the more people thought that they didn't know, and the more they would compromise.

DEAN WILLIAM SCHWARTZ: Let me throw out an alternative to you that is common to your theme and to Dr. Lederberg's theme of eugenic sterilization. What about the procedure that has evolved in Massachusetts in the sterilization of the retarded. When a person is incompetent, we have a substituted judgment procedure in which the court appoints a guardian. Is that procedure appropriate to both fetal research and sterilization?

MR. CHARLES H. BARON: I think that the courts are the appropriate place to decide sterilization questions. As to whether they are an appropriate place to decide fetal experimentation questions, the state of Massachusetts has already spoken on that. This friendly bill that was drafted by Jim Smith and Dave Nathan was later amended on the request of the medical community to include a procedure for prior court review. If you, the researcher, have doubts about whether you can really do your research, you just go first to your institutional review board and have them approve it. Then you go to the courts of Massachusetts or to the disctrict attorney; you've got your choice. Either the district attorney can say, "I'm not going to prosecute you because this is acceptable," or you can ask the court to render a declaratory judgment in advance that this is acceptable. And for reasons that I have articulated at great length in other places, I think this is a terrific way to do it. It's really hard to know in advance what the answers are in general terms, but when you have a specific case, somehow or other, because you've got to come up with an answer, you negotiate the answer and gradually you develop principles.

DR. AUBREY MILUNSKY: I am responding to Mr. Baron. I think that this is an abysmal situation. What has happened in Massachusetts is absolute devastation. The Massachusetts Fetal Research Law has had not a chilling effect on fetal research, but a killing effect on fetal research. The consequence, for example, in one small avenue, is that fetoscopy is not possible in Massachusetts today. Citizens of the Commonwealth leave Massachusetts to go to Yale or elsewhere to have these studies done. Two things have occurred as a consequence of the bill that Mr. Baron talks about. I am not at all impressed by the process or the activity. I think you exaggerate David Nathan's pleasure in the process. I was part of that process, too. We were not at all happy in any dimension, because what has occurred is what was predicted: Women whose fetuses (and ultimately whose children) could benefit from the intercession of therapy by the use of fetoscopy, intrauterine transfusion, remedy through fetoscopy, and so forth do not benefit. All of that progress has been stilled in this state. It is not satisfactory to say, well, it can be done elsewhere. That is certainly not an answer.

MR. CHARLES H. BARON: Can I answer in order to say that things have been slightly exaggerated? It's perfectly acceptable to do fetoscopy in Massachusetts under the statute. The problem is that you can't experiment when you don't know how to do it on some fetus that's scheduled for abortion in order to be able to develop the capability to do it. That's all.

DR. AUBREY MILUNSKY: That's a complete absurdity to say you can do fetoscopy. You cannot do fetoscopy in Massachusetts because no one can perfect the technique to do it.

MR. CHARLES H. BARON: But they can perfect it at Yale and move to Massachusetts.

DR. GISELLE TOTH (Creative Strategies International): I would like to make a comment in defense of industry. I have spent 17 years in industry, and I can tell you that, had it not been for industry, we wouldn't have been able to see some genetic engineering products coming to the marketplace in such a rapid time. Dr. Perpich, we have about 200 small genetic-engineering firms across the country. Most of these small companies are dependent on corporations for financial support, corporations that have substantial equity shares in time. Do you see any tendency for these small firms to become part of the large corporations, either by becoming subsidiaries or by being completely engulfed by them? This would mean that corporations would have control over research projects more or less performed on a contract basis by the smaller companies.

DR. JOSEPH G. PERPICH: My quick answer is yes. The nature of the private markets and the system in this country is that the small are often gobbled by the big, and that the big are even gobbled by the bigger. You see a lot of that these days in the Wall Street press. But for every one of those, you've got scores of other little companies being created by venture capital and other equity investments. Genex, where I was for two years, is still standing on its own two feet. It has many equity investments, but it is getting enough revenue through a variety of devices to continue as it is. The question will always be whether a large company will take it over. It depends a lot on the private markets, but my view is that that's healthy and good for that kind of exchange and that there will be a lot of others coming in. I've come to know about the entrepreneurs, and they don't like large organizations, and if they do sell out, they frequently go and create other companies of their own. You also see that in Silicon Valley in California. So I'm not too troubled by that. But you're right. That's always a problem if you're a small company chairperson and president. You're always a little nervous about this, particularly if it's your company, but you've gone public and are subject to the whims of Wall Street. In the main, it's a healthy system.

DEAN WILLIAM SCHWARTZ: I would supplement, however. I think that the venture capital market system does protect the small company. It does enable it to raise capital that would otherwise be unavailable. The danger of the swallowing up by the conglomerate, though (and I have served in some conglomerates and some subsidiaries—sometimes a law school is a subsidiary of a university), gives overemphasis to "ethical imperative number one," namely, profit to the detriment of other factors like safety.

MR. TERRY GOLDBERG (Executive Director, Committee for Responsible Genetics): Dr. Perpich, you noted that we're involved in a biological revolution of an unprecedented scale. The new industry will have its impact across all of the industries—and therefore, the consumers of the products of those industries—with the prospect of wide-ranging impacts. We have a regulatory system of the NIH and guidelines of the Recombinant DNA Advisory Committee (RAC). As you and Dr. Martin Alexander have noted, the membership of the RAC does not include those who can comment on potential problems, such as agronomists and ecologists, who may have some perspective on environmental problems related to releasing newly modified organisms. I find that the continued regulation of the industry on a voluntary basis by the RAC presents serious problems from the perspective of protecting the public health. I would like you to comment on the Industrial Biotechnology Association's perspectives on the need to create another structure that will encompass a broader representation than the RAC, such as that proposed by the report recently published by Rep. Albert Gore's Subcommittee on Investigation and Oversight of Science and Technology Committee, which recently published a report on environmental release of modified organisms, suggesting that the recombinant DNA Advisory Committee not continue to regulate in that area, and that another structure be formed.

DR. JOSEPH G. PERPICH: You always ask tough questions. Let me give you three quick responses. One is that it's voluntary compliance for research and development; it is not voluntary compliance for products. Once you get a product, you come under the relevant regulatory agencies: the FDA and particularly the EPA. Therefore, all the pharmaceutical products come under the aegis of the FDA and are regulated.

You raise a very important point that I touched on briefly, and that is the question of the system for products in the environment. That is a tough one, and as you point out, the RAC does not have that confidence. The question from my point of view is: Should it play a role here? The NIH is examining that question based on the kinds of issues you raised. People say that perhaps there should be a committee in the Environmental Protection Agency and that the NIH should not have a role here. My view is—and I can't speak for the EPA although I'm on their task force—that the NIH should expand that committee and continue in its role because the system has worked superbly from my perspective, thus far. We've had a national monitoring system. I think that, if we add those people, the committee can continue, particularly in the area of field testing, and that the EPA will be implementing regulations akin to those of the FDA. Then we'll see if that system works, and if it doesn't, or if there are problems in assessments and the like, then the EPA has sufficient authority for regulation in this area. It is one that I think Congress, the executive branch, and public and private groups have given a lot of thought to. I would like to see the present model, which works in the pharmaceutical area, work in the environmental area. But I realize that's an open question.

Ms. ROBIN BLATT (Massachusetts Department of Public Health): I have a few very easy questions. First, I wonder if any or all of the panelists could give the audience some examples of the kind of research that is done on fetuses or the kind that medical professionals might like to do. Second, when a woman gives informed consent, is she told what the research is? Third, if the physician who performs an elective abortion does obtain informed consent from the woman to do research on the fetus, but the physician himself or herself does not have a research protocol in progress, are the fetuses sent to another institution? The last question I wanted to ask is: How are the fetuses disposed of in Massachusetts?

MR. CHARLES H. BARON: With respect to the kind of experimentation that researchers either are doing or would like to be done, I've had some difficulty finding out from the researchers whom I have spoken to what it is that they have been frustrated from doing. Dr. Milunsky mentions one thing, fetoscopy, and this new chorionic villus biopsy is also questionable. There has not been an awful lot that I have been able to get out of researchers that they have been frustrated from doing. Maybe there are some things that they would like to do. There were things that were done before 1973. Second, most of that is being done in one place or another. Concerning how fetuses are disposed of in Massachusetts, the requirement is that they be disposed of in some sanitary fashion; presumably they are incinerated.

DR. AUBREY MILUNSKY: Burial and death certificates, if 20 weeks and above, are required, and a common grave is acceptable after that. Otherwise, cremation is available before that time. Fetal research is not done. It's the law. There are all kinds of other possibilities besides fetoscopy. For example, the pharmacokinetics of drugs. You can't find out if you can remedy and help the fetus in Massachusetts through pharmacokinetic studies, for example, find out drug concentrations in the fetal liver. That's called grave robbing in Massachusetts law.

DR. SEYMOUR LEDERBERG: Neither can you detect mutagens or teratogens that might be present in the amniotic sac, which you would like to determine for the protection of the mother.

DEAN WILLIAM SCHWARTZ: In response to your question about supposing that the mother does not know that the fetus is going to be used for research, by definition there would be no informed consent under those circumstances.

DR. LEE ROGERS (Attorney, Washington, DC): Dr. Perpich, you mentioned the biological weapons convention. Was it your suggestion that, because of the convention, recombinant DNA research does not present the possibility of developing biological warfare weapons?

DR. JOSEPH G. PERPICH: No, I didn't mean to imply that. What I was saying was that the U.S. Defense Department's sponsorship of such research and any use of this technology for these purposes is prohibited under that convention. I should also make the point that, currently, there are much more effective, naturally occurring agents that can be used than those that could be developed by the use of this technology, for purposes of biological warfare. But yes, there is that potential with this technology, and therefore, it is very important that our government say what it said.

DR. LEE ROGERS: Well, the point is that, right now, there's approved research by the Defense Department, some of it classified and some of it not classified. Whether or not it is used for biological weapons purposes or for some innocuous purpose depends on the intent of the holder of those research data and not on the innate nature of the research and the recombinant DNA research going on in that area.

DR. JOSEPH G. PERPICH: Yes, the Defense Department supports a great deal of that research. As far as I am aware, all of it is open and unclassified.

DR. LEE ROGERS: You don't know that.

DEAN WILLIAM SCHWARTZ: I think I can best express the sentiments of everyone in the audience by telling one very brief anecdote. A person once walked into a store and encountered an angel sales clerk and asked, "What do you have on sale here?" The angel said the customer could have anything he wanted for nothing. Just ask. And the customer asked, "If I can have anything I want, I want freedom from fear, want, hunger, and poverty for the entire world." The angel responded, "Sir, we don't sell the fruits here, just the seeds." Given the strictures of time, we may not have given you the fruits, but hopefully, we've given you the seeds.

Monitoring and Screening for Genetic Risks

MODERATOR: GEORGE J. ANNAS

33

How Can We Best Evaluate, and Compensate for, Genetic Hazards in the Environment and Workplace

James V. Neel, M.D., Ph.D.
Lee R. Dice University Professor
Department of Human Genetics
Kresge I, Room 4560
University of Michigan Medical School
Ann Arbor, MI 48109

Introduction

Much of this conference has been concerned with issues created by the "New Genetics," however that be defined. We have turned in this closing session to a much less spectacular issue, but an issue that, in the aggregate, will probably impact, directly or indirectly, on just as many people as any of the other issues covered at this meeting. I refer to the question of the genetic implications of a wide variety of potentially mutagenic exposures in the workplace and the environment.

Much of the early concern about environmental and workplace exposures was directed toward the somatic consequences, primarily cancer and lung disease; out of this concern has arisen a wide array of legislation protecting workers and providing for compensation when it is deemed appropriate. More recently, genetic considerations have been beginning to enter into legislation and regulation, and legal actions based on genetic considerations are being initiated. Public concerns (to which geneticists have contributed rather freely), coupled with inadequate knowledge, are finding expression in a variety of ways. My general thesis is that, for lack of appropriate data, this public concern may force—is forcing—inappropriate actions; with current technology, major steps can be taken to acquire the data necessary to more intelligent courses of action.

Some Recent Legal Developments

It will set the stage for my later comments if at the outset we consider briefly some of the recent legislative or administrative actions in which genetic considerations figure.

1. The U.S. Congress has recently enacted legislation (the Nuclear Waste Policy Act, P.L. 97-425) requiring a plan for the disposal of high-level radioactive waste by 1985. The responsibility for developing this plan has been assigned to the Environmental Protection Agency (EPA), whose proposal [40 CFR Part 191 (Proposed)], as modified by an appropriate review process, is now almost ready for implementation. The perceived health effects of the stored waste, both somatic and genetic, are the driving consideration in the preparation of this proposal. Clearly, such a plan is timely (some would say, overdue), but I am struck by the fact that, in reaching an assessment of the potential genetic effects, the EPA, drawing principally on the so-called BEIR I report (1972), has been forced to resort to linear extrapolation three orders of magnitude beyond the existing data, which data, in their genetic aspects, are primarily derived from experiments with mice. As the EPA (20/4-80-014) estimates that the geological repositories for the waste will each cost somewhere between $8 billion and $10 billion[1] and that the situation will require 8–10 repositories, large sums are involved. It is essential that these repositories be planned with an adequate margin of safety. The exposures to the public from these repositories are, however, projected to be only a fraction of the "normal" exposure from background radiation, and, in fact, at this stage in the fuel cycle, the radiation that the public will receive from this material, with present storage plans, is projected to be less than it would receive if the material had never been mined.

2. A second example pertains to the presumed "health effects" (including the genetic effects) of the low-level exposures of military veterans who participated in the testing of nuclear weapons in the American Southwest in the 1950s, as well as of civilians living in the vicinity of the test sites. Although most of the concern is currently directed toward an increased risk of neoplasms, legal actions are also being brought with respect to the genetic aspects of the exposure (e.g., Civil Action No. 79-29 in the U.S. District Court for the Eastern District of Pennsylvania). The U.S. Congress has very recently responded to the concerns expressed by military veterans about the delayed effects of these exposures by mandating a study of health effects that it is understood will be directed toward the genetic as well as the somatic effects of the exposures (Public Law 98-160). The Veterans Administration has requested a committee to make suggestions concerning a possible protocol. The average exposure of these veterans, whose exposure was monitored by film badges, is estimated to be less than 1 rem. As one involved, as a consultant to the Veterans Administration, in the design of an appropriate study, I suggest that extreme care must be exercised in the discharge of this mandate. Radiation biologists, with few exceptions, accept at low dose levels some version of the linear hypothesis of radiation effects. Accordingly, we must accept the probability that, among those veterans, there are some who have sustained a mutation in consequence of this exposure, a mutation that could find expression in their offspring. By an extension of current practices, this could be termed a service-connected disability. If, however, our current estimates of the sensitivity of human genetic material to radiation are even approximately correct (see below), then these relatively few mutations will increment those occurring spontaneously in a very minor way and will be impossible to identify individually as radiation-produced. Now, a very real and well-recognized danger in an epidemiological study wherein the agent of

concern is at such a low level (assuming the correctness of the calculations concerning exposure) is that, if a sufficient number of indicators of an exposure effect are pursued, by chance one or several among them will appear to indicate a positive effect at a statistically significant level. These will receive attention, whereas those equally deviating in the opposite (antihypothesis) direction will be ignored. The result will be an acceptance of a much larger effect than exists (i.e., a "false positive" error[2]), a result of service neither to the veterans nor to the public, and almost certainly leading to legal action with reference to indemnification.

3. A third recent example of a legal action stemming in part from the perceived genetic effects of radiation involves exposure to radionuclides. In June 1981, the Sierra Club filed suit in the U.S. District Court for the Northern District of California, alleging that the EPA had failed to discharge a nondiscretionary duty to propose standards for exposure to radionuclides under Section 112 of the Clean Air Act, inasmuch as the EPA had, in November 1979, listed radionuclides as a hazardous air pollutant. In September 1982, that district court ordered the EPA to propose standards by March 29, 1983. The agency promulgated such standards in the *Federal Register* of April 6, 1983 (pp. 15076–15091) [40 CFR Part 61 (AH-FRL 2324-3) Standards for Radionuclides]. These regulations have been resoundingly challenged by the FMC Corporation, in apparent consequence of which Administrator William Ruckelshaus has requested the Science Advisory Board of the EPA to review "the process by which the Agency estimates human cancer and genetic risk due to radionuclides in the environment." The EPA's calculations of "health effects" follow the format employed in dealing with the risks created by the proposed geological repositories for high-level radioactive waste. Again, the extrapolations are three orders of magnitude beyond the present imperfect base of knowledge, and again, the costs of implementing the regulations based on such imperfect knowledge entail large sums of money (Memorandum, Office of Management and Budget, December 1983: EPA's Standard-Setting for Toxic Pollutants), although well below the sums involved in the disposal of high-level radioactive waste.

These three examples, with which I happen to have had some personal involvement, serve to make the point that concerns about the genetic consequences of a variety of environmental exposures are increasingly finding expression in regulations and legal actions. Now, let us briefly consider the genetic knowledge on which these actions are based.

The Present State of the Data Base on the Genetic Effects of Radiation

The primary data base on which to base legislation concerning the genetic effects of the exposure of humans to radiation is derived from extensive experiments with mice. These are carefully and meticulously performed experiments that, by the very rigor with which they were performed, have made clear the complexity of the problem and the issues inherent in extrapolating from one species to another (cf. particularly the various reports of the Committee on the Biological Effects of Ionizing Radiation of the U.S. National

Academy of Sciences and of the United Nations Scientific Committee on the Effects of Atomic Radiation). Based primarily on the studies of the Russell group at the Oak Ridge National Laboratory and the Lyon group at Harwell, it has been estimated that, in round terms, the amount of *acute* gamma radiation that will produce the same frequency of mutation in mice as occurs spontaneously is approximately 40 rem units. In the most recent extrapolations of the former committee from these data to the human situation, it has been suggested that for low-level *chronic* or intermittent exposures (the more usual human experience), the doubling dose is to be found within the range of 50 and 250 rem. However, the experimental data have been collected for the most part at acute doses ranging from 50 r to (for some end points) over 1,000 r, and although the genetic response is linear (or linear quadratic) within this range (until the highest doses are reached), the potential for error in extrapolating from these findings to the results of the exposures from properly stored high-level waste or ambient radionuclides is clear. Furthermore, in recent years, the growing appreciation of differences among genetic loci, strains, and mammalian species regarding mutation rates has raised numerous questions concerning the error to be attached to that estimate of 40 r and the limits to extrapolation from mouse to human, reviewed by Denniston,[3] Neel,[4] Kohn,[5] and Lyon.[6]

Human data concerning the genetic effects of radiation stem predominantly from follow-up studies in Hiroshima and Nagasaki. The early data dealt with "complex" indicators of a genetic effect, primarily the frequency of congenital defects and death prior to the age of reproduction in the children of survivors within the zone of increased radiation. These are very "impure" end points; an increased mutation rate would be only one possible explanation were the frequency of these events to be elevated in the children of survivors within the zone of increased radiation. For this reason, the studies have required collecting a considerable number of data on extraneous variables, such as socioeconomic status and inbreeding, which must then be considered in the analysis. Furthermore, to develop an estimate of the doubling dose from these indicators, assumptions must be made concerning the extent to which mutation in the preceding generation contributes to the frequency of these indicators. More recently, as the appropriate cytogenetic and biochemical techniques have become available, studies have been initiated on the frequency of sex chromosome aneuploids and reciprocal translocations and of mutations altering the electrophoretic behavior of proteins or the activity of enzymes. These indicators lend themselves to more clear-cut interpretations. The number of children ever to be born to parents receiving significant amounts of radiation is 25,000, but by no means all these children are available for study. As doses are currently calculated (see below), the conjoint parental gonad exposure is approximately 60 rem.

Several years ago, in a reanalysis of all the relevant human data accumulated since the study was initiated shortly after the cessation of World War II, we estimated that the doubling dose of acute radiation for humans was approximately 160 rem.[7] (The dose must be expressed in rem units [roentgen-equivalent-man] because of the mixed [gamma and neutron] nature of the radiation exposure.) The error of that estimate was indeterminate, but its lower (5%) bound undoubtedly overlapped with the upper bound of the 40-rem figure quoted earlier for mice. The data are not adequate for any test of the linearity of the relationship between exposure and genetic effects at low doses. Unfortunately, even as that estimate became available, serious questions were being raised concerning the radiation exposures that had been assigned to the survivors by consultants to the organization (the Radiation Effects Research Foundation) under whose aegis the genetic studies have been performed. A thorough reappraisal of the organ doses sustained by survivors is in progress; it is clear that the estimates of exposure will ultimately be revised downward, but the uncertainties at this time preclude any meaningful revision of the doubling-dose estimate given above.

The Prospects for Improving That Data Base

Relatively little work is in progress on the genetic effects of the radiation of mice at present. With respect to humans, the types of studies in Japan just mentioned continue and will result in a substantial improvement in that data base.

In addition, the human data base can be improved in at least two different ways. The first is by an extension of studies such as those carried out in Hiroshima and Nagasaki to additional populations; the second is by the development of new technologies that will render the study of each child in a series more informative.

With respect to the first of these objectives, the Nuclear Regulatory Commission has sponsored a compilation of groups receiving unusually high radiation exposures (NUREG/CR-1728). This report suggests that within the United States, some of the principal candidate cohorts would be the children born to (1) persons engaged in the development and testing of nuclear weapons; (2) uranium miners; or (3) workers in nuclear shipyards or at power reactors. A group of unusual interest, although small and disadvantageously dispersed for study, are the children born to individuals who have received abdominopelvic radiation and chemotherapy for malignant disease. The size of these cohorts of children and the total radiation exposures of their parents are unknown but are almost surely smaller than the size of the Hiroshima–Nagasaki cohorts. Thus, the information yielded by any one of these cohorts will be so limited that any decision to undertake a study will probably (and should) be motivated as much by sociopolitical as by scientific considerations.

With respect to the second of the ways of improving the data base, at least two promising new technologies are in sight. A technique termed *two-dimensional polyacrylamide gel electrophoresis*, coupled with sensitive staining procedures, permits visualizing the protein contents of a cell in a detail impossible until recently. Our group has for several years been attempting to apply this technique to the study of mutation.[8,9] In this setting, a mutation would manifest itself as a protein moiety not present in comparable preparations from the parents. The principal alternative to mutation as an explanation for such a moiety would be a discrepancy between legal and biological parentage, a possibility that can be detected with high accuracy with current procedures. A particular effort is being made to develop computer algorithms that will lighten the tedium of scoring the gels.[10,11] Should the effort prove successful, the amount of information that can be gathered from each person in a study cohort might be increased by an order of magnitude over what is currently possible.

The other possible improvement on the scientific horizon, but somewhat further off, involves the study of mutation at the ultimate (the DNA) level. The principle is very simple: as in the approach focusing on proteins, one seeks for a DNA characteristic in a child that is not present in either parent. At present, such a search appears to be a quite laborious procedure, and technical developments are necessary before the approach will become practical.

These new technologies can, of course, be applied to experimental organisms, such as the mouse. They should permit carrying the study of the genetic effects of radiation to levels well below those employed in the past. They have the additional important feature that the indicators of a radiation effect can now be identical in mice and humans. Even so, I rather doubt whether, for the foreseeable future, society is prepared to support the massive studies necessary to test the linear hypothesis in a critical fashion at very low doses of radiation, of the order of up to 5 r. Thus, unless studies at doses of, say, 10–20 r conclusively reveal departures from linearity of the regression of effect on dose, radiation geneticists will continue to make the assumption of linearity as the most conservative approach to this difficult question.

TORT LAW AND GENETIC RISKS

With or without the improvements in the data base that could result from the techniques that have just been so briefly described, it seems very probable that tort law will have to deal increasingly with the question of genetic risks in the next decade. Genetic considerations will continue to enter into regulations designed to protect the public, and those whose exposures exceed certain specified levels and who later encounter a possibly genetic problem in their offspring will undoubtedly, on occasion, seek legal redress.

A precedent for proceeding in this difficult situation may be provided by developments with respect to indemnification for malignant disease that might be attributed to radiation exposures. Bond[12–14] and Oftedal et al.[15] have suggested that, in the event of the development of a variety of possibly radiation-related malignancies, the prototype for which is chronic myelogeneous leukemia, one compute a "probability of causation," using Bayes theorem. This approach requires an empirically derived estimate of the probability of developing the tumor under consideration per person year per rem exposure, as well as accurate baseline data on the "spontaneous" frequency of the event. Compensation would be initiated at some arbitrarily defined, probability-of-causation level and would increase with increasing probability up to some level at which full compensation is reached. This principle has been incorporated into proposed legislation for indemnifying for the somatic effects of radiation (e.g., S. 921, 98th Congress, Radiogenic Cancer Compensation Act of 1983), and Section 6 of the Orphan Drug Act of 1982 (P.L. 97-414) directs the Secretary of Health and Human Services to devise and publish radioepidemiological tables that estimate the likelihood that persons who have or have had any of the radiation related cancers and who have received specific doses prior to the onset of such disease developed cancer as a result of these doses.

There are at this moment two very practical difficulties in implementing the genetic equivalent of the approach that I have just described. First, as the reader should by now have gathered from this chapter, we cannot at present estimate the genetic doubling dose of radiation for humans with the same accuracy with which we can estimate the cancer doubling dose (and even for the latter, the uncertainties, especially at low levels of exposure, remain uncomfortably large). As I have emphasized, studies now in progress in Japan should result in significant advances in our understanding of the issue, but there is an urgent need for additional studies employing new technologies.

The second difficulty is more vexatious. The circumstance under which it is most likely that genetic damage will be claimed is a congenital defect in a child. From the etiological standpoint, major congenital defect constitutes a very mixed bag indeed. To a first approximation, perhaps 10% of major defects can be attributed to fresh mutation (all types) in a germ cell of one parent or the other in the preceding generation. This is the fraction that would respond simply and directly to an increased mutation rate. It includes syndromes due to an array of chromosomal abnormalities and such dominantly inherited syndromes as achondroplasia, Marfan syndrome, neurofibromatosis, and retinoblastoma. The remaining 90% of such defects either are nongenetic, are related to the action of a teratogen or maternal disease, or result from the interaction of a complex genetic predisposition and poorly understood factors of the maternal environment. Some, such as a variety of malformations of the skeletal system, are inherited in a recessive fashion. Although radiation-induced mutations will contribute to the frequency of these latter, etiologically more complex entities, it is not in any simple or direct way. Applying the principle of proportionate risk to the clearly genetic entities will be straightforward, but not so for the others. Because, depending on the definitions employed and the care with which a cohort of children is studied, at least 2%–3% of children have *serious major* defects (including mental retardation and handicapping deficiencies of vision or hearing), a rather considerable potential group for consideration is at issue.

It seems unwise at this point—given the uncertainties in the data base, uncertainties to some extent to be dispelled in the near future as more data come in—to open the discussion of an actual indemnification schedule. On the other hand, as it seems unlikely that the genetic doubling dose of radiation, which is *gonadal* dose, is less than the average of the doubling doses for the various radiation-related malignancies, and as the lifetime expectancy of a malignancy in a population is considerably greater than that of congenital defect as this is usually defined, it can be predicted that, on any reasonable schedule, indemnifiable claims for genetic damage will be much less frequent than for somatic (cancer) damage.

The Cost of Improving the Data Base versus the Cost of Not Improving It

I cannot put a price tag on the studies that have been suggested, but it will be high. In this context, it is of some importance to consider the cost of not doing studies. The studies to be performed would be of two principal types, one consisting of large experimental and epidemiological studies of the type that I have mentioned, and the other of studies elucidating the basis for the many congenital malformations. The latter will occur in due course with reasonable funding, but the former will require special encouragement.

Without further studies, we can be certain of a continuation of the current atmosphere of uncertainty. With appropriate studies, I would suggest that, within the next 10 years, we might reduce by one half the range of uncertainty regarding the human genetic doubling dose of radiation. I would hope that, during the discussion period, the members of the legal profession at this meeting will express an opinion about the usefulness of such clarification. It could be that, in practice, it would not be as useful as I believe. I hasten to add that, useful or not, I would advocate further studies for their value to radiation genetics—but the funding issue would undoubtedly be simplified if there were practical goals as well.

Some Particular Difficulties in Evaluating the Genetic Implications of Chemical Exposures

Thus far, we have been exclusively concerned with the issue of the genetic consequences of radiation in the workplace and the environment. Difficult though this issue be, it does not compare with the issue of potentially mutagenic chemicals. With exposures to ionizing radiation, because attenuation by the tissues follows rather simple physical laws, it is possible to estimate gonad doses with some accuracy. This is not the case with the chemical exposures.

One of the most publicized recent chemical exposures in this country was the Love Canal situation, where residence in an area that was a former chemical-waste dump was alleged to be associated with an increased frequency of congenital defect and illness among the children born to the residents. Without passing any judgment on the situation, I point out that attempts to characterize the exposure levels of these individuals and the cytological consequences to their somatic cells can only be described as chaotic,[16,17] and the responsibility for this situation rests far more with the official handling of the situation than with the scientists concerned. Although this may be an extreme example, I do believe that establishing with any accuracy the gonadal doses of a potentially mutagenic chemical encountered by an individual in the environment or the workplace is going to be well nigh impossible.

In the face of these uncertainties, I suggest that the only way to proceed in evaluating this problem is by an extension of the "worst-cases" approach advocated with reference to radiation exposures. That is to say, properly designed studies should be carried out on the highest risk groups that can be identified before political pressures force studies of much less appropriate groups whose study is also intrinsically more difficult because of such factors as dispersion and poorly documented exposures. Whereas, however, with radiation one can establish radiation categories and so conduct (more powerful) regression-type statistical analyses of the data, with the chemicals it will be simply a matter of "exposed" versus "nonexposed." If an apparent effect emerges in a group of children whose parents are drawn from a variety of chemical exposure categories, I would not underestimate the difficulty of trying to rank the chemicals in the order of their risk. If, on the other hand, no apparent effect emerges under the most adverse circumstances that society can define, in a combined sample of the appropriate size, the public should be appropriately reassured.

In considering studies of the effects of chemical mutagens, we tend to seek out exotic exposures. This may not be necessary. In 1977, Yamakasaki and Ames[18] reported that an extract of the urine of persons who smoked between 15 and 44 cigarettes a day increased the rate of mutation of bacteria in the Ames test on the average of about threefold. Urine from nonsmokers revealed no such effect. Cigarette smoke condensate has been shown to produce many dose-related lesions in the cellular DNA of cultured human lymphocytes, as measured by sister chromatid exchange (SCE) induction.[19] Heavy smokers show an increase in chromosomal aberrations in blood lymphocytes relative to nonsmokers.[20] Finally, there is evidence that cigarette smokers show an increase in SCEs,[21-23] although there is not complete agreement on this point.[24] Thus, heavy smokers may be one of the genetic "high-risk" subpopulations—and there is still a sufficient number of them for a rather extensive study.

THE ISSUE OF CREDIBILITY WITH A SUSPICIOUS AND CYNICAL PUBLIC

The final topic that I would like to touch on is the issue of credibility in this arena. The sums of money necessary for proper studies will almost certainly have to come from governmental sources, although the actual study may be performed either by a government laboratory or by a group based in a university or a consulting firm. The fact of ultimate government sponsorship, even if no governmental laboratory or center is directly involved in the study, will unfortunately render the findings, especially if they are basically nonfindings, suspect in the eyes of many who, rightly or wrongly, perceive a past lack of sensitivity of government to the issues involved.

I would hope that, in the discussion period, those of you who represent the legal profession would suggest the administrative framework that would render the findings of extensive studies most acceptable to the public. Let me raise a possibility, which I suspect will elicit strong responses, pro and con. From time to time, the President of the United States appoints so-called blue ribbon committees or commissions. Is something of this nature needed, to sift conflicting claims, promulgate guidelines, or perhaps even sponsor certain critical observations? Or is it sufficient for a position to evolve slowly, on a case-by-case basis, over the next decade?

References

1. Engle, R. L., and White, M. K., *Fiscal Implementations of a Mil/Kilowatt Hour Waste Management Fee*, Battelle Pacific Northwest Laboratory (1982), Document 4513.
2. Land, C. E., Estimating cancer risks from low doses of ionizing radiation, *Science* 209:1197–1203 (1980).
3. Denniston, C., Low level radiation and genetic risk estimation in man, *Ann. Rev. Genet.* 16:329–55 (1982).
4. Neel, J. V., Frequency of spontaneous and induced "point" mutations in higher eukaryotes, *J. Hered.* 74:2–15 (1983).
5. Kohn, H. I., Radiation genetics: The mouse's view. *Rad. Res.* 94:1–9 (1983).
6. Lyon, M. F., Problems in extrapolation of animal data to humans, in *Utilization of Mammalian Specific Locus Studies in Hazard Evaluation and Estimation of Genetic Risk* (F. J. deSerres and W. Sheridan, eds.), Plenum Press, New York (1983), 289–305.
7. Schull, W. J., Otake, M., and Neel, J. V. A reappraisal of the genetic effects of the atomic bombs: Summary of a thirty-four year study, *Science* 213:1220–7 (1981).
8. Neel, J. V., Nishimoto, Y., Goriki, K., Satoh, C., Fujita, M., and Yoshimoto, Y., Epidemiological studies of germ cell mutation in human populations, with particular reference to groups with unusual chemical exposures, in *Methods for Estimating Risk of Chemical Injury: Human and Non-human Biota and Ecosystems* (V. B. Vouk, G. L. Butler, D. G. Hoel, and D. B. Peakall, eds.), Wiley & Sons, Sussex (1985), 327–342.
9. Neel, J. V., Rosenblum, B. B., Sing, C. F., Skolnick, M. M., Hanash, S. M., and Sternberg, S., Adapting two-dimensional gel electrophoresis to the study of human germ-line mutation rates, in *Methods and Applications of Two-Dimensional Gel Electrophoresis of Proteins* (J. E. Celis, ed.), Academic Press, New York (1984), 259–306.
10. Skolnick, M. M., Sternberg, S. R., and Neel, J. V., Computer programs for adapting two-dimensional gels to the study of mutation, *Clin. Chem.* 28:969–78 (1982).
11. Skolnick, M. M., An approach to completely automatic comparison of two-dimensional electrophoresis gels, *Clin. Chem.* 28:979–86 (1982).
12. Bond, V. P., The medical effects of radiation, in *Proceedings, Thirteenth Annual Convention, National Association Claimant's Counsel of America*, W. H. Anderson, Cincinnati, (1959), 117–28.
13. Bond, V. P., The cancer risk attributable to radiation exposure: Some practical problems, *Hlth. Phys.* 40:108–11 (1981).
14. Bond, V. P., Statement. Hearings on Radiation Exposure Compensation Act of 1981 (S. 1483). GPO, Washington (1982), 242–257.
15. Oftedal, P., Kunt, M., and Torlief, H., On the probability of radiation being the cause of cancer, *Br J Radiol.* 41:711–2 (1968).
16. Kolata, G. B., Love Canal: False alarm caused by botched study, *Science* 208:1239–42 (1980).
17. Picianno, D., Comment on Love Canal, *Science* 209:754–5 (1980).
18. Yamasaki, E., and Ames, B. N., Concentration of mutagens from urine by absorption with the nonpolar resin XAD-2: Cigarette smokers have mutagenic urine. *Proc. Nat. Acad. Sci. USA* 74:3555–9 (1977).
19. Hopkin, J. M., and Evans, H. J., Cigarette smoke condensates damaged DNA in human lymphocytes, *Nature* 279:241–2 (1979).
20. Obe, G., and Herha, J., Chromosomal aberrations in heavy smokers, *Hum. Genet.* 41:259–63 (1978).
21. Lambert, B., Linblad, A., Nordenskjold, M., and Werelius, B., Increased frequency of sister chromatid exchanges in cigarette smokers, *Hereditas* 88:147–9 (1978).
22. Hopkin, J. M., and Evans, H. J., Cigarette smoke-induced DNA damage and lung cancer risks, *Nature* 283:388–90 (1980).
23. Livingston, G. K., Cannon, L. A., Bishop, D. T., Johnson, P., and Fineman, R. M., Sister chromatid exchange: Variation by age, sex, smoking, and breast cancer status, *Cancer Genet. Cytogenet.* 9:289–98 (1983).
24. Hollander, D. H., Tockman, M. S., Liang, Y. W., Borgaonkar, D. S., and Frost, J. K., Sister chromatic exchanges in the peripheral blood of cigarette smokers and in lung cancer patients; and the effects of chemotherapy, *Hum. Genet.* 44:165–171 (1978).

34

JUST WHEN YOU THOUGHT IT WAS SAFE
An Update on the Risks of Recombinant DNA Technology

DAVID OZONOFF, M.D., M.P.H.
Associate Professor of Public Health
Chief, Environmental Health Section
Boston University School of Public Health
80 East Concord Street
Boston, MA 02118

It is now just a bit more than a decade since the thoughts of scientists and policy makers were preoccupied with the recombinant DNA controversy. We are now told that this was a tempest in a teapot—that "without doubt, almost all fears and concerns over recombinant DNA expressed in the early days of its advent have been laid to rest."[1] The needless alarm notwithstanding, the manner in which the affair was handled is also portrayed as a proud moment for science, when scientists recognized their social responsibilities and voluntarily suspended potentially valuable work until secure that it could be pursued safely.

I would like to suggest that neither of these propositions is true, that, on the contrary, this is a doubly dangerous mythology, for it has not been demonstrated that recombinant DNA technology is either benign or without danger, nor is it clear that scientists have yet learned the lessons of Hiroshima and Nagasaki: having looked their social obligations squarely in the eye, scientists were the first to blink.

Concerning the question of the alleged safety of recombinant DNA technology, I would preface my remarks by acknowledging that it represents a major and revolutionary technology whose importance cannot be underestimated. One cannot be even slightly familiar with the details of this work without becoming excited and enthusiastic about its potential, and I am no exception to this general rule. By means of this technique, we have learned an immense amount about cellular biology and, in particular, about the cancer problem. It is quite clear that we have already benefited enormously from using these techniques. These facts neither contradict nor interfere with my main theses, which question the seriousness and thoroughness with which we have evaluated the risks of this technology.

RISK AND THE CLASH OF PROFESSIONAL VALUES

If we put the issue of conflict of interest aside for the moment, it is important to recognize that we all approach matters of risk with a certain bias. Mine are derived from the public health and medical professions rather than from the legal and laboratory professions. Let me explain.

The disciplinary biases that I am most concerned about here are the ones that involve differing tolerances for the various consequences of uncertainty or error. In the legal and laboratory professions, there is a low tolerance for what statisticians call the *Type I error* (what some call a *false positive*). Thus, for the legal professions, a person is innocent until proven guilty, and it is better to let a guilty person go free than to punish an innocent one. Likewise, for the laboratory scientist, it is better to leave the state of the art as it was than to accept a false proposition. Both of these disciplines employ elaborate safeguards to prevent Type I errors. In the legal profession, these safeguards use the entire judicial machinery, including constitutional guarantees, rules of evidence, and so forth, and in the laboratory professions, they are embodied in the system of controls, experimental procedures, and statistical tests that prevent the acceptance of results that could have been due to chance.

In medicine and public health, by contrast, the tolerance for Type I errors is considerably lower than tolerance for the reverse, the Type II, for false negative, error. An individual who presents with an acute pain in the belly is presumed to have an appendicitis until the physician is shown otherwise because the downside risks of missing this diagnosis are even more serious than the complications of major surgery. Likewise, in the public health profession, it is deemed more desirable to err on the side of safety and health than the reverse.

The relevance of all this to the recombinant DNA controversy is that the concerns expressed were, at least in part, those of public health and safety, whereas the standards of evidence were those of the laboratory and legal professions. It is understandable that we should have a clash of values. What is most interesting is whose values won out.

ENTER THE TECHNOLOGICAL FIX

The question of whether the safety of this technology has been demonstrated now becomes "To whose satisfaction?" It has certainly not been demonstrated to the level required by the established conventions of the medical and public health professions; it has only not yet conclusively been shown to be harmful. Moreover, contrary to common belief, few data pertinent to the original concerns have been developed. What exists does nothing to lessen our concerns, and indeed, if this technology does not turn out to have major negative consequences when it becomes widely disseminated, it will be unlike most other technologies. Thus, it will be doubly revolutionary—in its substance, and also by virtue of being an unmixed blessing.[2] A number of new problems have arisen that are of even greater concern but that are going unaddressed by the scientific and regulatory communities.

The details of the recombinant DNA controversy have been reviewed many times.[3] They include a heady brew of political activism, antiwar sentiment, and nuclear-age soul-searching by scientists.[4] But from the beginning, the participants in the research concentrated their attention on the potential biohazards. Briefly, the recombinant DNA technique involved splicing together portions of DNA from disparate sources, often from species widely separated taxonomically, and then reinserting the hybrid, or recombinant, DNA into a host organism, where the DNA might function through the genetic apparatus of the host cell. A major concern was that organisms would be created with novel genotypes that would have unpredictable or harmful properties that could threaten human health or the environment. Such novel agents, for example, might result in new pathways for the spread of disease or might produce animal tumor viruses that might be introduced into the human intestinal tract, with uncertain results.[5]

Most of the interest focused on a particular host organism, E. coli, the common gut bacterium. Because E. coli is a resident of the intestines of most warm-blooded animals, concern was expressed that, once E. coli organisms with a possibly harmful or unpredictable genotype were released into the environment, it would be impossible to retrieve them. Virtually all of the early work in recombinant DNA was done with E. coli, in particular a laboratory strain called K-12, which was thought by many scientists to be so enfeebled by multiple passages in a laboratory environment that it could not easily survive outside the test tube. To ensure further that E. coli containing recombinant DNA molecules would not get into the environment, it was initially required that many experiments be done in an even "safer" strain of E. coli K-12, called chi-1776, which had been engineered to have multiple safeguards to prevent it from living outside a laboratory environment. This kind of safeguard, called biological containment, was supplemented by a variety of physical barriers and work practices and was codified in successive sets of guidelines issued by NIH and required of all investigators funded by the National Institutes of Health (NIH).[6]

The adoption of the strategy embodied in the NIH Guidelines came relatively early in the recombinant DNA controversy. By the time this stage was reached, the slight breach that had occurred in the tradition of having the conditions of science controlled by scientists had been closed again. By redefining the social problems posed by the recombinant DNA technique in terms of biohazard, pure and simple, the scientific community had excluded many other questions of social concern, such as those involving genetic engineering, eugenics, and the control of science from outside. At the same time, this strategy allowed the use of a classic solution to problems of this type, the "technological fix," which, of course, permitted the solution to be designed and controlled by the scientists themselves.

SCIENCE: POLITICS AND DATA

Once having redefined the problem, scientists quickly seized control of the regulatory mechanism used to deal with it as well. The body chosen to oversee recombinant DNA research was the NIH, although as an agency it had no previous regulatory experience and, in fact, was promoting such work.[7] The NIH moved quickly to establish a formidable administrative framework to regulate its sponsored research involving recombinant DNA molecules. The NIH's Office of Recombinant DNA Activities (ORDA) was guided by its principal technical advisory group, the Recombinant DNA Advisory Committee (the RAC), which had the responsibility for drafting the guidelines and, when it deemed appropriate, recommending substantial revisions. Even though the RAC had expanded its membership in 1979 to include individuals knowledgeable about legal, social, environmental, and occupational issues, such representation was not required to constitute more than 20% of the RAC's membership, and indeed, the committee was dominated by scientists who had a direct stake in the outcome of the RAC's deliberations. There followed successive revisions of the NIH Guidelines that drastically reduced the scope of experiments covered, and at the same time, the technology and the work became more widespread and the techniques easier and ever more powerful.

Most of the revisions were based on little scientific evidence and a good deal of wishful thinking. One of the first attempts at systematic risk assessment was the Falmouth Conference held in June 1977.[8] This was a meeting of scientists, held by invitation only, that convened to discuss whether E. coli K-12 could be made into "an epidemic pathogen" by genetic manipulation. A detailed analysis of the results of the Falmouth Conference has been given elsewhere.[9] Although the conference suggested further risk-assessment work, its tone was decidedly "up beat," and it was frequently cited by the NIH as a reason for relaxing the guidelines.

Already, several of the major premises of the Falmouth group have proved false. First was the conclusion that K-12 could not be converted to a pathogen by genetic manipulations in the laboratory. I have previously pointed out that the weight of scientific evidence did not support this conclusion, and since then, the conversion of K-12 to a pathogenic Shigella-like organism has been accomplished by means of classical genetic techniques.[10]

Second, the belief of many scientists today that K-12 cannot survive outside the laboratory has also been shown to be false by some of the little risk-assessment work that has been done since Falmouth. In particular, it has been shown that K-12 will do very nicely in the environment, surviving in a viable state for 24–48 hours on laboratory benches, stainless steel, and a variety of other environments, and that there is significant dispersal of organisms during normal laboratory procedures.[11]

Third, K-12 and even its supposedly exquisitely fragile substrain, chi-1776, will pass in a viable state in a high percentage through both primary and secondary sewage-treatment plants and, from there, can be released to the environment.[12]

Fourth, K-12—and certainly the wild-type (natural) strains—will colonize animals and human beings under antibiotic pressure. Because common plasmid vectors used in recombinant DNA work, like pBR322, contain resistance-producing genes for antibiotics such as tetracycline on them, it is of great significance that antibiotic pressure can affect the residence of these strains in the human and animal gut.[13] Although recombinant DNA workers are not supposed to work while taking antibiotics, most places do not have such adequate and conscientious surveillance that they know whether their employees are taking antibiotics on an outpatient basis. Moreover, even chi-1776 survived in the intestines 500 times better than mandated by the guidelines, and its survivability was increased by the presence of the vector pBR322.[14] Just what effect a variety of other recombinant plasmids would have on *E. coli* survivability is unknown.

Fifth, organisms can increase tremendously in host range as a result of recombinant DNA manipulations. For example, the experiments of Rowe and Martin involved producing a hybrid between a bacterial virus and an animal tumor virus.[15] The result was a virus that could infect both bacteria—in this case, *E. coli*—and mammalian cells. Thus, each of the genomes was able to find new niches in nature. When cleaved by suitable restriction enzymes, the polyoma DNA segments now in *E. coli* were still capable of causing tumors in hamsters.[16]

Sixth, the concern that recombinant techniques might convert nonpathogens into pathogens has been demonstrated for two nonpathogenic organisms. In this case, an attempt to move genes from bacteria into a fungus symbiotic on trees to enhance the fungus's nitrogen-fixing ability resulted in a new organism pathogenic to tree seedlings. Neither of the original organisms involved in the hybridization showed any such pathogenicity.[17]

Many questions, of course, are still open and, with so little assessment work being done, are bound to remain open for some time. Commenting on the rapid relaxation of the NIH Guidelines in the face of little evidence demonstrating the safety of the technique, Roy Curtiss, the originator of the chi-1776 strain, remarked that the revisions were "based on the politics of science, not the data of science."[18]

THE FOX AND THE CHICKEN COOP

What actually occurred, of course, is that the biologists themselves had seized control of the levers of regulatory power and were running the show in much the same fashion as other regulated communities have done in similar circumstances: the Interstate Commerce Commission and the railroads, the Atomic Energy Commission and the nuclear industry, and so forth. This reassertion of control did not come easily; it required some hard work on the part of scientists, who learned the hard way what it meant to lose their grip on former prerogatives. RAC member and virologist Wallace Rowe expressed it this way:

> [The scientific community was naive], particularly in not foreseeing the inevitable, relentless movement from voluntary moratoria to external regulations. When the first guidelines were drawn up, in 1975, we on the committee were operating with a number of tacit assumptions in mind. Some of these were critical to the entire subsequent unfolding of events. 1) We assumed that by severely restricting the scope of

recombinant DNA research to a few extremely well understood laboratory organisms as hosts, and permitting work to proceed under only extremely stringent conditions, both scientific and administrative, we would buy time and allow a more informed, rational, data-based set of guidelines to be developed; 2) We thought we were writing guidelines, meaning guidance, for local decision-making bodies; and 3) we assumed we had the freedom to amend, alter, and undo what we had done. On the latter two points we were completely wrong. We watched shocked and paralysed as a variety of forces moved the decision making away from the scientists, the RAC and the local biohazard committees and into the hands of lawyers and bureaucrats. For a period of two and a half years, virtually all decisions under the guidelines, by NIH staff, by ORDA [Office of Recombinant DNA Research], and by the IBCs [Institutional Bio-safety Committees] have been made solely on the basis of what constitutes compliance and literal interpretation.[19]

By 1978, control had been reestablished. Today, by virtue of scientific dominance on the RAC, it is virtually absolute.

I don't blame the biological community for this. As an epidemiologist, I, too, am regulated by government bodies in the form of institutional review boards that oversee experiments involving human subjects. In my rather parochial view, many of the regulations are burdensome and do not contribute meaningfully to the protection of human subjects. If I had the chance to frame the regulations myself, there are many things I would eliminate. I also believe that it's a good thing that I can't frame those regulations because, as an interested party, I view the problem with intellectual blinders on.

New Problems

Finally, a variety of new problems have arisen in the area of recombinant DNA techniques that are going unaddressed by policymakers and the scientific community. Because the original NIH guidelines were designed with containment in mind, they did not deal with the problem of the deliberate release of organisms into the environment for beneficial purposes. Workers who are engaged in improving plants, designing organisms to consume toxic wastes or oil spills, or enriching the food supply now want to release genetically engineered organisms into the environment for these purposes.[20] At the moment, there is no regulatory framework to deal with these problems. Although the EPA has signaled its interest in regulating some of these applications under FIFRA (Federal Insecticide, Fungicide and Rodenticide Act) and TSCA (Toxic Substances Control Act), we have seen little actual activity in this area. Furthermore, the important problem of waste materials' emanating from biotechnology facilities has gone unaddressed by the EPA in its hazardous waste regulations.[21] Right now, there is nothing to prevent the release into the environment of high volumes of materials containing organisms with recombinant DNA molecules, purely as waste products. Although I have been addressing recombinant DNA techniques in this short chapter, everything I have written about the lack of a regulatory framework for recombinant techniques holds as well for other techniques that involve genetic manipulations, such as cell fusion and deliberate chemical mutagenesis.

I realize that this is a harsh and somewhat bitter interpretation of what has been portrayed in many circles as a great and proud success story for the scientific conscience. Recombinant DNA techniques have been remarkably successful and have already fulfilled their early promise. But it is important to treat any powerful technology with the greatest respect for the harm it can do. It serves neither the interests of science nor the public interest to mythologize the past and to blind ourselves to the dangers of the present.

Other than the many scientific advances fostered by recombinant DNA techniques, there has also emerged another very beneficial by-product: a new cadre of professionals versed in and adept at biosafety and risk analysis. Let us hope that this new professional discipline grows quickly enough and is aggressive enough to mitigate the almost certain negative consequences to be expected from a widespread and powerful technology like recombinant DNA techniques.

References and Notes

1. Levine, M. M., Kaper, J. B., Lockman, H., Black, R. E., Clements, M. L., and Falkow, S., Recombinant DNA risk assessment studies in man: Efficacy of poorly mobilizable plasmids in biologic containment, *Recombinant DNA Technical Bulletin* 6:89–97 (1983).
2. One could say that the profound changes that this technology has wrought in the ecology of academic biology departments and their relationship to industry is itself a major unforeseen and untoward event. But this matter has already been discussed by Dr. Krimsky in an earlier chapter.
3. Cf. Krimsky, S., *Genetic Alchemy*, MIT Press, Cambridge (1983); Lear, J., *Recombinant DNA: The Untold Story*, Crown, New York (1978); and Wade, N., *The Ultimate Experiment*, Walker, New York (1977).
4. See Krimsky, *supra*, chap. 1.
5. Cf. King, J., New diseases in new niches, *Nature* 276:4–7 (1978); and King, J., Recombinant DNA and autoimmune disease, *J. Inf. Diseases* 137:663–5 (1978).
6. For a review of the early regulatory strategy, see Krimsky, S., and Ozonoff, D., Recombinant DNA research: The scope and limits of regulation, *Am. J. Public Health* 69:1252–9 (1979).
7. The inherent conflict of having the agency that was the largest public supporter of biomedical research in the United States also regulating this work was commented on at the time by, among others, Wright, S., Setting science policy: The case of recombinant DNA, *Environment* 20:7–41 (1978).
8. Proceedings were published in *The Journal of Infectious Diseases*, vol. 137 (1978).
9. Krimsky, *supra* note 3, chap. 16.
10. Sansonetti, P. J., Hale, T. L., Dammin, G. J., Kapfer, C., Collins, H. H., Jr., and Formal, S. B., Alterations in the pathogenicity of *Escherichia coli* K-12 after transfer of plasmid and chromosomal genes from *Shigella flexneri*, *Infection and Immunity* 39:1392–1402 (1983).
11. Chatigny, M. A., Hatch, M. T., Wolochow, H., Adler, T., Hresko, J., Macher, J., and Besemer, D., Studies on release and survival of biological substances used in recombinant DNA laboratory procedures, *Recombinant DNA Technical Bulletin* 2:62–7 (1979).
12. Sagik, B. P., and Sorber, C. A., The survival of host-vector systems in domestic sewage treatment plants, *Recombinant DNA Technical Bulletin* 2:55–61 (1979).
13. Cohen, P. S., Pilsucki, R. W., Myhal, M. I., Rosen, C. A., Laux, D. C., and Cabelli, V. J., Fecal *E. coli* strains in the mouse GI tract, *Recombinant DNA Technical Bulletin* 2:106–13 (1979); cf. also Levine *et al.*, *supra* note 1.
14. Cf. Newman, S. A., The "scientific" selling of rDNA, *Environment* 24:21–3, 53–7 (1982); and also Levy,

S. B., and Marshall, B., Survival of *E. coli* host-vector systems in the human intestinal tract, *Recombinant DNA Technical Bulletin* **2**:77–80 (1979).

15. Israel, M. A., Chan, H. W., Rowe, W. P., and Martin, M. A., Molecular cloning of polyoma virus DNA in *Escherichia coli:* Lambda phage vector system, *Science* **203**:887–92 (1979).

16. Israel, M. A., Chan, H. W., Martin, M. A., and Rowe, W. P., Molecular cloning of polyoma virus DNA in *Escherichia coli:* Oncogenicity testing in hamsters, *Science* **205**:1140–2 (1979).

17. Giles, K. L., and Whitehead, H. C. M., Reassociation of a modified mycorrhiza with the host plant roots (*Pinus radiata*) and the transfer of acetylene reduction activity, *Plant and Soil* **48**:143–52 (1977).

18. Curtiss, R., Letter to D. Fredrickson, Oct. 4, 1979, reprinted in U.S. DHEW-NIH, *Recombinant DNA Research*, vol. 5, (March 1980), 339–40.

19. Rowe, W. P., Statement to the NIH recombinant DNA advisory committee, May 21–23, 1979, RAC Meeting Item #671.

20. For a review of this area, see *The Environmental Implications of Genetic Engineering*, Staff Report of the Sub-Committee on Investigations and Oversight, Committee on Science and Technology, U.S. House of Representatives, 98th Congress, 2nd Session, Feb. 1984.

21. There is a reserved section in the regulations promulgated under the RCRA (Resource Conservation and Recovery Act) for infectious wastes, but no regulations covering these wastes have yet appeared, nor are they likely to be issued in the near future.

35

Charting the Future Course for Corporate Management of Genetic and Other Health Risks

Michael S. Baram, LL.B.
Professor of Public Health Law
Boston University School of Public Health
80 East Concord Street
Boston, MA 02118

Responsibility for Health Risk Management

Corporations engage in technological activities of benefit to society and thereby also create new health risks for workers, consumers, and communities. Government regulatory agencies deal with this chronic problem by conducting risk analyses and imposing various duties on private firms. Despite agency efforts and corporate compliance, health risks continue to arise and to take their toll. To what extent will private firms voluntarily assume greater responsibility for preventing these risks? This question is of increasing social importance because the limitations of regulatory efforts are now obvious, whereas health risks are now being identified at what appears to be an increasing rate. This question is also of considerable importance to industry because of the economic impact on private firms of toxic tort actions, workers' compensation claims, and other "losses" that follow from the health risks.

The corporate role in health risk management is part of the larger issue of corporate social responsibility and is therefore influenced by changing values and policies that relate to the larger issue. Thus, the corporate role will not be advanced if we adhere to the narrow view that "there is one and only one social responsibility of business—to use its resources and engage in activities designed to increase its profits so long as it . . engages in open and free competition. . . ."[1] On the other hand, the corporate role would be dramatically changed if we adopt the broad view that it is absurd to regard the corporation simply as an enterprise established for the sole purpose of allowing profit-making. . . . Every corporation should be thought of as a social enterprise whose existence and decisions can be justified only insofar as they serve public or social purposes.[2]

The issue of corporate social responsibility is not likely to be fully resolved around either of these polar views and will therefore remain uncertain and ambiguous. Consequently, the corporate role in health risk management will continue to be largely a matter of corporate discretion, influenced by economic factors and public pressures, and governed by laws, which set forth the duties of directors and managers. Major firms that are now considering voluntary approaches to improved health-risk prevention and economic loss control face a complex situation, because risk and loss are dynamic problems. They result from technological innovation and new products and services that are valued and promoted by our society and that are essential to corporate growth. New and unforeseen risks are continuously identified because of advances in instrumentation and analysis. Public values and behavior become ever more risk-averse in proportion to our affluence, as in other Western nations.[3]

Thus, we can rephrase our central question: How will corporate discretion be used to cope with technological risks and the economic losses that attend inadequate management decisions and regulatory controls? The answer that is emerging is that new risk-assessment techniques and health-risk-prevention strategies will be put to use by managers and health professionals in the corporate sector as important supplements to traditional engineering approaches to risk and loss control.[4]

The risk assessment techniques are those that involve models and computer systems to integrate all relevant health-risk factors and data to produce quantified but probabilistic results. The strategies involve seeking new data and putting them to various uses for risk prevention and health promotion, and they include applications of biological monitoring, health screening, and medical surveillance, for example. The health professionals and consultants include experts from the fields of occupational and environmental medicine, epidemiology, toxicology, industrial hygiene, computer systems, and biostatistics.[5]

The new health strategies involve considerable technical uncertainties and legal issues and are laden with economic implications. In pursuing these complex strategies, the functions of health professionals are further complicated because they are subject to at least three systems of accountability: (1) *organizational accountability* to meet management needs (e.g., cost effectiveness) and corporate goals (e.g., avoidance of corporate liability); (2) *personal and professional accountability* (e.g., compliance with professional standards and ethics, avoidance of personal liability for negligence); and (3) *social accountability* (e.g., compliance with various constitutional and statutory requirements). No panaceas are at hand for corporate health professionals; and their careful exercise of judgment on the basis of adequate technical, legal, and economic information, infused with a strong sense of personal and professional ethics, is the only answer.[6]

GENETIC AND HEALTH RISK CONTROVERSIES: LEGAL AND ECONOMIC CONSIDERATIONS FOR THE CORPORATION

Corporations now face a dramatic increase in controversies over genetic and health risks to workers, consumers, and the environment, despite several decades of federal regulation. Some controversies are confined to the regulatory process, but most now take place in the courts and in workers' compensation board proceedings as private rights are asserted against corporations or particular corporate personnel and against insurers, under state common law and health protection statutes.

Many of these controversies arise from new scientific findings of health hazards and from rising public concerns over chemical, radiological, and biological substances. But fuel for these controversies has been provided by the Carter and Reagan administrations' Executive Orders and other "regulatory reform" efforts, which have brought about a dramatic loss of public confidence in federal regulation.[7] The results include an increase in product liability and toxic tort litigation by consumers, community residents, and workers; a spiral of disease claims under state workers' compensation laws by workers; and more negligence actions against medical and other corporate personnel. Other outcomes include a proliferation of new state laws and local ordinances to protect workers and others at health risk from industrial processes and hazardous wastes; new legal obstacles to the siting of waste facilities and industrial plants; and the filling of bills to establish new victims' compensation insurance programs, to be funded by industrial contributions, for injured or diseased workers and citizens.

Because of the special features of health risk disputes, such as the long time frames between exposure and injury, the evidentiary difficulties regarding fault and causation, the multiple plaintiffs and defendants involved, and the allegedly significant hazards to health involved, the courts have responded in flexible fashion to "do justice." The courts have construed statutes of limitation to run from the later time of discovery of the injury rather than from the earlier time of exposure and have adopted concepts of strict (no-fault) liability and joint and several liability to reduce barriers to recovery of compensation by plaintiffs. They have also adopted various presumptions about causation to reduce evidentiary problems and have permitted claims involving emotional distress to proceed even in the absence of measurable biological harm.[8] Juries have responded with high awards of actual damages and very high awards of punitive damages, with the latter a recent phenomenon of great economic significance.[9] And the courts have forced large settlements in cases involving "Agent Orange" and various hazardous waste problems.

Finally, we are witnessing a renaissance of turn-of-the-century common-law doctrines, which set forth three key corporate duties, a rudimentary "three commandments" to manage risk: (1) the duty to identify and know latent health and safety risks; (2) the duty to warn workers and others likely to be exposed to such risks; and (3) the duty to take timely and positive steps to reduce such risks.[10]

The dimensions of these duties were relatively easy to discern at the turn of the century, when accidents (e.g., boiler explosions) were of most concern; today, the dimensions are much less definite, with chronic health risks (e.g., mutagenicity) now of central concern. Thus, we have no clear guidelines as to how intensive and costly the corporate search to identify latent health risks should be, other than it must at least be consistent with relevant regulatory requirements, if any, and it probably must go beyond regulatory requirements to prevent liability.[11] Nor are any reliable guidelines available as to what degree of conclusiveness of results is required to trigger the second and third duties.

Similarly, there is uncertainty about the dimensions of the duty to warn workers, consumers, and community residents. Compliance with product labeling requirements has been found to be inadequate in some cases. Whether compliance with the "hazard communication rule" of the Occupational Safety and Health Administration (OSHA)[12] and with the "right-to-know" laws of the various states[13] is sufficient as a corporate defense against claims by injured workers is an issue awaiting judicial resolution.[14]

In tort litigation, corporations have sought to use defenses such as compliance with the state of the art, industry custom, and standards and government regulations; but this defense has not proved successful in many state jurisdictions, particularly in product liability actions, which can be brought by injured consumers and workers who used the products in their occupations.[15] These controversies have significant economic implications for the corporate sector, as well as health implications for all society. Compensatory and punitive damage awards against corporations are the most obvious economic losses for the corporate sector to absorb, the latter type of damages now running at such high award levels that they can have very serious effects on a firm of any size.[16]

Corporations must also absorb a variety of other economic losses arising from the health risks that they create and from the controversies over real and imagined risks. For example, insurance premiums for workers' compensation and other potential losses are increasing because they are often set on a claims-made basis; and attorney's fees and expert witness fees incurred as a result of litigation are not trivial economic considerations. To the extent that the health risks are real and manifest in injuries to workers, collective bargaining for wage increases and better protective systems follow; worker medical absences and lost productivity are incurred; and the costs of company medical-benefits programs increases.

A similar "loss experience" may be encountered when community health risks are involved, and suits are brought by victims of plant emissions and hazardous wastes. Government inspection, monitoring, clean-up, and standard-setting actions may then impose additional costs on corporations. Consumers put off by the adverse publicity shrink from company products; Securities and Exchange Commission reporting requirements further publicize these controversies and can lead to reductions in the market value of shares of company stock.

THE CORPORATE RESPONSE

New Strategies Involving Risk Assessment

To cope with these problems, major firms are now turning to an increased reliance on health-based intervention strategies and the use of health risk assessment techniques, which provide new opportunities for corporations to simultaneously reduce or prevent both health risks and economic losses. Many firms are developing new health-risk-assessment procedures and risk-management strategies to reduce risks and to contain costs. Health risk assessment is an analytic process that promotes the systematic identification of the hazard attributes of a proposed activity and the measurement of the potential adverse impacts on human health and the environment. The hazard attributes may stem from accident events, continuing emission events, or mixed accident and continuous events. To measure such impacts, the assessors must determine the human-population and environmental features at risk, estimate their exposure potential, and reach a judgment on their biological response to exposure at various doses or levels. [17]

Health risk assessment deals quantitatively and probabilistically with possible future events and their consequences and therefore involves inputs from medical and hygiene personnel, safety engineers, health scientists, environmental professionals, statisticians, and other experts, including decision theorists and systems analysts. [18] But health risk assessment cannot provide precise and conclusive results in most cases, because of technical uncertainties arising from incomplete data, analytic limitations, unforeseen exogenous factors, and other considerations that can confound any attempt to determine future conditions. Thus, it remains an art form, albeit at a somewhat advanced but not completely developed status. [19] Various efforts are being made to formalize and improve the quality of health risk assessment. Recommendations have been made, for example, to designate "commonly accepted data collections," "commonly accepted methods for estimating chemical properties," widely recognized systematic approaches to calculate safe . . . levels for pollutants," and the development of "a pool of accredited experts."[20]

Despite its present limitations, health risk assessment provides the analytic input into the larger task of corporate risk management. In risk management, the assessment results are used by management to determine risk control options, to choose the optimal set of options, and to implement them. The risk control options may include the redesign of processes and products, the careful siting of facilities, and other initiatives, including the development of screening, monitoring, and surveillance procedures for workers.

Many firms have viewed these strategies as *defensive options* in that they provide new facts, and corporate control of these facts can lead to more success in defending against litigants and regulatory officials. This view maintains the corporation's traditional position of responding to external developments, such as litigation and regulatory activity. It tends to contain some costs, but to reduce few health risks. But some firms now view new assessment procedures as a *positive opportunity* for management to take the initiative, at early planning and decision-making levels, to prevent the generation of health risks and their economic consequences. This perspective entails a greater investment but can put the firm out front on future problems to better prevent health risks and economic losses.

Because both approaches are manageable and can lead to legal compliance with regulatory requirements, the key issue for management is which is more cost-effective. [21] The usual response is that voluntary investments in health risk prevention do not lead to increased consumer preference or markets and therefore involve expenditures but no increased revenues; and that any economic advantages from improved loss control (e.g., less agency intervention and fewer lawsuits and compensation claims) would be realized only over a very long time and would not benefit current management, which is evaluated and rewarded for increased profitability and loss control over a far shorter time (e.g., from one to five years at most). Obviously, this "rational" approach for a manager is not necessarily rational for the firm over time, and it should be a more closely examined issue in each firm facing the prospects of health risk controversies and their costs over the long term. [22]

As firms consider using new health strategies, the threshold issue is therefore one of corporate perspective: defensive or positive. Firms that plan to use new, more probative, forms of prejob screening, monitoring, and surveillance for defensive cost-control purposes could run into substantial problems that lead to litigation, regulatory costs, and other inefficiencies. For example, screening to reject job applicants who are more likely to use medical benefits programs (e.g., diabetics) in order to reduce the costs of such programs, but who are otherwise well qualified for the job, raises legal and policy issues about new forms of discrimination and violation of privacy rights and leads to protective legislation and to litigation by the rejected applicants under federal and state statutes. [23]

Medical Screening and Other Initiatives

Biological monitoring and medical surveillance to identify workers at risk for defensive purposes of terminating their employment to reduce the possibility that they later may file workers' compensation or medical insurance claims against the firm lead to similar legal problems. Courts in many states have started to restrict corporate freedom to terminate employees at will, and the trend in the courts is now running against terminations on medical-cost and claims-reduction grounds. [24] Also, the data resulting from such tests are accessible by the workers and their unions under OSHA's "Access to Medical and Exposure Records" rule [25] and can be used by workers who later choose to file workers' compensation claims and tort suits for injuries and diseases incurred as a result of occupational exposures: a boomerang effect.

Genetic Screening

Probably the most controversial development has been the growing interest in genetic screening. Advances in molecular biology and the health sciences have led to a greater understanding of human genetic traits and their relevance to an individual's susceptibility to hazards in the workplace and the community. According to David Ozonoff:

> There may be thousands of genetic traits that are relevant [to individual susceptibility]. Only a few are suspected at this time. . . . These traits include the glucose-6-phosphate-dehydrogenase (G6PD) deficiency and the alpha-1-antitrypsin (AAT) deficiency (sickle cell trait). . . . G6PD deficiency can be found in blacks and Mediterranean Jews and is thought to predispose to hemolytic crises when the worker is exposed to . . . naphthalene. AAT deficiency *disease* . . . results in a severe emphysema, which may be aggravated when the lung is exposed to pulmonary irritants. . . . AAT

deficiency *trait* . . . is much more common [and] afflicts approximately .15% of black children. . . . These individuals can be precipitated into serious and painful hemolytic crises by a variety of conditions, including a decrease in blood oxygen.[26]

Much more has yet to be learned about traits and susceptibilities. Nevertheless, several employers have sought to use the available information on traits and health implications for the work force—incomplete as it is at the present time—to control occupational diseases and their economic consequences to the firm in various ways. A 1982 survey by the Office of Technology Assessment (OTA) of the U.S. Congress found that, of the 366 large firms that responded (out of 500 surveyed), 6 were conducting either genetic screening of job applicants or cytogenetic monitoring of workers, 17 had used such tests in the prior 12 years, 12 anticipated using genetic testing on job applicants and workers in the next 5 years, and 55 stated that they would possibly use such tests in the next 5 years.[27]

Such testing has many consequences for the firms and the workers involved, as the information provides a new basis for making decisions to control disease and corporate costs. The OTA survey reported that 18 of the 23 companies that were or had been engaged in genetic testing had taken some actions: 8 had informed the employees of potential problems, and 5 had transferred employees deemed to be at risk.[28] For example, DuPont has tested black employees for sickle-cell trait for the education and personal use of the employees on a voluntary and confidential basis.[29]

Beyond the scope of the OTA report may lie many other uses of genetic testing by other employers. For example, the U.S. Armed Forces have had a long-standing policy of prohibiting carriers of sickle-cell trait from assignment as pilots, co-pilots, submariners, or frogmen; and the U.S. Air Force has also excluded such carriers from the Air Force Academy.[30]

Finally, many companies use the most obvious of genetic differences to exclude women of childbearing years from certain occupations that will involve workplace exposure to known or suspected teratogens, in order to prevent the risk of harm to a fetus and the consequent tort litigation and company liability that could ensue. This policy has led to estimates that up to 100,000 jobs are closed to women because of teratogenic risks to the fetus; major firms, such as American Cyanamid, Johnson and Johnson, Monsanto, and General Motors employ such exclusionary policies.[31]

Thus, we stand at the beginning of a significant development with many moral, legal, economic, and human implications: the use of genetic and other information about biological diversity and human susceptibility to workplace disease by employers for purposes of controlling disease risks to workers and economic risks to employers. The consequences for classes of "susceptibles" and individuals with the risk traits include economic and career limitations, social categorization and stigmatization, and emotional distress. The consequences for society include the creation of new categories of discrimination based on genetic traits. Thus, advances in science and industrial risk management collide with the social trend of several decades toward equal treatment without discrimination, irrespective of sex, race, age, or handicap.

At the present time, no overall or generic social policy or law governs this development. The courts have narrowly permitted firms to discriminate against women because of possible teratogenic risks to a fetus if the firms provide a "business necessity defense"[32]; and presumably, this option will be available to firms employing discriminatory policies in less controversial or less legally defined areas od discrimination. The courts and OSHA have further found that certain risks arising from employee attempts to avoid corporate discrimination and to secure or retain jobs, such as self-imposed sterilization by women to avoid "fetal exclusion" policies, do not constitute hazards cognizable or governed by the Occupational Safety and Health Act, thereby reinforcing corporate uses of certain discriminatory policies.[33]

These recent decisions by the courts demonstrate the unpreparedness of the legal system and legal theories to deal with what promises to become a significant aspect of occupational disease control and management–labor relationships. Other legal issues and controversies abound and await judicial resolution on a case-by-case basis. One of these issues concerns the role of the examining physician as corporate employee or consultant, as well as his or her responbilities for disclosing information about traits to the job applicant, to management, to insurers, to medical and health promotion programs, and to other interested parties.

Responses to these problems outside the courts are now beginning to emerge, as several states legislate to protect job applicants from discrimination, loss of privacy, and other abuses arising from genetic and medical testing, but the resulting pattern of protection is irregular and fails to provide clear guidance to companies engaged in commerce on a national scale.[34] Until a national policy is adopted by Congress, or until occupational physicians and management adopt uniform self-regulation, events that may not be readily forthcoming, the major check on any abuses is the less-than-satisfactory one of fear of liability by companies and their doctors. The new information can be used by persons, if hired and subsequently diseased, to more readily establish causation and corporate responsibility and liability under state workers' compensation and tort law systems. Doctors face malpractice litigation and loss of licensure for improper disclosures and failures to treat "patients" under the variable criteria of the laws of 50 separate states. These concerns about liability therefore provide some sort of check on corporate uses of genetic testing when the corporate uses violate the rights of employees.[35]

But of course, these constraints are inadequate; and the full range of moral and policy considerations arising from these advances, illuminated by recent congressional hearings chaired by Representative Albert Gore, will hopefully provide a basis for action by Congress and by the private sector.[36]

SOME CONCLUSIONS

The medical and hygiene personnel involved in defensive-genetic and health-risk strategies are on the horns of a dilemma: whether to act as extensions of management and expose themselves to litigation for violating job applicant or worker interests in privacy, or for failing to warn workers of risk or to otherwise act in accordance with various state licensure laws; or whether to act as semi-independent professionals, consistent with the tenets and legal duties imposed on their professions. Doctors enjoy a certain amount of autonomy from corporate management control in such matters because of state medical licensure laws that impose certain duties on doctors regarding the diagnosis and treatment of their patients: to disclose relevant information to their "patients," to otherwise meet professional standards of practice, and to hold medical information confidential.

Industrial hygienists do not enjoy such autonomy under the law, although they run some of the same legal risks as their medical colleagues that they will be held legally accountable for unwarranted dissemination of personal health information, for failing to meet professional state of the art, and for failing to properly warn employees or otherwise act to prevent employee injury.[37] Professional associations for practitioners of occupational medicine and for industrial hygienists face the delicate task of establishing protocols that will assure the autonomy and the responsible actions of doctors and hygienists without endangering their important roles in corporate health programs.

The positive view of health-risk-prevention strategies gives primacy to the well-being and the health of those who may be at risk by developing a systematic approach to risk reduction that will be cost-effective for the firm over the long time.[38] This view tends to abide by the company doctor's credo, which holds that the needs of the organization can best be met by giving precedence to the needs and interests of the employees and others at risk, because "the benefit to the company is the aggregate good that we do for individuals."[39]

This view also enables epidemiologists and other health scientists to efficiently structure valid scientific studies that will yield more useful and credible results. They can therefore avoid being reactive, "continually trying to evaluate the health of . . . employees by bits and pieces in response to the chemical crises of the month."[40]

Some corporate initiatives now reflect the positive view and are apparently surviving the cost-effectiveness test. Allied Chemical has embarked on product liability profiling. Arthur D. Little and others provide new environmental audit services to corporate clients.[41] DuPont reports that its efforts have led to a construction safety record "three to four times better than the industry average," which, if replicated in other firms, could lead to cost savings of $2.75 billion a year; and that its program has "significantly reduced not only human suffering, but the cost of doing business."[42] Shell has described its new risk-assessment program as a procedure that "offers a way of improving workplace [health] without necessarily having to wait for the regulatory process to act."[43] Standard Oil (Indiana) now employs 23 industrial hygienists, 4 toxicologists, and other health professionals; does toxicological testing at its own laboratory; and has developed "product stewardship" committees and continuous monitoring, education, and other risk-reduction programs. It reports the "internalization of safety and health concern and responsibility throughout the line management" and "greater employee involvement through health and safety committees."[44]

These voluntary initiatives by large companies with vision, expertise, and financial resources may demonstrate that the positive approach to health risk is cost-effective and that it will eventually be reducible to practice in other, smaller firms. If these initiatives take root and demonstrate societal and human benefits as well as corporate cost control and improved profitability, still a utopian vision, we may finally be able to check the chronic problem of technological risk.

References and Notes

1. Friedman, M., *Capitalism and Freedom*, University of Chicago Press, Chicago (1962), 133–6.
2. Dahl, R., A prelude to corporate reform, in *Corporate Social Policy* (R. Heilbroner and P. London, eds.), Addison-Wesley, Lexington, MA (1975), 18–19.
3. See generally, Herman, E., *Corporate Control, Corporate Power*, Cambridge University Press, New York (1981), 242–301.
4. See Freeman, A., *Industry Response to Health Risk*, Rpt. 811, the Conference Board (1981).
5. *Id.*
6. See Ch. 2, "Corporate Social Responsibility," in *Ethical Theory and Business* (T. Beauchamp and N. Bowie, eds.), Prentice-Hall, Englewood Cliffs, NJ.
7. Executive Orders 12044 and 12291 have imposed cost–benefit analysis as the ultimate decision framework for regulatory rule-making and have provided special *ex parte* procedures, which industry has used to influence the Office of Management and Budget and the agencies. See Green, M., and Waitzman, N., *Business War against the Law*, Corporate Accountability Research Group, Washington, D.C. (1981); Baram, M., *Federal Regulation of Health, Safety and Environmental Quality and the Use of Cost-Benefit Analysis*, Report to Administrative Conference of the United States, Washington, D.C. (1979), with Recommendations (79-4).
8. Courts in New Jersey, for example, have adopted all of these reforms to reduce barriers to recovery by litigants in cases involving toxic torts. See, for example, *Ayers v. Jackson Township*, 19 ERC 24, L-5808-80 (Dec. 2, 1983). Also, see *Report of Proceedings on Toxic Torts*, American Bar Association Standing Committee on Environmental Law, published in *Environmental Law Reporter*, V. XIV, n.3, p. 100098, *et seq.*
9. *ABA Report, Id.*
10. See, for example, Buswell, H., *The Civil Liability for Personal Injuries Arising out of Negligence* (2d ed.), Little, Brown, Boston, MA (1899); Prosser, W., *Handbook of the Law of Torts* (4th ed.), West Pub. Co., St. Paul, MN (1971); and Toxic Substances Litigation, Practising Law Institute, New York (1983).
11. See *Borel v. Fibreboard Paper Products Corp.*, 493 F.2d 1076 (th Cir. 1973), in which the court established a "manufacturer's status as expert," with duties "to keep abreast of scientific knowledge [and] to test and inspect his product."
12. *Federal Register*, 48:53280 (Nov. 25, 1983).
13. See Baram, M., The right to know and the duty to disclose hazard information, *American Journal of Public Health* 74:385 (Apr. 1984).
14. For example, manufacturers of hazardous chemicals who comply with the OSHA rule stand on uncertain ground, as "downstream" industries that purchase their products and inform workers of health hazards may still experience occupational diseases. Given the inadequacies of workers' compensation, the injured employees of such downstream firms may resort to product liability law to sue the original manufacturer on the grounds that it failed to adequately inform the downstream firms or failed to monitor the adequacy of how the downstream firms actually implemented the OSHA rule to protect workers. Also, see *Restatement of Torts*, Sections 413 and 416.
15. See, e.g., *Beshada v. John Manville Corp.*, 90 N.J. 191 (1982); Comment, Product liability reform proposals: The state of the art defense, *Alb. L. Rev.* 43:941 (1979).
16. As demonstrated in litigation against the Johns-Manville Corporation, in which international breach of the duty to warn has been repeatedly argued. Also, see *Silkwood v. Kerr McGee*, 104 S.Ct. 615 (1984), for example, discussed in Annas, G. J. The case of Karen Silkwood, *American J. Public Health* 74:516 (1984).
17. *Risk Assessment Techniques*, (1st ed.), Defense Systems Management College, Fort Belvoir, VA (July 1983).
18. *Id.*
19. See, generally, House, P., and Shull, R., *Rush to Policy: Using Analytic Techniques in Public Sector*

Decision Making, U.S. National Science Foundation (draft) (1984), for analysis of public agency uses of risk assessment.

20. The name of the game, Environmental Science and Technology, 18(2):394 (Feb. 1984); editorial by D. Rosenblatt, U.S. Army Medical Bioengineering Research and Development Laboratory, Fort Detrick, MD.

21. Richards, E., and Silvers, A., Risk management theory: Reducing liability in corporate and medical environments, Houston L. Rev. 19:251 (1982). Long-term costs arising from collective bargaining of health provisions, like rising insurance costs, can be estimated. See, for example, Basic patterns in safety and health provisions in collective bargaining agreements, OSH Rptr., BNA, Inc. (May 19, 1983), 1092.

22. Id.

23. See Wright v. Olin Corp., 697 F.2d 1172 (4th Cir. 1982); Rothstein, J., Employee selection based on susceptibility to occupational illness, Mich. L. Rev. 81:1379 (1983). Also, see Mass. G.L., Ch.533 of Acts of 1983, which limits preemployment inquiries.

24. Silbergeld, A., Wrongful discharge and the "at-will" employee, National Law Journal (May 21, 1984), 14; and (Aug. 29, 1983), 20.

25. 29 CFR Part 1910.20; and Part 1904; also, see 42 CFR 85.3(b)(5).

26. D. Ozonoff, Roles for Genetic Screening and Biological Monitoring, unpublished report (Oct. 1983), Boston University Medical School. Genetic predispositions to heart disease, hypertension, and schizophrenia have also been suggested by various researchers.

27. The Role of Genetic Testing in the Prevention of Occupational Diseases, U.S. Congress, Office of Technology Assessment (1983), 33–40.

28. Id.

29. Severo, R., Screening of blacks by DuPont sharpens debate on gene test, New York Times (Feb. 4, 1980).

30. Air force challenged on sickle cell trait, Science 211:257 (1981).

31. Rothstein, M., Medical Screening of Workers, BNA, Inc. (1984), 77.

32. Wright v. Olin, 697 F.2d 1172 (4th Cir.); Hayes v. Shelby Memorial Hospital, N. 82-7296 52 U.S.L.W. 2560 (March 16, 1984).

33. Oil, Chemical and Atomic Worker's Int'l Union v. American Cyanamid, N. 81-1687 (D.C. Cir.) (Aug. 24, 1984).

34. New York, Massachusetts, and Connecticut have recently legislated on various aspects of these problems.

35. See, Baram, M., and Field, R., Screening and monitoring data as evidence in legal proceedings, presented at NIOSH Conference on Medical Screening and Biological Monitoring for the Effects of Exposure in the Workplace, Cincinnati, Ohio (July 12, 1984).

36. See the three reports of the Subcommittee on Investigations and Oversight, Committee on Science and Technology, U.S. House of Representatives; e.g., Genetic Screening in the Workplace (Oct. 6, 1982).

37. See Baron, F., Piercing the compensation veil: Third party remedies for job-related injuries, Occupational Disease Litigation, Practising Law Institute, New York (1983), 78–80; and state court decisions such as Okerblom v. Baskies, Massachusetts Superior Court, Middlesex County, No. 74-2570 (March 8, 1983), involving a malpractice claim by employee and family against a company psychiatrist and social worker. Also, see Legal and Professional Liability of Industrial Hygienists Employed by Insurance Companies, J. Biancheri, CNA Insurance Co., presented at the American Industrial Hygiene Conference, Detroit, Michigan (May 24, 1984).

38. In the design of such testing programs, some firms set forth certain criteria to minimize legal problems for medical and hygiene personnel. These include criteria that the program be designed to meet all legal requirements, to have substantial value to employees, to be consistent with the state of scientific and medical knowledge, to be cost-effective and manageable, and to be amenable to computerization. Personal communication, Robert Wheaton, Digital Equipment Corporation, April 1984.

39. Walsh, D., Strategic Planning for Corporate Health, Health Policy Research Institute, Boston University (1984).

40. Cook, R., et al., Dow Chemical Co., Epidemiology in Industry, paper presented at AIHC, Detroit, Michigan (May 23, 1984).

41. Some of these initiatives are discussed in Freeman, supra. note 5. Also, see materials in Baram, M., Corporate Management of Health Risks, (1983), course materials used at Boston University Schools of Law and Public Health.

42. Annual cost savings of $2.75 billion provide incentive for safety, meeting told, *OSH Rptr.*, BNA, Inc. (May 31, 1984).
43. New health protection procedure described by Shell official at AIHC, *OSH Rptr.*, BNA, Inc. (May 24, 1984), 1343.
44. Minter, S., Oil major's program targets changing needs, *Occupational Hazards* (May 1984), 63.

DISCUSSION

MR. GEORGE J. ANNAS: Dr. Baram, how effective do you think the advisory committee system has been in developing radiation standards to protect the public's health?

DR. MICHAEL S. BARAM: Advisory committees, such as the National Academy of Sciences, have inadequately protected public health. They have tended to wait too long, virtually until the bodies can be counted, before recommending any reduction in radiation exposure. They have also transgressed their scientific and medical mandate by giving great weight to the economic factors that promote the growth of the nuclear power industry.

DR. JAMES V. NEEL (University of Michigan Medical School): The first steps in this country to develop genetic standards were taken in 1956 by a committee of the National Academy of Sciences composed of very thoughtful and conscientious geneticists who concluded that some radiation is inevitable in our environment. The relevant question was: What is the largest amount that our consciences permit us to see human populations experience in return for the undoubted benefits that have come from the procedures that resulted in this radiation? Basically, out of that meeting, for nonmedical uses the committee recommended an annual exposure of 170 rem, which has been commonly accepted as the standard. We all accepted the straight-line hypothesis for lack of data at lower exposure levels. That is to say, there is no dose that is completely safe.

There are real difficulties in human epidemiological studies that would permit us to progress in this field in setting better estimates of effects than we have at the present time. In particular, although we can demonstrate chromosome breaks in somatic cells, we have no present method of extrapolating from those findings in somatic cells to true transmitted genetic damage. So that doesn't help us very much in arriving at a real risk–benefit analysis in this complex setting. I, for one, am certainly pushing that we develop more sensitive ways to proceed just as rapidly as they can be brought on-line. I don't think that we can eliminate radiation. We will have, for the foreseeable future, to live with it and really to understand the trade-off.

DR. MICHAEL S. BARAM: Radiation protection history is not edifying. I served on the second BEIR committee, "BEIR II," which followed "BEIR I," and which was itself succeeded by "BEIR III." There is a lot of dispute outside the BEIR committees about how one should set radiation standards, and for what health effects. There are fairly conclusive and defensible findings of fact. I found the BEIR committee a "Wonderland," with members who had long been serving together on these committees, many for years without a breath of fresh air. A shorthand language was used back and forth across the table, like "$1,000 a man rem" for the value of life, used in the cost–benefit analysis approach of the BEIR Committee for radiation-standard setting. I found all this mystifying, how such important issues as the value of health and life with regard to radiation had been reduced to a shorthand that nobody else in the whole world knew except the same body of people who had been working in these committees for years. I think this has contributed to some of the credibility problems that the nuclear enterprise has today. I am not going to express any opinions on the nuclear energy dispute, but I think it's clear that this closed process has tended, ultimately, to hurt the nuclear energy program and other uses of nuclear material.

DR. AUBREY MILUNSKY (Boston University School of Medicine): Dr. Neel, is there any solid foundation for Canada's law allowing women to take paid leave during pregnancy when they are working with mutagens?

DR. JAMES V. NEEL: Would that we really knew. There is some evidence that the very young are more susceptible to the impact of a carcinogen and, presumably, a mutagen. In the Japanese follow-up studies, for instance, the rate of excess malignancy is a factor two or three times higher in those exposed to the A-bomb in the 0–9 category than in those exposed in their 20s or 30s. So we do have some reason to think that the developing fetus might be particularly susceptible to some sort of mutagenic, teratogenic, or carcinogenic insult. On the other hand, we simply can't quantify this issue in any very respectable fashion at the present time.

DR. AUBREY MILUNSKY: Does that mean that, when you are now asked by a woman working with chemical solvents that are clearly known mutagens, you will tell her to not work when she is planning pregnancy because you have theoretical concerns for which there isn't yet a true foundation in fact?

DR. JAMES V. NEEL: Now, let's distinguish between the genetic and the teratogenic here. I'll try both. If we think we have trouble evaluating the genetic impact of radiation in a realistic way, chemicals are a far, far greater problem. With radiation, we can at least get the gonad doses. We know how X rays penetrate tissue. We know very, very little about the extent to which chemical mutagens reach the germ line. At the risk of sounding academic, I can't think of a more important issue into which to put a lot of epidemiological money right now because the sums involved, in terms of regulation, are tremendous. I wish to protect, but on the basis of information, not on a "guess-estimate." Now, you asked me what I would do with the individual woman who might come to me as a patient. I would, I'm sure, say, "I can't advise any chemical exposures during your pregnancy, but I would like to know more about those chemical exposures." Does she get a whiff of benzene as she passes a certain laboratory 200 yards from where she works, or does she have a real chemical exposure? I don't see how to give you a generic answer.

Ms. SYLVIA RUBIN (Columbia Presbyterian Medical Center): I cannot leave without extending my personal thanks to you, Dr. Milunsky, and your whole staff for what everyone here will agree with me was a superb, innovative, and well-organized three days. I myself have been to all three of these symposia and agree with Margery Shaw, who looks forward to the fourth. I am going to go home with many, many more questions than answers, but I fully expected that. I hope we never stop asking the questions we have asked today. That's the most important thing. As Dr. Baram said, the bottom line is "There is no bottom line." I hope we never forget that. Thank you again.

DR. AUBREY MILUNSKY: You are most gracious. We set out to explore the interface between genetics, ethics, and the law and to continue the dialogue. I think we succeeded in some part. Thank you.

MR. GEORGE J. ANNAS: On that pleasant note, let me bring this session and this conference to a close and thank you all for your thoughtful and constructive participation.

Selected Additional Bibliography[*]

Books

Anderson, J. K., *Genetic Engineering, The Ethical Issues*, Zondervan, Grand Rapids, MI (1982).

Applied Genetics, A Booming Industry, Business Communications Co., Inc., Stanford, CT (1981).

Atkinson, B. G., *Changes in Gene Expression in Response to Environmental Stress*, Academic Press, New York (1985).

Ball, C., *Genetics and Breeding of Industrial Microorganisms*, Chemical Rubber Co., Boca Raton, FL (1984).

Beier, H. M., and Lindner, H. R. (eds.), *Fertilization of the Human Egg in Vitro: Biological Basis and Clinical Application*, Springer-Verlag, Berlin (1983).

Berg, K., *Genetic Damage in Man Caused by Environmental Agents*, Academic Press, Inc., San Diego (1979).

Berg, K., and Tranoy, K. E. (eds.), *Research Ethics*. Alan R. Liss, New York, 1983.

Blank, R. H., *The Political Implications of Human Genetic Technology: Special Studies in Science, Technology and Public Policy*, Westview, Boulder, CO (1981).

Calabrese, E. J., *Ecogenetics, Genetic Variation in Susceptibility to Environmental Agents*, Wiley-Interscience, London (1984).

Chahakrabarty, A. M., *Genetic Engineering*, Chemical Rubber Co., Boca Raton, FL (1978).

Chase, A., *The Legacy of Malthus, The Social Costs of the New Scientific Racism*, Knopf (1977).

Clements, C. D., *Medical Genetics Casebook: A Clinical Introduction to Medical Ethics Systems Theory*, Humana, Clifton, NJ (1982).

Crosignani, P. G., and Rubin, B. L., *In Vitro Fertilization and Embryo Transfer*, Grune & Stratton, New York (1983).

Dean, D. H., *Gene Structure and Expression*, Ohio State University Press, Columbus, OH (1980).

DeSerres, J., *Utilization of Mammalian Specific Locus Studies in Hazard Evaluation and Estimation of Genetic Risk*, Plenum Press, New York (1983).

Dobbing, J. (ed.), *Prevention of Spina Bifida and Other Neural Tube Defects*, Academic Press, New York (1983).

Glover, D. M., *Genetic Engineering*, Methuen, New York (1980).

Haller, M. H., *Eugenics, Hereditarian Attitudes in American Thought*, Rutgers (1983).

Hamer, D. H., and Rosenberg, M. J. (eds.), *Gene Expression*, Alan R. Liss, New York (1983).

Herrmann, K., *Amino-Acid Biosynthesis and Genetic Regulation*, Addison-Weslay Publishing Co., Inc., Reading, MA (1983).

Hollaender, A., *Genetic Engineering, Principles and Methods*, Plenum Publishers, New York (1979).

Ishihara, T., Sasaki, M. S. (eds.), *Radiation-Induced Chromosome Damage to Man*, Alan R. Liss, New York (1983).

---

[*] See *Genetics and Law II* (1980) for earlier references.

Kevles, D. J., *In the Name of Eugenics, Genetics and the Uses of Human Heredity*, Knopf, New York (1985).

Langone, J., *Human Engineering, Marvel or Menace*, Little, Boston (1978).

Lebacz, K., *Genetics, Ethics and Parenthood*, Pilgrim, New York (1983).

Menditto, J., *Genetic Engineering, DNA and Cloning: A Bibliography in the Future of Genetics*, Whitston Publishing, Troy, NY (1982).

Mertens, T. R., *Human Genetics: Readings on the Implications of Genetic Engineering*, Wiley (1975).

Milunsky, A. (ed.), *Genetic Disorders and the Fetus, Diagnosis, Prevention, and Treatment*, Plenum Press, New York (1979).

Milunsky, A., and Annas, G. J. (eds.), *Genetics and the Law* (Vol. 2), Plenum Press, New York (1980).

Moraczewski, A. S., *Genetic Medicine and Engineering, Ethical and Social Dimensions*, Cath-Health, Catholic Health Association, St. Louis (1983).

Motulsky, A. G., *Human Genetic Variation in Response to Medical and Environmental Agents: Pharmacogenetics and Ecogenetics*, Springer-Verlag, Berlin (1979).

O'Connor, T. E., and Rauscher, F. J. *Oncogenes and Retroviruses: Evaluation of Basic Findings and Clinical Potential (Progress in Clinical and Biological Research*, (Vol. 119), Alan R. Liss, New York (1983).

Office of Technology Assessment, U.S. Congress, *Genetic Technology, A New Frontier*, Westview, Boulder, CO. (1982).

Old, R. W., *Principles of Gene Manipulation: An Introduction to Genetic Engineering*, University of California Press, Berkeley (1982).

Oliverio, A., *Genetics, Environment and Intelligence*, Elsevier, Amsterdam (1977).

Packard, V., *The People Shapers*, Little, Boston (1977).

Persuad, T. F., *Genetic Disorders, Syndromology and Prenatal Diagnosis: Advances in the Study of Birth Defects* (Vol. 5). Alan R. Liss, New York (1982).

Pierce, C. W., Cullen, S. E., Kapp, A., Schwartz, B. D., Shreffler, D. C. (eds.), *Genes: Past, Present, and Future. (Experimental Biology and Medicine)*. Humana Press, Clifton, NJ (1983).

Purdy, J. M., *Methods for Fertilization and Embryo Culture in Vitro, In Human Conception in Vitro*, edited by R. G. Edwards and J. M. Purdy. Academic Press, London (1983).

Reilly, P., *Genetics, Law, and Social Policy*, Harvard University Press, Cambridge (1977).

Rowley, J. D., and Ultmann, J. E. (eds.), *Chromosomes and Cancer from Molecules to Man*, Academic Press, Orlando (1983).

Sebek, O. K., *Genetics of Industrial Microorganisms*, American Society of Microbiology (1979).

Setlow, J. K., *Genetic Engineering: Principles and Methods*, Plenum Publishers, (1979).

Smith, G. P., *Genetics, Ethics and the Law: New Studies on Law and Society*, Associated Faculty Press (1981).

Sokoloski, J. E., and Wolf, D. P., Laboratory details in an in vitro fertilization and embryo transfer program, in *Human in Vitro Fertilization and Embryo Transfer*, edited by D. P. Wolf and M. D. Quigley. Plenum Press, New York (1984).

Testart, J., Lassalle, B., and Frydman, R., Success of human in vitro fertilization in spontaneous or stimulated cycles and technical procedures used, in *Proceedings of the 4th Reiner De Graaf Symposium, Follicular Maturation and Ovulation, Nijmegen, The Netherlands*, edited by R. Rolland, E. V. van Hall, S. G. Miller, I. C. P. McNatty, and J. Schoemaker, Excerpta Medica, Amsterdam (1982).

Timmis, K. N., *Plasmids of Medical Environmental and Commercial Importance*, Elsevier, Amsterdam (1979).

Warr, R. F., *Genetic Engineering in Higher Organisms*, E. Arnold, Baltimore (1984).

Williams, A. R., *Ultrasound: Biological Effects and Potential Hazards*, Academic Press, London (1983).

Williamson, R., *Genetic Engineering*. Academic Press, New York (1982).

Wood, C., and Trounson, A., *Clinical in Vitro Fertilization*, Springer-Verlag, Berlin (1984).

SELECTED ADDITIONAL BIBLIOGRAPHY[*]

Journals

PRENATAL DIAGNOSIS, GENETIC COUNSELING, AND SCREENING

Adams, M. M., Finley, S., Hansen, H., Jahiel, R. I., Oakley, G. P., Jr., Sanser, W., Wells, G., and Wertelecki, W., Utilization of prenatal genetic diagnosis in women 35 years of age and older in the United States, 1977 to 1978, *Am. J. Obstet. Gynecol.* **139**:673–7 (1981).

Anionwu, E. N., Sickle cell disease: Screening and counselling in the antenatal and neonatal period, Part 2, *Midwife Health Visit. Community Nurse* **19**:440–4 (1983).

Annas, G. J., Mandatory PKU screening: The other side of the looking glass, *Am. J. Public Health* **72**:1401–3 (1982).

Beer, A. E., Quebbeman, J. F., Ayers, J. W., and Haines, R. F., Major histocompatibility complex antigens, maternal and paternal immune responses, and chronic habitual abortions in humans, *Am. J. Obstet. Gynecol.* **141**:987–99 (1981).

Birnholz, J. C., Determination of fetal sex, *N. Engl. J. Med.* **309**:942–4 (1983).

Bixler, D., Boggs, W. S., Jorgenson, R. J., Salinas, C. F., Sanger, R. G., and Taichman, L. B., The role of genetics in the practice of dentistry, *Birth Defects* **16**:7–12 (1980).

Boehm, C. D., Antonarakis, S. E., Phillips, J. A., 3rd, Stetten, G., and Kazazian, H. H., Jr., Prenatal diagnosis using DNA polymorphisms: Report on 95 pregnancies at risk for sickle-cell disease or beta-thalassemia, *N. Engl. J. Med.* **308**:1054–8 (1983).

Buri, C. E., and Hecht, F., Tort liability in genetic diagnosis and genetic counseling, *Am. J. Hum. Genet.* **34**:353–6 (1982).

Cadkin, A. V., Ginsberg, N. A., Pergament, E., and Verlinski, Y., Chorionic villi sampling: A new technique for detection of genetic abnormalities in the first trimester, *Radiology* **151**:159–62 (1984).

Cao, A., Pintus, L., Lecca-U., Olla, G., Cossu, P., Rosatelli, C., and Galanello, R., Control of homozygous beta-thalassemia by carrier screening and antenatal diagnosis in Sardinians, *Clin. Genet.* **26**:12–22 (1984).

Capron, A. M., Autonomy, confidentiality, and quality care in genetic counseling, *Birth Defects* **15**:307–40 (1979).

Daniell, J. F., Sex-selection procedures, *J. Reprod. Med.* **18**:235–7 (1983).

Dmowski, W. P., Gaynor, L., Rao-R., Lawrence, M., and Scommegna, A., Use of albumin gradients for X and Y sperm separation and clinical experience with male sex preselection, *Fertil. Steril.* **31**:52–7 (1979).

Duca, D., Cioltei, A., Ioan, D., and Maximilian, C., The importance of cytogenetic investigation of the

---

[*]See *Genetics and Law II* (1980) for earlier references.

couples with multiple spontaneous abortions and malformed offspring, *Endocrinologie* **17**:17–22 (1979). (Review)

Ducos, J., and Gortz, R., Importance of precise identification of haplotypes of the Gm system in medico-legal expert opinions on paternity exclusion, *Arch. Belg. Med. Soc.* **37**:248–53 (1979).

Dunne, M. D., and Cunat, J. S., Sonographic determination of fetal gender before 25 weeks gestation, *Am. J. Radiology* **140**:741–3 (1983).

Elles, R. G., Williamson, R., Niazi, M., Coleman, D. V., and Horwell, D., Absence of maternal contamination of chorionic villi used for fetal-gene analysis, *N. Eng. J. Med.* **308**:1433–5 (1983).

Faden, R., Chwalow, A. J., Holtzman, N. A., and Horn, S. D., A survey to evaluate parental consent as public policy for neonatal screening, *Am. J. Public Health* **72**:1347–52 (1982).

Faden, R. R., Holtzman, N. A., and Chwalow, A. J., Parental rights, child welfare, and public health: The case of PKU screening, *Am. J. Public Health* **72**:1396–400 (1982).

Feil, R. N., Largey, G. P., and Miller, M., Attitudes toward abortion as a means of sex selection, *J. Psychol.* **116**(2nd half):269–72 (1984).

Fisher, N. L., Starr, E. D., Greene, T., and Hoehn, H., Utility and limitations of chromosome banding in pre- and postnatal service cytogenetics, *Am. J. Med. Genet.* **5**:285–94 (1980).

Fletcher, J. C., Ethical issues in genetic screening and antenatal diagnosis, *Clin. Obstet. Gynecol.* **24**:1151–68 (1981). (Review)

France, J. T., Graham, F. M., Gosling, L., and Hair, P. I., A prospective study of the preselection of the sex of offspring by timing intercourse relative to ovulation, *Fertil. Steril.* **41**:894–900 (1984).

Fraser, F. C., Introduction: The development of genetic counseling, *Birth Defects* **15**:5–15 (1979).

Friesen, H., and Nishiokia, Y., A molecular method for detecting the presence of the human Y chromosome, *Am. J. Med. Genet.* **18**:289–94 (1984).

Genetic registers (editorial), *Lancet* **1**:253 (1979).

Glaser, G., Karsai, A., Karem, H., Yarkoni, S., and Rachmilewitz, E., Prenatal diagnosis of beta-thalassemia using genetic engineering techniques, *Harefuah* **103**:293–4 (1982).

Goerth, C. R., Genetic screening and the law: Question waiting for an answer, *Occup. Health Saf.* **52**:49–51 (1983).

Gosden, J. R., Mitchell, A. R., Gosden, C. M., Rodeck, C. H., and Morsman, J. M. Direct vision chorion biopsy and chromosome-specific DNA probes for determination of fetal sex in first-trimester prenatal diagnosis, *Lancet* **2**:1416–9 (1982).

Gosden, J. R., Gosden, C. M., Christie, S., Cooke, H. J., Morsman, J. M., and Rodeck, C. H. The use of cloned Y chromosome-specific DNA probes for fetal sex determination in first trimester prenatal diagnosis, *Human Genetics* **66**:347–51 (1984).

Gosden, J. R., Gosden, C. M., Christie, S., Morsman, J. M., and Rodeck, C. H., Rapid fetal sex determination in first trimester: prenatal diagnosis by dot hybridisation of DNA probes, *Lancet* **1**:540–1 (1984).

Gray, C., Prenatal diagnosis: The demand is increasing, *Can. Med. Assoc. J.* **126**:64,66,70–1 (1982).

Harper, P. S., Genetic counselling and prenatal diagnosis, *Br. Med. Bull.* **39**:302–9 (1983).

Hartley, S. F., and Pietraczyk, L. M., Preselecting the sex of offspring: Technologies, attitudes, and implications, *Soc. Biol.* **26**:232–46 (1979).

Hassold, T., and Matsuyama, A. Origin of trisomies in human spontaneous abortions, *Hum. Genet.* **46**:285–94 (1979).

Hassold, T., Chen, N., Funkhouser, J., Jooss, T., Manuel, B., Matsuura, J., Matsuyama, A., Wilson, C., Yamane, J. A., and Jacobs, P. A., A cytogenetic study of 1000 spontaneous abortions, *Ann. Hum. Genet.* **44**:151–78 (1980).

Hassold, T., Chiu, D., and Yamane, J. A., Parental origin of autosomal trisomies, *Ann. Hum. Genet.* **48**:129–44 (1984).

Headings, V. E., Comprehensive counseling for prenatal diagnosis of hemoglobinopathies, *Prog. Clin. Biol. Res.* **98**:143–50 (1982).

Hobbins, J. C., Determination of fetal sex in early pregnancy (editorial), *N. Eng. J. Med.* **309**:979–80 (1983).

Hockey, A., Michael, C. A., and Bain, J. G., Genetic screening in Western Australia, *Med. J. Aust.* **1**:363–5 (1979).

Holzsreve, B., Holzsreve, W., and Golbus, M. S., The relevance of pre-amniocentesis pedigree analysis and genetic counseling, *Clin. Genet.* **24**:429–33 (1983).

Hook, E. B., Genetic triage and genetic counseling, *Am. J. Med. Genet.* **17**:535–8 (1984).

Hook, E. B., and Schreinemachers, D. M., Trends in utilization of prenatal cytogenetic diagnosis by New York State residents in 1979 and 1980, *Am. J. Public Health* **73**:198–202 (1983).

Hook, E. B., Woodbury, D. F., and Albright, S. G., Rates of trisomy 18 in livebirths, stillbirths, and at amniocentesis, *Birth Defects* **15**:81–83 (1979).

Hsu, L, Y., Prenatal cytogenetic diagnosis: A mini-review, *Prog. Clin. Biol. Res.* **44**:3–25 (1980).

Hunter, A. G., and Cox, D. M., Counseling problems when twins are discovered at genetic amniocentesis, *Clin. Genet.* **16**:34–42 (1979).

Johnson, V., Indications and techniques for genetic amniocentesis, *H. Reprod. Med.* **27**:557–9 (1982).

Kaback, M. D., The control of genetic disease by carrier screening and antenatal diagnosis: Social, ethical, and medicolegal issues, *Birth Defects* **18**:243–54 (1982).

Kaback, M. M., Screening for reproductive counseling: Social, ethical, and medicolegal issues in the Tay-Sachs disease experience, *Prog. Clin. Biol. Res.* **103**:447–59 (1982).

Kalousek, D. K., and Dill, F. J., Chromosomal mosaicism confined to the placenta in human conception, *Science* **221**:665–7 (1983).

Kapp, R. W., Jr., Detection of aneuploidy in human sperm, *Environ. Health Perspect.* **31**:27–31 (1979).

Karp, L. E., The arguable propriety of preconceptual sex determination, *Am. J. Med. Genet.* **6**:185–7 (1980).

Katz, A. H., Genetic counseling in chronic disease, *Health Soc. Work* **5**:14–9 (1980).

Kenen, R. H., Genetic counseling: The development of a new interdisciplinary occupational field, *Soc. Sci. Med.* **18**:541–9 (1984).

Kessler, S., The psychological paradigm shift in genetic counseling, *Soc. Biol.* **27**:167–85 (1980).

Kopelman, L., Genetic screening in newborns: Voluntary or compulsory? *Perspect. Biol. Med.* **22**:83–9 (1978).

LaRochelle, D., Prenatal genetic counseling: Ethical and legal interfaces with the nurse's role, *Issues Health Care Women* **4**:77–92 (1983).

Lau, Y. F., Huang, J. C., Dozy, A. M., and Kan, Y. W., A rapid screening test for antenatal sex determination, *Lancet* **1**:14–6 (1984).

Laurence, K. M., Prevention of neural tube malformation by genetic counselling, and prenatal diagnostic surveillance, *J. Genet. Hum.* **27**:289–99 (1979).

Levine, C., Genetic counseling: The client's viewpoint, *Birth Defects* **15**:123–35 (1979).

Lundberg, M., Jerominski, L., Livingston, G., Kochenour, N., Lee, T., and Fineman, R., Failure to demonstrate an effect of in vivo diagnostic ultrasound on sister chromatid exchange frequency in amniotic fluid cells, *Am. J. Med. Genet.* **11**:31–5 (1982).

Lynch, H. T., Lynch, P. M., Kimberling, W. J., and Lynch, J. F., Medical genetics, Huntington's chorea, and legal questions pertaining to autopsy, *Am. J. Med.* **75**:157–60 (1983).

Martinez, F., Cheung, S. W., Crane, J. P., and Arias, F., Use of trophoblast cells in tissue culture for fetal chromosomal studies, *Am. J. Obstet. Gynecol.* **147**:542–7 (1983).

Marion, J. P., Kassam, G., and Fernhoff, P. M., Brantley, K. E., Carroll, L., Zacharias, J., Klein, L., Priest, J. H., and Elsas, L. J., 2d, Acceptance of amniocentesis by low-income patients in an urban hospital, *Am. J. Obstet. Gynecol.* **138**:11–5 (1980).

Markova, I., Forbes, C. D., and Inwood, M., The consumer's views of genetic counseling or hemophilia, *Am. J. Med. Genet* **17**:741–52 (1984).

McCormack, M. K., Medical genetics and family practice, *Am. Fam. Physician* **20**:142–54 (1979).

Modell, B., and Mouzouras, M., Social consequences of introducing antenatal diagnosis for thalassemia, *Birth Defects* **18**:285–91 (1982).

Pembrey, M. E., Genetic registers, *Arch. Dis. Child.* **54**:169–70 (1979).

Pernoll, M. L., King, C. R., and Prescott, G. H., Genetics for the clinical obstetrician-gynecologist, *Obstet. Gynecol. Annu.* **9**:1–53 (1980).

Polani, P. E., Alberman, E., Alexander, B. J., Benson, P. F., Berry, A. C., Blunt, S., Daker, M. G., Fenson, A. H., Garrett, D. M., McGuire, V. M., Roberts, J. A., Seller, M. J., and Singer, J. D., Sixteen years' experience of counselling, diagnosis, and prenatal detection in one genetic centre: Progress, results, and problems, *J. Med. Genet.* **16**:166–75 (1979).

Prenatal diagnosis for sex choice, *Hastings Cent. Rep.* **10**:15–20 (1980).

Reed, S. C., A short history of human genetics in the USA, *Am. J. Med. Genet.* **3**:282–95 (1979).

Rett, A., Genetic counselling and human handicap, *Wien. Klin. Wochenschr.* **94**:315–7 (1982).

Robinson, F. C., Robinson, S. W., and Williams, L. J., Eugenic sterilization: Medico-legal and sociological aspects, *J. Natl. Med. Assoc.* **71**:593–8 (1979).

Roblin, R., Genetic disease as seen on a continuum, *Birth Defects* 15:47–56 (1979).

Rosner, F., The Biblical and Talmudic secret for choosing one's baby's sex, *Isr. J. Med. Sci.* 15:784–7 (1979).

Rowley, P. T., Genetic screening: Marvel or menace? *Science* 225:138–44 (1984).

Rozovsky, L. E., and Rozovsky, F. A., Genetic screening: Public health and the law, *Can. J. Public Health* 72:15–6 (1981).

Rubin, S. P., Malin, J., and Maidman, J., Genetic counseling before prenatal diagnosis for advanced maternal age: An important medical safeguard, *Obstet. Gynecol.* 62:155–9 (1983).

Schechter, D., Genetic screening in the workplace, *Occup. Health Saf.* 52:8–12 (1983).

Seidenfeld, M. J., Braitman, A., and Antley, R. M., The determinants of mothers' knowledge of the Down syndrome before genetic counseling, Part II, *Am. J. Med. Genet.* 6:9–23 (1980).

Seller, M. J., Ethical aspects of genetic counselling, *J. Med. Ethics* 8:185–8 (1982).

Simoni, G., Brambati, B., Danesino, C., Rossella, F., Terzoli, G. L., Ferrari, M., and Fraccaro, M., Efficient direct chromosome analysis and enzyme determinations from chorionic villi samples in the first trimester of pregnancy, *Hum. Genet.* 63:349–357 (1983).

Simpson, J. L., Genes, chromosomes, and reproductive failure, *Fertil. Steril.* 33:107–16 (1980).

Simpson, J. L., Antenatal diagnosis of cytogenetic abnormalities, *Clin. Obstet. Gynecol.* 24:1023–39 (1981).

Simpson, J. L., Elias, S., Gatlin, M., and Margin, A. O., Genetic counseling and genetic services in obstetrics and gynecology: Implications for educational goals and clinical practice, *Am. J. Obstet. Gynecol.* 140:70–80 (1981).

Singh, D. N., Hara, S., Foster, H. W., and Grimes, E. M., Reproductive performance in women with sex chromosome mosaicism, *Obstet. Gynecol.* 55:608–11 (1980).

Srensen, S. A., and Hasholt, L., Attitudes of persons at risk for Fabry's disease towards predictive tests and genetic counselling, *J. Biosoc. Sci.* 15:89–94 (1983).

Trotzis, M. A., The defective child and the actions for wrongful life and wrongful birth, *J. Leg. Med.* 2:85–111 (1980).

Tsuan, M. T., Genetic counseling for psychiatric patients and their families, *Am. J. Psychiat.* 135:1465–75 (1978).

Turner, J. H., Hayashi, T. T., and Pogoloff, D. D., Legal and social issues in medical genetics, *Am. J. Obstet. Gynecol.* 134:83–99 (1979). (Review)

Van-Resemorter, N., Dodion, J., Druart, C., Hayez, F., Vamos, E., and Rodesch, F., Major congenital malformations in 5448 newborns: Comments on genetic counseling and prenatal diagnosis, *Acta Paediat. Belg.* 34:73–81 (1981).

Van-Regemorter, N., Dodion, J., Druart, C., Hayez, F., Vamos, E., Flament-Durand, J., Perlmutter-Cremer, N., and Rodesch, F., Congenital malformations in 10,000 consecutive births in a university hospital: Need for genetic counseling and prenatal diagnosis, *J. Pediat.* 104:386–90 (1984).

Vergnaud, G., Kaplan, L., Weissenbach, J., Dumez, Y., Berger, R., Tiollais, P., and Guellaen, G., Rapid and early determination of sex using trophoblast biopsy specimens and Y chromosome specific DNA probes, *Br. Med. J. (Clin. Res.)* 289:73–6 (1984).

Warren, W. C., Participation of the dentist in the Genetic Services Act, *Birth Defects* 16:191–5 (1980).

Williamson, N. E., Lean, T. H., and Vengadasalam, D., Evaluation of an unsuccessful sex preselection clinic in Singapore, *J. Biosoc. Sci.* 10:375–88 (1978).

Wright, E. E., The legal implications of refusing to provide prenatal diagnosis in low-risk pregnancies or solely for sex selection, *Am. J. Med. Genet.* 5:391–7 (1980).

Wright, E. E., and Shaw, M. W., Legal liability in genetic screening, genetic counseling, and prenatal diagnosis, *Clin. Obstet. Gynecol.* 24:1133–49 (1981). (Review)

GENETICS, INDUSTRY, AND LAW

Abbott, M. H., Abbey, H., Bollins, D. R., and Murphy, E. A., The familial component in longevity—a study of offspring of nonagenarians: III. Intrafamilial studies, *Am. J. Med. Genet.* 2:105–20 (1978).

Andersson, H. C., Tranberg, E. A., Uggla, A. H., and Zetterberg, G., Chromosomal aberrations and sister-chromatid exchanges in lymphocytes of men occupationally exposed to styrene in a plastic-boat factory, *Mutat. Res.* 73:387–401 (1980).

Bauchinger, M., Schmid, E., Dresp, J., Kolin-Gerresheim, J., Hauf, R., and Suhr, E., Chromosome changes in lymphocytes after occupational exposure to toluene, *Mutat. Res.* 102:439–45 (1982).

Blank, C. E., Cooke, P., and Potter, A. M., Investigations for genotoxic effects after exposure to crude 2,4,5-trichlorophenol, *Br. J. Ind. Med.* 40:87–91 (1983).

Brandom, W. F., Bloom, A. D., Archer, P. G., Archer, V. E., Biltline, R. W., and Saccomanno, G., Somatic cell genetics of uranium miners and plutonium workers: A biological dose-response indicator. In: Late biological effects of ionizing radiation, Vol. 1, Vienna, International Atomic Energy Agency 1:507–18 (1978).

Bridges, B. A., Bochkov, N. P., and Jansen, J. D., Genetic monitoring of human populations accidentally exposed to a suspected mutagenic chemical, *Mutat. Res.* 64:57–60 (1979).

Camurri, L., Codeluppi, S., Pedroni, C., and Scarduelli, L., Chromosomal aberrations and sister-chromatid exchanges in workers exposed to styrene. *Mutat. Res.* 119:361–9 (1983).

Dalpra, L., Tibiletti, M. G., Nocera, G., Giulotto, P., Auriti, L., Carnelli, V., and Simoni, G., SCE analysis in children exposed to lead emission from a smelting plant, *Mutat. Res.* 120:249–56 (1983).

Diamond, A. L., Genetic testing in employment situations: A question of worker rights. *J. Leg. Med.* 4:231–56 (1983).

Ehrenberg, L., Anderstam, B., Hussain, S., and Hamnerius, Y., Statistical aspects of the design of biological tests for the detection of low genotoxic activity, *Hereditas* 98:33–41 (1983).

Evans, H. J., Buckton, K. E., Hamilton, G. E., and Carothers, A., Radiation-induced chromosome aberrations in nuclear-dockyard workers, *Nature* 277:531–4 (1979).

Forni, A., Sciame, A., Bertazzi, P. A., and Alessio, L., Chromosome and biochemical studies in women occupationally exposed to lead, *Arch. Environ. Health* 35:139–46 (1980).

Fredga, K., Davring, L., Sunner, M., Bengtsson, B. O., Elinder, C. G., Sistryggsson, P., and Berlin, M., Chromosome changes in workers (smokers and nonsmokers) exposed to automobile fuels and exhaust gases, *Scand. J. Work Environ. Health* 8:209–21 (1982).

Gamow, R. I., The many facets of bioengineering, *Biomed. Sci. Instrum.* 20:5–8 (1984).

Goldsmith, J. R., Potashnik, G., and Israeli, R., Reproductive outcomes in families of DBCP-exposed men, *Arch. Environ. Health* 39:85–9 (1984).

Gonzalez Cid, M. D., and Matos, E., Sister chromatid exchange in workers of a chemical industry, *Medicina* (B. Aires) 43:513–6 (1983).

Grandjean, P., Wulf, H. C., and Niebuhr, E., Sister chromatid exchange in response to variations in occupational lead exposure, *Environ. Res.* 32:199–204 (1983).

Green, J., Detecting the hypersusceptible worker: Genetics and politics in industrial medicine, *Int. Health Serv.* 13:247–64 (1983).

Haglund, U., Jundberg, I., and Zech, L., Chromosome aberrations and sister chromatid exchanges in Swedish paint industry workers, *Scand. J. Work Environ. Health* 6:291–8 (1980).

Hatch, M., Parental occupation and cytogenetic studies in abortuses, *Prog. Clin. Biol. Res.* 160:475–83 (1984).

Hogstedt, B., Colnig, A. M., Mitelman, F., and Skerfving, S., Cytogenetic study of pesticides in agricultural work, *Hereditas* 92:177–8 (1980).

Horne, S. L., Tennent, R., Lovegrove, A., Dosman, J. A., and Cockcroft, D. W., Pi type MZ and an increased risk of pneumonia, *Clin. Invest. Med.* 7:85–8 (1984).

Husum, B., Wulf, H. C., and Niebuhr, E., Sister chromatid exchanges in humans exposed to inhalation anaesthetics, *Prog. Clin. Biol. Res.* 109:465–70 (1982).

Husum, B., Niebuhr, E., Wulf, H. C., and Nrgaard, I., Sister chromatid exchanges and structural chromosome aberrations in lymphocytes in operating room personnel, *Acta Anaesthesiol. Scan.* 27:262–5 (1983).

Kolata, G. B., Love Canal: False alarm caused by botched study. *Science* 208:1239–42 (1980).

Lambert, B., Bredberg, A., McKenzie, W., and Sten, M., Sister chromatid exchange in human populations: The effect of smoking, drug treatment, and occupational exposure, *Cytogenet. Cell Genet.* 33:62–7 (1982).

Laurent, C., Frederick, J., and Marechal, F., Increased frequency of sister chromatid exchange in persons occupationally exposed to ethylene oxide, *Ann. Genet.* (Paris) 26:138–42 (1983).

Linnainmaa-K., Sister chromatid exchanges among workers occupationally exposed to phenoxy acid herbicides 2,4,-D and MCPA, *Teratogenesis Carcinog. Mutagen.* 3:269–79 (1983).

Lower, W. R., Drobney, V. K., Aholt, B. J., and Politte, R., Mutagenicity of the environments in the vicinity of an oil refinery and a petrochemical complex, *Teratogenesis Carcinog. Mutagen.* 3:65–73 (1983).

Mabille, V., Roels, H., Jacquet, P., Leonard, A., and Lauwerys, R., Cytogenetic examination of leucocytes of workers exposed to mercury vapour, *Int. Arch. Occup. Environ. Health* 53:257–60 (1984).

Maki-Paakkanen, J., Husgafvel-Pursiainen, K., Kalliomaki, P. L., Tuominen, J., and Sorsa, M., Toluene-exposed workers and chromosome aberrations, *J. Toxicol. Environ. Health* **6**:775–81 (1980).

Miller, H. I., Designer genes for producing drugs: Will they wash? (editorial), *DNA* **1**:101–2 (1982).

Mitelman, F., Nilsson, P. G., and Brandt, L., Fourth International Workshop on Chromosomes in Leukemia 1982: Correlation of karyotype and occupational exposure to potential mutagenic/carcinogenic agents in acute nonlymphycytic leukemia, *Cancer Genet. Cytogenet.* **11**:326–31 (1984).

Murray, T. H., Genetic screening in the workplace: Ethical issues, *J. Occup. Med.* **25**:451–4 (1983).

Neidleman, S. L., and Cape, R. E., Genetics of industrial microorganisms: Look how far we have come! *Riv. Biol.* **75**:351–71 (1982).

Nordenson, I., and Beckman, L., Chromosomal aberrations in lymphocytes of workers exposed to low levels of styrene, *Hum. Hered.* **34**:178–82 (1984).

Nordenson, I., Sweins, A., and Beckman, L., Chromosome aberrations in cultured human lymphocytes exposed to trivalent and pentavalent arsenic, *Scand. J. Work Environ. Health* **7**:277–81 (1981).

Nordenson, I., Nordstrom, S., Sweins, A., and Beckman, L., Chromosomal aberrations in lead-exposed workers, *Hereditas* **96**:265–8 (1982).

Norppa, H., Vainio, H., and Sorsa, M., Chromosome aberrations in lymphocytes of workers exposed to styrene, *Am. J. Ind. Med.* **2**:299–304 (1981). (Review)

O'Brien, M. W., Assessment of reproductive and genetic monitoring in occupational settings—legal/labor viewpoint, *Proc. Clin. Biol. Res.* **160**:551–5 (1984).

Oftedal, P., The control of genetic hazards of radiation, *Hereditas* **92**:297–301 (1980).

O'Riordan, M. D., Hughes, E. G., and Evans, H. J., Chromosome studies on blood lymphocytes of men occupationally exposed to cadmium, *Mutat. Res.* **58**:305–11 (1978).

Pass, F., Biotechnology, a new industrial revolution (editorial), *J. Am. Acad. Dermatol.* **4**:476–7 (1981).

Perocco, P., Pane, G., Bolosnesi, S., and Zannotti, M., Increase of sister chromatid exchange and unscheduled synthesis of deoxyribonuclic acid by acrylonitrile in human lymphocytes in vitro, *Scand. J. Work Environ. Health* **8**:290–3 (1982).

Perpich, J. G., Biotechnology programs between government and industry, *Recomb. DNA Tech. Bull.* **7**:53–9 (1984).

Popescu, H. I., Negru, L., and Lancranjan, I., Chromosome aberrations induced by occupational exposure to mercury, *Arch. Environ. Health* **34**:461–3 (1979).

Reilly, P., Keynote address: Screening workers: Privacy, procreation, and prevention, *Prog. Clin. Biol. Res.* **106**:1–11 (1984).

Rissler, J. F., Research needs for biotic environmental effects of genetically-engineered microorganisms, *Recomb. DNA Tech. Bull.* **7**:20–30 (1984).

Rossner, P., Sram, R. J., Novakova, J., and Lambl, V., Cytogenetic analysis in workers occupationally exposed to vinyl chloride, *Mutat. Res.* **73**:425–7 (1980).

Sandberg, A. A., Chromosomes and carcinogenesis: Public health application, *Prog. Clin. Biol. Res.* **132C**:295–309 (1983).

Schmid, E., Bauchinger, M., and Dresp, J., Chromosome analyses of workers from a pentachlorophenol plant, *Prog. Clin. Biol. Res.* **109**:471–7 (1982).

Schull, W. J., Chronic disease in the workplace and the environment. Reproductive problems: Fertility, teratogenesis, and mutagenesis, *Arch. Environ. Health* **39**:207–12 (1984).

Smedley, H. M., Sikora, K., and Ciclitira, P. J., Medical monitoring of genetic engineering research in Cambridge, the first five years, *J. Soc. Occup. Med.* **32**:167–70 (1982).

Sorsa, M., Maki-Paakkanen, J., and Vainio, H., Identification of mutagen exposures in the rubber industry by the sister chromatid exchange method, *Cytogenet. Cell Genet.* **33**:68–73 (1982).

Sorsa, M., Falck, K., Maki-Paakkanen, J., and Vainio, H., Genotoxic hazards in the rubber industry, *Scand. J. Work Environ. Health* **9**:103–7 (1983).

Tobin, M. J., Cook, P. J., and Hutchison, D. C., Alpha-1-antitrypsin deficiency: The clinical and physiological features of pulmonary emphysema in subjects homozygous for Pi type Z. A survey by the British Thoracic Association, *Br. J. Dis. Chest.* **77**:14–27 (1983).

Tuschl, H., Kovac, R., and Altmann, H., USA and SCE in lymphocytes of persons occupationally exposed to low levels of ionizing radiation, *Health Phys.* **45**:1–7 (1983).

Vainio, H., and Sorsa, M., Application of cytogenetic methods for biological monitoring, *Ann. Rev. Public Health* **4**:403–7 (1983).

Wade, N., Cloning gold rush turns basic biology into big business, *Science* 208:688–92 (1980).

Wolff, S., Problems and prospects in the utilization of cytogenetics to estimate exposure at toxic chemical waste dumps, *Environ. Health Perspect.* 48:25–7 (1983).

Yager, J. W., Hines, C. J., and Spear, R. C., Exposure to ethylene oxide at work increases sister chromatid exchanges in human peripheral lymphocytes, *Science* 219:1221–3 (1983).

Zauss, R. H., and Swarz, J. R., Industrial use of applied genetics and biotechnologies, *Recomb. DNA Tech. Bull.* 5:7–13 (1982).

Zinder, N. D., and Winn, J., A partial summary of university-industry relationships in the United States, *Recomb. DNA Tech. Bull.* 7:8–19 (1984).

GENETICS, GOVERNMENT, AND LAW

Betz, F., Levin, M., and Rogul, M., Safety aspects of genetically-engineered microbial pesticides, *Recomb. DNA Tech. Bull.* 6:135–41 (1983).

Brahams, D., Warnock report on human fertilization and embryology, *Lancet* 2:238–9 (1984).

Capron, A. M., Ethical and social issues in the application of genetic engineering to human beings. Statement to Subcommittee on Investigations and Oversight Committee on Science and Technology, United States House of Representatives. *Recomb. DNA Tech. Bull.* 6:3–10 (1983).

Carmi, A., Genetic engineering, *Med. Law* 2:181–92 (1983).

Fischinger, P. J., and DeVita, V. T., Jr., Governance of science at the National Cancer Institute: Perceptions and opportunities in oncogene research, *Cancer Res.* 44:4693–6 (1984).

The Food and Drug Administration's Points to Consider in Recombinant DNA Technology, *Recomb. DNA Tech. Bull.* 7:38–9 (1984).

Grobstein, C., and Flower, M., Gene therapy: Proceed with caution, *Hastings Cent. Rep.* 14:13–7 (1984).

Larsen, K. H., Brash, D., Cleaver, J. E., Hart, R. W., Maher, V. M., Painter, R. B., and Sega, G. A., DNA repair assays as tests for environmental mutagens. A report of the U.S. EPA Gene-Tox Program, *Mutat. Res.* 98:287–318 (1982).

Meeting of the large-scale review working group of the recombinant DNA Advisory Committee, *Recomb. DNA Tech. Bull.* 5:192–8 (1982).

Milewski, E., RAC discussion of the construction of biological weapons, *Recomb. DNA Tech. Bull.* 5:188–91 (1982).

Milewski, E., Congressional hearing on the environmental implications of genetic engineering, *Recomb. DNA Tech. Bull.* 6:103–10 (1983).

Milewski, E. A., Evolution of the NIH guidelines, *Recomb. DNA Tech. Bull.* 4:160–5 (1981).

Miller, H. I., Gene therapy: Overregulation may be hazardous to our health (editorial), *Gene* 17:1–2 (1984).

Omenn, G. S., Genetics and epidemiology: Medical interventions and public policy, *Soc. Biol.* 26:117–25 (1979).

Opt-Hof, J., and Rouxm, J. PL., Genetic services in the State Health Department of the RSA: Development and structure, *S. Afr. Med. J.* 64:43–8 (1983).

Proposal to add a new Section III-A-4 to the Guidelines and a footnote to Section III-B-4-b, *Recomb. DNA Tech. Bull.* 7:83–4 (1984).

Proposal to add a new section III-A-4 to the guidelines and to devise mechanisms to review proposals involving genetic engineering in humans, *Recomb. DNA Tech. Bull.* 7:34–5 (1984).

Recommendations of the Warnock Committee, *Lancet* 2:217–8 (1984).

Robb, J. W., Reflections: Ethics and the recombinant DNA debate, *J. Craniofac. Genet. Dev. Biol.* 2:51–63 (1982).

Rozovsky, L. E., and Rozovsky, F. A., Human fertility controls in Canada, *Can. J. Pub. Health* 73:158–9 (1982).

Summary from "Splicing life": A report on the social and ethical issues of genetic engineering with human beings. President's Commission for the Study of Ethical Problems in Medicine and Biomedical and Behavioral Research, *Recomb. DNA Tech. Bull.* 6:10–2 (1983).

Szybalski, W., Changes in the NIH guidelines for recombinant DNA research (appendix 4: May 1980–April 1981), *Gene* Vol. **13**:423–6 (1981).

Talbot, B., Congressional hearings on "Human Applications of Genetic Engineering," *Recomb. DNA Tech. Bull.* **6**:1–3 (1983).

Williamson, R., Genetic manipulation advisory group (CMAG) and the environment for genetic engineering in Britain, *Biochem. Soc. Symp.* **44**:119–21 (1979).

Biotechnology

Abelson, P. H., Biotechnology: An overview, *Science* **219**:611–3 (1983).

Adler, R. G., Biotechnology as an intellectual property, *Science* **224**:357–63 (1984).

Basic biology of new developments in biotechnology, *Basic Life Sci.* **25**:1–579 (1983).

Boone, C. K., Splicing life, with scalpel, and scythe, *Hastings Cent. Rep.* **13**:8–10 (1983).

Cooper, A., Patentability of genetically engineered microorganisms, *JAMA* **249**:1553–4 (1983).

Crespi, S., Patenting nature's secrets and protecting microbiologists' interests, *Nature* **284**:590–1 (1980).

Davis, B. D., The two faces of genetic engineering in man (editorial), *Science* **219**:1381 (1983).

Editorial: Key biotechnology patent delayed, *Nature* **298**:409 (1982).

Evans, H. J., Biotechnology and medicine, *Health Bull.* **40**:34–8 (1982).

Ferrandiz, Garcia-F., Biotechnology: Genetic engineering (Chemico-pharmaceutical area), *Rev. Esp. Fisiol.* **38**:353–66. (Review)

Goldstein, J. A., A footnote to the Cohen-Boyer patent and other musings, *Recomb. DNA Tech. Bull.* **5**:180–8 (1982).

Karny, G. M., Patenting biotechnology, *Recomb. DNA Tech. Bull.* **6**:145–8 (1983).

Keen, H., Microbial biotechnology in industry and medicine, *Trans. Med. Soc. Lond.* **98**:53–8 (1981–82).

Marcus, I., International patent procedures, *In Vitro* **17**:1086–8 (1981).

Pharis, M. E., and Manosevitz, M., Parental models of infancy: A note on gender preferences for firstborns, *Psychol. Rep.* **47**:763–8 (1980).

Response to the "Report on the social and ethical issues of genetic engineering with human beings," *Recomb. DNA Tech. Bull.* **6**:154–5 (1983).

Rutter, J. M., Gene manipulation and biotechnology, *Vet. Rec.* **109**:192–4 (1981).

Weir, R., Truthtelling in medicine, *Perspect. Biol. Med.* **24**:95–112 (1980).

Williamson, B., Gene therapy, *Nature* **298**:416–8 (1982).

Woodruff, H. B., and Miller, B. M., Patenting of hybridomas and genetically engineered microorganisms, *In Vitro* **17**:1078–80 (1981).

Ethics, Philosophy, Law and Genetics

Annas, G. J., Medical paternity and "wrongful life," *Hastings Cent. Rep.* **9**:15–7 (1979).

Berg, K., Ethical problems arising from research progress in medical genetics, *Prog. Clin. Biol. Res.* **128**:261–75 (1983).

Callahan, D., The moral career of genetic engineering, *Hastings Cent. Rep.* **9**:9–21 (1979).

Callahan, S., An ethical analysis of responsible parenthood, *Birth Defects* **15**:217–38 (1979).

Carter, C. O., Developments in human reproduction and their eugenic, ethical implications: Eugenic implications of new techniques, *Proc. Annu. Symp. Eugen. Soc.* **19**:205–11 (1983).

Childress, J. F., and Casebeer, K., Public policy issues in genetic counseling, *Birth Defects* **15**:279–90 (1979).

Cusine, D. J., Developments in human reproduction and their eugenic, ethical implications; Legal implications, *Proc. Annu. Sump. Eugen. Soc.* **19**:227–36 (1983).

Developments in human reproduction and their eugenic, ethical implications. Proceedings of the nineteenth annual symposium of the Eugenics Society, London 1982. *Proc. Annu. Symp. Eugen. Soc.* **19**:1–240 (1983).

Dunstan, G. R., Developments in human reproduction and their eugenic, ethical implications: Social and ethical aspects, *Proc. Annu. Symp. Eugen. Soc.* **19**:213–26 (1983).

Engels, W. R., Evolution of altruistic behavior by kin selection: An alternative approach, *Proc. Nat. Acad. Sci. USA* **80**:515–8 (1983).

Feinman, M. A., Getting along with the genetic genie, *Leg. Aspects Med. Pract.* 7:37–41 (1979).

Fletcher, F. C., Ethical and social aspects of risk predictions, *Clin. Genet.* 25:25–32 (1984).

Fletcher, J. C., Ethics and amniocentesis for fetal sex identification, *N. Eng. J. Med.* 301:550–3 (1979).

Fletcher, J. C., Genetic decision making and pastoral care: Clergy involvement relating practice to principle, *Hosp. Pract.* 18:38F,38K-38L,38P (1983).

Fletcher, J. C., Is sex selection ethical? *Prog. Clin. Biol. Res.* 128:333–48 (1983).

Goodman, M. J., and Goodman, L. E., The overselling of genetic anxiety, *Hastings Cent. Rep.* 12:20–7 (1982).

Grant, M. A. Genetic control and the law, *Med. Trial. Tech. Q.* 24:306–27 (1978).

Hamerton, J. L., Ethical considerations in newborn chromosome screening programs, *Birth Defects* 15:267–78 (1979).

Holtzman, N. A., Public interest in genetics and genetics in the public interest, *Am. J. Med. Genet.* 5:383–9 (1980).

Jones, G. E., and Perry, C., Can claims for "wrongful life" be justified? *J. Med. Ethics* 9:162–4, 174 (1983).

Karp, L. E., Should God take out a patent? (editorial), *Am. J. Med. Genet.* 8:1–3 (1981).

Kass, L. R., Change and permanence: Reflections on the ethical-social contract of science in the public interest, *In Vitro* 17:1091–9 (1981).

Lappe, M., Humanizing the genetic enterprise, *Hastings Cent. Rep.* 9:10 (1979).

Lebel, R. R., Ethical issues arising in the genetic counseling relationship, *Birth Defects* 14:1–46 (1978).

Mazumdar, P. M., The eugenists and the residuum: The problem of the urban poor, *Bull. Hist. Med.* 54:204–15 (1980).

Motulsky, A. G., Bioethical problems in pharmacogenetics and ecogenetics, *Hum. Genet.* (Suppl.) 1:185–92 (1978).

Murphy, E. A., Eugenics, An ethical analysis, *Mayo Clin. Proc.* 53:655–64 (1978).

Robertson, M., Towards a medical eugenics? (editorial), *Br. Med. J. (Clin. Res.)* 288:429–30 (1984).

Rosenberg, L. E., New genetics and old values, *Pharos* 46:13–9 (1983).

Storey, P., Ethical implications of genetic practice, *S. Afr. Med. J.* 58:781–3 (1980).

The Supreme Court and patenting life, *Hastings Cent. Rep.* 10:10–5 (1980).

Thomas, S., Ethics of a predictive test for Huntington's chorea, *Br. Med. J. (Clin. Res.)* 284:1383–5 (1982).

Towers, B., Medical involvement in procreation: How far? *J. Med. Ethics* 8:100–1 (1982).

Twiss, S. B., The genetic counselor as moral advisor, *Birth Defects* 15:201–12 (1979).

Twiss, S. B., Problems of social justice in applied human genetics, *Birth Defects* 15:255–77 (1979).

Young, I. D., Ethical dilemmas in clinical genetics, *J. Med. Ethics* 10:73–6

ARTIFICIAL INSEMINATION BY DONOR

Annas, G. J., Artificial insemination: Beyond the best interests of the donor, *Hastings Cent. Rep.* 9:14–5, 43 (1979).

Beck, W. W., Jr., Artificial insemination and preservation of semen, *Urol. Clin. North. Am.* 5:593–605 (1978).

Beck, W. W., Jr., Two hundred years of artificial insemination (editorial), *Fertil. Steril.* 41:193–5 (1984).

Behrman, S. J., Artificial insemination and public policy (editorial), *New Eng. J. Med.* 300:619–20 (1979).

Clayton, C. E., and Kovacs, G. T., A.I.D.—A pretreatment social assessment, *Aust. NZ J. Obstet. Gynaecol.* 20:208–10 (1980).

Corson, S. L., Batzer, F. R., and Baylson, M. D., Donor insemination, *Obstet. Gynecol. Ann.* 12:283–309 (1983).

Curie-Cohen, M., Luttrell, L., and Shapiro, S., Current practice of artificial insemination by donor in the United States, *N. Eng. J. Med.* 300:585–90 (1979).

Czeizel, A., Szentesi, I., and Horvath, L., Results of genetic screening of donors for artificial insemination, *Clin. Genet.* 24:113–6 (1983).

Dandrea, K. G., The role of the nurse practitioner in artificial insemination, *J.O.G.N. Nurs.* 13:75–8 (1984).

Fraser, F. C., and Forse, R. A., On genetic screening of donors for artificial insemination, *Am. J. Med. Genet.* 10:399–405 (1981).

Friedman, S., and Broder, S., Homologous artificial insemination after long-term semen cyropreservation, *Fertil. Steril.* 35:321–4 (1981).

Howards, S. S., and Bergman, S., Analysis of the feasibility of storing human semen for future artificial insemination, *Trans. Am. Assoc. Genitourin-Surg.* 71:45–6 (1979).

Hulka, J. F., Donor insemination: Guidelines for uncharted territory (editorial), *Fertil. Steril.* 35:500–1 (1981).

Johnson, W. G., Schwartz, R. C., and Chutorian, A. M., Artificial insemination by donors: The need for genetic screening: Late-infantile GM2-gangliosidosis resulting from this technique, *N. Eng. J. Med.* 304:755–7 (1981).

Karp, L. E., A.I.D. and genetics: Some further thoughts (editorial), *Am. J. Med. Genet.* 9:271–3 (1981).

Kovacs, G. T., Clayton, C. E., and McGowan, P., The attitudes of semen donors, *Clin. Reprod. Fertil.* 2:73–5 (1983).

Leeton, J., and Backwell, J., A preliminary psychosocial follow-up of parents and their children conceived by artificial insemination by donor (AID), *Clin. Reprod. Fertil.* 1:307–10 (1982).

McCormack, M. K., Leiblum, S., and Lazzarini, A., Attitudes regarding utilization of artificial insemination by donor in Huntington disease, *Am. J. Med. Genet.* 10:399–405 (1981).

Meijer, A. M., Hamerlynck, J. V., and Schagen, S., Psychological aspects of donor insemination, *Ned. Tijdschr. Geneeskd.* 124:592–9 (1980).

Newton, J. R., The present status of AID in the United Kingdom, *Proc. Ann. Symp. Eugen. Soc.* 16:165–82 (1981).

Rowland, R., Attitudes and opinions of donors on an artificial insemination by donor (AID) programme, *Clin. Reprod. Fertil.* 2:249–59 (1983).

Samuels, A., Artificial insemination and genetic engineering: The legal problems, *Med. Sci. Law* 22:261–8 (1982).

Simpson, J. L., Genetic screening for donors in artificial insemination (editorial), *Fertil. Steril.* 35:395–6 (1981).

Smith, G. P., 2d, Artificial insemination redivivus: Permutations within a penumbra, *J. Leg. Med.* (Chicago) 2:113–30 (1981).

Strong, C., and Schinfeld, J. S., The single woman and artificial insemination by donor, *J. Reprod. Med.* 29:293–9 (1984).

Suggested code of practice for artificial insemination by donor (AID), *S. Afr. Med. J.* 58:781–3 (1980).

Teper, S., and Symonds, E. M., Artificial insemination by donor: Problems and perspectives, *Proc. Ann. Symp. Eusgn. Soc.* 19:19–52 (1983). (Review)

Thompson, W., and Boyle, D. D., Counselling patients for artificial insemination and subsequent pregnancy, *Clin. Obstet. Gynaecol.* 9:211–25 (1982).

Timmons, M. C., Rao, K. W., Sloan, C. S., Kirkman, H. N., and Talbert, L. M., Genetic screening of donors for artificial insemination, *Fertil. Steril.* 35:451–6 (1981).

Tyler, J. P., Nicholas, M. K., Crockett, N. G., and Driscoll, G. L., Some attitudes to artificial insemination by donor, *Clin. Reprod. Fertil.* 2:151–60 (1983).

Waltzer, H., Psychological and legal aspects of artificial insemination (A.I.D.): An overview, *Am. J. Psychother.* 36:91–102 (1982).

Whelan, D., The law and artificial insemination with donor semen (aid), *Med. J. Aust.* 1:56–8 (1978).

Worsnop, D., Mack, H., Robbie, M., Pick, A., Sons, L. Y., and McGuire, P., Human artificial insemination: Donors in Melbourne, *Aust. Fam. Physician* 11:218, 220–4 (1982).

Surrogate Motherhood

Davis, J. H., and Brown, D. W., Artificial insemination by donor (AID) and the use of surrogate mothers, *West. J. Med.* 141:127–30 (1984).

Gorovitz, S., On surrogate mothers, *Prog. Clin. Biol. Res.* 139:141–3 (1983).

Greenberg, L. J., and Hirsh, H. L., Surrogate motherhood and artificial insemination: Contractual implications, *Med. Trial Tech. Q.* 29:149–66 (1982).

Keane, N. P., Pirslin, N. A., and Chadwick, C. S., Surrogate motherhood: Past, present, future, *Prog. Clin. Biol. Res.* 139:155–64 (1983).

Krimmel, H. T., The case against surrogate parenting, *Hastings Cent. Rep.* 13:35–9 (1983).

Mady, T. M., Surrogate mothers: The legal issues, *Am. J. Law Med.* 7:323–52 (1981).
Parker, P. J., Motivation of surrogate mothers: Initial findings, *Am. J. Psychiat.* 140:117–8 (1983).
Parker, P. J., Surrogate motherhood, psychiatric screening and informed consent, baby selling, and public policy, *Bull. Am. Acad. Psychiat. Law* 12:21–39 (1984).
Robertson, J. A., Surrogate mothers: Not so novel after all, *Hastings Cent. Rep.* 13:28–34 (1983).
Surrogate mothering: Case for discussion. *Prog. Clin. Biol. Res.* 139:141–3 (1983).
Weil, B. J., Introduction: Surrogate mothering, *Prog. Clin. Biol. Res.* 139:137–9 (1983).

In Vitro Fertilization

Brahams, D., Medicine and the law: In-vitro fertilization and related research: Why Parliament must legislate, *Lancet* 2:726–9 (1983).
Dandeker, P. V., and Quigley, M., Laboratory setup for human in vitro fertilization, *Fertil. Steril.* 42:1–12 (1984).
Hirsh, B. D., Parenthood by proxy, *JAMA* 249:2251–2 (1983).
Jones, H. W., Jr., Acosta, A. A., Gracia, J. E., Sandow, B. A., and Veeck, L. L., On the transfer of conceptuses from oocytes fertilized in vitro, *Fertil. Steril.* 39:241 (1983).
Kolata, G., In vitro fertilization goes commercial, *Science* 221:1160 (1983).
Lopata, A., Johnston, I. W. H., Hoult, I. J., and Speirs, A. L., Pregnancy following intrauterine implantation of an embryo obtained by in vitro fertilization of a preovulatory egg, *Fertil. Steril.* 33:117 (1980).
Trounson, A. O., Leeton, J. F., Wood, C., Webb, J., and Kovacs, G., The investigation of idiopathic infertility by in vitro fertilization, *Fertil. Steril.* 34:431 (1980).
Warren, D. G., The law of human reproduction: An overview, *J. Leg. Med.* 3:1–57 (1982).
Wortham, J. W. E., Jr., Veeck, L. L., Witmyer, J., Sandow, B. A., and Jones, H. W., Jr., Vital initiation of pregnancy (VIP) using human menopausal gonadotropin and human chorionic gonadotropin ovulation induction: Phase II-1981, *Fertil. Steril.* 40:170 (1983).

DEATH AND DYING IN THE NEWBORN PERIOD

After the trial at Leicester (editorial), *Lancet* 2:1085–6 (1981).
Angell, M., Handicapped children: Baby Doe and Uncle Sam (editorial), *N. Eng. J. Med.* 309:659–61 (1983).
Annas, G. J., Disconnecting the Baby Doe hotline, *Hastings Cent. Rep.* 13:14–6 (1983).
Atkinson, G. M., Ambiguities in "killing" and "letting die," *J. Med. Philos.* 8:159–68 (1983).
Berseth, C. L., A neonatologist looks at the Baby Doe Rule: Ethical decisions by edict, *Pediatrics* 72:428–9 (1983).
Black, P. M., Selective treatment of infants with myelomeningocele, *Neurosurgery* 5:334–8 (1979).
Brahams, D., Acquittal of paediatrician charged after death of infant with Down Syndrome, *Lancet* 2:1101–2 (1981).
Brahams, D., and Brahams, M., Symposium 1: The Arthur case—A proposal for legislation, *J. Med. Ethics* 9:12–5 (1983).
Bridge, P., and Bridge, M., The brief life and death of Christopher Bridge, *Hastings Cent. Rep.* 11:17–9 (1981).
Britton, J. R., Baby Doe rulings—Review and comment, *West. J. Med.* 140:303–7 (1984).
Coburn, R. C., Morality and the defective newborn, *J. Med. Philos.* 5:34–57 (1980).
Cohen, D., The right to live and the right to die, *Med. J. Aust.* 140:59–61 (1984).
Cordner, S. M., The Leicester case, *Med. J. Aust.* 1:313–4 (1982).
Death without concealment (editorial), *Br. Med. J. (Clin. Res.)* 283:1629–30 (1981).
Dunea, G., Letter from Chicago: Squeal rules in the nursery, *Br. Med. J. (Clin. Res.)* 287:1203–4 (1983).
Ellis, T. S., 3d, Letting defective babies die: Who decides? *Am. J. Law Med.* 7:393–423 (1982).
Gray, P., Euthanasia and clinical practice: The report of a working party of the Linacre Centre, *Arch. Dis. Child* 58:837–8 (1983).

Hardman, M. D., and Drew, C. F., Parent consent and the practice of withholding treatment from the severely defective newborn, *Ment. Retard.* 18:165–9 (1980).

Harvard, J., Symposium: 3. Legislation is likely to create more difficulties than it resolves, *J. Med. Ethics* 9:18–20 (1983).

In the matter of the treatment and care of Infant Doe: Declaratory judgment: Circuit court for the County of Monroe, State of Indiana, *Conn. Med.* 47:409–10 (1983).

Klitsch, M., Mercy or murder? Ethical dilemmas in newborn care, *Fam. Plan. Perspect.* 15:143–6 (1983).

O'Rourke, K. D., Lessons from the Infant Doe case, *Conn. Med.* 47:411–2 (1983).

Paris, J. F., and Fletcher, A. B., Infant Doe regulations and the absolute requirement to use nourishment and fluids for the dying infant, *Law Med. Health Care* 11:210–3 (1983).

Paris, J. J., Terminating treatment for newborns: A theological perspective, *Law Med. Health Care* 10:120–4, 144 (1983).

Rasatz, S. C., and Ellison, P. H., Decisions to withdraw life support in the neonatal intensive care unit, *Clin. Pediatr.* (Phila.) 22:729–35 (1983).

The right to live and the right to die (editorial), *Br. Med. J. (Clin. Res.)* 283:569–70 (1981).

Robertson, J. A., Dilemma in Danville, *Hastings Cent. Rep.* 11:5–8 (1981).

Rozovsky, L. E., and Rozovsky, F. A., Law reform and euthanasia, *Can. J. Public Health* 73:431–2 (1982).

Slack, A., Killing and allowing to die in medical practice, *J. Med. Ethics* 10:82–7 (1984).

Statement of the American Medical Association to the Department of Health and Human Services RE: Handicapped infants, April 14, 1983, *Conn. Med.* 47:413–6 (1983).

Strain, J. E., The American Academy of Pediatrics comments on the "Baby Doe II" regulations, *New Eng. J. Med.* 309:443–4 (1983).

Strain, J. E., The decision to forgo life-sustaining treatment for seriously ill newborns, *Clin. Pediatr.* (Phila.) 22:729–35 (1983).

Taub, S., Legal problems of medical practice: Withholding treatment from defective newborns, *Law Med. Health Care* 10:4–10 (1982).

Taub, S., Medical decision-making for defective infants by the Federal government, *Conn. Med.* 47:411–2 (1983).

Veatch, R. M., Maternal brain death: An ethicist's thoughts (editorial), *JAMA* 248:1102–3 (1982).

Weir, R. F., The government and selective nontreatment of handicapped infants, *New Eng. J. Med.* 309:661–3 (1983).

Index